Recent Advancements in Biomarkers and Detection of Gastrointestinal Cancers

Recent Advancements in Biomarkers and Detection of Gastrointestinal Cancers

Editor: Mikhael Kular

AMERICAN
MEDICAL PUBLISHERS
www.americanmedicalpublishers.com

AMERICAN
MEDICAL PUBLISHERS
www.americanmedicalpublishers.com

Cataloging-in-Publication Data

Recent advancements in biomarkers and detection of gastrointestinal cancers / edited by Mikhael Kular.
p. cm.
Includes bibliographical references and index.
ISBN 979-8-88740-419-6
1. Gastrointestinal system--Cancer. 2. Gastrointestinal system--Cancer--Diagnosis. 3. Biochemical markers.
4. Gastrointestinal system--Cancer--Treatment. 5. Digestive organs--Cancer. I. Kular, Mikhael.
RC280.D5 R43 2023
616.994 33--dc23

American Medical Publishers,
41 Flatbush Avenue,
1st Floor, New York,
NY 11217, USA

ISBN 979-8-88740-419-6 (Hardback)

Contents

Preface

The purpose of the book is to provide a glimpse into the dynamics and to present opinions and studies of some of the scientists engaged in the development of new ideas in the field from very different standpoints. This book will prove useful to students and researchers owing to its high content quality.

A biomarker is a biological molecule present in the blood, other body fluids or tissues that indicates normal or abnormal process, condition or a disease. It can act as an alternative tool and is helpful in selecting accurate treatment in various diseases. Gastrointestinal cancer is a malignant condition affecting gastrointestinal tract and organs of the digestive system, including the stomach, pancreas, esophagus, small and large intestine, biliary system, rectum, and anus. In the case of esophageal cancer, methylation of DNA can be used as a biomarker for early detection because methylation patterns appear in the initial stages. Protein biomarkers are utilized as markers for gastric tumor for effective diagnosis, prognosis and checking for recurrence of cancer after treatment. Various biomarkers that are utilized in case of stomach cancer include antigens like CA12-5 and CA72-4 as well as alpha-fetoprotein. This book provides comprehensive insights on biomarkers. The topics covered herein deal with the core aspects of the detection of gastrointestinal cancers through biomarkers. This book will serve as a reference to a broad spectrum of readers.

At the end, I would like to appreciate all the efforts made by the authors in completing their chapters professionally. I express my deepest gratitude to all of them for contributing to this book by sharing their valuable works. A special thanks to my family and friends for their constant support in this journey.

Editor

1

uc.77- Downregulation Promotes Colorectal Cancer Cell Proliferation by Inhibiting FBXW8-Mediated CDK4 Protein Degradation

Zhijian Zheng[1†], Dan Hong[1†], Xiaodong Zhang[2†], Yixin Chang[1], Ning Sun[1], Zhenni Lin[1], Hongyan Li[1], Shirui Huang[3], Ruirui Zhang[1], Qipeng Xie[3], Haishan Huang[1] and Honglei Jin[1*]*

[1] *Zhejiang Provincial Key Laboratory of Medical Genetics, Key Laboratory of Laboratory Medicine, Ministry of Education, School of Laboratory Medicine and Life Sciences, Wenzhou Medical University, Wenzhou, China,* [2] *Department of Colorectal Anal Surgery, The First Affiliated Hospital of Wenzhou Medical University, Wenzhou, China,* [3] *Department of Clinical Laboratory, The Second Affiliated Hospital & Yuying Children's Hospital of Wenzhou Medical University, Wenzhou, China*

***Correspondence:**
Honglei Jin
jhlbmd@163.com
Haishan Huang
haishan_333@163.com

[†]*These authors have contributed equally to this work*

Transcribed ultraconserved regions (T-UCRs) are a new type of long non-coding RNA, and the UCR has 481 segments longer than 200 base pairs that are 100% conserved between humans, rats, and mice. T-UCRs involved in colorectal cancer (CRC) have not been studied in detail. We performed T-UCR microarray analysis and found that uc.77- was significantly downregulated in CRC tissues and cell lines. Ectopic expression of uc.77- significantly inhibited the proliferation of CRC cells *in vitro* and the growth of xenograft tumors in nude mice *in vivo*. Mechanistic studies showed that uc.77- competed with FBXW8 mRNA for binding to microRNA (miR)-4676-5p through a competing endogenous RNA mechanism and inhibited the proliferation of CRC cells by negatively regulating CDK4. The present findings highlight the role of the uc.77-/miR-4676-5p/FBXW8 axis in CRC and identify uc.77- as a potential novel target for the treatment of CRC.

Keywords: uc.77-, miR-4676-5p, FBXW8, CDK4, colorectal cancer

INTRODUCTION

Colorectal cancer (CRC) is the third most common cancer worldwide. Approximately 1.93 million new cases of CRC were reported in 2020, with an incidence rate of 10.0% and a mortality rate of 9.4% (1). In China, CRC is the third most common malignant tumor and the fourth leading cause of cancer-related death (2). Elucidating the pathogenesis of CRC and identifying diagnostic markers are urgent needs.

Ultraconserved regions (UCRs) are non-coding gene sequences composed of 481 segments that are 100% conserved among mammals such as humans, rats, and mice. These segments can be located on exons or introns of the coding gene. RNAs transcribed from the UCR region are called T-UCRs or ultra-conserved (uc) RNAs. Non-coding RNAs transcribed from UCRs may regulate gene expression (3).T-UCRs are a new type of long non-coding RNAs (lncRNAs) that can function as oncogenes or tumor suppressors in different tumor types (4). uc.338 is highly expressed in liver cancer cells, and it promotes cell proliferation by affecting cell cycle progression (5). uc.338 is also expressed at high levels in CRC, and it promotes metastasis and invasion of CRC (6). On the other hand, uc.160+ is expressed at low levels in gastric cancer, where it plays a tumor suppressor role (7). The role of T-UCRs in tumor development is not well understood.

Cyclin-dependent kinase 4 (CDK4) is an important regulator of the cell cycle that forms a complex with CDK6 and cyclin D1, and phosphorylates retinoblastoma (Rb) protein. Inactivated Rb releases E2F, thereby promoting the transition from G0/G1 phase to S phase of the cell cycle (8, 9). CDK4 is frequently dysregulated in cancer, and the development of CDK4-targeted therapies is important. However, the development of CDK inhibitors is challenging, and several clinical trials have shown disappointing results (10, 11). uc.77-, a new lncRNA that was identified as a potential target for the treatment of CRC, is involved in the regulation of CDK4. In this study, we show that uc.77- competes with FBXW8 mRNA for binding to microRNA (miR)-4676-5p, thereby promoting the expression of FBXW8 and the ubiquitination of CDK4, which inhibits the proliferation of CRC cells.

MATERIALS AND METHODS

T-UCR Microarray

This study was previously detected by our team at Kangcheng Bio (Shanghai, China). The total RNA of each sample was quantified with NanoDrop ND-1000 (Thermo Fisher Scientific), and RNA integrity was evaluated by standard denaturing agarose gel electrophoresis. For microarray analysis, the Agilent array platform (Agilent Technologies, Santa Clara, California) was employed. Sample preparation and microarray hybridization were performed according to the manufacturer's standard protocol. In short, the purified mRNA and LncRNA were amplified by random primer method (Arraystar Flash RNA Labeling Kit, Arraystar) and transcribed into fluorescent cRNA along the full length of the transcript. The labeled cRNA was hybridized to human T-UCR array (8×60K, Arraystar). After cleaning the slides, the array was scanned by the Agilent scanner G2505C (Agilent Technologies). The extracted data was normalized using Agilent GeneSpring GX v12.1 software. Use GeneSpring GX v12.1 and a signal processing algorithm called Otsu method for further data analysis. Finally, the differentially expressed T-UCRs between the samples were identified by fold change filtering.

Plasmids, Antibodies, and Reagents

The plasmid overexpressing uc.77- and the corresponding control plasmid were purchased from TsingKe Biological Technology (Beijing, China). The CDK4 plasmid was constructed and used in a previous study (12). Mimics for miR-4676-5p and miR-3605-5p were purchased from Ruibo Biotechnology (Guangzhou, China). The wild-type and mutant luciferase reporter genes for the predicted miR-4676-5p binding sites at uc.77- and at the FBXW8 3′ untranslated region (3′-UTR) were purchased from TsingKe Biological Technology.

Short hairpin RNAs (shRNAs) against FBXW8 and the control plasmid were purchased from Open Biosystems (Thermo Fisher Scientific, NY, USA). Antibodies against CDK2 (sc-6248), CDK4 (sc-260), CDK6 (sc-177), cyclin D1 (sc-20044), cyclin E2 (sc-481), and FBXW8 (sc-514385) were purchased from Santa Cruz Biotechnology (Santa Cruz, CA, USA). Antibodies against cyclin E2 (sc-481), FBXW11 (13149-1-AP), and HECTD3 (11487-1-AP) were purchased from Proteintech (Chicago, IL, USA). Antibody against α-tubulin (ab7291) was purchased from Abcam (Cambridge, UK). Cycloheximide (CHX) and MG132 were purchased from Calbiochem (San Diego, CA, USA).

Cell Culture and Transfection

The human CRC cell lines HCT116, HT-29, LoVo, and SW620 were purchased from the Shanghai Chinese Academy of Sciences. SW480 and CCD-18Co cells were purchased from American Type Culture Collection. HCT116 cells were cultured in M5A medium (PM150710; Procell) supplemented with 10% fetal bovine serum (FBS; 42Q8982K; Gibco), and SW620 cells were cultured in RPMI 1640 (11875–093, Gibco) supplemented with 10% FBS. The Polyjet Transfection Reagent (SL100688, SignaGen Laboratories) was used for stable transfection. According to the different antibiotic resistance plasmids transfected, selection was performed using puromycin (4–6 μg/mL; J593; Amresco Inc.) or G418 (1000–1500 μg/mL; sc-29065;Santa Cruz, Dallas, TX, USA) for 3–4 weeks.

Lentiviral Infection

The 293T cells were inoculated into 6-well plates in 2 mL DMEM containing 10% FBS and grown until reaching a density of 60–70%. A combination of 1.2 μg pMD2.G (12259, Addgene), 1.2 μg psPAX.2 (12260, Addgene), and 2 μg plasmid was mixed with 50 μL serum-free DMEM containing 6 μL Polyjet. The mixture was incubated at room temperature for 15 min and added to 293T cells in 6-well plates, which were placed in a 5% CO_2 incubator at 37°C for 6–8 h. After replacing the medium with fresh DMEM containing 10% FBS, the plates were incubated for 48 h. Then, 2 mL of supernatant containing virus was collected, centrifuged at 3000 rpm for 30 min, and passed through a 0.45 μm filter with a syringe. The virus supernatant was added to the cell culture medium at a ratio of 1:1, and stable cell lines were selected with puromycin.

Anchorage-Independent Growth

To examine the anchorage-independent growth of CRC cells, a suspension culture containing 10^4 stably transfected HCT116 (uc.77-) or SW620 (uc.77-) cells and their control carrier cells was placed in a 6-well plate containing 0.33% agar and 10% FBS basal medium. The plates were incubated at 37°C and 5% CO_2 for 2–3 weeks, and the number of colonies was counted under a DMi1 microscope (Leica Microsystems, Buffalo Grove, IL, USA). The result is presented as the mean ± SD of colonies/10,000 inoculated cells (13).

Cell Proliferation

Approximately 1500 HCT116 (vector), HCT116 (uc.77-), SW620 (vector), or SW620 (uc.77-) cells were seeded into 96-well plates in 200 μL of complete medium/well. After the cells adhered to the wall, the complete medium was replaced with 0.1% FBS medium, and cells were starved for 12 h to synchronize the cycle. The medium was then replaced with fresh complete medium, and cells were incubated for the indicated number of days. The cell proliferation index was determined using the CellTiter-Glo Luminescent Cell Viability Assay Kit (G7572; Promega). Briefly, the culture medium from 96-well plates was discarded, and 25 μL PBS mixed with 25 μL of the reagents provided in the kit were added to the cells. The plates were shaken for 2 min and incubated at room temperature for 10 min. Luminescence was detected using the Centro LB 960 luminometer (Berthold, Bad Wildbad, Germany) (14, 15).

Cell Cycle

The stably transfected HCT116 (uc.77-) and SW620 (uc.77-) cells and control vector cells seeded in 6-well plates were washed with PBS, digested with 0.25% EDTA trypsin, and then fixed in 70% ethanol at 4°C overnight. The cells were then washed with pre-cooled PBS and treated with 500 μL RNase A (KGA511; KeyGen Biotech, Nanjing, China) and propidium iodide at a ratio of 1:9. The plates were incubated at room temperature for 30–60 min and analyzed using the CytoFlex flow cytometer (Beckman Coulter, Brea, CA, USA) and CytExpert software.

qRT-PCR

Total RNA was isolated from cells using Trizol (15596018, Invitrogen), and cDNA was synthesized using the SuperScript™ First Strand Synthesis System (18091200, Invitrogen). The qRT-PCR analysis was performed using the Q6 real-time PCR system (Thermo Fisher Scientific, Waltham, MA, USA) and the fast SYBR Green Master Mix kit (4385614, Applied Biosystems). Real-time PCR primers for uc.77- (forward, 5′-CTGTCACACTGCTCCCAAGAA-3′; reverse, 5′-GGGAGAACTCA GCCAAAGATG-3′) were purchased from Sunny Biotechnology (Shanghai, China). Other primers used in this study were synthesized by TsingKe Biological Technology, including FBXW8 (forward, 5′-CTACAGCCTGGATGAG TTCCG-3′; reverse, 5′-TGCAATCACCTTCCACGTCT-3′) and GAPDH (forward, 5′-GACTCATGACC ACAGTCCATG C-3′; reverse, 5′-CAGGTCAGGTCCACCACTGA-3′). GAPDH was used as an endogenous control.

Western Blot Analysis

Protein was extracted from cells using boiling buffer (1% SDS, 1 mM Na3VO4, 10 mM Tris-HCl [pH 7.4]) on ice. The samples were heated at 100°C for 5 min, and nucleic acid fragments were sonicated. The protein samples were separated by polyacrylamide gel electrophoresis and transferred to a PVDF membrane (Bio-Rad, Hercules, CA, USA). The membrane was blocked with 5% skim milk in TBST for 1 h, incubated with the indicated primary antibodies at 4°C overnight, and then incubated with alkaline phosphatase-conjugated secondary antibody at 4°C for 3 h. Films were processed with ECF (RPN5787; GE Healthcare, PA, USA) for signal detection, and images were captured on the Typhoon FLA 7000 scanner (GE Healthcare) (16).

Dual Luciferase Reporter Assay

Luciferase assays were performed using a dual luciferase reporter system (Promega) according to the manufacturer's instructions. The wild-type and mutant uc.77- and FBXW8 3′-UTR fragments cloned into the pmirGLO vector were purchased from TsingKe Biological Technology. The wild-type or mutant FBXW8 3′-UTR vector and miR-4676-5p mimic were co-transfected with pRL-TK using the RiboFECT CP Transfection Kit (C10511-05, Ruibo Biotechnology). Cells were cultured for 48 h before addition of cell lysis buffer and incubation at room temperature for 15 min. Then, 20 μL aliquots were pipetted into a 96-well plate and treated with 40 μL Luciferase Assay Reagent II in the dark. The luciferase activity in each well was measured in a Centro LB 960 luminometer (Berthold). After adding 40 μL Stop&Glo reagent to the same well, the luciferase activity value was analyzed again.

Xenotransplantation Model in Nude Mice

Female BALB/c athymic nude mice (3–4 weeks old) were purchased from Jiangsu Jicui Yaokang Biotechnology Co., Ltd. Animal experiments were performed in the Animal Center of Wenzhou Medical University according to the protocol approved by the Experimental Animal Ethics Committee. After 1–2 weeks of adaptive culture, 12 nude mice were randomly divided into two groups of six mice each. A volume of 100 μL HCT116 (vector) or HCT116 (uc.77-) cell suspension in PBS containing 4×10^6 cells was subcutaneously injected into the right ventral side. After 3–4 weeks, the mice were sacrificed, and the tumors were surgically removed, photographed, and weighed. One half of each tumor was fixed in 4% paraformaldehyde for immunohistochemistry (IHC). The remaining half was frozen and stored at -80°C and used for RNA extraction (17).

Protein Degradation Experiment

HCT116 (vector) and HCT116 (uc.77-) cells were seeded in 6-well plates containing complete medium. When the cell density reached 80%, the medium was replaced with fresh medium containing 0.1% FBS, and cells were starved for 12 h. Then, the medium was replaced with fresh medium containing 10 μM MG-132 and 10% FBS for 5 h. After replacing the medium with fresh medium containing 50 μg/mL CHX, the plates were placed in a 37°C incubator with 5% CO_2. Cells were collected at 0, 3, 6, and 12 h. The CDK4 degradation rate was assessed by western blotting (18).

RNA Antisense Purification (RAP)

Cell suspensions were prepared according to the instructions of the RAP kit (Bersinbio, Guangzhou, China). Briefly, a biotin-labeled 50 bp antisense probe (detailed information is provided in **Table S1**) was added to the lysis solution. After denaturation and hybridization, streptavidin magnetic beads were added, and the eluate was obtained after washing to remove non-specifically bound RNA. The RNA interacting with the lncRNA was collected, transcribed into cDNA, and analyzed by qRT-PCR.

Immunohistochemistry (IHC)

Ki67 expression was detected by IHC in formalin-fixed paraffin-embedded specimens from mice using a specific primary antibody against Ki67 (ab16667, Abcam). IHC staining was performed using a kit from Boster Bio-Engineering Company (SA1022; Wuhan, China). Immunostained images were captured using the Nikon Eclipse Ni microsystem (DS-Ri2), and the integrated optical density of each stained area was calculated.

Clinical Specimens

Approved by the Ethics Committee of Wenzhou Medical University, a total of 150 pairs of samples of human CRC tissue and corresponding adjacent normal tissues were isolated from patients in the First Affiliated Hospital of Wenzhou Medical University, which has been described in the accepted article (Frontiers in Oncology Manuscript ID: 668743). Each sample was quick-frozen in liquid nitrogen during separation. One third of each sample was used for RNA extraction, and synthesized cDNA was stored at -80°C. The remaining sample was fixed with 4% paraformaldehyde, embedded into a wax block, and stored at room temperature.

Statistical Analysis

GraphPad Prism 7 was used for graph production and data analysis. Experimental data are expressed as the mean ± standard deviation (mean ± SD). The significance of differences between groups was determined using the Student's t-test. Significance was accepted at $P < 0.05$.

RESULTS

uc.77- Screening and Expression in CRC Tissues and Cells

To investigate the roles T-UCRs in CRC development, we analyzed T-UCR microarray data (GSE167326) published by our group. The top two downregulated T-UCRs, uc.77- and uc.166-, were identified by real-time PCR in 150 pairs of clinical tissues (tumor/normal tissue), of which uc.77- was the most significantly downregulated transcript in CRC (**Figure 1A**). Therefore, uc.77- was selected for further analysis, and its biological functions and mechanisms were examined *in vivo* and *in vitro*. Analysis of uc.77- in CRC cell lines (HT-29, HCT116, LoVo, SW480, and SW620) showed that uc.77- expression was significantly lower in HCT116 and SW620 cells than in the human normal colon tissue cell line CCD-18Co cells (**Figure 1B**). The coding potential calculator CPC2.0 (http://cpc2.gao-lab.org/) was used to determine whether uc.77- is a non-coding RNA, we found that the coding potential of uc.77- is significantly lower than the coding genes (GAPDH;ACTB and ACTA1) and typical non-coding RNAs (Malatl and Hotair) (**Figure 1C**) (19). The results showed that uc.77- is an exon from the Zinc Finger E-Box binding homeobox 2 (ZEB2) transcript (**Figure 1D**).

Ectopic Overexpression of uc.77- Inhibits the Proliferation of CRC Cells *In Vivo* and *In Vitro*

To further investigate the role of uc.77- in the development of human CRC, real-time PCR was performed to detect the relationship between uc.77- and tumor size. As shown in **Figure 2A**, the uc.77- level was lower in big size tumor than in small size tumor. To ensure the biological function of uc.77- in CRC, an uc.77- overexpression plasmid was constructed and stably transfected into HCT116 and SW620 cells, and the overexpression efficiency was tested (**Figure 2B**). Overexpression of uc.77- inhibited the monolayer proliferation ability of HTC116 and SW620 cells (**Figures 2C, D**). Consistently, the anchorage-independent growth of HTC116 (uc.77-) and SW620 (uc.77-) cells was inhibited compared with that of control vector cells (**Figures 2E, F**). To determine whether uc.77- inhibits the growth of CRC cells *in vivo*, a xenograft tumor nude mouse model was used to examine the effect of uc.77- on the tumorigenicity of HTC116 and SW620 cells. The results showed that overexpression of uc.77- significantly reduced tumor growth compared with that in vector control-injected mice (**Figures 2G–I**). The expression of uc.77- in xenograft tumors was also confirmed by real-time PCR (**Figure 2J**). Immunohistochemical (IHC) staining of xenograft tumor samples was also showed that Ki67 expression was significantly lower in tumor tissues of mice injected with HCT116 (uc.77-) than in control vector tumors (**Figures 2K, L**). Taken together, these results indicated that uc.77- inhibits the growth of CRC cells.

CDK4 Acts as a Downstream Effector of uc.77- to Regulate CRC Cell Proliferation

To explore the mechanism underlying the inhibition of CRC cell growth by uc.77-, the effect of uc.77-on cell cycle progression was detected in HCT116 and SW620 cells by flow cytometry. As shown in **Figures 3A, B**, uc.77- caused cell cycle arrest at the G0/G1 phase, suggesting that uc.77- inhibits CRC cell growth by blocking the cell cycle at G0/G1. The effect of uc.77- on G0/G1 cell cycle transition was further examined by assessing the expression of G0/G1 phase-related proteins (CDK2, CDK4, CDK6, cyclin D1, and cyclin E2). The results showed that overexpression of uc.77- downregulated CDK4 in HCT116 and SW620 cells consistently (**Figure 3C**). The results showing that uc.77- inhibits CRC cell proliferation and blocks G0/G1 transition suggested that CDK4 is a downstream effector of uc.77-.

uc.77- Inhibits CRC Cell Proliferation by Accelerating the Degradation of CDK4

To determine whether CDK4 is necessary for the uc.77-mediated inhibition of CRC growth, a CDK4 overexpression plasmid was stably transfected into HCT116 (uc.77-) cells to restore CDK4 expression (**Figure 4A**). The results showed that overexpression of CDK4 rescued the anchorage-independent growth of cells compared with that in HCT116 uc.77-/pEGFP cells (**Figures 4B, C**). Consistently, analysis of the cell cycle showed that overexpression of CDK4 promoted G0/G1 cell cycle transition compared with that in control HCT116 (uc.77-/pEGFP) cells (**Figure 4D**). These data indicate that CDK4 is the downstream effector of uc.77-.

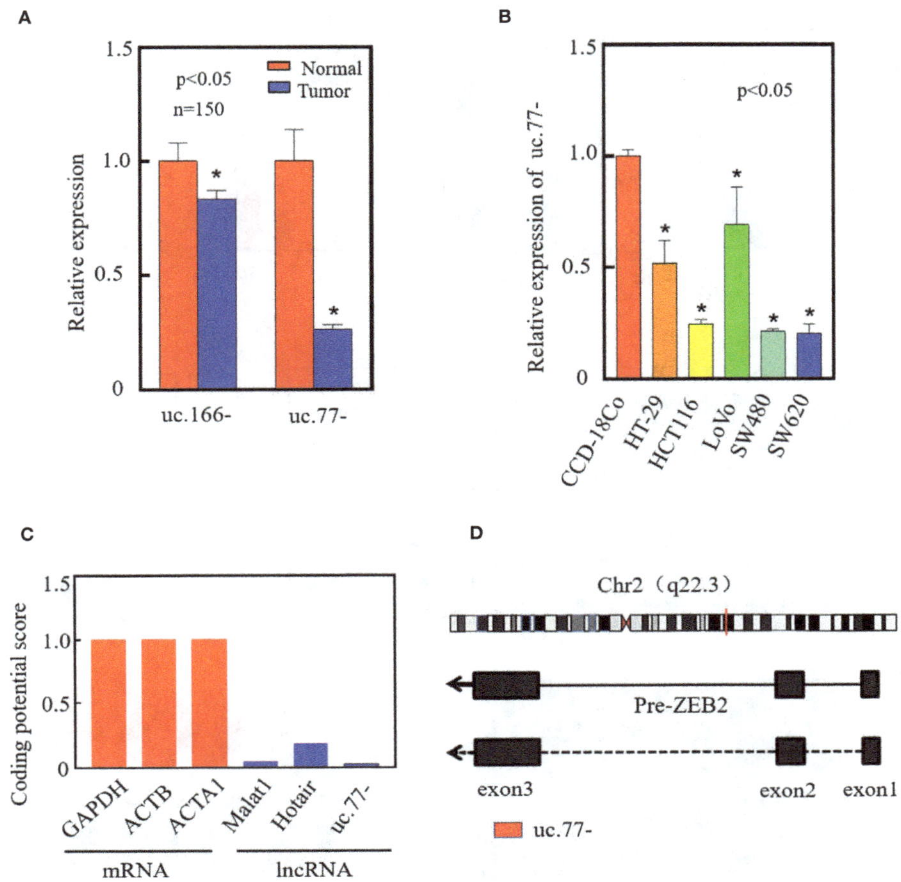

FIGURE 1 | uc.77- is downregulated in human CRC tissues and cell lines. **(A)** The expression of top two downregulated T-UCRs in CRC tissues was detected by qRT-PCR ($P < 0.05$). **(B)** Expression of uc.77- in human colorectal cancer cell lines (HT-29, HCT116, LoVo, SW480, and SW620) and human normal colorectal epithelial cells (CCD-18Co) detected by qRT-PCR. **(C)** Coding potential score of uc.77- measured by CPC2.0. **(D)** Genome structure of uc.77- from the third exon of ZEB2 located in chromosome 2q22.3. Data are presented as the mean ± SD, *$P < 0.05$.

Next, we sought to determine whether uc.77- regulates the expression of CDK4 at the mRNA level or the protein level. First, the effect of uc.77- on the level of CDK4 mRNA was examined by real-time PCR (**Figure 4E**). CDK4 mRNA levels did not differ significantly between uc.77-overexpressing cells and control vector-transfected cells, suggesting that uc.77- did not affect the expression of CDK4 at the mRNA level. We hypothesized that uc.77- modulates the expression of CDK4 at the protein level. Consistent with this hypothesis, the protein level of CDK4 decreased in a time-dependent manner. As shown in **Figure 4F**, the rate of CDK4 protein degradation was faster in uc.77-overexpressing cells than in control plasmid transfected cells, suggesting that uc.77- affects the ubiquitination level of CDK4 by regulating an E3 ligase.

uc.77- Directly Binds miR-4676-5p and Upregulates FBXW8 in CRC Cells

To explore the downstream regulatory mechanism of uc.77-, we used RegRNA2.0 (http://regrna2.mbc.nctu.edu.tw/detection.html) to predict potential miRNAs related to uc.77- (**Figure 5A**). RAP experiments indicated that the binding specificity of miR-3605-5p and miR-4676-5p for uc.77- was significantly higher than that of the control sequence probe (**Figure 5B**), which suggested that uc.77- has a binding relationship with miR-3605-5p and miR-4676-5p. Next, we searched for potential E3 ligases using the TargetScan and Ubibrowser databases. The results identified HECTD3 as a potential E3 for miR-3605-5p, and FBXW8 and FBXW11 as potential E3s for miR-4676-5p, indicating that these ligases might affect the degradation of the CDK4 protein (**Figures 5C, D**). Further analysis showed that FBXW8 was the only ligase expressed at higher levels in both HCT116 (uc.77-) and SW620 (uc.77-) cells than in control plasmid transfected cells (**Figure 5E**). These results suggest that FBXW8 acts downstream of miR-4676-5p to affect the degradation of the CDK4 protein. The potential binding sites between uc.77- and miR-4676-5p were analyzed (**Figure 5F**), and a dual luciferase reporter assay was performed to detect the interaction between uc.77- and miR-4676-5p. Co-transfection of uc.77-wild-type vector and miR-4676-5p mimic significantly decreased luciferase activity (**Figure 5G**), indicating that uc.77- interacts directly with miR-4676-5p.

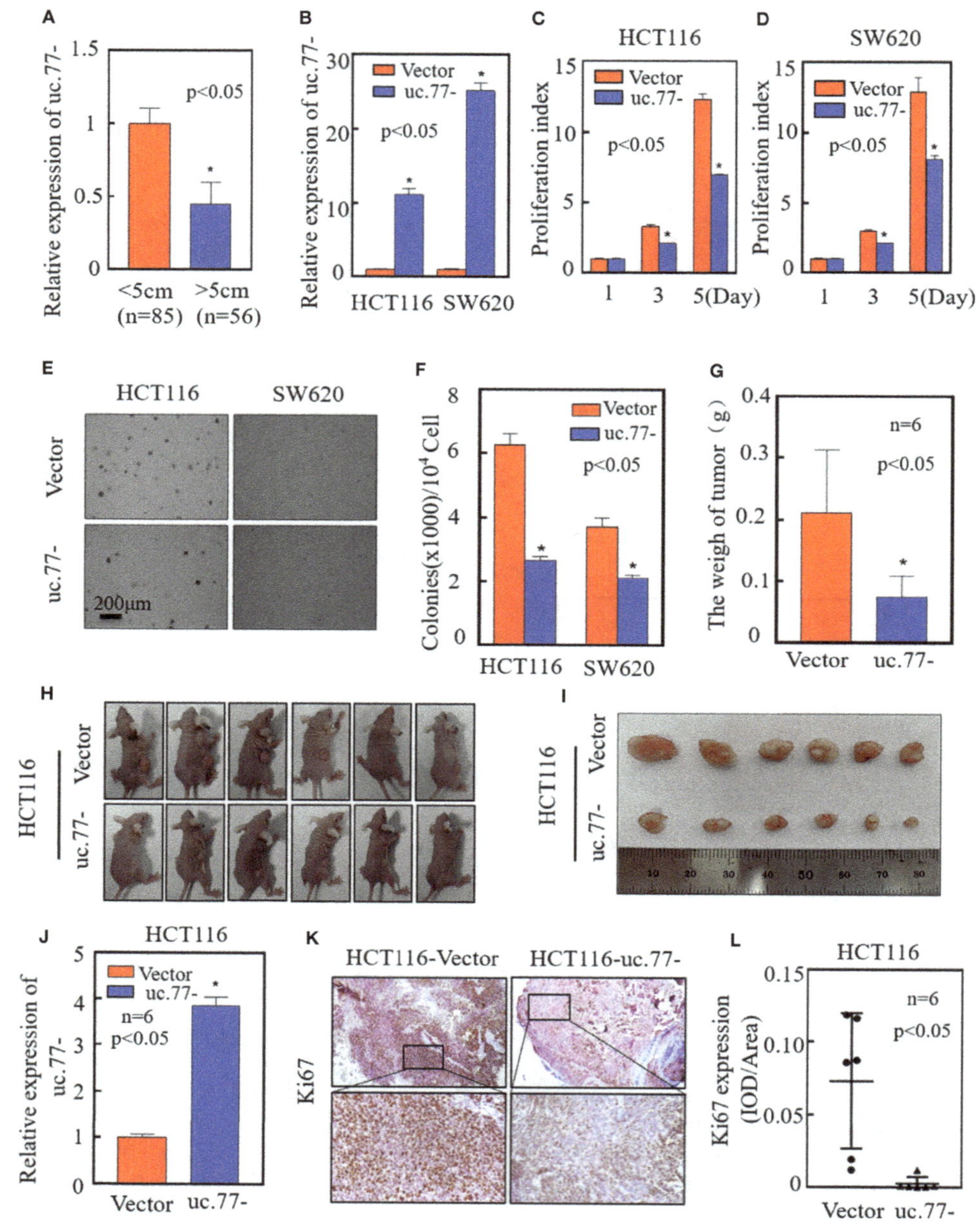

FIGURE 2 | uc.77- promotes the growth of CRC cells *in vivo* and *in vitro*. **(A).** Real-time PCR was used to detect the expression of uc.77-in fresh clinical cancer tissues. **(B)** Detection of uc.77- stable overexpression by real-time PCR. **(C, D)** Effect of uc.77- on the proliferation of HCT116 **(C)** and SW620 **(D)** cells detected by ATP assays. **(E, F)** Effect of uc.77- on anchorage-independent growth in HCT116 and SW620 cells detected by soft agar assays. **(E)** Representative microscope images and **(F)** number of colonies per 10^4 cells. **(G–I)** HCT116 (uc.77-) and control vector cells were injected into the right lower abdomen of athymic nude mice. After 3–4 weeks, the mice were euthanized, and the tumors were surgically removed, weighed, and photographed. **(J)**Total RNA was extracted from mouse exnograft tumor tissue, and real-time PCR was used to detect the expression of uc.77-. **(K)** Representative IHC images showing the expression of Ki67 in tumor tissues of mice injected with HCT116 (uc.77-) and control vector cells. **(L)** Optical density of Ki67 IHC staining in mouse tumor tissues. Data are presented as the mean ± SD and analyzed by the Student's t-test, *P < 0.05.

FBXW8 Is a Direct Target of miR-4676-5p and Mediates CDK4 Protein Stabilization and CRC Cell Growth

To test the role of FBXW8 in mediating the regulatory effect of uc.77- on CRC cell growth, we established stable FBXW8 knockdown HCT116 (uc.77-) cells using a specific shRNA from Open Biosystems (**Figure 6A**). As shown in **Figures 6B–D**, knockdown of FBXW8 significantly reversed the inhibitory effect of uc.77- on HCT116-anchor-independent growth and G0/G1 cell cycle arrest. To examine whether FBXW8 causes CDK4 protein

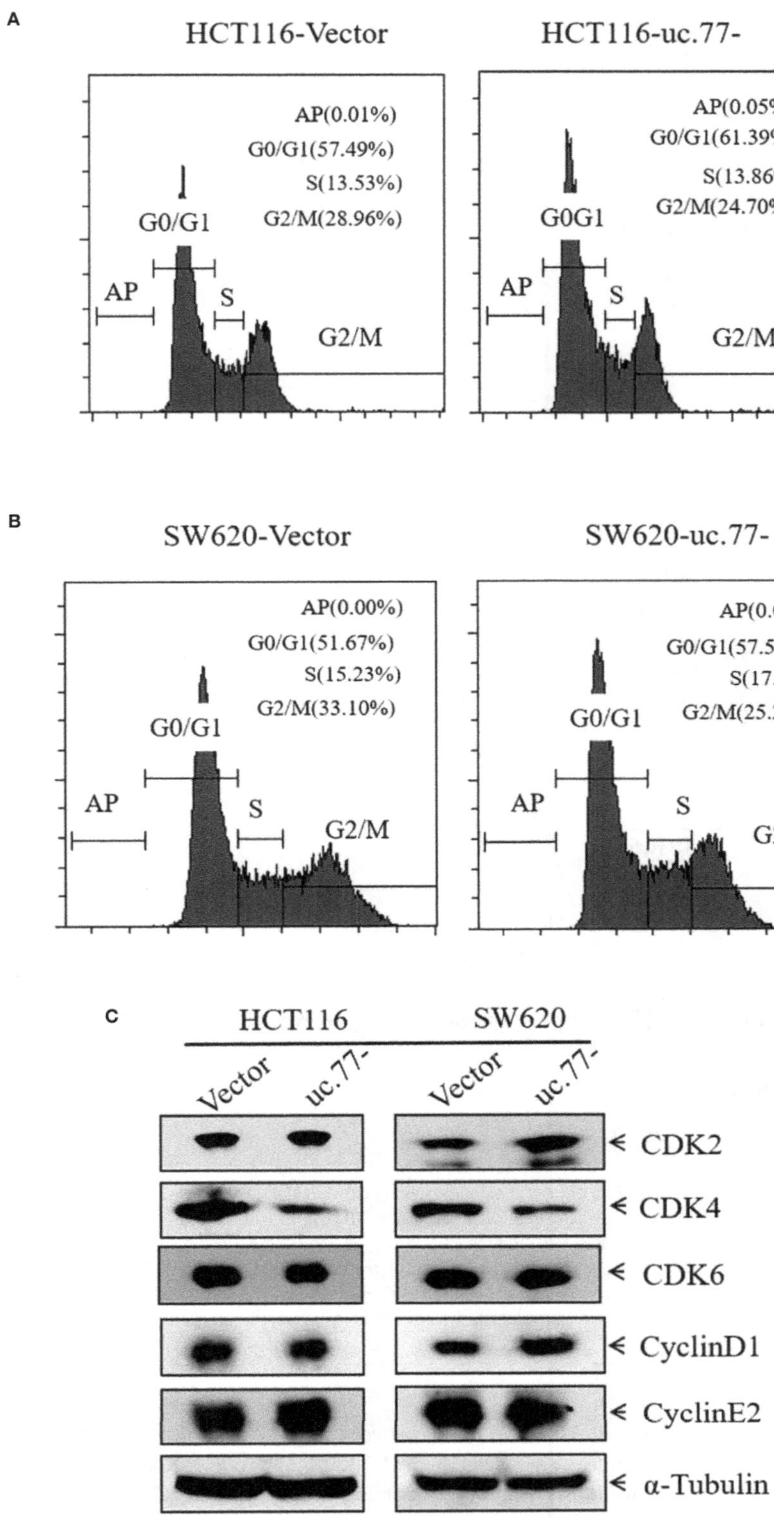

FIGURE 3 | CDK4 acts as a downstream effector of uc.77-. **(A, B)** HCT116 **(A)** and SW620 **(B)** cells as indicated were cultured in 6-well plates, and cell cycle progression was analyzed. **(C)** Expression of CDK2, CDK4, CDK6, cyclin D1, and cyclin E2 in cell lysates detected by western blotting; α-Tubulin was used as a control.

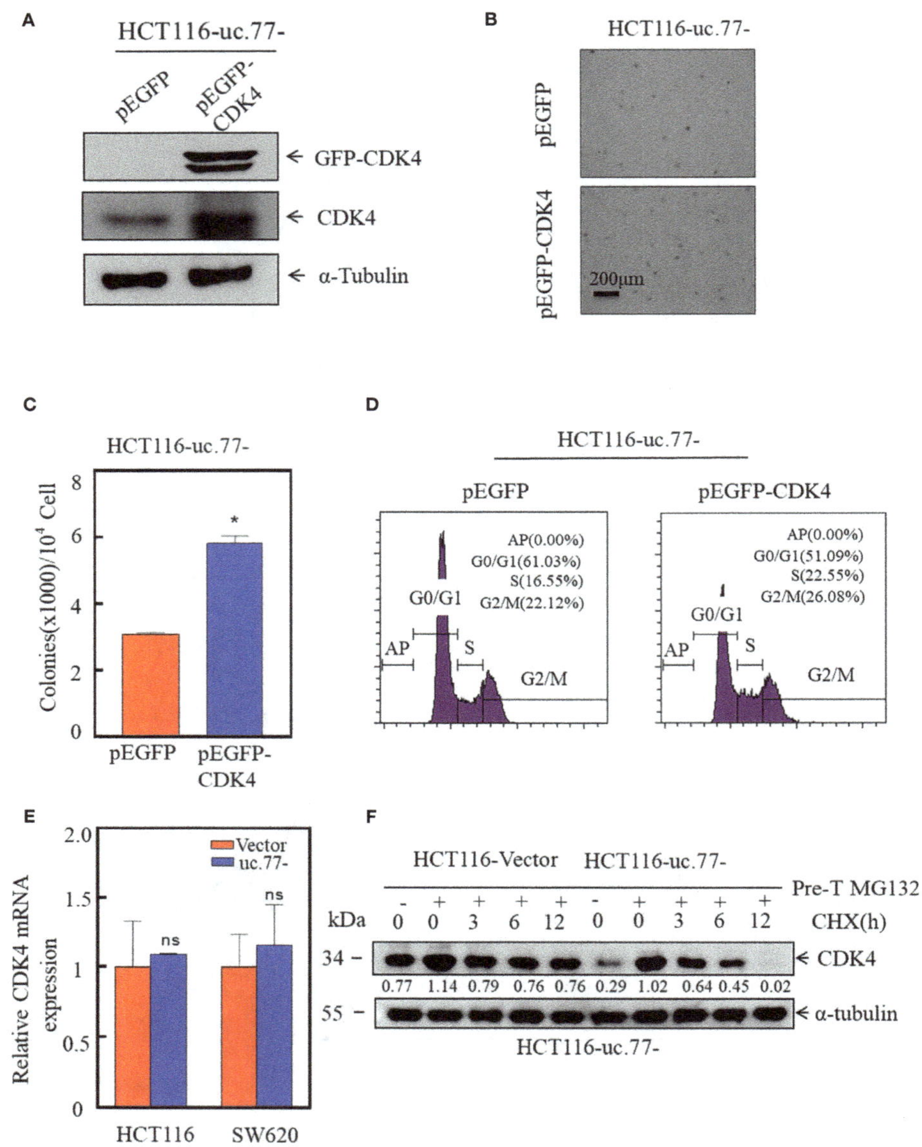

FIGURE 4 | CDK4 promotes the growth of CRC, and uc.77- promotes the degradation of CDK4. **(A)** A CDK4 overexpression vector was stably transfected into HCT116 (uc.77-) cells, and the overexpression efficiency was evaluated by western blotting. **(B, C)** Effect of CDK4 overexpression on the anchorage-independent growth of HCT116 (uc.77-) cells determined by the soft agar assay. **(B)** Representative images and **(C)** number of colonies per 10^4 cells. **(D)** HCT116 (uc.77-/pEGFP-CDK4) and control cells were cultured in 6-well plates, and cell cycle analysis was performed. **(E)** Detection of CDK4 mRNA expression in HCT116 (uc.77-) and SW620 (uc.77-) cells and the corresponding control vector cells by real-time PCR. **(F)** HCT116 (uc.77-) and control carrier cells were treated with MG132 for 8 h, followed by treatment with CHX for the indicated times. CDK4 degradation was detected by western blotting. Data are presented as the mean ± SD and analyzed by the Student's *t*-test, *P < 0.05, ns p > 0.05.

degradation, we performed a protein degradation test. As shown in **Figure 6E**, knockdown of FBXW8 in HCT116 (uc.77-) cells significantly reduced the CDK4 degradation rate. miRNAs bind to the 3′-UTR of a target gene, causing RNA degradation or inhibiting protein translation. IHC staining of xenograft tumor samples was also showed that FBXW8 expression is significantly higher in tumor tissues of mice injected with HCT116 (uc.77-) than in control vector tumors (**Figure S1**). The potential relationship between miR-4676-5p and FBXW8 was examined by analyzing the 3′-UTR of FBXW8 mRNA, including potential miR-4676-5p binding sites (**Figure 6F**). Wild-type and mutant FBXW8 3′-UTR plasmids were co-transfected with miR-4676-5p mimics, and a dual luciferase reporter assay was performed (**Figure 6G**). Mutation of the FBXW8 3′-UTR increased luciferase activity significantly. These results we predicted that miR-4676-5p interacts with the 3′-UTR of FBXW8 mRNA to inhibit FBXW8 protein translation.

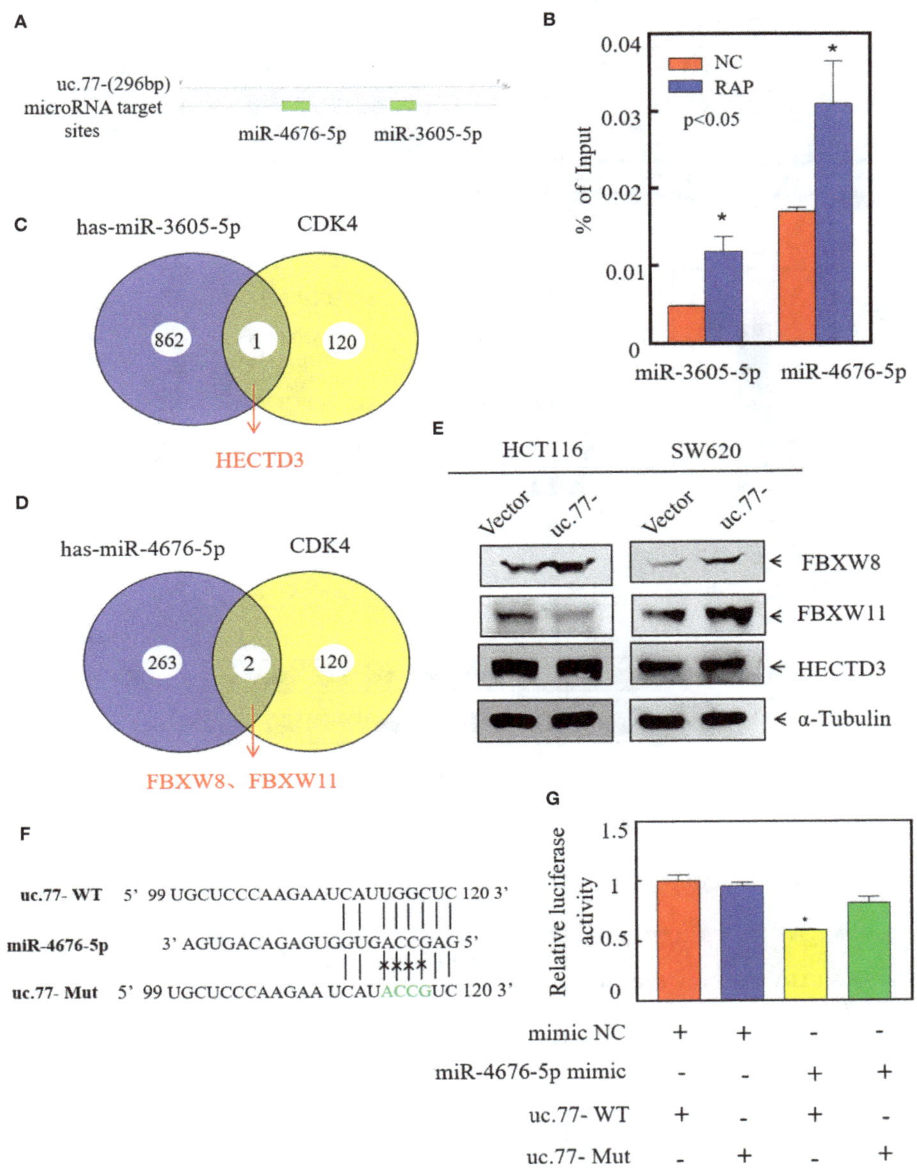

FIGURE 5 | uc.77- binds to miR-4676-5p and indirectly affects downstream CDK4 E3 ligases. **(A)** Potential interacting miRNAs were predicted using (http://regrna2.mbc.nctu.edu.tw/detection.html). **(B)** RNA antisense purification technology was used to detect the binding of uc.77- to selected miRNAs. **(C, D)** E3 ligases were predicted by TargetScan and Ubibrowser. **(E)** FBXW8, FBXW11, and HECTD3 expression was evaluated by western blotting. **(F)** Alignment between miR-4676-5p and the uc.77-seed sequence. WT and Mut represent the wild-type and mutant sequences of uc.77-. **(G)** Luciferase activity of pmirGLO-uc.77–wt and pmirGLO-uc.77–mut upon cotransfection with miRNA mimics NC or miR-4676-5p mimics in 293T cells.Data are presented as the mean ± SD and analyzed by the Student's *t*-test, *P < 0.05.

DISCUSSION

CRC is a common malignancy worldwide, and the number of new cases and deaths is increasing. It is estimated that the number of new cases of CRC may reach 2.5 million by 2035 (20). Surgery and chemotherapy are the primary treatments for cancer patients. Biomarkers are important for the detection and treatment of cancer, and the identification of new and sensitive biomarkers is therefore essential (21–23). In this study, we found that uc.77- is downregulated in CRC tissues, and inhibition of CDK4 ubiquitination and degradation mediated by the miR-4676-5p-FBXW8 axis leads to CRC cell growth. These data indicate that uc.77- may serve as a new biomarker and therapeutic target for CRC.

Increasing evidence suggests that T-UCRs play an important role in human diseases, and studies indicate that T-UCRs are

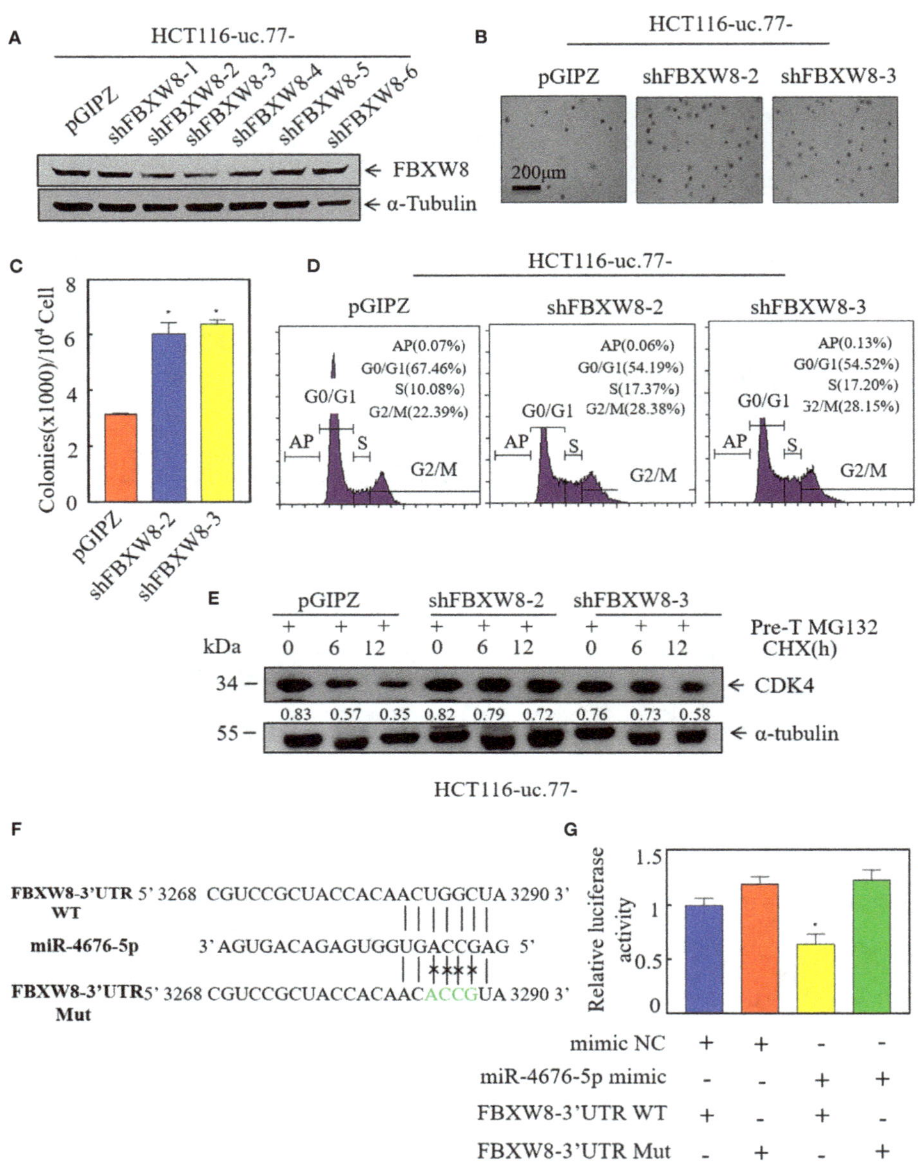

FIGURE 6 | FBXW8 is a direct target of miR-4676-5p, and is involved in CDK4 protein stabilization and CRC cell growth. **(A)** Western blot detection of the knockdown efficiency of FXBW8 in HCT116 (uc.77-) cells. α-Tubulin was used as an internal reference. **(B, C)** Effect of FBXW8 knockdown on anchorage-independent growth detected by soft agar assays; representative microscope images are shown **(B)**, and the number of colonies per 10^4 cells was counted **(C)**. **(D)** HCT116 (uc.77-/shFBXW8-2), HCT116 (uc.77-/shFBXW8-3), and the corresponding controls were cultured in 6-well plates, and cell cycle analysis was performed. **(E)** HCT116 (uc.77-/shFBXW8-2), HCT116 (uc.77-/shFBXW8-3), and control vector HCT116 (uc.77-/pGIPZ) cells were treated with MG132 for 5 h, and then treated with CHX for the indicated times. CDK4 degradation was detected by western blotting. **(F)** Alignment between miR-4676-5p and the FXBW8 3′-UTR seed sequence. WT and Mut represent wild-type and mutant sequences of the FXBW8 3′-UTR. **(G)** Luciferase activity of pmirGLO-FXBW8 3′-UTR-wt and pmirGLO-FXBW8 3′-UTR-mut upon cotransfection with miRNA mimics NC or miR-4676-5p mimics in 293T cells. Data are presented as the mean ± SD and analyzed by the Student's *t*-test, *P < 0.05.

involved in the pathogenesis of cancer (24–28). Carlin et al. reported that the expression of T-UCRs is altered in human cancers and that they play vital roles in cancer progression (4). uc.73 and uc.338 are upregulated in CRC and play oncogenic roles in CRC development (4, 5). In the present study, a T-UCR microarray of CRC identified uc.77- as a markedly downregulated T-UCR, suggesting that it could be a potential molecular target in CRC. uc.77 is upregulated in lung cancer cells and plays an oncogenic role in lung cancer by inducing EMT (29). Interestingly, our research found that ZEB2 may not be a key factor in uc77- regulation of human CRC cell proliferation (**Figure S2**). In this study, we demonstrated that uc.77- was significantly downregulated in CRC tissues and cells, and functional experiments *in vivo* and *in vitro* showed that overexpression of uc.77- inhibited the proliferation of CRC cells. This suggests that uc.77- plays a tumor suppressor role in the development of CRC.

The regulatory role of T-UCRs can be mediated by its sponge function through interaction with miRNAs. T-UCRs can bind to miRNAs and decrease the inhibitory effect of miRNAs on the target mRNA, similar to many lncRNAs that interact with miRNAs (30, 31). miRNAs regulate many important physiological functions, and the combination of miRNAs and T-UCRs can alter the function of cells (32). For example, uc.8+ is upregulated in bladder cancer and promotes the development of bladder cancer by interacting with miR-596 (33). uc.173 interacts with pri-miR-195 transcripts to promote the renewal of the intestinal mucosa (34). uc.416+ promotes the development of gastric cancer by interacting with miR-153 (35). uc.339 is highly expressed in non-small cell lung cancer and acts as a sponge for miR-339-3p, miR-663b-3p, and miR-95-5p, which upregulates cyclin E2, the common target of the three miRNAs, thereby promoting cancer growth (36). In this study, we identified the potential miRNA of uc.77- using the RegRNA2.0 software and confirmed it by dual luciferase reporter experiments. The results suggested that uc.77- binds directly to miR-4676-5p. However, a previous study showed that uc.77 regulates ZEB2 in human lung cancer (29). To the best of our knowledge, this study is the first to show that miR-4676-5p acts as an oncogene in CRC. miRNAs bind to the 3′-UTR of target genes to regulate translation or stability (37–39). In this study, dual luciferase reporter experiments showed that miR-4676-5p directly binds to the 3′-UTR of FBXW8 to inhibit its expression. These results not only reveal the function and mechanism of miR-4676, but also provide a potential therapeutic target for the treatment of CRC.

The cell cycle is regulated by the activity of cyclins and the chaperone kinases CDKs. CDKs that induce cell division are often active in cancer, and sustained proliferation signals are recognized as malignant tumor markers (40). Pharmacological inhibitors of CDKs have been researched extensively. However, many compounds lack potency or selectivity. Therefore, controlling the cell cycle remains an unmet goal (8, 41). In the present study, we found that uc.77- promoted the ubiquitination of CDK4 by regulating the E3 ubiquitin ligase FBXW8. The present findings indicate that uc.77- may be a target for the treatment of CRC. FBXW8-mediated ubiquitination and degradation of MRFAP1 is important for the regulation of cell cycle progression (30). However, the role of FBXW8 in CRC remains unclear. This study is the first to propose a mechanism underlying the role of FBXW8 in CRC, and to show that inhibition of FBXW8 reduces the formation of CRC cell colonies. The expression and regulation of FBXW8 and CDK4 in clinical tissues need further study.

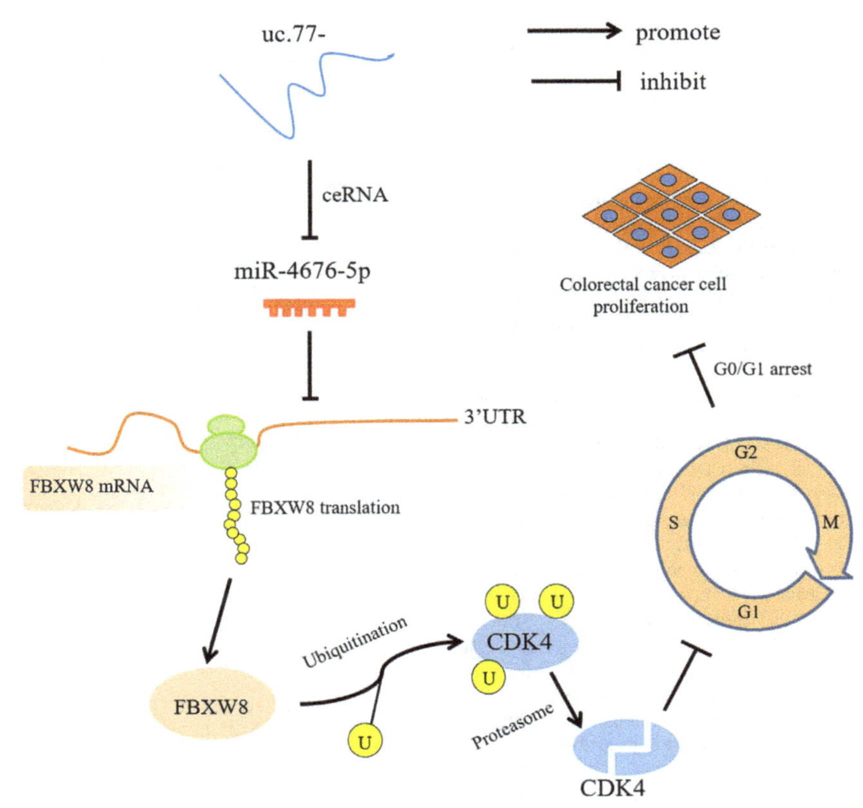

FIGURE 7 | uc.77- schematic diagram of the molecular mechanism underlying the regulation of CRC cell proliferation.

In summary, we showed that uc.77- is downregulated in human CRC and may represent an unfavorable prognostic factor for CRC. Overexpression of uc.77- inhibited the proliferation of CRC cells *in vivo* and *in vitro*. A schematic diagram in **Figure 7** shows that uc.77- competes with FBXW8 to bind miR-4676-5p through a ceRNA mechanism, thereby suppressing the inhibitory effect of miR-4676-5p on the 3′-UTR of FBXW8. The resulting increase in FBXW8 expression and CDK4 ubiquitination results in the downregulation of CDK4 and a block of the G0/G1 transition, thereby inhibiting the proliferation of CRC cells. The findings of this study provide evidence supporting the important role of T-UCRs in CRC, and indicate that uc.77- and its downstream effectors may serve as potential targets for the treatment of CRC.

ETHICS STATEMENT

The studies involving human participants were reviewed and approved by Ethics Committee of Wenzhou Medical University. Written informed consent for participation was not required for this study in accordance with the national legislation and the institutional requirements. The animal study was reviewed and approved by Experimental Animal Ethics Committee of Wenzhou Medical University.

AUTHOR CONTRIBUTIONS

ZZ, HJ, and HH conceived and designed the study. ZZ, DH, RZ, and XZ detected the cells′ biological function, performed the RT-PCR assays, carried out the soft agar, ATP assay, Western blot, and luciferase reporter assays, and conducted the statistical analyses. YC, SH, QX, and HL analyzed clinical samples. ZZ, HJ, and HH drafted the manuscript. NS and ZL performed immunohistochemistry assay and the statistical analysis. All authors contributed to the article and approved the submitted version.

REFERENCES

1. Sung H, Ferlay J, Siegel RL, Laversanne M, Soerjomataram I, Jemal A, et al. Global cancer statistics 2020: GLOBOCAN estimates of incidence and mortality worldwide for 36 cancers in 185 countries. *CA: Cancer J Clin* (2021). doi: 10.3322/caac.21660
2. Chen W, Zheng R, Zeng H, Zhangand S, He J. Annual report on status of cancer in China, 2011. *Chin J Cancer Res* (2015) 27:2–12. doi: 10.3978/j.issn.1000-9604.2015.01.06
3. Bejerano G, Pheasant M, Makunin I, Stephen S, Kent WJ, Mattick JS, et al. Ultraconserved elements in the human genome. *Science* (2004) 304:1321–5. doi: 10.1126/science.1098119
4. Calin GA, Liu CG, Ferracin M, Hyslop T, Spizzo R, Sevignani C, et al. Ultraconserved regions encoding ncRNAs are altered in human leukemias and carcinomas. *Cancer Cell* (2007) 12:215–29. doi: 10.1016/j.ccr.2007.07.027
5. Zhang Y, Wang S, Qian W, Ji D, Wang Q, Zhang Z, et al. uc.338 targets p21 and cyclin D1 via PI3K/AKT pathway activation to promote cell proliferation in colorectal cancer. *Oncol Rep* (2018) 40:1119–28. doi: 10.3892/or.2018.6480
6. Wang C, Wang Z, Zhou J, Liu S, Wu C, Huang C, et al. TUC.338 promotes invasion and metastasis in colorectal cancer. *Int J Cancer* (2017) 140:1457–64. doi: 10.1002/ijc.30542
7. Honma R, Goto K, Sakamoto N, Sekino Y, Sentani K, Oue N, et al. Expression and Function of Uc.160+, a Transcribed Ultraconserved Region, in gastric cancer. *Gastric Cancer* (2017) 20:960–9. doi: 10.1007/s10120-017-0714-9
8. Malumbres M, Barbacid M. Cell cycle, CDKs and cancer: a changing paradigm. *Nat Rev Cancer* (2009) 9:153–66. doi: 10.1038/nrc2602
9. Sherr CJ, Beachand D, Shapiro GI. Targeting CDK4 and CDK6: From Discovery to Therapy. *Cancer Discovery* (2016) 6:353–67. doi: 10.1158/2159-8290.CD-15-0894
10. Asghar U, Witkiewicz AK, Turnerand NC, Knudsen ES. The history and future of targeting cyclin-dependent kinases in cancer therapy. *Nat Rev Drug Discovery* (2015) 14:130–46. doi: 10.1038/nrd4504
11. Dickson MA. Molecular pathways: CDK4 inhibitors for cancer therapy. *Clin Cancer Res* (2014) 20:3379–83. doi: 10.1158/1078-0432.CCR-13-1551
12. Yan H, Ren S, Lin Q, Yu Y, Chen C, Hua X, et al. Inhibition of UBE2N-dependent CDK6 protein degradation by miR-934 promotes human bladder cancer cell growth. *FASEB J Off Publ Fed Am Soc Exp Biol* (2019) 33:12112–23. doi: 10.1096/fj.201900499RR
13. Zhu J, Li Y, Tian Z, Hua X, Gu J, Li J, et al. Atg7 Overexpression is Crucial for Tumorigenic Growth of Bladder Cancer In Vitro and In Vivo by Targeting the ETS2/miRNA196b/FOXO1/p27 Axis. *Mol Ther Nucleic Acids* (2017) 7:299–313. doi: 10.1016/j.omtn.2017.04.012
14. Jin H, . Sun W, Zhang Y, Yan H, Liufu H, Wang S, et al. Microrna-411 Downregulation Enhances Tumor Growth by Upregulating Mllt11 Expression in Human Bladder Cancer.Molecular Therapy. *Nucleic Acids* (2018) 11:312–22. doi: 10.1016/j.omtn.2018.03.003
15. Xie Q, Chen C, Li H, Xu J, Wu L, Yu Y, et al. miR-3687 Overexpression Promotes Bladder Cancer Cell Growth by Inhibiting the Negative Effect of FOXP1 on Cyclin E2 Transcription. *Mol Ther J Am Soc Gene Ther* (2019) 27:1028–38. doi: 10.1016/j.ymthe.2019.03.006
16. Sun W, Li S, Yu Y, Jin H, Xie Q, Hua X, et al. Microrna-3648 Is Upregulated to Suppress Tcf21, Resulting in Promotion of Invasion and Metastasis of Human Bladder Cancer. *Mol Ther Nucleic Acids* (2019) 16:519–30. doi: 10.1016/j.omtn.2019.04.006
17. Li X, Tian Z, Jin H, Xu J, Hua X, Yan H, et al. Decreased c-Myc mRNA Stability via the MicroRNA 141-3p/AUF1 Axis Is Crucial for p63α Inhibition of Cyclin D1 Gene Transcription and Bladder Cancer Cell Tumorigenicity. *Mol Cell Biol* (2018) 38:e00273-18. doi: 10.1128/mcb.00273-18
18. Chang Y, Jin H, Li H, Ma J, Zheng Z, Sun B, et al. MiRNA-516a promotes bladder cancer metastasis by inhibiting MMP9 protein degradation via the AKT/FOXO3A/SMURF1 axis. *Clin Trans Med* (2020) 10:e263. doi: 10.1002/ctm2.263
19. Kong L, Zhang Y, Ye ZQ, Liu XQ, Zhao SQ, Wei L, et al. CPC: assess the protein-coding potential of transcripts using sequence features and support vector machine. *Nucleic Acids Res* (2007) 35:W345–9. doi: 10.1093/nar/gkm391
20. Dekker E, Tanis PJ, Vleugels JLA, Kasiand PM, Wallace MB. Colorectal cancer. *Lancet (London England)* (2019) 394:1467–80. doi: 10.1016/s0140-6736(19)32319-0
21. Ludwig JA, Weinstein JN. Biomarkers in cancer staging, prognosis and treatment selection. *Nat Rev Cancer* (2005) 5:845–56. doi: 10.1038/nrc1739
22. Coghlin C, Murray GI. Biomarkers of colorectal cancer: recent advances and future challenges. *Proteomics Clin Appl* (2015) 9:64–71. doi: 10.1002/prca.201400082
23. Mármol I, Sánchez-de-Diego C, Pradilla Dieste A, Cerradaand E, Rodriguez Yoldi MJ. Colorectal Carcinoma: A General Overview and Future Perspectives in Colorectal Cancer. *Int J Mol Sci* (2017) 18:197. doi: 10.3390/ijms18010197

24. Mestdagh P, Fredlund E, Pattyn F, Rihani A, Van Maerken T, Vermeulen J, et al. An integrative genomics screen uncovers ncRNA T-UCR functions in neuroblastoma tumours. *Oncogene* (2010) 29:3583–92. doi: 10.1038/onc.2010.106
25. Esteller M. Non-Coding RNAs in Human disease. *Nat Rev Genet* (2011) 12:861–74. doi: 10.1038/nrg3074
26. Hudson RS, Yi M, Volfovsky N, Prueitt RL, Esposito D, Volinia S, et al. Transcription signatures encoded by ultraconserved genomic regions in human prostate cancer. *Mol Cancer* (2013) 12:13. doi: 10.1186/1476-4598-12-13
27. Braconi C, Valeri N, Kogure T, Gasparini P, Huang N, Nuovo GJ, et al. Expression and functional role of a transcribed noncoding RNA with an ultraconserved element in hepatocellular carcinoma. *Proc Natl Acad Sci United States America* (2011) 108:786–91. doi: 10.1073/pnas.1011098108
28. Sana J, Hankeova S, Svoboda M, Kiss I, Vyzulaand R, Slaby O. Expression levels of transcribed ultraconserved regions uc.73 and uc.388 are altered in colorectal cancer. *Oncology* (2012) 82:114–8. doi: 10.1159/000336479
29. Sun H, Chen J, Qian W, Kang J, Wang J, Jiang L, et al. Integrated long non-coding RNA analyses identify novel regulators of epithelial-mesenchymal transition in the mouse model of pulmonary fibrosis. *J Cell Mol Med* (2016) 20:1234–46. doi: 10.1111/jcmm.12783
30. Li DZ, S.F L, Zhu L, Wang YX, Chen YX, Liu J, et al. FBXW8-dependent degradation of MRFAP1 in anaphase controls mitotic cell death. *Oncotarget* (2017) 8:97178–86. doi: 10.18632/oncotarget.21843
31. Ebert MS, Sharp PA. Emerging roles for natural microRNA sponges. *Curr Biol CB* (2010) 20:R858–61. doi: 10.1016/j.cub.2010.08.052
32. Ballantyne MD, McDonaldand RA, Baker a.H. lncRNA/MicroRNA interactions in the vasculature. *Clin Pharmacol Ther* (2016) 99:494–501. doi: 10.1002/cpt.355
33. Olivieri M, Ferro M, Terreri S, Durso M, Romanelli A, Avitabile C, et al. Long non-coding RNA containing ultraconserved genomic region 8 promotes bladder cancer tumorigenesis. *Oncotarget* (2016) 7:20636–54. doi: 10.18632/oncotarget.7833
34. Xiao L, Wu J, Wang JY, Chung HK, Kalakonda S, Rao JN, et al. Long Noncoding RNA uc.173 Promotes Renewal of the Intestinal Mucosa by Inducing Degradation of MicroRNA 195. *Gastroenterology* (2018) 154:599–611. doi: 10.1053/j.gastro.2017.10.009
35. Goto K, Ishikawa S, Honma R, Tanimoto K, Sakamoto N, Sentani K, et al. The transcribed-ultraconserved regions in prostate and gastric cancer: DNA hypermethylation and microRNA-associated regulation. *Oncogene* (2016) 35:3598–606. doi: 10.1038/onc.2015.445
36. Vannini I, Wise PM, Challagundla KB, Plousiou M, Raffini M, Bandini E, et al. Transcribed ultraconserved region 339 promotes carcinogenesis by modulating tumor suppressor microRNAs. *Nat Commun* (2017) 8:1801. doi: 10.1038/s41467-017-01562-9
37. Shi D, Zhang Y, Luand R, Zhang Y. The long non-coding RNA MALAT1 interacted with miR-218 modulates choriocarcinoma growth by targeting Fbxw8. *Biomed Pharmacother = Biomed Pharmacother* (2018) 97:543–50. doi: 10.1016/j.biopha.2017.10.083
38. Wang JY, Yang Y, Ma Y, Wang F, Xue A, Zhu J, et al. Potential regulatory role of lncRNA-miRNA-mRNA axis in osteosarcoma. *Biomed Pharmacother = Biomed Pharmacother* (2020) 121:109627. doi: 10.1016/j.biopha.2019.109627
39. Dong X, Yang Z, Yang H, Liand D, Qiu X. Long Non-coding RNA MIR4435-2HG Promotes Colorectal Cancer Proliferation and Metastasis Through miR-206/YAP1 Axis. *Front Oncol* (2020) 10:160. doi: 10.3389/fonc.2020.00160
40. Hanahan D., Weinberg RA. Hallmarks of cancer: the next generation. *Cell* (2011) 144:646–74. doi: 10.1016/j.cell.2011.02.013
41. Goel S, DeCristo MJ, McAllisterand SS, Zhao JJ. CDK4/6 Inhibition in Cancer: Beyond Cell Cycle Arrest. *Trends Cell Biol* (2018) 28:911–25. doi: 10.1016/j.tcb.2018.07.002

2

Coiled-Coil Domain-Containing 68 Downregulation Promotes Colorectal Cancer Cell Growth by Inhibiting ITCH-Mediated CDK4 Degradation

Cong Wang[1†], Hongyan Li[1†], Lei Wu[2†], Xueli Jiao[1], Zihui Jin[1], Yujie Zhu[1], Ziling Fang[1], Xiaodong Zhang[3], Haishan Huang[1] and Lingling Zhao[1*]*

[1] Key Laboratory of Laboratory Medicine, Ministry of Education, School of Laboratory Medicine and Life Sciences, Wenzhou Medical University, Wenzhou, China, [2] Department of General Surgery, Heze Municipal Hospital, Heze, China, [3] Department of Colorectal anal surgery, The First Affiliated Hospital of Wenzhou Medical University, Wenzhou, China

***Correspondence:**
Lingling Zhao
zhaolingling@wmu.edu.cn
Haishan Huang
haishan_333@163.com

†These authors have contributed equally to this work

Coiled-coil domain-containing 68 (CCDC68) plays different roles in cancer and is predicted as a tumor suppressor in human colorectal cancer (CRC). However, the specific role of CCDC68 in CRC and the underlying mechanisms remain unknown. Here, we showed that CCDC68 expression was lower in CRC than that in corresponding normal tissues, and CCDC68 level was positively correlated with disease-free survival. Ectopic expression of CCDC68 decreased CRC cell proliferation *in vitro* and suppressed the growth of CRC xenograft tumors *in vivo*. CCDC68 caused G0/G1 cell cycle arrest, downregulated CDK4, and upregulated ITCH, the E3 ubiquitin ligase responsible for CDK4 protein degradation. This increased CDK4 degradation, which decreased CDK4 protein levels and inhibited CRC tumor growth. Collectively, the present results identify a novel CDK4 regulatory axis consisting of CCDC68 and ITCH, which suggest that CCDC68 is a promising target for the treatment of CRC.

Keywords: CCDC68, colorectal cancer, CDK4 degradation, ITCH, cell proliferation

INTRODUCTION

Colorectal cancer (CRC), one of the three most common cancers worldwide, has the third highest incidence rate (10%) and the second highest mortality rate (9.4%), and is therefore a considerable threat to human life and health (1). Currently, approximately one in ten CRC patients die from the disease each year despite undergoing treatment (1). Understanding the molecular mechanisms underlying the occurrence and development of CRC and exploring new approaches to the treatment of CRC are important research objectives.

The occurrence and development of CRC are mediated by a complex process that involves multiple pathways (2, 3), such as the EGFR, Wnt/β-catenin, TGF-β, and Sonic Hedgehog pathways. The factors and/or genes involved in these pathways may be potential therapeutic targets in CRC (4, 5). The combination of panitumumab, a human monoclonal antibody against EGFR, with supportive therapy is a common strategy for the treatment of metastatic CRC (6). Several inhibitors of the Wnt/β-catenin signaling pathway have been developed for the treatment of

CRC (7). Identifying and understanding the factors and/or genes implicated in CRC occurrence and development would facilitate the early diagnosis or treatment of CRC patients.

Coiled-coil domain-containing (CCDC) proteins are a large family of proteins possessing a unique α-helical coiled coil that mediates multiple functions, including cytoskeleton formation, regulation of cell polarity and movement, transportation of intracellular substances, molecular recognition, and signal transduction (8). Many members of this family are involved in the progression of multiple cancers, such as CCDC43 in gastric cancer (9), CCDC8 in lung cancer (10), and CCDC34 in bladder cancer (11). CCDC68, a member of the CCDC family, is an important component of mother centriole subdistal appendages; it is a centrosome protein and is thus involved in cell cycle progression (12–14). CCDC68 also plays a role in cancer. Radulovich et al. found that CCDC68 is downregulated and acts as a tumor suppressor in pancreatic ductal adenocarcinoma (15). However, CCDC68 is upregulated in non-small cell lung cancer (NSCLC) and promotes cell proliferation (16). Therefore, the role of CCDC68 in cancer remains controversial. There is only one article reporting that CCDC68 is downregulated in 89% of patients with primary CRC, suggesting that CCDC68 might be a new candidate tumor suppressor gene in CRC (17). The specific biological role of CCDC68 in CRC and the underlying mechanism remain largely unclear.

In this study, we demonstrated that CCDC68 suppresses CRC cell proliferation *in vitro* and *in vivo* by promoting ITCH transcription. This was mediated by upregulation of the transcription factor RXRα and alterations of cyclin-dependent kinase (CDK)-4 protein degradation. We showed that CCDC68 downregulation promoted the growth of CRC cells through the RXRα/ITCH/CDK4 axis, thereby identifying a new mechanism underlying the development of CRC and providing a theoretical basis for targeted therapy for CRC.

MATERIALS AND METHODS

Plasmids, Antibodies, and Reagents

The HA-CCDC68 plasmid, a set of shRNA plasmids specifically targeting ITCH, and the Flag-RXRα plasmid were purchased from MiaoLingBio (Wuhan, China). The pEGFP-CDK4 plasmid was constructed as described in our previous study (18). The luciferase reporter driven by the ITCH promoter was constructed by inserting the ITCH promotor sequence into the pGL3-basic vector (E1751; Promega) with the primers (F) 5′;-TCTATC GATAGGTACCTGACTTTCCAGATGGCAAAATACT-3′; and (R) 5′;-CCGGAATGCCAAGCTTTTCGCCCACGGGGGT TTA-3′;. Antibodies against CDK2 (sc-6248), CDK4 (sc-260), CDK6 (sc-177), cyclinD1 (sc-20044), P21 (sc-397), and P27 (sc-1641) were purchased from Santa Cruz Biotechnology (Santa Cruz, CA, USA). Antibodies against CDC37 (4793S), cyclin E2 (4132S), HA (3724S), BTRC (11984S), and RXRα (3085S) were purchased from Cell Signaling Technology (Boston, MA, USA). Antibodies against α-Tubulin (ab7291), FBXO4 (ab230302), and SOCS7 (ab224589) were purchased from Abcam (Cambridge, UK). Antibodies against CCDC68 (PA5-61687) and FZR1 (34-2000) were purchased from Invitrogen (Grand Island, NY, USA). Antibody against ITCH (20920-1-AP) was purchased from Proteintech (Chicago, IL, USA). The chemicals cycloheximide (CHX) and MG132 were purchased from Calbiochem (San Diego, CA, USA).

Clinical Specimens

This study was approved by the Ethics Committee of Wenzhou Medical University. Tumor tissues and corresponding adjacent normal tissues were obtained from patients with colorectal cancer treated at the First Affiliated Hospital of Wenzhou Medical University (Zhejiang, China). A total of 150 pairs of tumor and normal tissues were collected and confirmed by histological and pathological diagnosis (**Table S1**). Each specimen was divided into two parts: RNA was extracted from one third of the material, and cDNA was synthesized and stored at -80°C until analysis. Two thirds of the material were fixed in formalin, embedded in paraffin, and stored at room temperature.

Cell Culture and Transfections

The human CRC cell lines HCT116 and HT29 were obtained from the Cell Bank of Shanghai Institute of Biochemistry and Cell Biology, Chinese Academy of Sciences. SW480 cells were bought from ATCC. HCoEpiC and RKO cells were bought from Cobioer (Nanjing, China). HCT116 and HT29 cells were maintained in McCoy's 5A medium supplemented with 10% fetal bovine serum (FBS); RKO and SW480 cells were cultured in 1640 medium (Gibco, 11875–093) containing 10% FBS; and HCoEpiC cells were cultured in minimum essential medium (MEM; Gibco, 11095–080) containing 10% FBS. All cells were grown in a 5% CO_2 cell culture incubator at 37°C. For stable cell line construction, HCT116 and RKO cells were transfected with plasmids using PolyJet™ DNA In Vitro Transfection Reagent (SignaGen Laboratories, SL100688). After 48 h, cells were subjected to selection with puromycin (4–6 μg/mL; J593, Amresco Inc) or G418 (1000–1500 μg/mL; sc-29065, Dallas, TX, USA) according to the antibiotic resistance of different transfected plasmids.

Lentivirus Packaging and Infection

Lentivirus packaging and infection experiments were performed as described previously (18). HA-CCDC68 stable expression cells and vector control cells were constructed by lentivirus infection. Briefly, two packaging vectors, 1.2 μg pMD2.G (12259, Addgene) and 1.2 μg psPAX2 (12260, Addgene), and 2.0 μg HA-CCDC68-PLVX-puro or HA- PLVX-puro plasmid, were transfected into 293T cells. The viral supernatants were then collected after 48 h, filtered, and used to infect HCT116 and RKO cells. Stable cell lines were screened by puromycin.

Immunohistochemistry (IHC)

IHC assays were performed to detect CCDC68 expression in formalin fixed paraffin embedded CRC specimens obtained from humans. An antibody specific against CCDC68 (PA5-61687; Invitrogen, Grand Island, NY, USA) was used for IHC staining, which was performed using a kit from Boster Bio-

Engineering Company (SA1022; Wuhan, China). Immunostained images were captured with the Nikon Eclipse Ni microsystem (DS-Ri2) and analyzed with Image-Pro Plus version 6.0 (Media Cybernetics, Rockville, MD, USA) by calculating the integrated optical density (IOD) of each stained area (IOD/area). At least five images per specimen were counted.

Western Blotting

The cells were lysed with a lysis buffer containing 10 mM Tris-HCl, 1 mM Na_3VO_4, and 1% SDS (pH 7.4) on ice. The samples were then collected and heated at 100°C for 5 min, and nucleic acids were broken with ultrasound. Protein samples were separated on SDS-PAGE gels, followed by transfer to polyvinylidene fluoride membranes (Bio-Rad, Hercules, CA, USA). The membranes were blocked with 5% non-fat milk and probed with the indicated primary antibodies overnight at 4°C, and then incubated with AP-conjugated secondary antibody. The ECF western blotting system (RPN5787; GE Healthcare, PA, USA) was used to detect the protein signal, and images were captured using a phosphorimager (Typhoon FLA 7000, GE Healthcare) (19).

Anchorage-Independent Growth Assay

The potential inhibitory effect of CCDC68 on the anchorage-independent growth of human CRC cells was assessed in the HCT116 and RKO cell lines. First, 0.5% agar in Basal Medium Eagle (BME) containing 10% FBS was used to cover the bottom layer of 6-well plates. Then, 1×10^4 HCT116 (Vector), HCT116 (CCDC68), RKO (Vector), and RKO (CCDC68) stable transfectants were suspended in 1 mL of 0.33% agar in 10% FBS-BME and seeded on the bottom layer. After culturing in a 5% CO_2 incubator for 2–4 weeks, the number and size of cell colonies were determined under a microscope (DMi1; Leica Microsystems, Germany) (20).

Cell Proliferation

A Cell Titer-Glo Luminescent Cell Viability Assay kit (G7572; Promega) was used to determine the effect of CCDC68 on the proliferation of CRC cells. The assay was performed as described previously (18). Briefly, 2000 HCT116 (Vector), HCT116 (CCDC68), RKO (Vector), and RKO (CCDC68) cells were seeded into each well of 96-well plates. After adherence, the cells were synchronized for 12 h by exposure to 0.1% FBS medium and then cultured in complete medium for the indicated days. Cell viability was detected at 1, 3, and 5 days using a Centro LB 960 luminometer (Berthold Technologies, Berthold, Germany). Cell proliferation rate was defined as the relative absorbance of cells cultured for 3 and 5 days versus that of cells cultured for 1 day. Each experiment was repeated at least three times.

Cell Cycle Analysis

Cell Cycle Analysis was performed by flow cytometry (FCM). Cells were collected and fixed with 70% ethanol at 4°C overnight, and then washed and stained with a mixed solution of propidium iodide and RNase A (9:1) (KGA511; KeyGen Biotech, Nanjing, China) for 1 h at room temperature. Immediately thereafter, the cell cycle was detected by CytoFLEX (Beckman Coulter, San Diego, CA, USA), and the results were analyzed with the CytExpert software.

Quantitative Real-Time PCR (qRT-PCR)

Total RNA was extracted using TRIzol (15596018, Invitrogen), and cDNAs were synthesized using the SuperScript™ First-Strand Synthesis system (18091200, Invitrogen). qRT-PCR assays were performed using the Fast SYBR Green Master Mix kit (4385614, Applied Biosystems) in the Q6 real-time PCR system (Thermo Fisher Scientific, Waltham, MA, USA). The primers used in this assay were as follows: human CCDC68 (forward, 5′-TCTGCCTTGTATGAGTCTACGTCC-3′; reverse, 5′- A GGATCCATTTCAGAATCAGAGCC-3′), human CDK4 (forward, 5′-CTACAGCTACCAGATGGCACTTAC-3′; reverse, 5′-CAAAGATACAGCCAACACTCCACA-3′), human ITCH (forward, 5′-GGAAGCAACCCCTTACAGTTATC-3′; reverse, 5′-CTAATGCAGCAGTTCCCAACAA-3′), and human GAPDH (forward, 5′-GACTCATGACCACAGTCCATGC-3′; reverse, 5′-CAGGTCAGGTCCACCACTGA-3′).

Dual-Luciferase Reporter Assay

HCT116 (Vector), HCT116 (CCDC68), RKO (Vector), and RKO (CCDC68) cells were transiently co-transfected with the ITCH promoter-driven luciferase reporter and pRL-TK for 24 h. After washing twice with PBS, cells were lysed with passive lysis buffer for 10 min at room temperature. Then, 20 μL cell lysate was transferred to a 96-well plate, and 40 μL Luciferase Assay Reagent II was added to detect ITCH promoter activity. Thereafter, Stop & Glo Buffer (Promega, USA) was added to each well to detect TK activity, which was measured in a Centro LB 960 luminometer (Berthold).

Protein Degradation Assay

To evaluate the potential effects of CCDC68 on the degradation of CDK4 in CRC cells, 5×10^5 stably transfected HCT116 (Vector) and HCT116 (CCDC68) cells were added into each well of a 6-well plate and cultured in complete medium at 37°C in a 5% CO_2 incubator. The medium was replaced by 0.1% FBS medium after the cell density reached 50–60%, and cells were then starved for 12 h, followed by culture in 10% FBS medium for 12 h. Thereafter, cells were treated with medium containing 10 μM MG132 for 5 h before exposure to CHX (50 μg/mL) for 0, 3, 6, and 12 h. The protein stability of CDK4 was evaluated by western blotting at each time point.

Immunoprecipitation

293T cells were transiently transfected with GFP-CDK4 plasmid. At 36 h after transfection, cells were harvested, and total cell lysates were extracted using cell lysis buffer (9803, Cell Signaling Technology, USA) containing a complete protein inhibitor cocktail (04693116001, Roche, Germany) on ice. The obtained lysates were incubated with rotation at 4°C for 30 min. After centrifugation, the supernatant (1000 μL) was divided into two aliquots: 450 μL (50 μL was removed, denatured, and stored to check the input by western blotting) was incubated with 2 μg anti-CDK4 antibody (sc-260); and 450 μL (50 μL was removed, denatured, and stored to check the input by western blotting) was incubated with a nonspecific antibody (rabbit IgG, sc-2749). After incubation overnight at 4°C, 30 μL protein A/G-coated magnetic beads (Thermo Fisher Scientific) were added to each sample and incubated for 2–4 h at 4°C. Extracts were sequentially washed five times with 1× Cell Lysis Buffer using a magnetic stand. Finally, 60 μL protein elution buffer and 0.6 μL DTT were added, and samples were heated at 37°C for 2 h to denature and separate the magnetic beads. The samples without magnetic beads were subjected to western blotting analysis.

Xenograft Model in Nude Mice *In Vivo*

Animal experiments were performed in the animal institute of Wenzhou Medical University according to the protocols approved by the Laboratory Animal Center of Wenzhou Medical University and the Laboratory Animal Ethics Committee of Wenzhou Medical University, as described in our previous publication (21). Female BALB/c athymic nude mice (3 or 4 weeks old) were purchased from Shanghai Silaike Experimental Animal Company (license no. SCXK, Shanghai 2010-0002). After 1–2 weeks of acclimatization, mice were randomly allocated to one of two groups (five mice/group) and then subcutaneously injected into the right flank with 5×10^6 HCT116 (Vector) or HCT116 (CCDC68) cells suspended in 100 μL Serum-free medium McCoy's 5A. After 4 weeks, mice were sacrificed, and tumors were surgically removed, imaged, and weighed. Two third of the tumor was fixed in 4% paraformaldehyde for IHC, and the remaining third was frozen at -80°C to extract RNA if necessary.

Bioinformatic Analysis

UbiBrowser database was used to screen possible E3 ligases related to CDK4 (http://ubibrowser.ncpsb.org/). The potential transcription factors binding to the ITCH promoter were predicted by the JASPAR database (http://jaspar.genereg.net/), with a profile score threshold of 95%.

Statistical Analysis

All experimental data are expressed as the mean ± standard deviation (mean ± SD). Graphs and statistical analyses were performed using GraphPad Prism 6 (GraphPad Software, San Diego, CA, USA). The Kaplan–Meier method was used to draw the survival curve, and the log-rank test was used to compare the differences between groups. Comparisons between the control group and the experimental group were performed using the Student's *t*-test. $P < 0.05$ was considered statistically significant.

RESULTS

CCDC68 is Downregulated in CRC and Related to Patient Prognosis

To investigate the potential role of CCDC68 in human CRC progression, the Cancer Genome Atlas (TCGA) database was used to analyze the expression levels of CCDC68 in 41 pairs of cancerous and normal tissues from CRC patients. The results showed that CCDC68 was markedly downregulated in CRC (**Figure 1A**). Furthermore, we analyzed the expression levels of CCDC68 in 150 fresh CRC samples and matched adjacent (normal) colorectal tissues by qRT-PCR and IHC assays. The results showed that CCDC68 was significantly downregulated in tumor tissues, which was consistent with TCGA data (**Figures 1B–D**).

To assess the role of CCDC68 in CRC, we analyzed the relationship between CCDC68 expression levels and disease-free survival (DFS) data from the TCGA database. Kaplan–Meier survival analysis revealed that CCDC68 downregulation was associated with a poor prognosis in CRC patients (**Figure 1E**). In addition, CCDC68 expression was lower in human CRC cell lines (HCT116, HT29, RKO, and SW480) than that in the human immortalized normal colorectal epithelial cell line HCoEpiC (**Figure 1F**).

CCDC68 Overexpression Suppresses Human CRC Cell Growth *In Vitro* and *In Vivo*

To evaluate whether CCDC68 is involved in the development of CRC, we constructed four stable transfectants, HCT116 (CCDC68), HCT116 (Vector), RKO (CCDC68), and RKO (Vector), which were examined by western blotting (**Figure 2A**). CCDC68 overexpression significantly decreased the monolayer growth of HCT116 and RKO cells compared with that of control vector transfectants (**Figures 2B, C**). CCDC68 overexpression also significantly decreased the anchorage-independent growth of CRC cells (**Figures 2D, E**). These data indicate that CCDC68 inhibited CRC cell growth *in vitro*.

To extend our findings *in vivo*, a xenograft nude mouse model was established by subcutaneous injection of equal numbers of HCT116 (Vector) and HCT116 (CCDC68) cells into nude mice. Tumor size was measured periodically, and a tumor growth curve was drawn (**Figure 2F**). The results showed that the weight and size of the subcutaneous tumors were significantly reduced in mice injected with HCT116 (CCDC68) cells than that in the HCT116 (Vector) control group (**Figures 2G, H**). These data confirmed that overexpression of CCDC68 decreased the growth ability of CRC cells.

Overexpression of CCDC68 Induces G0/G1 Phase Arrest in CRC Cells and Downregulates the Expression of the CDK4 Protein

Uncontrolled cell cycle progression and cell proliferation are two important biological characteristics of tumor cells (22). We therefore used FCM to analyze cell cycle progression in HCT116 (Vector or CCDC68) and RKO (Vector or CCDC68) cells, and to explore the potential molecular mechanism underlying the effect of CCDC68 on inhibiting CRC cell growth. As shown in **Figures 3A, B**, CCDC68 overexpression induced cell cycle G0/G1 arrest, suggesting that the inhibition of CRC cell growth by CCDC68 is related to its ability to induce G0-G1 growth arrest.

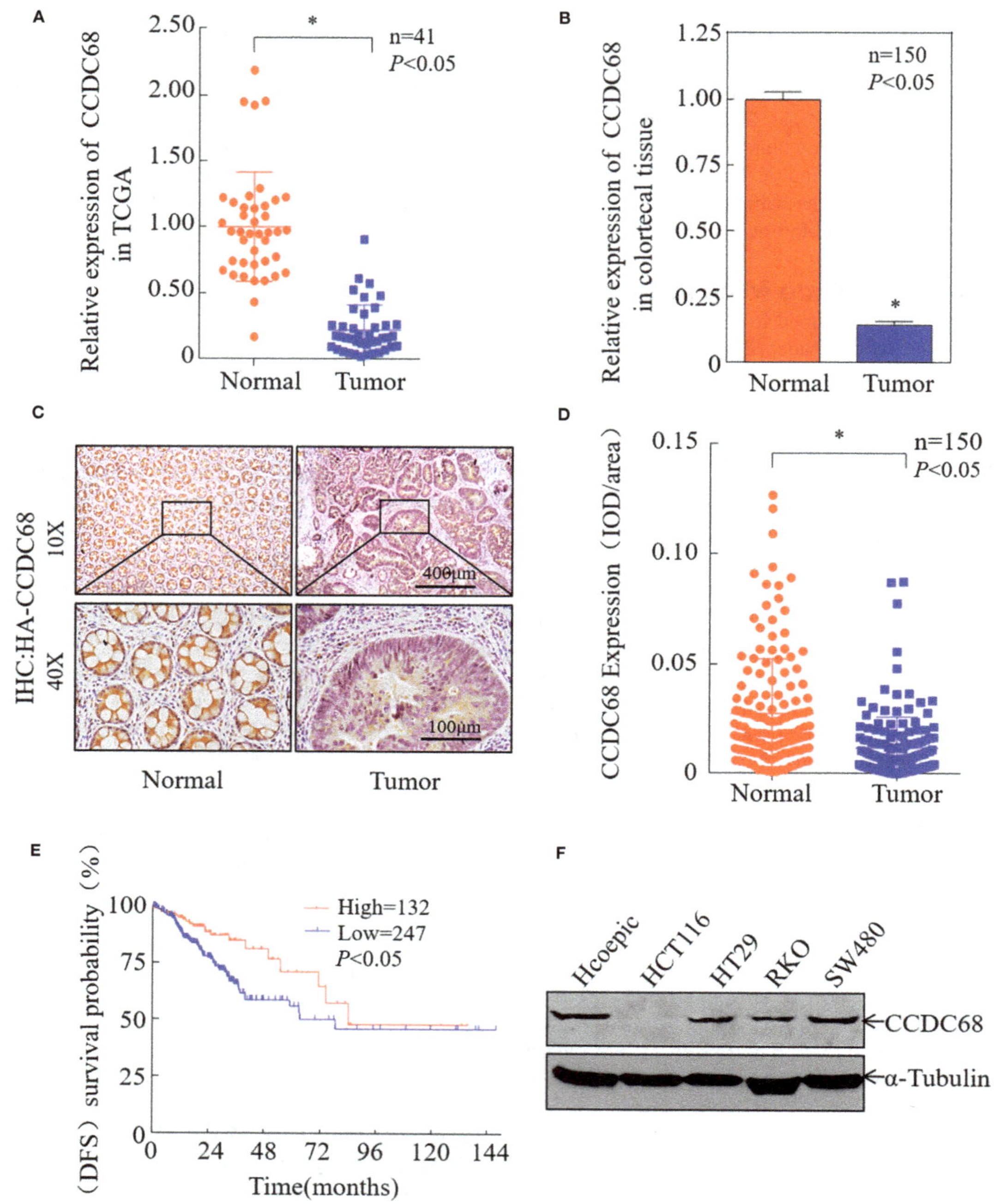

FIGURE 1 | CCDC68 is downregulated in CRC tissues and cells. **(A)** CCDC68 mRNA levels in CRC according to the Cancer Genome Atlas (TCGA) data. **(B)** The mRNA expression level of CCDC68 in 150 pairs of CRC tissues and paracancerous tissues (normal). **(C)** Representative IHC images of CCDC68 protein expression in CRC tissues and adjacent normal tissues. **(D)** Quantification of CCDC68 expression in 150 pairs of CRC tissues and adjacent normal tissues. **(E)** CCDC68 mRNA expression levels and disease-free survival of patients from TCGA CRC data. **(F)** Expression of CCDC68 in human CRC cell lines (HCT116, HT29, RKO, and SW480) and in the normal colorectal epithelial cell line HCoEpiC. Data are presented as the mean ± SD, $^{*}P < 0.05$.

To elucidate the molecular mechanism underlying the effect of CCDC68 on inducing G0/G1growth arrest in CRC cells, the expression of G0/G1 phase-related proteins was detected in HCT116 and RKO cells by western blotting. Ectopic expression of CCDC68 did not significantly affect the expression of the cell cycle regulatory proteins CDK2, CDK6, cyclin D1, cyclin E2, P21, and P27 (**Figure 3C**). However, CDK4 expression was lower in HCT116 (CCDC68) and RKO (CCDC68) cells than in the

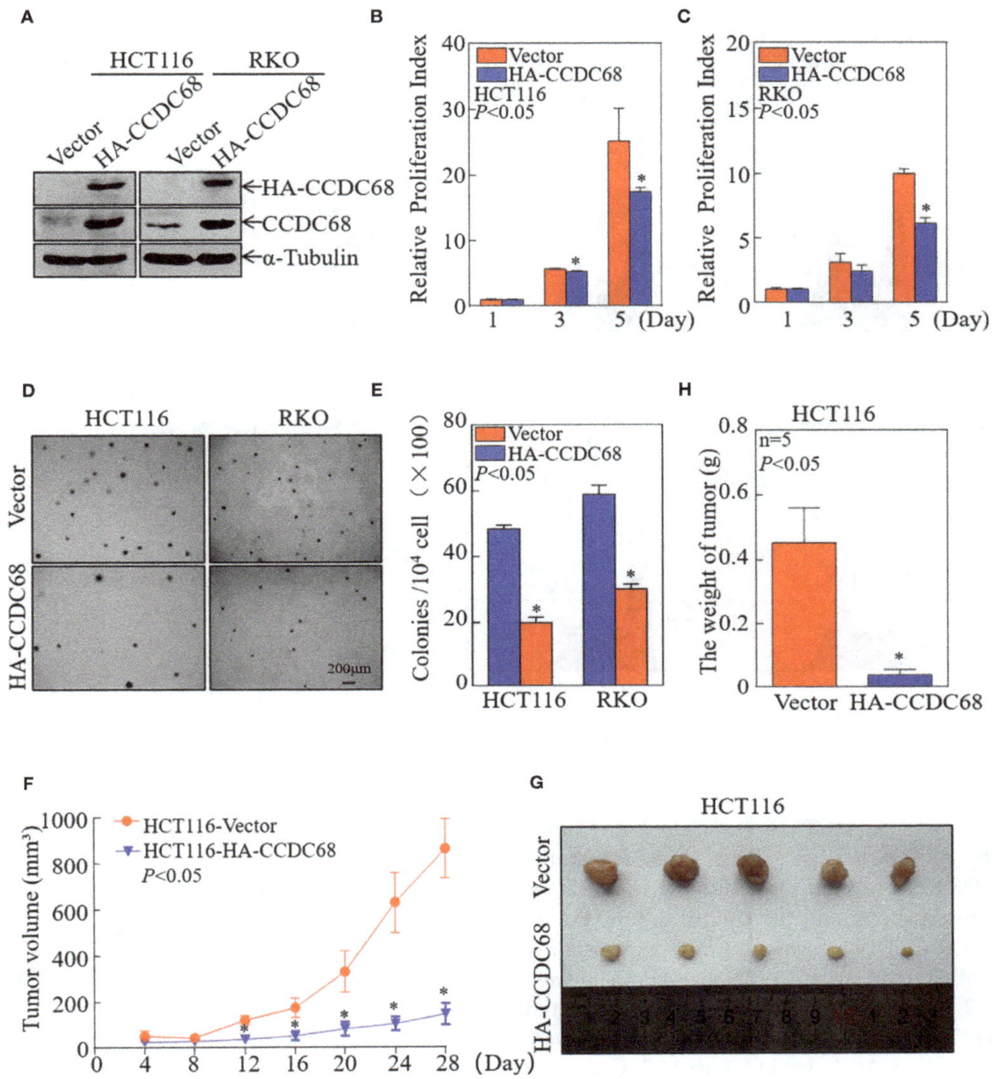

FIGURE 2 | CCDC68 overexpression inhibits CRC cell growth in vitro and in vivo. **(A)** Stable transfectants of HCT116 (Vector) vs. HCT116 (HA-CCDC68) and RKO (Vector) vs. RKO (HA-CCDC68) were identified by western blotting. **(B, C)** Cell proliferation was detected by ATP assay. Data were analyzed Student's *t*-test. **(D, E)** Anchorage-independent growth was examined by soft agar assay. Cell colonies were counted, and data were presented as colonies per 10,000 cells and analyzed by Student's *t*-test. **(F)** Tumor growth curve for each group. Data were analyzed by Student's *t*-test. **(G)** Representative images of tumors in each group. **(H)** Statistical analysis of tumor mass in each group; n = 5, Student's *t*-test. Data are presented as the mean ± SD. $^*P < 0.05$.

corresponding control cells. These results suggest that CDK4 is a key downstream molecule associated with the inhibition of CRC cell proliferation by CCDC68.

CCDC68 Inhibits the Proliferation of CRC Cells by Targeting CDK4

To further explore the role of CDK4 as a downstream effector of CCDC68, CDK4 was ectopically expressed in HCT116 (CCDC68) and RKO (CCDC68) cells (**Figures 4A, D**). The effect of CDK4 overexpression on the anchorage-independent proliferation of HCT116 (CCDC68) and RKO (CCDC68) cells was examined by soft agar assay. As shown in **Figures 4B, C, E, F**, ectopic expression of GFP-CDK4 increased anchorage-independent growth. The results of FCM analysis confirmed that CCDC68-induced G0/G1 growth arrest was reversed by CDK4 overexpression compared with that in the control vector (**Figures 4G, H**). Collectively, these results suggest that CDK4 is a downstream regulator mediating the inhibition of CRC cell proliferation by CCDC68.

ITCH might Serve as an E3 Ubiquitin Ligase Targeting CDK4 for Degradation

To elucidate the molecular mechanism underlying the effect of CCDC68 on downregulating CDK4 expression, the mRNA levels

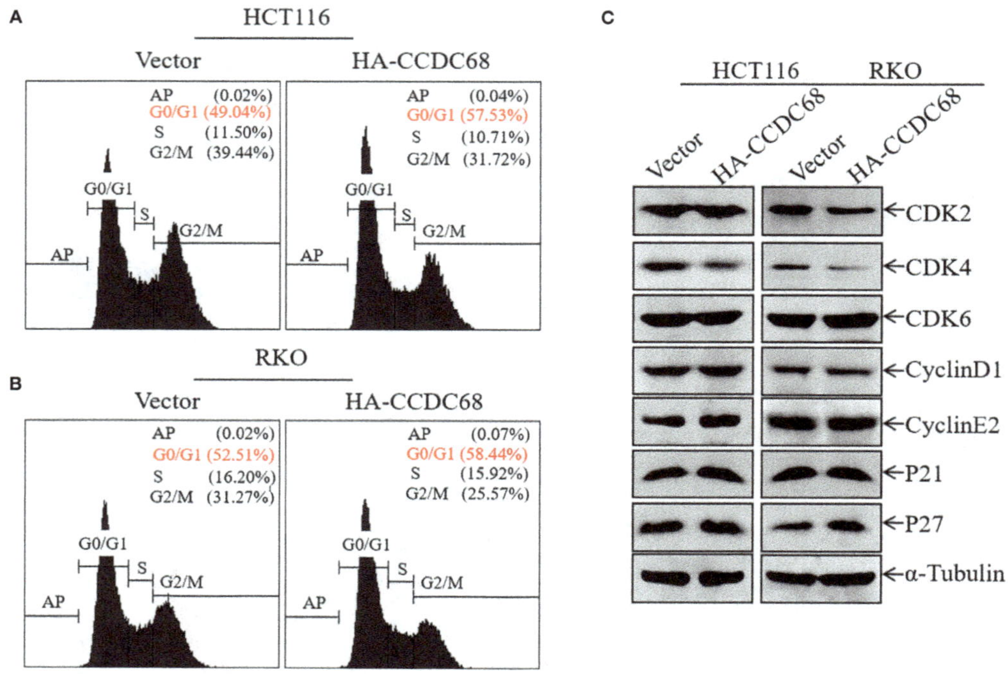

FIGURE 3 | Overexpression of CCDC68 induces G0/G1 phase arrest and downregulates CDK4 in CRC cells. **(A, B)** Cell cycle of HCT116 (Vector/HA-CCDC68) and RKO (Vector/HA-CCDC68) cells examined by flow cytometry. **(C)** Expression of positive cell cycle regulators in the G0/G1 phase of HCT116 (Vector/HA-CCDC68) and RKO (Vector/HA-CCDC68) cells.

of CDK4 were measured in HCT116 (CCDC68) and RKO (CCDC68) cells by qRT-PCR. The results showed that the mRNA levels of CDK4 did not differ significantly between the CCDC68 overexpression group and the control group (**Figure 5A**). This suggests that CCDC68 regulates CDK4 expression at the protein level rather than at the mRNA level. Cells were treated with MG132 (10 μM) and CHX (50 μg/mL) (23), and harvested at different time points, and CDK4 protein levels were detected by western blotting. As shown in **Figures 5B, C**, the rate of degradation of the CDK4 protein was significantly higher in HCT116 cells overexpressing CCDC68 than in the control group. These results indicate that CCDC68 downregulates CDK4 by promoting its ubiquitination.

Next, we examined the mechanism by which CCDC68 regulates the ubiquitination of CDK4. FBXO4 is an E3 ubiquitin ligase for CDK4 (24), and cell division cycle 37 (Cdc37), a partner of heat stress protein 90 (HSP90), enhances CDK4 stability and promotes CRC cell survival (25). In addition, we used the UbiBrowser database to screen for possible E3 ligases related to CDK4 degradation (**Figure 5D**). Potential E3 enzymes acting as tumor suppressors in CRC and related to cell growth were selected from the top 20 E3 enzymes identified (**Figure 5E**), and the expression levels of these proteins were examined in HCT116 and RKO cells overexpressing CCDC68 by western blotting. The results showed that the expression of ITCH was significantly higher in the HCT116 (CCDC68) and RKO (CCDC68) transfectants than in the control groups, whereas other enzymes showed no significant differences in expression (**Figure 5F**). We speculated that CCDC68 may accelerate the degradation rate of CDK4 through ITCH, ultimately inhibiting the malignant proliferation of CRC cells.

CCDC68 Promotes the Degradation of CDK4 by Upregulating ITCH Expression

To verify the role of ITCH in CCDC68-regulated cell growth, four stable ITCH knockdown clones of HCT116 (CCDC68) cells were established (**Figure 6A**). The effect of ITCH knockdown on cell proliferation and cell cycle progression was examined by soft agar assay and FCM in HCT116 (CCDC68) cells. The results showed that ITCH knockdown markedly reversed the inhibitory effects of CCDC68 on HCT116 anchorage-independent growth and G0/G1cell cycle arrest (**Figures 6B–D**).

To further investigate whether ITCH mediates CDK4 degradation, the effect of ITCH knockdown on CDK4 expression was examined by western blotting in HCT116 (CCDC68) cells; a protein degradation assay and IP assay were also performed. As shown in **Figures 6E, F**, knockdown of ITCH in HCT116 (CCDC68) cells significantly upregulated CDK4 and dramatically decreased the rate of CDK4 protein decay. The results of IP with an antibody that specifically pulls down the CDK4 protein showed that ITCH was present in the immune complex (**Figure 6G**), suggesting that ITCH binds to and interacts with CDK4 to trigger its degradation. These results suggest that CCDC68 promotes CDK4 protein degradation by regulating ITCH protein expression, thereby inhibiting the malignant proliferation of CRC cells.

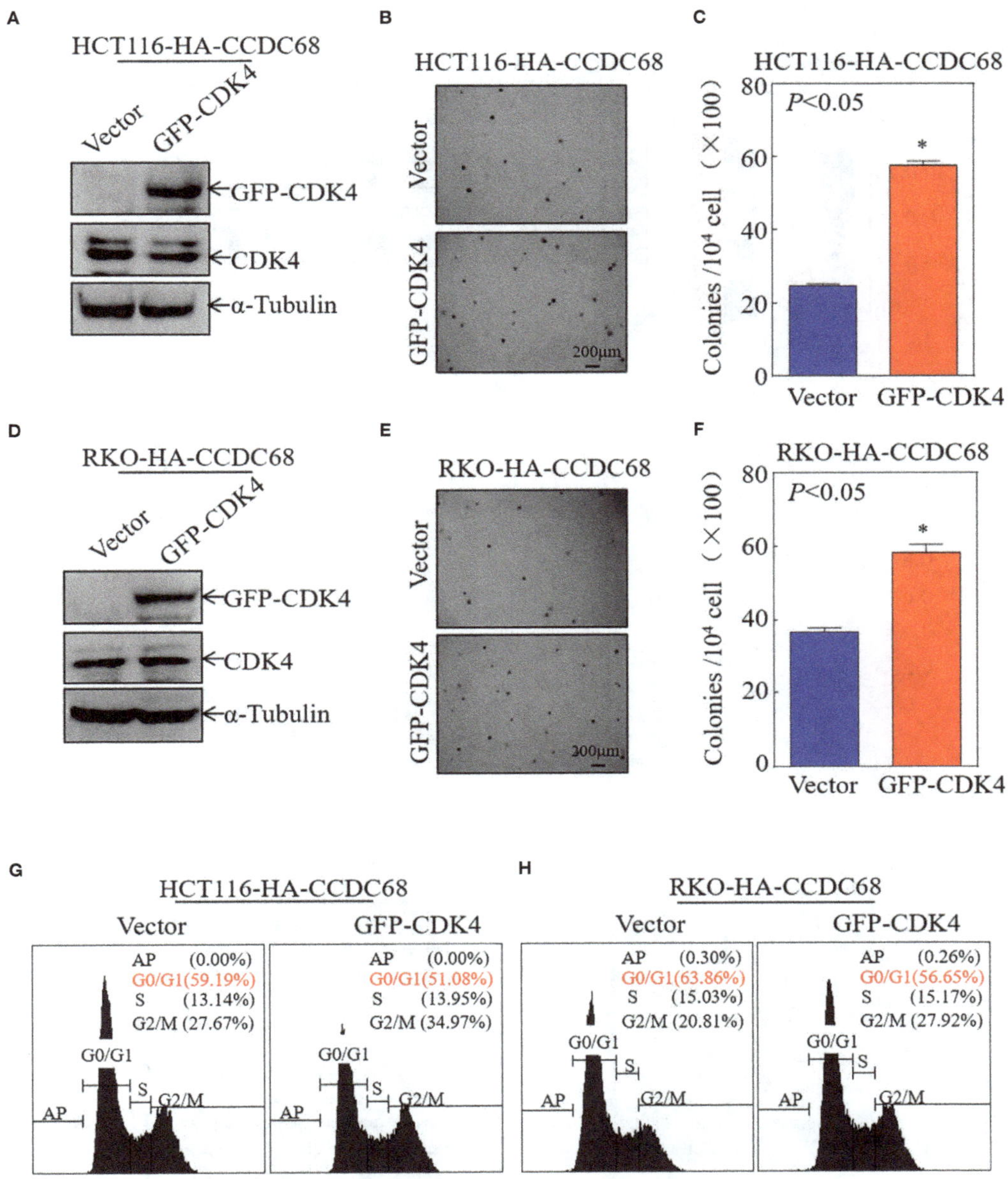

FIGURE 4 | CCDC68 inhibits malignant CRC cell proliferation by downregulating CDK4. **(A, D)** Stable transformation efficacy was assessed by western blotting in HCT116 (CCDC68) and RKO (CCDC68) cells overexpressing GFP-CDK4. **(B, E)** A soft agar colony formation assay was used to detect the effect of CDK4 on the proliferation of CRC cells. **(C, F)** Diagrams comparing the number of cell clones between the control and experimental groups. **(G, H)** Effect of CDK4 on the G0/G1 phase in HCT116 (CCDC68) and RKO (CCDC68) cells. Data are presented as the mean ± SD and analyzed by Student's *t*-test, $^{*}P < 0.05$.

CCDC68 Promotes ITCH Transcription by Upregulating RXRα Protein Expression

To elucidate the potential mechanisms underlying the upregulation of ITCH by CCDC68 in CRC cells, the mRNA expression level of ITCH was measured in transfectants. As shown in **Figure 7A**, ITCH mRNA levels were markedly higher in CCDC68-overexpressing stable transfectants than in vector transfectants, suggesting that the upregulation of ITCH occurs at the transcriptional level or by modulating mRNA stability.

To determine whether CCDC68 regulates ITCH promoter activity, we detected the promoter activity of ITCH in HCT116 (CCDC68) and RKO (CCDC68) cells, and in the corresponding control groups using a dual-luciferase reporter assay. The results showed that CCDC68 overexpression significantly promoted the transcriptional activity of the ITCH promoter (**Figure 7B**), indicating that CCDC68 upregulates ITCH expression at the transcriptional level. Transcription factors regulate the expression of target genes by binding to the promoter region. Therefore, we predicted the

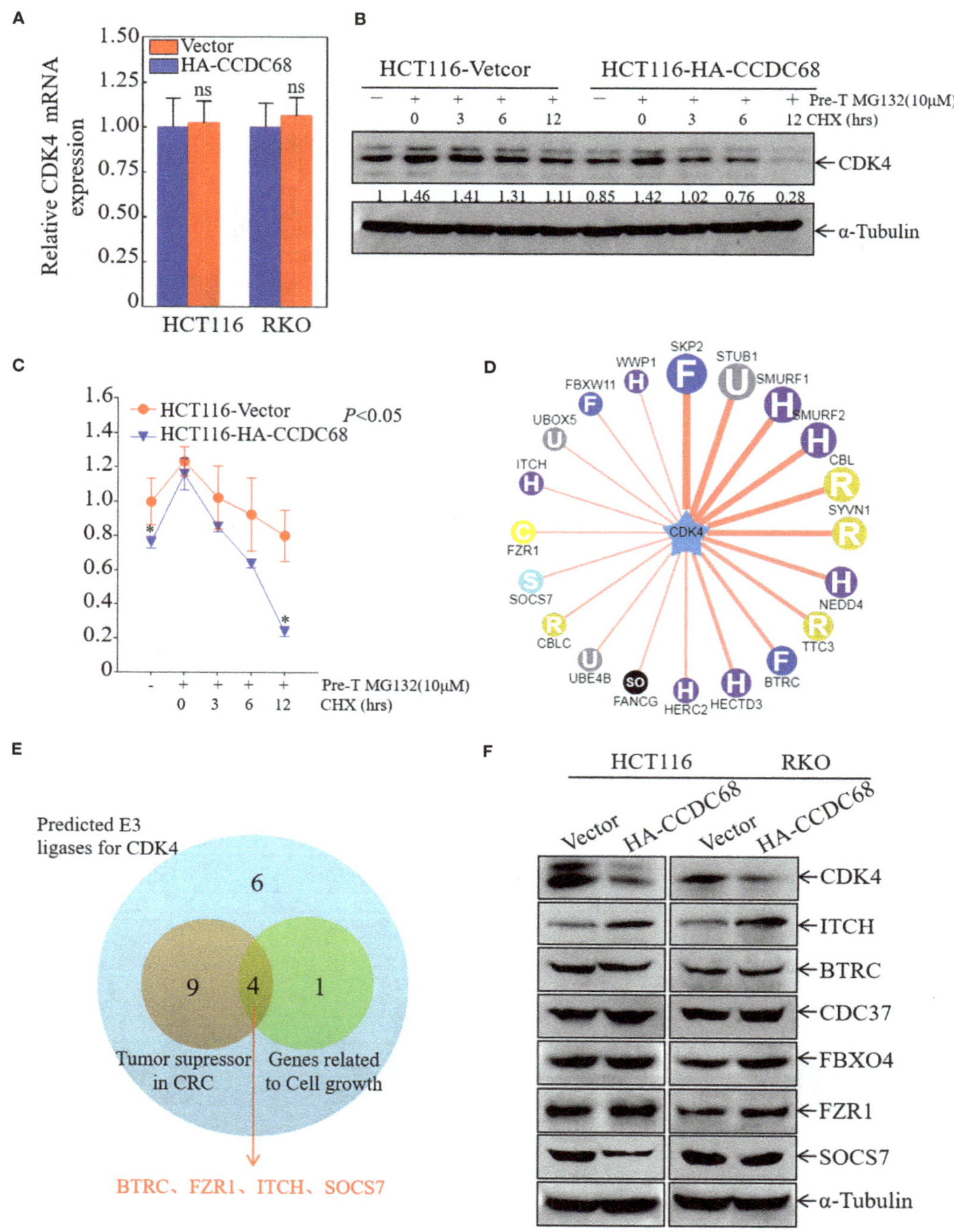

FIGURE 5 | ITCH may function as an E3 ubiquitin ligase targeting CDK4 for degradation. **(A)** Relative CDK4 mRNA expression in HCT116 (Vector/HA-CCDC68) and RKO (Vector/HA-CCDC68) cells. Student's *t*-test, ns, not significant. **(B)** CDK4 protein degradation was monitored in HCT116 (CCDC68) and HCT116 (Vector) cells pretreated with MG132 for 5 h followed by CHX for various times. **(C)** CDK4 protein degradation rates in HCT116 (CCDC68) and HCT116 (Vector) cells. Three independent degradation experiments were performed, and the results were analyzed using ImageJ software and analyzed by Student's *t*-test. $^*P < 0.05$. **(D)** Molecules potentially involved in the regulation of CDK4 protein degradation were predicted by the UbiBrowser database. **(E)** Venn diagram screening the E3 enzymes involved in the regulation of CDK4 protein degradation. **(F)** Expression of CDK4, ITCH, BTRC, CDC37, FBXO4, and SOCS7 in HCT116 (Vector/HA-CCDC68) and RKO (Vector/HA-CCDC68) cells.

transcription factors that may bind to the ITCH promoter using the JASPAR dataset with a profile score threshold of 95%.

Next, quantitative proteomics analysis was performed to identify the transcription factor involved in the regulation of ITCH expression by CCDC68. The transcription factors that play an inhibitory role in CRC were identified, and the data were combined with the results of website prediction and proteomics analysis. The results indicated that RXRα might be involved in the

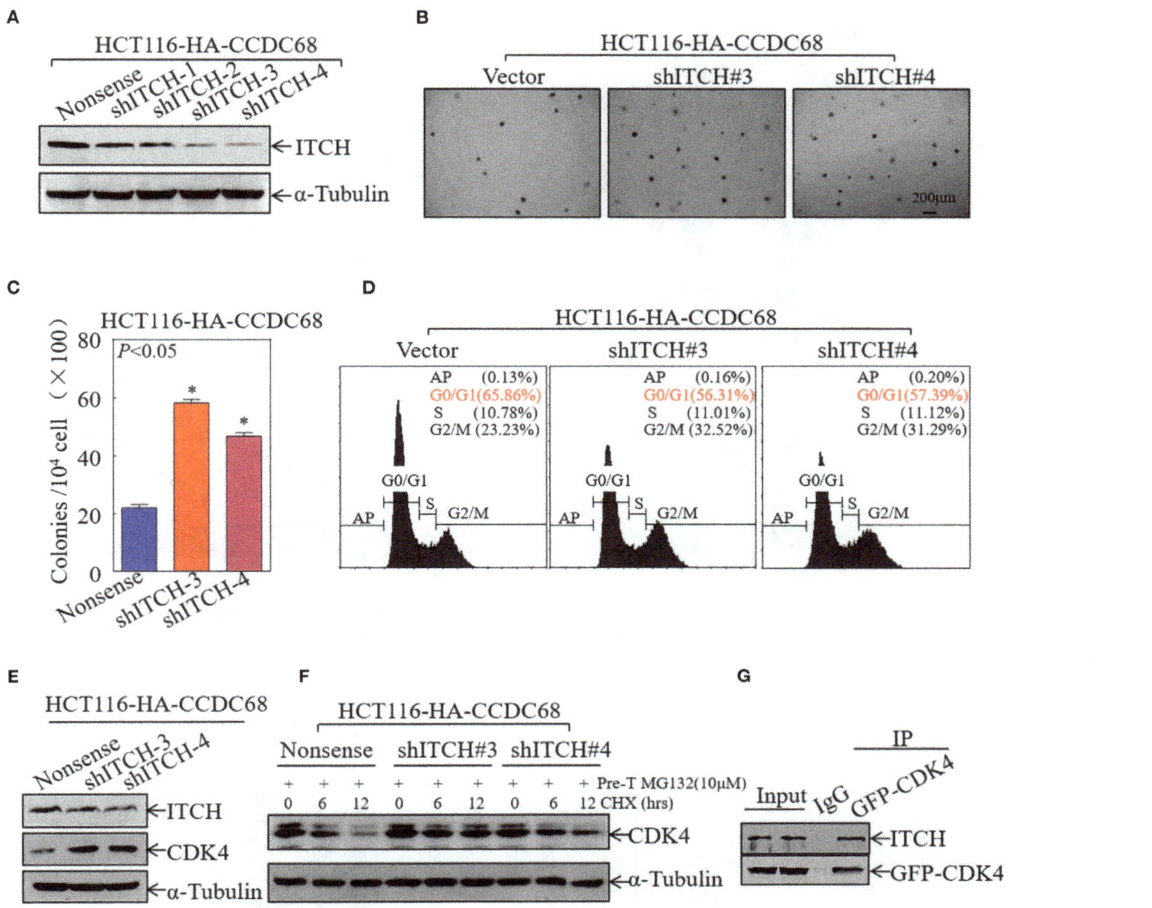

FIGURE 6 | CCDC68 accelerates the degradation of CDK4 by regulating ITCH expression. **(A)** Western blotting analysis of the efficacy of HCT116 (CCDC68) transfection with shITCH lentivirus or Nonsense lentivirus. **(B, C)** HCT116 (CCDC68/shITCH#3, #4) and HCT116 (CCDC68/Nonsense) cells were tested for anchorage-independent growth. Cell colonies were counted, and the results are presented in the diagram. Data are presented as the mean ± SD and analyzed by Student's *t*-test, **P* < 0.05. **(D)** Analysis of HCT116 (CCDC68/shITCH#3, #4) and HCT116 (CCDC68/Nonsense) cell cycles by flow cytometry. **(E)** Western blotting analysis of CDK4 levels in HCT116 (CCDC68/shITCH #3 and #4), and HCT116 (CCDC68/Nonsense) cells. **(F)** Effect of ITCH knockdown on CDK4 degradation rate in HCT116 (CCDC68) cells detected by western blotting. **(G)** The interaction between CDK4 and ITCH was analyzed by co-immunoprecipitation in 293T cells transfected with the GFP-CDK4 plasmid.

regulation of ITCH expression by CCDC68 at the transcriptional level (**Figure 7C**). Analysis of RXRα expression in HCT116 (CCDC68) and RKO (CCDC68) cells and control cells by western blotting showed that RXRα was upregulated in CCDC68-overexpressing cells (**Figure 7D**). RXRα was overexpressed in HCT116 cells, and the mRNA level, promoter activity, and protein levels of ITCH were analyzed. RXRα overexpression significantly increased ITCH mRNA levels, promoter activity, and the expression of the ITCH protein (**Figures 7E–G**). Collectively, these results identified RXRα as a critical transcription factor involved in the regulation of ITCH transcription by CCDC68.

DISCUSSION

CCDC68 is upregulated in NSCLC, and downregulating CCDC68 expression decreases cell proliferation and increases apoptosis, suggesting that CCDC68 is a candidate biomarker for the detection of malignant transformation in lung cancer (16). However, CCDC68 plays a tumor-inhibitory role in pancreatic cancer (15), which is inconsistent with the tumor-promoting function of CCDC68 in NSCLC. This suggests that CCDC68 plays different roles in various human cancers. CCDC68 copy number is decreased in CRC (17), although its specific biological function and underlying molecular mechanism remain unclear. In this study, we confirmed the role of CCDC68 in inhibiting the growth of human CRC cells, and clarified the molecular mechanism underlying the effect of CCDC68 on the progression of CRC. The results showed that CCDC68 expression was lower in human CRC than in paired non-tumor tissues, and analyses of a human CRC database and cell lines supported the low expression of CCDC68 in CRC. The data suggested that CCDC68 acts as a tumor suppressor in CRC and has a potential prognostic role in predicting survival.

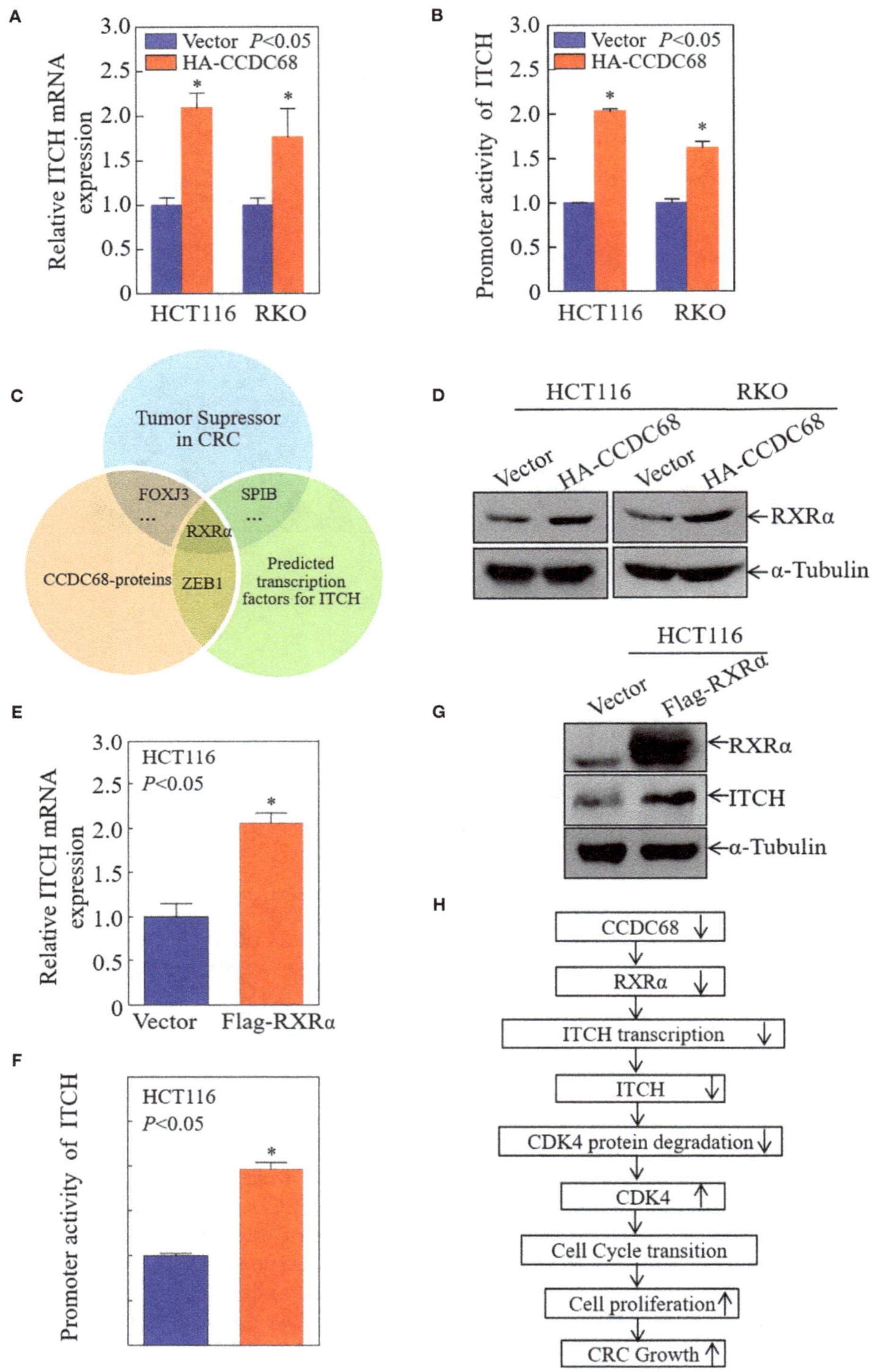

FIGURE 7 | CCDC68 promotes ITCH transcription by upregulating RXRα expression. **(A)** CCDC68 overexpression increased the mRNA levels of ITCH. **(B)** ITCH promoter activity in CCDC68 overexpression cells compared with vector control cells. **(C)** Bioinformatics and proteomics analysis of transcription factors potentially involved in the regulation of ITCH transcription. **(D)** RXRα expression levels in HCT116 (Vector/HA-CCDC68) and RKO (Vector/HA-CCDC68) cells. **(E)** ITCH mRNA levels in HCT116(RXRα) and HCT116(Vector) cells. **(F)** ITCH promoter activity in HCT116 (RXRα) and HCT116 (Vector) cells. **(G)** Expression levels of ITCH in HCT116 (RXRα) and HCT116 (Vector) cells. **(H)** Schematic diagram of the molecular mechanism underlying the effect of CCDC68 on regulating the proliferation of colorectal cancer cells. Data are presented as the mean ± SD and analyzed by Student's *t*-test. *P < 0.05.

Overexpression of CCDC68 inhibited the monolayer growth and adhesion-independent growth of CRC cells *in vitro*, and the growth of transplanted tumors *in vivo*. In addition, CCDC68 promoted the transcription of ITCH by upregulating the transcription factor RXRα, and increased levels of ITCH downregulated CDK4 expression by inducing its degradation. Thus, CCDC68 inhibits the malignant transformation of cells by inhibiting G0/G1 cell cycle phase transition, thereby playing an important role in inhibiting the growth of CRC. These findings provide important insight into the role of CCDC68 in the development of human CRC. Consistent with the inhibitory function of CCDC68 in pancreatic cancer, it plays a tumor suppressor role in CRC, providing a potential new target for early diagnosis and treatment of CRC.

CDKs are endogenous cell cycle regulators that modulate cell division and proliferation (26). CDK4 is an important regulator of the G1 phase of the cell cycle. CDK4/6 bind to cyclin D to form a kinase-active complex, which phosphorylates retinoblastoma protein and drives the progression from G1 to S phase (27). Several studies have demonstrated that CDK4 is upregulated in cancer (28–33) and inhibiting CDK4 expression increases the efficacy of clinical treatments for breast cancer, melanoma, liposarcoma, and mantle cell lymphoma (34–37). This indicates that CDK4 could be a target for the treatment of malignant tumors. However, current CDK4 inhibitors are not clinically effective in treating CRC. Therefore, looking for specific inhibitors that regulate CDK4, developing highly selective drugs for CDK4, and preparing reasonable and effective combined strategies for specific patients are of great significance for improving the clinical treatment effect of CRC patients (38). However, the mechanism underlying the regulation of CDK4 protein degradation in human CRC has not been fully elucidated. Ubiquitin-mediated degradation is essential for controlling CDKs. Studies have shown that PAQR4 controls the steady-state level of CDK4 by regulating the Skp2-mediated ubiquitination of CDK4 (24). In CRC, Cdc37 activates the RB1 signaling pathway by increasing the stability of CDK4, which plays a key role in promoting the survival of CRC cells (25). In addition, Bury et al. showed that DUX4, a direct inhibitor of CDK1 activity, can also bind to CDK4, but it is unclear whether DUX4 inhibits CDK4 activity (39). The present results indicate that CCDC68 is a key upstream regulator of CDK4 in CRC. CCDC68 overexpression accelerated the degradation rate of the CDK4 protein. A bioinformatics screening of E3 ubiquitin ligases interacting with CDK4 showed that ITCH was involved in CDK4 degradation mediated by CCDC68.

Ubiquitination is a post-translational modification involved in the regulation of signaling pathways (40), and E3 ubiquitin ligases catalyze the ubiquitination of target proteins (41). ITCH is a member of the Nedd4 family of HECT-type E3 ligases, which mediate the ubiquitination of multiple targets (42–44). ITCH acts as a cancer-promoting factor in breast cancer, pancreatic cancer, hepatocellular carcinoma, and chronic lymphocytic leukemia (45–47). However, studies analyzing the expression and function of ITCH in CRC show that ITCH is downregulated in CRC and acts as a tumor suppressor by inhibiting the Wnt/β-catenin pathway (48, 49). In addition, Kathania et al. found that ITCH can inhibit IL-17-mediated colon inflammation and tumorigenesis through ROR-γt ubiquitination (50), and Ko et al. reported that ITCH can form a destruction complex to antagonize tumor necrosis factor receptor I (TNFRI), thereby inhibiting TNF-NF-κB signal transduction and tumorigenesis (51). In this study, we found that overexpression of CCDC68 significantly upregulated ITCH and downregulated CDK4 in CRC cells, resulting in G0/G1 phase arrest. Knockdown of ITCH in HCT116 (CCDC68) cells decreased the degradation rate of the CDK4 protein, thereby promoting the formation and proliferation of CRC cell colonies. Co-immunoprecipitation assays confirmed the interaction between ITCH and CDK4, revealing a new mechanism underlying the role of CCDC68 in regulating CDK4 protein degradation through ITCH. The results indicated that ITCH acts as a downstream effector of CCDC68 to inhibit the growth of CRC, which is consistent with reports that ITCH plays a negative regulatory role in the progression of CRC (48, 49). Taken together, these findings indicate that upregulating ITCH may provide therapeutic benefits for CRC patients.

The regulation of ITCH expression has not been studied extensively. Studies show that ITCH expression is regulated by microRNAs in cancer (46–52). We showed that CCDC68 upregulated the expression of ITCH at the transcriptional level. RXRα is a member of the nuclear receptor (NR) superfamily, which functions in the regulation of transcription, and in controlling the development, homeostasis, and metabolism of organisms (53). RXRα is downregulated in cervical cancer and inhibits its progression (54). In this study, proteomics analysis and bioinformatics prediction showed that the ITCH promoter contains a DNA binding site for RXRα, and ITCH and RXRα were consistently upregulated. Western blotting experiments indicated that CCDC68 overexpression significantly increased the levels of RXRα, suggesting that RXRα is involved in the transcription of ITCH. Low expression levels of RXRα are closely related to the pathogenesis and progression of CRC (55). Volate et al. reported that low concentrations of green tea are sufficient to de-silence RXRα and inhibit intestinal tumorigenesis in the $Apc^{Min/+}$ mouse (56). Therefore, epigenetic regulation of RXRα may be a new strategy for the prevention and treatment of CRC. However, the exact mechanisms underlying the regulation of RXRα by CCDC68 need to be further studied.

In summary, as shown in **Figure 7H**, the present study identified a new CCDC68/RXRα/ITCH/CDK4 regulatory axis involved in CRC progression. CCDC68 was downregulated in CRC, and functional experiments showed that CCDC68 inhibited CRC cell growth *in vitro* and tumor formation *in vivo*. CCDC68 overexpression increased the transcription and expression of ITCH by upregulating RXRα, thereby promoting the binding of ITCH to CDK4 and the degradation of CDK4. This led to the inhibition of G0/G1 phase transition and cell growth in human CRC cells. The present results indicate that CCDC68 is an important tumor suppressor molecule in CRC, and CCDC68 and its downstream effectors may become potential targets for the early diagnosis and/or treatment of CRC.

ETHICS STATEMENT

The studies involving human participants were reviewed and approved by Ethics Committee of Wenzhou Medical University. Written informed consent for participation was not required for this study in accordance with the national legislation and the institutional requirements. The animal study was reviewed and approved by Institutional Animal Care and Use Committee of Wenzhou Medical University.

AUTHOR CONTRIBUTIONS

CW, LZ and HH conceived and designed the study. CW, HL, ZJ, YZ, ZF and XJ detected the cells' biological function, performed the RT-PCR assays, carried out the soft agar, ATP assay, Western blotting, and luciferase reporter assays, and conducted the statistical analyses. XZ and LW analyzed clinical samples. CW, LZ and HH drafted the manuscript. All authors contributed to the article and approved the submitted version.

ACKNOWLEDGMENTS

Bioinformatics results announced here based on data produced by the TCGA research network (http://cancergenome.nih.gov/). We thank the participants, specimen donors and research groups who participated in the data set of the TCGA CRC data set to contribute to the database construction.

REFERENCES

1. Sung H, Ferlay J, Siegel RL, Laversanne M, Soerjomataram I, Jemal A, et al. Global Cancer Statistics 2020: GLOBOCAN Estimates of Incidence and Mortality Worldwide for 36 Cancers in 185 Countries. *CA Cancer J Clin* (2021). doi: 10.3322/caac.21660
2. Verma M, Sarfaty M, Brooks D, Wender RC. Population-Based Programs for Increasing Colorectal Cancer Screening in the United States. *CA Cancer J Clin* (2015) 65:497–510. doi: 10.3322/caac.21295
3. Khan K, Rata M, Cunningham D, Koh DM, Tunariu N, Hahne JC, et al. Functional Imaging and Circulating Biomarkers of Response to Regorafenib in Treatment-Refractory Metastatic Colorectal Cancer Patients in a Prospective Phase II Study. *Gut* (2018) 67:1484–92. doi: 10.1136/gutjnl-2017-314178
4. Takebe N, Miele L, Harris PJ, Jeong W, Bando H, Kahn M, et al. Targeting Notch, Hedgehog, and Wnt Pathways in Cancer Stem Cells: Clinical Update. *Nat Rev Clin Oncol* (2015) 12:445–64. doi: 10.1038/nrclinonc.2015.61
5. Gulbake A, Jain A, Jain A, Jain A, Jain SK. Insight to Drug Delivery Aspects for Colorectal Cancer. *World J Gastroenterol* (2016) 22:582–99. doi: 10.3748/wjg.v22.i2.582
6. Gravalos C, Cassinello J, García-Alfonso P, Jimeno A. Integration of Panitumumab Into the Treatment of Colorectal Cancer. *Crit Rev Oncol Hematol* (2010) 74:16–26. doi: 10.1016/j.critrevonc.2009.06.005
7. Cheng X, Xu X, Chen D, Zhao F, Wang W. Therapeutic Potential of Targeting the Wnt/β-Catenin Signaling Pathway in Colorectal Cancer. *BioMed Pharmacother* (2019) 110:473–81. doi: 10.1016/j.biopha.2018.11.082
8. Burkhard P, Stetefeld J, Strelkov SV. Coiled Coils: A Highly Versatile Protein Folding Motif. *Trends Cell Biol* (2001) 11:82–8. doi: 10.1016/s0962-8924(00)01898-5
9. Wang J, Wu X, Dai W, Li J, Xiang L, Tang W, et al. The CCDC43-ADRM1 Axis Regulated by YY1, Promotes Proliferation and Metastasis of Gastric Cancer. *Cancer Lett* (2020) 482:90–101. doi: 10.1016/j.canlet.2020.03.026
10. Jiang GY, Zhang XP, Zhang Y, Xu HT, Wang L, Li QC, et al. Coiled-Coil Domain-Containing Protein 8 Inhibits the Invasiveness and Migration of non-Small Cell Lung Cancer Cells. *Hum Pathol* (2016) 56:64–73. doi: 10.1016/j.humpath.2016.06.001
11. Gong Y, Qiu W, Ning X, Yang X, Liu L, Wang Z, et al. CCDC34 is Up-Regulated in Bladder Cancer and Regulates Bladder Cancer Cell Proliferation, Apoptosis and Migration. *Oncotarget* (2015) 6:25856–67. doi: 10.18632/oncotarget.4624
12. Bornens M. Centrosome Composition and Microtubule Anchoring Mechanisms. *Curr Opin Cell Biol* (2002) 14:25–34. doi: 10.1016/s0955-0674(01)00290-3
13. Huang N, Xia Y, Zhang D, Wang S, Bao Y, He R, et al. Hierarchical Assembly of Centriole Subdistal Appendages Via Centrosome Binding Proteins CCDC120 and CCDC68. *Nat Commun* (2017) 8:15057. doi: 10.1038/ncomms15057
14. Piel M, Nordberg J, Euteneuer U, Bornens M. Centrosome-dependent Exit of Cytokinesis in Animal Cells. *Science* (2001) 291:1550–3. doi: 10.1126/science.1057330
15. Radulovich N, Leung L, Ibrahimov E, Navab R, Sakashita S, Zhu CQ, et al. Coiled-Coil Domain Containing 68 (CCDC68) Demonstrates a Tumor-Suppressive Role in Pancreatic Ductal Adenocarcinoma. *Oncogene* (2015) 34:4238–47. doi: 10.1038/onc.2014.357
16. Hua T, Ding J, Xu J, Fan Y, Liu Z, Lian J. Coiled-Coil Domain-Containing 68 Promotes non-Small Cell Lung Cancer Cell Proliferation in Vitro. *Oncol Lett* (2020) 20:356. doi: 10.3892/ol.2020.12220
17. Sheffer M, Bacolod MD, Zuk O, Giardina SF, Pincas H, Barany F, et al. Association of Survival and Disease Progression With Chromosomal Instability: A Genomic Exploration of Colorectal Cancer. *Proc Natl Acad Sci U S A* (2009) 106:7131–6. doi: 10.1073/pnas.0902232106
18. Yan H, Ren S, Lin Q, Yu Y, Chen C, Hua X, et al. Inhibition of UBE2N-dependent CDK6 Protein Degradation by miR-934 Promotes Human Bladder Cancer Cell Growth. *FASEB J* (2019) 33:12112–23. doi: 10.1096/fj.201900499RR
19. Xie Q, Chen C, Li H, Xu J, Wu L, Yu Y, et al. Mir-3687 Overexpression Promotes Bladder Cancer Cell Growth by Inhibiting the Negative Effect of FOXP1 on Cyclin E2 Transcription. *Mol Ther* (2019) 27:1028–38. doi: 10.1016/j.ymthe.2019.03.006
20. Jin H, Sun W, Zhang Y, Yan H, Liufu H, Wang S, et al. Microrna-411 Downregulation Enhances Tumor Growth by Upregulating Mllt11 Expression in Human Bladder Cancer. *Mol Ther Nucleic Acids* (2018) 11:312–22. doi: 10.1016/j.omtn.2018.03.003
21. Jin H, Ma J, Xu J, Li H, Chang Y, Zang N, et al. Oncogenic Role of MIR516A in Human Bladder Cancer was Mediated by its Attenuating PHLPP2 Expression and BECN1-dependent Autophagy. *Autophagy* (2020), 1–15. doi: 10.1080/15548627.2020.1733262
22. Icard P, Fournel L, Wu Z, Alifano M, Lincet H. Interconnection Between Metabolism and Cell Cycle in Cancer. *Trends Biochem Sci* (2019) 44:490–501. doi: 10.1016/j.tibs.2018.12.007
23. Jung JH, Jung DB, Kim H, Lee H, Kang SE, Srivastava SK, et al. Zinc Finger Protein 746 Promotes Colorectal Cancer Progression Via c-Myc Stability Mediated by Glycogen Synthase Kinase 3β and F-box and WD Repeat Domain-Containing 7. *Oncogene* (2018) 37:3715–28. doi: 10.1038/s41388-018-0225-0
24. Wang L, Zhang R, You X, Zhang H, Wei S, Cheng T, et al. The Steady-State Level of CDK4 Protein is Regulated by Antagonistic Actions Between PAQR4 and SKP2 and Involved in Tumorigenesis. *J Mol Cell Biol* (2017) 9:409–21. doi: 10.1093/jmcb/mjx028

25. Zhu J, Yan F, Tao J, Zhu X, Liu J, Deng S, et al. Cdc37 Facilitates Cell Survival of Colorectal Carcinoma Via Activating the CDK4 Signaling Pathway. *Cancer Sci* (2018) 109:656–65. doi: 10.1111/cas.13495
26. Whittaker SR, Mallinger A, Workman P, Clarke PA. Inhibitors of Cyclin-Dependent Kinases as Cancer therapeutics. *Pharmacol Ther* (2017) 173:83–105. doi: 10.1016/j.pharmthera.2017.02.008
27. Narasimha AM, Kaulich M, Shapiro GS, Choi YJ, Sicinski P, Dowdy SF. Cyclin D Activates the Rb Tumor Suppressor by Mono-Phosphorylation. *Elife* (2014) 3(1):e02872. doi: 10.7554/eLife.02872
28. Feng T, Xu D, Tu C, Li W, Ning Y, Ding J, et al. MiR-124 Inhibits Cell Proliferation in Breast Cancer Through Downregulation of CDK4. *Tumour Biol* (2015) 36:5987–97. doi: 10.1007/s13277-015-3275-8
29. Aboushousha T, Hammam O, Aref A, Kamel A, Badawy M, Abdel Hamid A. Tissue Profile of CDK4 and STAT3 as Possible Innovative Therapeutic Targets in Urinary Bladder Cancer. *Asian Pac J Cancer Prev* (2020) 21:547–54. doi: 10.31557/apjcp.2020.21.2.547
30. Feng H, Ge F, Du L, Zhang Z, Liu D. MiR-34b-3p Represses Cell Proliferation, Cell Cycle Progression and Cell Apoptosis in non-Small-Cell Lung Cancer (NSCLC) by Targeting CDK4. *J Cell Mol Med* (2019) 23:5282–91. doi: 10.1111/jcmm.14404
31. Zhou Y, Shen JK, Yu Z, Hornicek FJ, Kan Q, Duan Z. Expression and Therapeutic Implications of Cyclin-Dependent Kinase 4 (CDK4) in Osteosarcoma. *Biochim Biophys Acta Mol Basis Dis* (2018) 1864:1573–82. doi: 10.1016/j.bbadis.2018.02.004
32. Peurala E, Koivunen P, Haapasaari KM, Bloigu R, Jukkola-Vuorinen A. The Prognostic Significance and Value of Cyclin D1, CDK4 and p16 in Human Breast Cancer. *Breast Cancer Res* (2013) 15:R5. doi: 10.1186/bcr3376
33. Wu A, Wu B, Guo J, Luo W, Wu D, Yang H, et al. Elevated Expression of CDK4 in Lung Cancer. *J Transl Med* (2011) 9:38. doi: 10.1186/1479-5876-9-38
34. O'Leary B, Finn RS, Turner NC. Treating Cancer With Selective CDK4/6 Inhibitors. *Nat Rev Clin Oncol* (2016) 13:417–30. doi: 10.1038/nrclinonc.2016.26
35. Curtin JA, Fridlyand J, Kageshita T, Patel HN, Busam KJ, Kutzner H, et al. Distinct Sets of Genetic Alterations in Melanoma. *N Engl J Med* (2005) 353:2135–47. doi: 10.1056/NEJMoa050092
36. Dickson MA, Tap WD, Keohan ML, D'Angelo SP, Gounder MM, Antonescu CR, et al. Phase II Trial of the CDK4 Inhibitor PD0332991 in Patients With Advanced CDK4-amplified Well-Differentiated or Dedifferentiated Liposarcoma. *J Clin Oncol* (2013) 31:2024–8. doi: 10.1200/jco.2012.46.5476
37. Leonard JP, LaCasce AS, Smith MR, Noy A, Chirieac LR, Rodig SJ, et al. Selective CDK4/6 Inhibition With Tumor Responses by PD0332991 in Patients With Mantle Cell Lymphoma. *Blood* (2012) 119:4597–607. doi: 10.1182/blood-2011-10-388298
38. Asghar U, Witkiewicz AK, Turner NC, Knudsen ES. The History and Future of Targeting Cyclin-Dependent Kinases in Cancer Therapy. *Nat Rev Drug Discovery* (2015) 14:130–46. doi: 10.1038/nrd4504
39. Bury M, Le Calvé B, Lessard F, Dal Maso T, Saliba J, Michiels C. Et AlNfe2l3 Controls Colon Cancer Cell Growth Through Regulation of DUX4, a CDK1 Inhibitor. *Cell Rep* (2019) 29:1469–81.e9. doi: 10.1016/j.celrep.2019.09.087
40. Hershko A, Ciechanover A. The Ubiquitin System. *Annu Rev Biochem* (1998) 67:425–79. doi: 10.1146/annurev.biochem.67.1.425
41. Lim SD, Hwang JG, Han AR, Park YC, Lee C, Ok YS, et al. Positive Regulation of Rice RING E3 Ligase OsHIR1 in Arsenic and Cadmium Uptakes. *Plant Mol Biol* (2014) 85:365–79. doi: 10.1007/s11103-014-0190-0
42. Rotin D, Kumar S. Physiological Functions of the HECT Family of Ubiquitin Ligases. *Nat Rev Mol Cell Biol* (2009) 10:398–409. doi: 10.1038/nrm2690
43. Bernassola F, Karin M, Ciechanover A, Melino G. The HECT Family of E3 Ubiquitin Ligases: Multiple Players in Cancer Development. *Cancer Cell* (2008) 14:10–21. doi: 10.1016/j.ccr.2008.06.001
44. Melino G, Gallagher E, Aqeilan RI, Knight R, Peschiaroli A, Rossi M, et al. Itch: A HECT-type E3 Ligase Regulating Immunity, Skin and Cancer. *Cell Death Differ* (2008) 15:1103–12. doi: 10.1038/cdd.2008.60
45. Salah Z, Itzhaki E, Aqeilan RI. The Ubiquitin E3 Ligase ITCH Enhances Breast Tumor Progression by Inhibiting the Hippo Tumor Suppressor Pathway. *Oncotarget* (2014) 5:10886–900. doi: 10.18632/oncotarget.2540
46. Luo ZL, Luo HJ, Fang C, Cheng L, Huang Z, Dai R, et al. Negative Correlation of ITCH E3 Ubiquitin Ligase and miRNA-106b Dictates Metastatic Progression in Pancreatic Cancer. *Oncotarget* (2016) 7:1477–85. doi: 10.18632/oncotarget.6395
47. Rathinam C, Matesic LE, Flavell RA. The E3 Ligase Itch is a Negative Regulator of the Homeostasis and Function of Hematopoietic Stem Cells. *Nat Immunol* (2011) 12:399–407. doi: 10.1038/ni.2021
48. Wei W, Li M, Wang J, Nie F, Li L. The E3 Ubiquitin Ligase ITCH Negatively Regulates Canonical Wnt Signaling by Targeting Dishevelled Protein. *Mol Cell Biol* (2012) 32:3903–12. doi: 10.1128/mcb.00251-12
49. Huang G, Zhu H, Shi Y, Wu W, Cai H, Chen X. cir-ITCH Plays an Inhibitory Role in Colorectal Cancer by Regulating the Wnt/beta-catenin Pathway. *PloS One* (2015) 10:e0131225. doi: 10.1371/journal.pone.0131225
50. Kathania M, Khare P, Zeng M, Cantarel B, Zhang H, Ueno H, et al. Itch Inhibits IL-17-mediated Colon Inflammation and Tumorigenesis by ROR-γt Ubiquitination. *Nat Immunol* (2016) 17:997–1004. doi: 10.1038/ni.3488
51. Ko KP, Jeong SI, Lim JS, Lee KW, Lee MG, Chi SG. NORE1A Directs Apoptotic Switch of TNF Signaling Through Reciprocal Modulation of ITCH-mediated Destruction of TNFRI and BAX. *Oncogene* (2020) 39:5675–89. doi: 10.1038/s41388-020-01392-y
52. Sun MX, An Q, Chen LM, Guo L. MIR-520f Regulated Itch Expression and Promoted Cell Proliferation in Human Melanoma Cells. *Dose Response* (2020) 18:1559325820918450. doi: 10.1177/1559325820918450
53. Xu Y, O'Malley BW, Elmquist JK. Brain Nuclear Receptors and Body Weight Regulation. *J Clin Invest* (2017) 127:1172–80. doi: 10.1172/jci88891
54. Shi Y, Liu M, Huang Y, Zhang J, Yin L. Promotion of Cell Autophagy and Apoptosis in Cervical Cancer by Inhibition of Long Noncoding RNA LINC00511 Via Transcription Factor RXRA-regulated Pld1. *J Cell Physiol* (2020) 235:6592–604. doi: 10.1002/jcp.29529
55. Zhang F, Meng F, Li H, Dong Y, Yang W, Han A. Suppression of Retinoid X Receptor Alpha and Aberrant β-Catenin Expression Significantly Associates With Progression of Colorectal Carcinoma. *Eur J Cancer* (2011) 47:2060–7. doi: 10.1016/j.ejca.2011.04.010
56. Volate SR, Muga SJ, Issa AY, Nitcheva D, Smith T, Wargovich MJ. Epigenetic Modulation of the Retinoid X Receptor Alpha by Green Tea in the Azoxymethane-Apc Min/+ Mouse Model of Intestinal Cancer. *Mol Carcinog* (2009) 48:920–33. doi: 10.1002/mc.20542

3

Advances of Tumorigenesis, Diagnosis at Early Stage and Cellular Immunotherapy in Gastrointestinal Malignancies

Haipeng Zhu[1,2*] *and Xiaojun Liu*[3]

[1] *Precision and Personalized Cancer Treatment Center, Division of Cancer Diagnosis & Therapy, Ciming Boao International Hospital, Boao Lecheng International Medical Tourism Pilot Zone, Qionghai, China,* [2] *Stem Cell and Biotherapy Technology Research Center, Xinxiang Medical College, Xinxiang, China,* [3] *Division of Cellular & Biomedical Science, Ciming Boao International Hospital, Boao Lecheng International Medical Tourism Pilot Zone, Qionghai, China*

Correspondence:
Haipeng Zhu
dr.haipengzhu@cimingboao.com;
dr.haipengzhu@hotmail.com

Globally, in 2018, 4.8 million new patients have a diagnosis of gastrointestinal (GI) cancers, while 3.4 million people died of such disorders. GI malignancies are tightly relevant to 26% of the world-wide cancer incidence and occupies 35% of all cancer-associated deaths. In this article, we principally investigated molecular and cellular mechanisms of tumorigenesis in five major GI cancers occurring at esophagus, stomach, liver, pancreas, and colorectal region that illustrate high morbidity in Eastern and Western countries. Moreover, through this investigation, we not only emphasize importance of the tumor microenvironment in development and treatment of malignant tumors but also identify significance of M2PK, miRNAs, ctDNAs, circRNAs, and CTCs in early detection of GI cancers, as well as systematically evaluate contribution of personalized precision medicine including cellular immunotherapy, new antigen and vaccine therapy, and oncolytic virotherapy in treatment of GI cancers.

Keywords: gastrointestinal cancers, tumor microenvironment, tumorigenesis, early detection, cellular immunotherapy

INTRODUCTION

Gastrointestinal (GI) malignant tumors generally cover esophagus, stomach, liver, pancreas, as well as colorectal region. Most primary cancers from those parts worldly covered 26% of cancer incidence and 35% of all deaths related to cancer, while 4.8 million new cases were yearly diagnosed and 3.4 million people lost their lives due to those malignancies, statistically in 2018 (1). Currently, clinical scientists are segmentally concentrated on contribution of the tumor microenvironment (TME) to tumorigenesis and resistance to anticancer therapy (2–4), feasibility of precise methodologies in detection of GI cancers at early stage based on tumor growth-associated serological and histochemical changes (5–12), as well as personalized application of biomedical therapies in reduction of tumor size and control of metastases (13–20). More importantly, through combating with cancers over several centuries, many clinicians eventually and principally come back to the nature of malignant tumor, in which an outside exhibition of malignant tumors is uncontrolledly growing but the inside mechanism shows primary inhibition of immune surveillance and cytotoxic activity locally and systematically.

TUMOR MICROENVIRONMENT AND TUMORIGENESIS IN GASTROINTESTINAL CANCERS

Tumor Microenvironment (TME)

Like Achilles, if we cannot lift him from the ground, he will be alive last long. The Achilles malignant tumors that depend on is the TME. The TME is more like a matrix, in which cancer cells communicate with non-transformed cells through a variety of cytokines, chemokines, growth factors, as well as inflammatory mediators, purposely to maintain a dynamic equilibrium in causing metastases and resisting to physical, chemical, and immune pressure (2, 21, 22). The following components principally play critical roles in tumorigenesis and metastasis, including dendrite cells (DCs), T lymphocyte, natural killer cells (NKs), tumor-associated macrophage cells (TAMs), cancer-associated fibroblast cells (CAFs), and myeloid-derived suppressor cells (MDSCs) as well as transform growth factor β (TGFβ).

Dendrite Cells (DCs)

DCs, as antigen-processing vehicles, are tightly communicating with tumor-infiltrating T cells in purpose of elimination of carcinogenic cells and prevention of local tumorigenesis and systematical metastases. Primarily, DCs are functional to activate $CD4^+$ and $CD8^+$ T cell *via* antigen presentation, in which immature DCs intake the antigen to promote DCs maturation (23–25). However, based on hypoxic and inflammatory conditions in the TME, T cells activated by tumor-associated antigens are much less produced due to reduction of DC maturation, accumulation of immature DCs, and specific DC-mediated impairment of T-cell response (26, 27). Thus utilizing immune checkpoint inhibitors (ICIs) not only decrease programmed cell death protein 1 (PD-1) activity on DCs but also increase DC activity promoted *via* amonophosphoryl lipid A produced by E. coli, both of which strongly improve efficiency and efficacy of cellular immunotherapy to GI cancers (28–34).

T Lymphocytes

T lymphocytes inside or around the TME are the majorly powerful enforce to fight with cancer cells, in which tumor-infiltrating lymphocytes (TILs) have been purposely used to treat GI cancers and TILs expressed in the TME are closely relevant to therapeutic efficacy (35–40). Generally, cytotoxic $CD8^+$-T cells are antigen-processed and have ability to eliminate tumor cells, whereas $CD4^+$ T helper 1 cells (Th1) activate cytotoxic T cells to secrete interleukin-2 (IL2), interferon gamma (IFNγ), and tumor necrosis factor (41). Thereby, the higher expression of cytotoxic $CD8^+$-TIL on biopsy, the better prognosis whether with cancer treatment or not (35–39). However, regulatory $CD4^+$ cells, such as Th2 and Th17 group, focus on promoting tumor growth (41). Furthermore, $CD4^+$ T regulatory cells (Tregs) with FOXP3 and CD25 expression release IL10, TGF-β, and cytotoxic T-lymphocyte antigen 4 (CTLA4), which tremendously diminish immune surveillance (42, 43). Expression of Treg cells in biopsy represents a negative prognosis (43). Interestingly, in Hodgkin's lymphoma, Treg cells inhibit malignant cell growing, which show a good prognosis (44–46). More interestingly, γδT cells stained in the TME directly destroy transformed cells and upregulate activity of DCs, cytotoxic T cells, and NK cells in most malignant tumors (47–50). Invertedly, *in situ* production of IL17 *via* γδT cells recruits MDSCs and increases program death protein-ligand 1 (PD-L1) expression that is beneficial for tumorigenesis and metastases (51, 52). Due to contradictory results, whether presentation of γδ TILs in the TME is an eligible biomarker to evaluate prognosis has always been investigated.

Natural Killer Cell (NKs)

NK cells, another category of TILs, are characterized with $CD16^{dim}CD56^{bright}$ subset mostly in circulation, whereas with $CD16^{bright}CD56^{dim}$ subset predominantly in mucosa, in which $CD56^{bright}$ NK cells have cytotoxic action directly on cancer cells independent of antigen presentation (53). Different from functionally killing tumor cells and cancer stem cells (CSCs) in the bloodstream, NK cells show reduced cytotoxicity on transformed cells in the TME with producing less IFNγ (54). Unsurprisingly, through combating with immune defense system, malignant cells also develop several tools to dodge NK cell-mediated elimination including activation of inhibitory receptor of NK cells and reduction of NK cell activity induced by platelets and TGFβ (55). However, due to NK-mediated induction of DC cells and increased activation of more NK cells *via* ICI treatment, the existence of NK cells in biopsy highly predicts a good prognosis in GI cancer therapy (54, 56–58).

Tumor-Associated Macrophage (TAMs)

Macrophage cells are essentially in regulation of individual immunity through activating adaptive immunity, healing the

Abbreviation: GI, gastrointestinal; TME, tumor microenvironment; DCs, dendrite cells; NKs, natural killer cells; TAMs, tumor-associated macrophage cells; CAFs, cancer-associated fibroblast cells; MDSCs, myeloid-derived suppressor cells; TGFβ, transform growth factor β; PD-1, programmed cell death protein 1; PD-L1, program death protein ligand 1; ICIs, immune checkpoint inhibitors; TIL, tumor-infiltrating lymphocytes; IL2, interleukin-2; IFNγ, interferon gamma; Tregs, T regulatory cells; CTLA4, cytotoxic T-lymphocyte antigen 4; CSCs, cancer stem cells; EMT, epithelial-mesenchymal transition; ECM, extracellular matrix; MAPK, mitogen-activated protein kinase; PI3K-Akt, phosphatidylinositol 3 kinase-Akt; STAT3, Signal Transducer and Activator of Transcription 3; EAC, Esophageal adenocarcinoma; ESCC, Esophageal squamous cell carcinoma; Hp, H. pylori; EBV, Epstein Barr Virus; HCC, hepatocellular carcinoma; PDAC, pancreatic duct adenocarcinoma; CRC, colorectal cancer; M2PK, M2 pyruvate kinase; FOBT, fecal occult blood test; CTCs, Circulating tumor cells; AUC, area under curve; ctDNAs, circulating tumor DNAs; miRNAs, microRNAs; circRNA, circular RNAs; BNCT, boron-neutron capture therapy; CIK, cytokine-induced killer cells; DC-CIK, dendritic cell-activated cytokine-induced killer cells; CAR-NK, chimeric antigen receptor-natural killer cells; and CAR-T, chimeric antigen receptor-T cells; OV, oncolytic virus.

wound, and kicking off infectious effectors, in which M1 type macrophages with $IL12^{bright}IL10^{dim}$ are majorly activated by IFNγ and lipopolysaccharide, whereas M2 type macrophages with $IL12^{dim}IL10^{bright}$ are typically activated by glucocorticoid and IL4/13 (59). M1 macrophages produce higher level of IL12 and drive the recruitment of Th1, which promotes antitumor activity, while M2 macrophage-mediated high secretion of IL10 largely sends votes to tumorigenesis. Within the TME, cytokines and inflammatory agents predominantly polarize M1 macrophage to M2 subtype, which produces TAMs (60). There are several receptors commonly expressing TAMs, such as the mannose receptor and scavenger receptor class A, in which blocking scavenger receptor class A *via* monoclonal antibody amplifies cytotoxicity of NK cells to transformed cells in the TME (61). In addition to immunosuppression, TAMs also notably increase tumor angiogenesis, especially at hypoxic area or hypoxia-induced tumor necrosis region where oligonucleotide microarray of aggregated TAMs shows extensive activation of the transcriptional zones encoding angiogenic factors such as vascular endothelial growth factor and endothelin (62). Furthermore, TAMs are strictly relevant with tumor invasion and metastases, and largely prevention of chemotherapy-induced apoptosis in GI cancers (63–65). These discoveries firmly identify high expression of TAMs in biopsy as a poor signal of prognosis in cancer therapy.

Myeloid-Derived Suppressor Cells (MDSCs)

MDSCs have two subpopulations including monocytic group and granulocytic group that are characterized through expression of different kinds of membrane markers and immunosuppressive components (66). MDSCs exhibit two directions in promotion of tumorigenesis and metastases including accelerating tumor angiogenesis (67) and inactivating innate and adaptive immune function through producing high concentration of reactive oxygen and nitrogen species (68), slowing down amino acid-mediated T-cell activation and proliferation by less production of arginine (69) and L-cysteine (70) within the TME and reducing intratumoral migration of cytotoxic T cells by peroxynitrite-modified chemoattractant CCL2 (71), as well as enlarging Treg cell-dependent immunosuppression *via* IL10, TGFβ, IFNγ, and CD40-CD40L interactions (72, 73).

Impressively, MDSCs have a triple communication with DCs, NK cells, and TAMs. In the TME, MDSC-TAM complex significantly regulates production of IL10 and IL12, in which IL10-knockdown animal model verifies that MDSC-dependent IL10 level is the key factor of reducing IL12 production through influencing IL12 transcription (74). But cytokine- and inflammatory mediator-induced production of MDSC-TAM complex directly leads to high level of IL10 and low level of IL12 in the TME, which promotes recruitment of Treg cells and predominantly inactivates antitumor function of cytotoxic T cells and NK cells (75). Moreover, higher IL10 production also increases IL4 expression, which basically supports more transformation of TAMs (76). Recent investigation found that granulocytic MDSC-induced inflammation decreased NKG2D expression, an activating receptor of NK cells, which reduced cytotoxicity in the TME (77), whereas monocytic MDSCs amplified expression of activating ligand Rae1 on NK cells to increase killing activity through NKG2D, which subsequently lysed MDSCs (78). Furthermore, combining with ICIs and N803, an IL15 superagonist, NK cell therapy increased cytolysis of MDSCs in squamous cell carcinoma (79). Also, another case in treatment of head and neck squamous cell carcinoma reported that orally bioagent SX-682, a small-molecule inhibitor of CXCR1 and CXCR2, tremendously abolished MDSC aggregation and amplified activity of infiltrating NK cells in the TME (80). These investigations strongly indicate that MDSCs suppress NK cell-mediated elimination of cancer cells in the TME. Through studying effects of MDSCs on DCs in melanoma patients, the evidence showed that MDSCs decreased antigen presentation of DCs, inhibited incubation of immature DCs, and blocked recruitment of DCs to cytotoxic T cells, all of which were activated *via* IL23-mediated Th17 cell pathway (78, 81, 82). More evidences showed that IL23-mediated Th17 cell proliferation damaged adaptive and innate immunity and significantly promoted tumor metastases (78, 83). Therefore, MDSCs primarily enhance TAM-induced immunosuppression and selectively downregulate DC and NK cell activity in promotion of tumor growth and metastases.

Cancer-Associated Fibroblast Cells (CAFs)

Healing tissue damage with scar essentially needs participation of fibroblast cells, in which paracrine signals transform residential fibroblasts to myofibroblasts that produce TGFβ and α-smooth muscle actin (84, 85). However, in the TME, myofibroblast cells independent from mutations in cancer cells or the epithelial-mesenchymal transition (EMT) are primarily recognized as CAFs that are abundantly expressed in most malignant tumors (86). In purpose of constantly activating proliferation and metastases, CAFs produce various kinds of growth factors such as hepatocyte growth factor, fibroblast growth factor, and insulin-like growth factor 1 (87). CAF secretion partially activates expression of vascular endothelial growth factor that highly causes angiogenesis (88). Cytokines and chemokines produced by CAFs are functional on cytotoxic T cells, Treg cells, and macrophages, which cause both immune enhancement and immunosuppression (89). Differently, CAF-secreted IL6, CXCL9, and TGFβ reduce T cell response to cancer cells, especially cytotoxic T cells (90), whereas CAF-mediated production of CXCL12 (91) and inactivation of focal adhesion kinase in cancer cells (92) amplify antitumor effects through diminishing stromal fibroblast activation. Moreover, CAFs in the TME also contribute to building up the extracellular matrix (ECM) that consists of fibrovascular cores and remodeling enzymes for increasing tumor density to resist selective pressure (90, 93), while TGFβ-activated CAFs crucially stop activity of anticancer medicine (94, 95). Collectively, CAFs promote tumorigenesis and metastasis through modifying the ECM, utilizing growth factors for angiogenesis, and preventing drug access to reduce therapeutic effects.

Transform Growth Factor β (TGFβ)

TGFβ almost regulates all types of human cells and acts as a double agent in the TME (96, 97). Generally, TGFβ secretion is locally responsible to maintain homeostasis, and higher level of TGFβ created by blood platelet and stromal components is responsible for healing the injury and regeneration; however, in the TME, not only stromal cells produce TGFβ through paracrine but also malignant cells autocrinally generate more TGFβ (98). Being a cytokine, TGFβ activates signal transduction through Smad-dependent or Smad-independent pathways, in which Smad-dependent signaling demonstrates that TGFβ-mediated phosphorylation of Smad family protein, Smad2 and Smad3, *via* TβR1 receptor interplays with the cofactor to form the complex that is subsequently translocated into the nucleus and binds with Smad binding element to activate gene transcription (99, 100); however, to Smad-independent signaling, TGFβ activity is amplified mostly through mitogen-activated protein kinase (MAPK) pathway that is activated *via* p38, c-Jun amino terminal kinase, extracellular signal-regulated kinase, and nuclear factor-κB as well as phosphatidylinositol 3 kinase-Akt (PI3K-Akt) (101, 102). The dual roles of TGFβ showing at early and advanced stage of cancers are not due to the change of TGFβ structure, but are mediated through mutant TGFβ receptors as well as interaction of cancer cell-secreted TGFβ with the whole stromal cells such as dendritic cells, T cells, NK cells, TAMs, CAFs, and MDSCs. To suppress tumor growth, TGFβ arrests cell cycle through inhibiting cyclin dependent kinase and c-Myc pathways (103), induces cell apoptosis through activating JNK and Fas pathway, and antagonizing Bcl-2, Bcl-X, and survivin (104), and eventually prevents cell immortalization through regulating reverse transcriptase activity of human telomerase (105). To support tumorigenesis and metastases, paracrinal and autocrinal TGFβ enhances immunosuppression through diminishing immune surveillance maintained by DCs, cytotoxic T cells, and NK cells as well as cytokines such as IL2 and INFγ (22), amplifies angiogenesis through activation of ALK1 and ALK5 pathway and more production of vascular endothelial growth factor and connective tissue growth factors in epithelial cells and fibroblasts (97), and induces the EMT for promoting metastases through Smad-dependent and Smad-independent pathway (98), as well as accelerates malignant cells invasiveness through remodeling the ECM and decreasing TβR2 signaling and miRNA-mediated protein regulation (99).

Furthermore, hyperactivation of TGFβ signaling in advanced-stage malignant tumors also swiftly decreases efficacy of ICI therapy in the TME (106), whereas malignant tissue insensitive to ICI treatment exhibits a high expression pattern of TGFβ1 (107). Neutralized monoclonal antibodies individually targeting on TGFβ or dual recognition of TGFβ and PD-1/PDL-1 have achieved significant antitumor effects in treatment of liver cancer, pancreatic cancer, lung cancer, and urethral cancer (108, 109). Therefore, once malignant cells finish the transition from locally seeding to angiogenesis, TGFβ ultimately abandons the antitumor arm and majorly serves to immunosuppression and metastases.

Tumorigenesis in Gastrointestinal Cancers

Esophageal Cancer

Esophageal adenocarcinoma (EAC) and esophageal squamous cell carcinoma (ESCC) are two major malignant exhibitions at esophagus. Epidemiological studies demonstrate that multiple factors cause EAC and ESCC, such as smoking, obesity, gastroesophageal reflex disorder, and Barrett's esophagus, as well as epithelial injury *via* frequently intaking hot solution, all of which indicate that chronic inflammation is mainly responsible for malignant transition (110). In chronic inflammation-mediated esophageal cancers, not only IL6-STAT3 (signal transducer and activator of transcription 3) pathway increases epithelial proliferation and apoptotic resistance in Barrett's esophagus and EAC but also neoplastic cells utilize STAT3 signaling to promote tumorigenesis, angiogenesis, and metastases (111, 112). To ESCC, increased production of IL6 causes a poor prognosis following neoadjuvant radiochemotherapy, while higher expression of STAT3 at surgical resection correlates to increased mortality; however, siRNA-activated inhibition of IL6/STAT3 signaling augments chemotherapy sensitivity, accelerates apoptosis, and reduces angiogenesis, as well as decreases the EMT formation for metastases (113, 114).

More importantly, in EAC and ESCC, high expression of CD38-positive MDSCs is abundantly found in the peripheral blood at advanced stage, while Daratumumab binding with CD38 expression reduces tumor growth (115). Previous studies reported that MDSCs increased recruitment of Treg cells in maintenance of immunosuppression in the TME (116). It is highly possible that MDSCs promote malignant invasion through increasing Treg cell activity, in which the higher level of Treg cells, the stronger prediction of tumor invasion, metastasis, disease severity, and reduced overall survival (114, 117). Furthermore, due to the TME in esophageal cancers, especially in ESCC, enormously supporting transition of M1 macrophages to TAMs, infiltrating TAM-based immunosuppression (113), and TAM-mediated upregulation of Treg cell activity tremendously promote the development of EAC and ESCC through STAT3 signaling (118). Additionally, TGFβ directly increases CAF production in the TME, because of which, CAF-based secretion of vascular growth factors accelerates metastases in ESCC, whereas inhibition of CAF activity in EAC notably improves overall survival associated with an excellent prognosis (119). Collectively, interplay of various chronic inflammation conditions activates tumorigenesis in esophageal cancer.

Gastric Cancer

Similar to esophageal cancers, most environmental issues are directly and indirectly functional on generating gastric malignancy including high-salt food, pickled food, smoking, nitrates, and food preservers (120). But malignant tumors occurring at cardia and gastroesophageal junction are mostly related to gastroesophageal reflux, intestinal mucosa transition, and chronic mucosal infection caused by H. pylori (Hp) (121). External factors and internal issues confirm the contribution of chronic inflammation in promotion of gastric cancer (122, 123). Two pathological categories in gastric cancer are intestinal type and diffuse type, in which intestinal type is closely related to Hp infection in older males and less morbidity in last several decades worldly, while diffuse type is characterized with loss of E-cadherin expression, frequently occurring in young people unisexually, and less correlating with precancerous lesion (124).

As extensively reported, microorganisms make a great contribution in stimulation of tumorigenesis through dysregulation of cycle progression, protein translation, and cell survival. Epstein Barr Virus (EBV) and Hp are frequently emphasized due to mostly triggering PI3K-Akt pathway and Wnt/β-catenin pathway, respectively (121, 125). Crucially, mutant PI3KAc, an oncogene encoding a catalytic subunit of $PI3K_{\alpha}$, is remarkably expressed in up to 42% EBV-associated gastric adenocarcinoma, which predominantly causes DNA hypermethylation, especially promoting tumor suppressive gene CDKN2A hypermethylation (125). Moreover, amplification of mutant PI3KAc swiftly increases angiogenesis stimulated by VEGF and EGF through TGFβ-CAFs pathway (125). Also blocking oncosuppressive gene, PTEN, activates Akt expression and phosphorylation of Akt, which strongly dysregulates cell apoptosis, tumor invasiveness, and radiosensitivity (126). miRNA-21 targeting on PTEN expression rises proliferation and invasiveness of gastric cancer (126). Dysfunction of Wnt/β-catenin pathway occurs in about 70% gastric cancer patients, in which two virulence factors of Hp, CagA and VacA, are mainly responsible for such dysregulation (127). CagA not only interplays with E-cadherin to increase β-catenin accumulation in cytoplasm and nucleus but also activates CDX1 and P21 genes also firmly responsible for transition of Hp-infected gastric epithelium to mesenchymal stemness such as CSCs (128). Interestingly, chronic inflammation induced *via* Hp infection reprograms SALL4 expression, which directly promotes intestinal metaplasia to neoplastic transformation (129), whereas increased interaction of SALL4 with Wnt/β-catenin signaling also accelerates lymphatic node metastases in gastric cancer patients (130). Furthermore, unsurprisingly, TGFβ is a valid sponsor in upregulation of Hp-induced EMT (131).

Activation of EGFR is responsible for up to 30% gastric cancer cases, in which increased EGFR expression or mutant EGFR is responsible for 5–10% patients and correlates with microsatellite instability molecular subtypes (132). Various coregulators binding with EGFR and TNFα recruit signaling cascades that activate MAPK and PI3K-Akt pathways (133). Nevertheless, HER-2 overexpression exists in 10–30% gastric cancer patients, in which mutant HER-2 occurs in 5% gastric cancer cases, and is more prevalent in 7% microsatellite instability cases and 12% EBV-positive ones (132). Thereby, overexpression of mutant EGFR and HER-2 is highly associated with metastases and poor prognosis in gastric cancer patients (132). Furthermore, specific categories of miRNAs functionally contribute to the development of gastric cancer through increased oncogene expression, reduced expression of oncosuppressive genes, and dysfunction of tumor suppressive proteins; therefore, depending on miRNAs, they are highly likely to become a practically clinical tool in detection of GI cancers and evaluation of prognosis (134).

Liver Cancer

Hepatocellular carcinoma (HCC) mostly is diagnosed at the late stage following viral infection, alcohol overconsumption, steatohepatitis, primary biliary cirrhosis, autoimmune hepatitis, and aflatoxin contamination, in which chronic viral infections, such as HBV and HCV, are responsible for 80% cases (135). More researchers believe that oncogenic background changes, dysregulation of up- and downstream molecular pathways, and interaction between stromal cells and cytokines in the TME are tightly connected with cancer cell transition, proliferation, angiogenesis, invasion, and metastasis in HCC.

Single-cell transcriptomic profiling of HCC patients identifies that TME reprogram mainly controls HCC biodiversity, and VEGF-A-mediated regulation of CAFs and TAMs activities is only exhibited in malignant cells, especially in high diversity tumors, but not found in non-malignant hepatocytes (136). This investigation also verifies that individual activation of VEGF-A pathway in HCC is completely responsible to immunosuppression, aggressiveness, and negative prognosis (136). Also, VEGF-A is a critical trigger of angiogenesis in HCC serving for invasion and metastases (137). In HBV- and HCV-mediated hepatitis, chronic infection leads to cirrhotic situation that causes a hypoxic environment, in which hepatocytes upregulate hypoxia-induced factor 1α expression, and consequently that causes overexpression of VEGF at transcriptional level, and finally promotes angiogenesis in HCC (138). Treatment using lenvatinib and sorafenib targeting on VEGFs notably significantly improves prognosis in HCC patients (139). As mentioned previously, TGFβ dysregulated VEGF expression in different kinds of cancers (99); however, TGFβ is a double agent in health and diseased liver. In health liver, Kupffer cells and stellate cells produce most TGFβ except for hepatocytes, while in an injured health liver, temporary activation of TGFβ is functional on nuclear Yes-associated protein and Smad2 phosphorylation (140) that induces the EMT formation dependent on activated hepatic stellate cells and hepatocytes-transformed myofibroblast cells. Moreover, stromal cells in the TME utilize the fibrosis process induced by EMT for metastases, which has been actually verified through miRNA-dependent inactivation of TGFβ pathway in reducing HCC tumorigenesis and improving prognosis (141, 142).

More importantly, overexpression of EGFR and insulin-like growth factor receptors enhances activation of PI3K/Akt/mTOR signaling in HCC, in which atypical PTEN activity upregulates activation of the PI3K/AKT/mTOR pathway (143). Previous researches demonstrated that mutant PTENTs were identified in 5% HCC patients, while reduced or deleted PTEN expression was associated with nearly 50% HCC cases (144, 145). Abnormal expression of PTEN in chronic HBV- and HCV-infected patients constantly stimulates overactivation of PI3K/AKT/mTOR pathway, which constitutively promotes tumor grades and advanced disease stage, and diminishes overall survival in HCC patients (144). Clinically, everolimus and mTOR inhibitor plus a PI3K inhibitor (BKM120), Akt inhibitor (MK-2206), and mTOR/PI3K inhibitor (BEZ235) significantly increase immune cytotoxic activity, especially in treatment of advanced HCC *via* everolimus, in which 40–73% patients quickly catch the disease stable state in a short-time study (146, 147).

Alternatively, in almost 50–70% HCC patients, immunostainings identify overexpression of β-actin in cytoplasm and nucleus especially for tumor cell proliferation and suppression of physiological differentiation; however, under nonmalignant situation, high accumulation of β-actin shows less contribution to HCC formation (148). Furthermore, the early-stage HCC demonstrates that β-actin mutation occurs in 17% HCC patients and these mutant regions cover some specific sites such as phosphorylated site of glycogen synthase kinase-3β (149). Investigation of clustering β-actin resource in HCC shows that mutant β-actins are responsible for 12–26% of patients, whereas mutations in Wnt/β-actin pathway contribute 8–13% cases, both of which predominantly occur in HCV-infected population (149). Clinically, genetic profiling of 603 HCC patients illustrates that either Wnt/β-actin pathway or Myc/Akt pathway is abnormally activated, which is parallel with TGFβ overexpression (150). Interestingly, through activation of Wnt/β-actin pathway, miRNAs regulate TGFβ-mediated ECM formation (151), and more evidences expose that due to the ECM transition, liver has generally become a common site not only for HCC metastasis but also for other solid tumors (152, 153).

Pancreatic Cancer

As a deadly disease, pancreatic cancer, like mountain Everest, has always been attractive to many physicians and surgeons in that 5-year survival rate is only 8% (154), in which 90% pancreatic cancer is pathologically defined as pancreatic duct adenocarcinoma (PDAC) and 10-year survival rate is less 4% (155, 156). Principally, in pancreatic cancer, the TME promotes tumor growth and angiogenesis, CSCs focus on anticancer therapy and increased tumor bulk, and interaction between CSCs and the EMT contributes to metastases.

One of pathological characteristics in PDAC is desmoplasia, a state of extensive fibrosis around the primary tumor region, in which the ECM proteins are overexpressed and myofibroblast cells are tremendously identified (157). Clinical evidences also demonstrate that desmoplasia displaying in lymphonodes of the PDAC patients predicts a poor prognosis (157). Desmoplasia occurring in PDAC tightly depends on the TME in that TME-associated secretion of connective tissue growth factors, fibroblast growth factor 2, and TGFβ stimulates desmoplasia formation, especially the absence of anticancer arm of TGFβ caused by reduced Smad4 function depending on RAS-mediated ERK pathway (158). Due to high fibrosis in desmoplasia, the TME exhibits hypovascular and hypoxic conditions, through which pancreatic cancer cells reprogram metabolic pathways, inactivate apoptosis, and amplify proliferation and anticancer resistance, as well as promote invasion and metastasis (159). In purpose of maintenance and enhancement of hypoxia, pancreatic cancer cells produce more angiostatin, endostatin, and pigment epithelium-derived factors, whereas the ECM creates more endostatin, both of which are eventually countering vessel growing (160, 161). Desmoplasia-induced hypoxia, especially *via* hypoxia-induced factor 1α and TGFβ, constantly stimulates production of activated pancreatic stellate cells, in which stellate cells with quiescent vitamin-A contents transform into myofibroblast-like type (162). Through this procedure, normal cellular framework in pancreatic microenvironment steps into the carcinogenic ECM, which is responsible for upregulating secretion of cytokines and chemokines such as matrix metalloproteinases, platelet-derived growth factor, epidermal growth factor, insulin-like growth factor 1, fibroblast growth factor, and stromal-derived factor 1, as well as small leucine-rich proteoglycans and collagen type I, all of which make a great contribution to cancer development and metastasis (162, 163). Moreover, activated pancreatic stellate cells notably participate into immunosuppression in the TME, in which activation of stellate cell-dependent IL6 secretion causes MDSC aggregation deliberately to reduce T-cell proliferation, and increases Treg cell infiltration *via* STAT3 pathway (164). In addition, activated stellate cells also cause more T-cell apoptosis and Th2 cytokine secretion in the TME through upregulating Galectin-1 expression (165). Recently, investigation identified that inhibiting heat-sensitive protein 90 restricted transformation of cancerous pancreatic stellate cells and diminished IL6 production in the TME, which significantly amplified effects of ICIs and increased cytotoxic T cells and Th1 cell infiltration through inactivation of JAK/STAT and MAPK signaling in PDAC (166).

Hypoxia in PDAC not only stimulates production of activated stellate cells but also promotes stemness, in which hypoxic environment indirectly and directly supports CSC creation (167, 168). Growing with pancreatic cancer cells *in vitro* simultaneously, activated stellate cells increase spheroid formation of malignant cells and upregulate expression of stemness markers such as ABCG2, Nestin, and LIN28, which strongly indicates the importance of activated stellate cells in generating CSC niches (169). Specially, TGFβ1 predominantly secreted by activated stellate cells in PDAC stimulates CSC production through negatively regulating L1 cell adhesion molecule expression by TGFβ-Smad2/3 pathway, which causes PDAC to be more progressive (170). More importantly, self-renewal CSCs have become a major barrier of conventional chemoradiotherapy, in which gemcitabine is unable to eradicate CSCs but rather increase the number of CSCs (171, 172). In purpose of maintaining the renewal, increasing the tumor bulk, and promoting metastases, CSCs dysregulate several signal pathways including Wnt/β-catenin, hedgehog, notch, NF-κB, PI3K/Akt, and PTEN (173). Unsurprisingly, CSCs also secret Actin and Nodal that interact with Alk4/7 receptors to form pancreatic cancer cell sphere; however, through reduction of Akl4/7 expression and inhibition of interplay with CSCs, pancreatic cancer cells are more sensitive to gemcitabine treatment and lead to a long overall survival (174).

For entirely understanding the procedure of metastases in PDAC as well as contribution of CSCs in metastases, more investigations evidently show that the EMT insidiously plays a pivotal role during invasion through inducing CSC production continuously (175, 176). The most critical event in forming the EMT is to transform epithelial cells from a normally mature condition into mesenchymal phenotype, which causes morphogenetic changes occurring in embryonic development, organ fibrosis, and tumor metastasis, as well as less expression of epithelial markers such as E-cadherin, desmoplakin, and plakoglobin and overexpression of mesenchymal markers including vimentin, fibronectin, and α-smooth muscle actin (177, 178). Interestingly, hypoxia-inducible factor 1α is functional on expression of SIP1, Snail, Twist1, and Zeb1 indirectly or directly, while hypoxia-inducible factor 2α directly regulates Twist1 expression, both of which enlighten the essential role of hypoxia in induction of the EMT formation (179–181). Impressively, Zeb1 suppresses E-cadherin expression to promote metastases through downregulating expression of stemness inhibitors such as miR-203 and miR-200, in which TGFβ directly causes upregulation of Zeb1 signaling in the EMT (176, 182). Furthermore, circulating tumor cells (CTCs) depending on the EMT-mediated extravascular invasion and migration occupy 100-fold increases of $CD24^+$ and $CD44^+$ expression that are highly exhibited in pancreatic CSCs associated with therapeutical resistance and negative prognosis (183, 184). That TGFβ predominantly secreted by activated stellate cells strongly enhances CSC production in desmoplasia indicates that interaction between CSCs and the EMT crucially supports metastatic infrastructure and pathological progression in PDAC.

Colorectal Cancer

Clinical practice using non-steroid anti-inflammable drugs such as COX-2 antagonists but not aspirin exhibits 40–50% reduction at risk of colorectal cancer (CRC), which strongly demonstrates that chronic inflammation initially promotes tumorigenesis in CRC (185, 186). Further evidences verify that COX-2-mediated prostaglandin E2 production is critically responsible for CRC invasion (187). However, recent researches substantially identified that prostaglandin E2 secreted by CAFs essentially correlates with immunosuppression, angiogenesis, and metastases in CRC, in which upregulation of COX-2 expression on CAFs promotes migration and invasiveness (188), reduction of COX-2-mediated miR-335 expression blocks CAF-induced carcinogenesis through restoring PTEN activity (189), and dysregulation of NK cell function by hepatocellular CAFs depends on prostaglandin E2 and indoleamine 2,3-dioxygenase activity (190). Therefore, transformation of normal fibroblasts to CAFs is a milestone in CRC formation, which purposely remodels the TME through reprogramming secretion of the ECM proteins (191). Moreover, CAFs in CRC strongly amplify immunosuppression in the TME through CAF-mediated enhancement of TAM and MDSC activities (192, 193), CAF-dependent promotion of Treg cell proliferation (194), and CAF-induced PDL-1 overexpression on cancer cells (195), as well as CAF-activated reduction of cytotoxic T cell activity (196). Furthermore, exosomes predominantly secreted by CAFs typically contain miR-21, miR-378e, and miR-143, most of which travel from CAFs to cancer cells in response to increased expression of the EMT markers and stemness to become more aggressive phenotype, which is parallel with results obtained from cancer cells transfected with miR-21, miR-378e, and miR-143 (197). Therefore, miR-21-contained vehicles majorly created by CAFs play an essential role in upregulation of cancer cell-based tissue damaging, especially causing more metastases to liver in CRC (198). Eventually, CAF-dependent exosome secretion is inherently in recruitment of CSCs to resist oxaliplatin or 5-fluorouracil treatment in CRC therapy; however, inhibition of exosome production significantly reduces such kind of behaviors (199). In addition, CAF-induced IL17a secretion also notably promotes self-renewal and invasiveness of CSCs and worthfully to know that chemotherapy of CRC unfortunately upregulates IL17a secretion (200).

CLINICAL APPROACHES IN DIAGNOSIS OF GASTROINTESTINAL CANCERS AT EARLY STAGE

Currently, conventional screening cancer tools including plasma-based tumor markers, barium enema, GI endoscopy, and computed tomography have been practiced extensively in asymptomatic population for decades of years in purpose of identifying malignant tumors at early stage, in which GI endoscopy is strongly recommended due to high accuracy of histology; however, invasive nature, unhappier feeling, and noticeable cost have conditionally slabbed this optimal practice for a large-scale of screening tests (201, 202). Most of serum tumor markers generally show less specific in early detection of GI malignancies except for αfetoprotein and CA19-9 with highly predictable value of hepatocellular cancer and pancreatic cancer, respectively (203, 204). According to diversity of cytokines, chemokines, and glycoproteins in the TME, it is necessary to comprehensively apply novel biomarkers for early diagnosis of GI malignancies, which are not independent from traditional cancer-screening tests.

M2 Pyruvate Kinase (M2PK)

Glutaminolysis and glycolysis almost exist in all kinds of solid tumors in that hypoxia in the TME significantly upregulates glycolysis d in malignant tissues (205, 206). Being a rate-limiting enzyme, M2PK plays a crucial role in regulation of glycolysis, in which tetrameric structure of M2PK exhibits high affinity to phosphoenolpyruvate, whereas a dimeric form, named tumor M2PK with low affinity to phosphoenolpyruvate, is predominantly expressed in malignant tumors (207). A large number of evidences demonstrate that increased expression of tumor M2PK in screening samples especially correlates with GI cancers and also has a pan-sensitive to malignancies in brain, thyroid, lung, breast, ovary, cervix, kidney, bladder, and prostate (205, 208–215).

As a meta-analysis study showed, tumor M2PK as a plasma marker had 62.1% sensitivity and 89% specificity in detection of gastric cancer and esophageal cancer (216). According to different stages of gastric cancer, tumor M2PK has 71% sensitivity to metastatic cases, whereas CA72-4 is 57%, while to the cases without metastases, tumor M2PK has 63% sensitivity, whereas CA72-4 is 25% (11). The study focusing on accuracy of tumor M2PK, CEA, CA19-9, and CA72-4 in diagnosis of GI cancers confirms that tumor M2PK is significantly higher in screening esophageal cancer, gastric cancer, and CRC than other three tumor markers, while in pancreatic cancer, tumor M2PK has a similar predictable rate as CA19-9, but more sensitive than CEA and CA72-4 (6). Furthermore, a comparable meta-analysis study found that screening pancreatic cancer through CA19-9 and M2PK together has 60% sensitivity and 95% specificity (11). More conveniently, testing tumor M2PK in fecal samples is significantly sensitive and reliable than fecal occult blood test (FOBT) due to intermittent bleeding or the absence of bleeding in CRC, in which tumor M2PK shows 68.8 to 91.0% sensitivity and 71.9 to 100% specificity, whereas FOBT has 40% sensitivity only or less (217). Therefore, combining with conventional plasma tumor markers and periodic endoscopy examination, tumor M2PK is practically selected as an earlier alert signal in detection of GI malignancies, especially in screening CRC.

Circulating Tumor Cell and Circulating Tumor DNA

CTCs are tumor cells that have broken away from primary tumors or metastatic sites, and then enter into the blood circulation in purpose of distal metastases (218). Comparing with other peripheral blood cells, the number of CTCs is extremely low, generally 10^{-7} to 10^{-8}, and lifetime mostly lasts for several hours (219–221). Currently, using CTCs to screen GI cancers in normal population is not actually realistic due to remarkably low fraction of CTC-positive patients, screening markers less specific for CTCs assessment, and tremendously lower level of CTCs detected at early-stage tumors (222–224). A cohort study of 138 CRC patients at stage I to III demonstrates that postoperative CTC-positive patients who were negative at preoperative CTC test independently predict a really poor prognosis, whereas preoperative CTC-positive patients have similar results as preoperative CTC-negative group in evaluation of prognosis (225). Therefore, CTC test may be highly valid to patients with extensive metastases, post-surgery relapse, or the high-risk population with family history of GI cancers as well as a good candidate in prediction of prognosis after chemoradiotherapy.

Circulating tumor DNA (ctDNA) is a kind of cell-free DNA originally traveling from primary cancer site, metastatic location, or CTCs to the bloodstream, in which the size of ctDNAs is generally shorter than normal cell-free DNAs, lifetime lasts for 16–150 min, and can be released into exosomes (226, 227). Different from CTC test, ctDNAs screening has employed tumor-specific genetic markers and epigenetic markers in discrimination of ctDNAs from normal cell-free DNAs (228), and sensitivity of ctDNA detection has exhibited microscale level through molecular barcoding techniques (229). Furthermore, identification of ctDNAs through low-coverage genome sequencing has not required genomic information of primary malignancy (230), and ctDNA detection using plasma samples is more accurate than in serum due to lower level of wild-type DNA released (231). Through combinative application of both ctDNAs and CTCs techniques as well as through detection of hypomethylation or hypermethylation of ctDNAs at promoter region of cancerous and oncosuppressive genes, ctDNAs have been extensively used in early diagnosis of GI cancers. However, due to few amounts of ctDNAs released into the circulation, ctDNA technique is encountering some challenges in detection of ultra-early stage of GI malignancies (232, 233).

In esophageal cancer, ctDNAs targeting CASZ1, CDH13, and ING2 genes show significant high level of hypermethylation in ESCC patients but mild level in healthy controls, whereas dysregulation of 5-hydroxymethylcytosine expression on ctDNAs also has remarkable sensitivity in screening ESCC; therefore, ctDNA detection based on these two different patterns is highly likely to identify the early-stage esophageal cancer (234, 235). Through screening methylation and hypermethylation of 14 genes in 1193 samples, ctDNA approach has 65% sensitivity and 95% specificity in diagnosis of gastric cancer, whereas in comparison with CEA, CA72-4, CA19-9, and CA50, the higher concentration of ctDNAs tested by *alu*-dependent branch DNA assessment, the more accuracy in early diagnosis of gastric cancer, which has 79% sensitivity and 91.8% specificity (236, 237). Therefore, combining hypermethylation of CASZ1, CDH13, and ING2 genes with increased ctDNA burden is a valuable approach for a large-scale screening of upper digestive cancers. Using somatic copy number aberration (SCNA) *via* low-depth whole genome sequencing technique demonstrates that increased ctDNA burden has area under curve (AUC) value of 0.874 in early diagnosis of HCC and 0.933 at advanced stage of HCC, whereas application of ctDNA panel focusing on eight targeted genes has 83.3% sensitivity and 90.5% specificity in screening HCC; thereby, screening people through a panel containing multiple ctDNAs with increased ctDNA burden comprehensively provides a specific method in diagnosis of HCC (238, 239). To detect pancreatic cancer, several investigations clarify that single ctDNA-mediated tests are not sensitive at the early-stage; however, through combining with conventional serum tumor markers, specific proteins expressed in the TME and methylation at protomer regions of cancer-related genes, ctDNA technique significantly increases sensitivity and specificity in diagnosis of pancreatic cancer (240, 241). Using ctDNAs to detect methylation expression at promoter regions of 17 genes exhibits 91.2% sensitivity and 90.8% specificity to discriminate PDAC patients from chronic pancreatitis group (242). Through examining methylation at both ADAMTS1 and BNC1 genes in screening PDAC, ctDNAs tests remarkably accomplish the accuracy with 94.8% sensitivity and 91.6% specificity (243). Moreover, detection of mutant KRAS through ctDNAs combined with other four protein markers notably has 64% sensitivity and 99.5% specificity in diagnosis of PDAC patients from healthy controls (244). Thereby, the methodology of integrating ctDNAs with KRAS mutation, methylation on targeted genes, and high expression level of tumor-specific proteins predominantly occupies a position in early diagnosis of pancreatic cancers. Similarly to detect early gastric cancer, increased ctDNA burden through *Alu*83 and *Alu*244 is also used to detect CRC, combination of which with methylation of specific gene achieved higher sensitivity in CRC diagnosis (245). Furthermore, using ctDNAs to examine B4GALT1 gene hypermethylation performs 50% sensitivity and 100% specificity in early diagnosis of CRC, whereas hypomethylation of LINE-1 gene tested by ctDNAs yields 65.8% sensitivity and 90.0% specificity in screening CRC (246). Therefore, testing M2PK-positive samples depending on increased ctDNA burden, hypermethylated B4GALT1 gene, and hypomethylated LINE-1 gene is a reliable methodology in early detection of CRC.

Circulating microRNA

microRNAs (miRNAs) generally composing of 19–24 nucleotides are functional on 3'-UTR of messenger RNA, which effectively regulates targeted protein expression (247). miRNAs are endurable in various physiological changes and resist to RNase activity, thereby circulating miRNAs extensively and stably present in 12 kinds of cell-free body fluids and excretions including serum, plasma, urine, and feces (248). Since downregulation of miR-15 and miR-16 expression was firstly recognized as a novel biomarker in diagnosis of B-cell chronic lymphocytic leukemia (249), clinical professionals have applied circulating miRNAs in detection of GI cancers considerably and identified several unique expression patterns in early diagnosis of esophageal cancer (250, 251), gastric cancer (252), liver cancer (253), pancreatic cancer (254), and CRC (255).

Comparing to healthy controls, the expression panel containing miR-16-5p, miR-197-5p, miR451a, and miR-92a-3p is specially associated with ESCC, whereas the group of miR-16-5p, miR-320c, miR-638, and miR-92a-3p is significantly higher in squamous dysplasia, a precancer pathology, especially miRNA-21 overexpression highly correlating with alcohol-induced ESCC (250, 251). In a cost-effective screening of gastric cancer, 12-miRNA panel shows 87% sensitivity and 68.4% specificity, which is remarkably higher than CEA and CA-19-9 (252). A meta-analysis study of circulating miRNA-mediated detection of HCC demonstrates that the higher expression group of circulating miR-21, miR-122, and miR-223 is more specific in diagnosis of HCC than in healthy, hepatitis, or cirrhosis group, in which confident rates of miR-21, miR-122, and miR-223 are 0.9293, 0.8128, and 0.8597, respectively, especially miR-21 expression in high priority (256). Screening of pancreatic cancer proves that the expression group containing miR-125a-3p, miR-5100, and miR-642b-3p achieves the most promising result in discrimination of cancer patients from healthy ones, which shows 98% sensitivity and 97% specificity (254). Moreover, in diagnosis of CRC, the expression pattern consisting of miR-15b, miR-17, miR-21, miR-26b, and miR-145 has the best predictable performance, especially miR-21 and miR-26b with maximal specificity (257). Recently, circulating exosomes were also considered as the early biomarkers in diagnosis of GI cancers; however, the reliability of this approach mainly depends on analysis of contents within the circulating exosomes, especially miRNAs and cell-free DNAs (258).

Finally, through reviewing 42 investigations significantly relevant to the diagnostic performance of circulating miRNAs in GI cancers, this meta-analysis study concludes that comparing to CEA and CA19-9, circulating miRNAs have become reliable biomarkers in early diagnosis, moderately with 75% sensitivity and 81% specificity, and multiple-miRNA screening assay significantly achieves more accurate result than a single-miRNA test, as well as plasma-dependent miRNAs assay is precisely used in diagnosis of gastric cancer, while serum-based miRNA test is more suitable for CRC detection (259).

Circular RNA

Circular RNAs (circRNA), non-coding RNA with closed circular form, have been discovered in mammalian cells for decades and structurally characterized through high-throughput sequencing over 10 years, in which circRNAs are functional on the axle of circRNA-miRNA-mRNA responsible for target gene expression, interplay with RNA-binding protein in regulation of target protein activities, and act as posttranscriptional regulators influencing parental gene transcription and splicing (260). Due to strongly resisting to exoribonuclease, circulating circRNAs are stably and extensively expressed in exosomes, serum, plasma, saliva, and urine (261). Since ciRS-7 firstly exhibited sponging action on miRNA-7 to promote carcinogenesis, different kinds of cancers have shown unique existing patterns of circRNAs that are practically applied in diagnosis of malignancy at early stage (261). Moreover, recent investigation demonstrated that artificial expression of circRNA targeting on miRNA21 eliminated miRNA-21-mediated promotion of gastric cancer (262). Therefore, examining expression pattern of circRNAs sponging on cancer-specific miRNAs is highly likely to become a more efficient methodology in early diagnosis of GI malignancies.

Using a pool of circRNAs to screen ESCC identifies that upregulation of circ-DLG1 and circ-TTC17 combining with downregulation of hsa_circ_0001946, hsa_circ_0062459 and circ-SMAD7 has 79% sensitivity and 85% specificity, in which positive samples in this pool test have 5-fold higher possibility in transition to ESCC than normal controls (263). Through analyzing 343 plasma circRNAs expressed in gastric cancer patients and healthy controls, downregulation of hsa_circ_0001017 and hsa_circ_0061276 has the best diagnostic performance with 95.5% sensitivity and 95.7% specificity (264). Another study shows that lower expression of plasma hsa_circ_0000181 has 99.0% sensitivity and 85.2% specificity in gastric cancer (265). Therefore, the expression group of hsa_circ_0001017 and hsa_circ_0061276 and hsa_circ_0000181 is practically becoming a novel biomarker for early diagnosis of gastric cancer. For HCC detection, upregulation of seven circRNAs expression plus downregulation of five circRNAs expression in serum shows the best combinative performance, in which the expression group covering hsa_circ_0004001, hsa_circ_0004123, and hsa_circ_0075792 has 90.5% sensitivity and 78.1% specificity (266). Furthermore, two independent studies identically discover that plasma circ-LDLRAD3 overexpression significantly correlates with pancreatic cancer, in which together with CA19-9, combinative test has 80.3% sensitivity and 93.6% specificity in early diagnosis of pancreatic cancer (267, 268). Thus, integrating conventional tumor markers with circRNA expression highly possibly obtains more precise diagnosis in screening of pancreatic cancer. Similar methodologies are also used in early diagnosis of CRC, in which combining with CEA and CA19-9, the group of downregulated expression of plasma circ-CCDC66, circ-ABCC1, and circ-STIL increases AUC value 0.780–0.855 (269). Another investigation focusing on early diagnosis of CRC shows that using upregulated expression group of hsa_circ_0001900, hsa_circ_0001178, and hsa_circ_0005927 precisely identifies CRC patients in the CEA-negative group with AUC value 0.859 (270). Therefore, combinative patterns of using circRNAs with CEA and M2PK will maximally increase the diagnostic accuracy in screening CRC.

CELLULAR IMMUNOTHERAPY IN TREATMENT OF GASTROINTESTINAL CANCERS

Cellular immunotherapy is a combinative methodology of applying cellular therapy and immunotherapy in personalized cancer treatment (271–273), in which personalized analysis to an individual cancer patient is the key strategy to achieve a clinically effective treatment (273). Personalized investigation in cancer therapy includes genomic DNA sequencing, genomic exons sequencing, cancer-specific mutant genes sequencing, dysfunction of signaling proteins analysis, neoantigen detection, loss of immune cytotoxicity, and diversity of the TME (274). However, following nearly one century training, oncological clinicians have been used to dogmatically applying conventional chemotherapy and radiotherapy in almost all cancer treatment. Whether therapy-induced immune alterations are responsible for an effective therapy is less attractive in main menu despite the critical role of cellular immunotherapy to malignancy having been successfully exhibited through Dr Coley's vaccine in 1893 (275). Actually, Coley's vaccine strongly indicates that turning cold tumor to hot through immune modulation is an essential conversion from treatable to clinically curable. Currently, cellular immunotherapy includes neoantigens and vaccines, adoptive cell therapy, CAR-T/NK techniques, and oncolytic virus (OV) in purpose to recover immune normalization, reduce immunosuppression in the TME, increase tumor-specific antigen expression, and locally rebuild inflammatory conditions, as well as rearrange tumor vasculature.

Combination of Conventional Chemotherapy and Radiotherapy With Cellular Immunotherapy

For many years, a number of investigations have demonstrated that using pan-cytotoxic chemotherapy in cancer treatment causes a direct immunosuppression (276, 277), PDL-1 overexpression (278), recruitment of CSC-mediated drug resistance (200), and increased VEGFR-1-activated metastases (279), as well as myelosuppression (280), all of which objectively and comprehensively indicate that conventional chemotherapy is not an approach of precise medicine in cancer treatment. Surprisingly, through combining with certain kinds of chemotherapeutic agents, cellular immunotherapy significantly increases overall survival than singly using chemotherapy (281, 282). Further analysis elucidates that chemotherapeutics specifically acting on MDSCs and CSCs to reduce immunosuppression in the TME remarkably amplify efficiency and efficacy of ICI treatment and adoptive cell therapy (282, 283). Previously, clinical professionals supposed that apoptotic cancer cells or chemotherapy-induced mutation should have expressed more neoantigens; however, this idea is highly likely a misconception (284), but through applying histone deacetylase inhibitors or radioactive treatments, neoantigens expressed on cancer cells are notably beneficial for cellular immunotherapy due to enormously increased antigenicity (285, 286). Moreover, boron-neutron capture therapy (BNCT) not only precisely and largely eliminates tumor volume but also produces a large amount of various neoantigens due to radiation-damaged DNAs extensively existing in survived cancer cells, which are specifically utilized by cellular immunotherapy for constantly attacking (287, 288).

Adoptive Cell Therapy

Adoptive cell therapy includes TILs, cytokine-induced killer cells (CIK), dendritic cell-activated cytokine-induced killer cells (DC-CIK), NK cells, CAR-NK (chimeric antigen receptor-natural killer cells), and CAR-T (chimeric antigen receptor-T cells), in which TIL methodology showed clinical effects firstly on patients with metastatic melanoma in 1983 (289), and currently, TIL (290), DC-CIK (291), NK (292), CAR-NK (293), and CAR-T (294) all have achieved convincing results in cancer treatment, especially through DC-CIK, NK, and CAR-NK approaches.

As given knowledge, DCs are the most powerful antigen presentation immunocytes, which directly command cytotoxic T lymphocytes to attack cancer cells; therefore, depending on DC-mediated recruitment of CIKs through tumor-associated antigens, DC-CIK therapy efficiently and specifically eliminates malignant cells (295). Through three meta-analysis studies of more than 8 thousand patients with gastric cancer and CRC, comparing to individual application of chemotherapy, CIK/DC-CIK plus chemotherapy significantly increases overall survival and progression-free survival in drug-resistant patients, and swiftly improves most adverse events caused by chemotherapy (28, 296, 297). Similar results are also exhibited in CIK/DC-CIK therapy of pancreatic cancer and HCC, especially in advanced-stage patients (298, 299). Interestingly, infusion of allogeneic CIKs has also demonstrated encouraging effects on hematological malignancies (300). Comparing to DC-CIK therapy, as innate immune system, NK cell treatment occupies a unique advantage, in which tumor-associated antigen presentation is not compulsory for NK cell cytotoxicity, cytokine release syndrome is less possible to occur, and human leukocyte antigen matching is not stringently required for donor NK cell infusion; therefore, despite autologous NK cells showing very limited clinical efficacy (301), allogeneic NK cells including semi-allogeneic NK cells, NK cells isolated from umbilical cord blood, and iPSC-derived NK cells all show extraordinary immune killing specificity to malignant tumors without graft-versus-host disease (53, 302). Multiple infusions of allogeneic NK cells to stage-III/IV pancreatic cancer patients significantly increase overall survival and progression-free survival to 13.6

months and 9.9 months, respectively (303), whereas to unresectable primary HCC, are 23.2 months and 15.1 months, respectively (304), both of which clinically identify allogeneic NK cell therapy as a novel and promising methodology in treatment of GI cancers. Recent investigations discovered that PD-1 and PDL-1 expressed on DCs and NK cells reduced DC-activated maturation of cytotoxic T lymphocytes (305, 306) and NK-mediated antigen presentation of DCs (307–312), but through applying ICIs, both DC-CIK and NK therapies exhibit the higher level of cytotoxic activity to cancer cells (313–315).

Through studying the principle of TILs, clinical scientists naively consider that arming T cells from cancer patients with Chimeric tumor-specific Antigen Receptors (CAR-T) is efficient to destroy cancer cells precisely, and CAR-T technique indeed achieves the success in treatment of some kinds of hematological malignancies (316). However, different from attacking an individual malignant cell with unique antigen expression in the bloodstream or in the lymphatic nodes, CAR-T therapy to solid tumors is like using the sharpness of a knife to fight with the thickness of a tank, disadvantages of which include immunosuppression of the TME in solid tumors always primarily focusing on T cells, loss of tumor-associated antigens at the surface of mature solid tumors, and high cell density of inside solid tumors stopping CAR-Ts entering into the bulk, as well as extremely lethal side effects caused by immunotoxicity to the normal cells co-expressing tumor-associated antigens (317, 318). Also, due to continuously selective pressure caused by specific CAR, cancer cells may highly possibly abandon unique antigen expression through endocytosis. Therefore, in purpose of promoting immune normalization but not enhancement (319), rebuilding normal immunity in cancer patients through cellular immunotherapy is far more essential than CAR expression. Due to specific cytotoxicity to malignant tumors and much less possibility of inducing cytokine storm, clinical scientists design CAR-NK technique through equipping NK cells with chimeric antigen receptors, and have applied CAR-NK in patients with relapsed and refractory acute myeloid leukemia to test safety and tolerance (320). Whether CAR-NK therapy has more therapeutical advantages in solid tumors than combinative treatment of DC-CIK plus allogeneic NK cells, clinicians still have a long way to go. Following identification of specific biomarkers of TAMs, MDSCs, CAFs and CSCs, CAR-NK therapy certainly makes a great contribution in breaking through immunosuppression in the TME and strongly provide a beneficiary immune infrastructure for other kinds of cancer therapies.

Vaccine and Oncolytic Virus

Vaccines used in cancer therapy mainly depend on transferring tumor-associated antigens to antigen presenting cells such as DCs, and then inducing $CD4^+$ helper T cells and $CD8^+$ cytotoxic T cells to eradicate cancer cells (321). Genetic vaccines including DNA and RNA vaccines are theoretically able to synthesize all sequences encoding targeted antigens; however, according to various levels of protein translation, immunogenicity produced by genetic vaccines is hard to control (322). Despite DNA vaccines achieving pathological regression in treatment of intraepithelial neoplasia caused by human papillomavirus infection (323), clinical trials have not shown effective results in solid tumors therapy such as breast cancer (324), CRC (325), prostate cancer (326), and melanoma (327). Similar to DNA vaccines, messenger RNA vaccines containing 20 epitopes inoculated for patients with advanced-stage GI cancers have not obtained clinical efficacy, although they are safe and have activated immune response to neoepitopes (328). Actually, DC vaccines are more appropriately applied for cancer therapy in that they are *ex vivo* induced through the whole cancer cells, tumor lysates, peptides, DNAs, and RANs, which are strongly functional on tumor-specific cytotoxic T cells to eliminate cancer cells. Therapeutic DC vaccines have been extensively used in treatment of GI cancers at phase II or III trials, in which DC vaccine combining with MAGE peptide safely promotes immune response to tumor-specific antigens and significantly reduces tumor marker expression in nearly 90% advanced GI cancer patients (329), but for accomplishment of more optimal prognosis, prior to using DC vaccines, it is critical to examine NK cell activity in the candidates (330). Furthermore, *in situ* vaccines generated through chemoradiotherapy show more beneficial to cancer patients than conventional vaccines in that there is no screening requisition of positive antigen expression (331, 332). Almost all clinical trials demonstrate that adding ICIs into vaccine therapy remarkably increase vaccine-mediated cytotoxicity, which partially explains why individually using vaccine therapy only achieves suboptimal impact in cancer treatment (333, 334). Currently, the challenges vaccine therapy needs to deal with are multiple immunogenic antigen expression, construction of highly potent vaccine vectors, and breakthrough of immunosuppression in the TME.

Oncolytic virotherapy includes various kinds of viruses targeting a large range of malignant tumors, in which cancer cells are vulnerable to viral infection due to absence of type I interferon system and mutations promoting attachment of viruses (335, 336). In cancer therapy, using adenoviruses as a platform to express tumor-specific antigens and tumor-suppressive proteins has exhibited the promising results in preliminary animal studies, and currently in human studies, telomelysin-targeted adenovirus is testing in treatment of esophageal cancer, whereas evaluation of ideal viral vectors is processing in gastric cancer therapy, as well as more clinical trials are manipulating in treatment of pancreatic cancer, primary HCC, and CRC (337). Currently, clinical scientists are also concentrated on myxoma virus due to absence of infection to human beings and extremely sensitive to cancer cells; however, there still have a distance for clinical application (338). Furthermore, in diagnosis of GI cancers, depending on specific expression of fluorescence and bioluminescence on infected cancer cells, OVs, being tracing signals, are used to accurately expose the border of malignant tissue in surgery, and precisely identify the primary tumor and metastatic microtumors through nuclear medical imaging techniques such as CT, MRI, SPECT, and PET-CT (339–343). Through practicing oncolytic virotherapy, some barriers clinicians have to quell include tumor heterogeneity, general immune elimination of OVs, and capability to hack into tumor bulk and induce more activated cytotoxic T cells in the TME.

CONCLUSION

To successfully apply personalized therapy in cancer treatment, it is crucial to set up an assessment of tumor heterogeneity (344). In this review, we seemly underrate the importance of tumoral heterogeneity, in fact, which has been broadly discussed in parts of diagnosis and cellular therapy. Due to high variability of single subclone- or multiple subclone-induced tumor evolution in the same tumor or metastatic regions of the same tumor, as well as in different types of GI cancers, intratumoral genomic heterogeneity is highly beneficial for early diagnosis *via* liquid biopsy (345–347), while intertumoral heterogeneity-mediated changes of temporal and spatial plasticity and stemness in the TME precisely support the significance of comprehensive therapeutic principle (348, 349). Complexity of tumor heterogeneity essentially reflects adaption of genomic heterogeneity to selective pressure and utility of angiogenesis and immunosuppression through the TME for distant metastasis (350–352). Tumor heterogeneity also strongly indicates that rebuilding immune normalization to block interaction of intertumoral heterogeneity with the TME is a practical methodology to alter cancer therapy to chronic disease management.

Through systematically discussing key contributions of various components in the TME to tumorigenesis and metastases, reliability of early diagnostic methodologies, and personalized application of cellular immunotherapy in GI malignancies, it has become more apparent that immunosuppression induced by TAMs, MDSCs, CAFs, and CSCs in the TME and autocrine-paracrine network supported by stromal cells and cytokines and growth factors, especially TGFβ, are critically responsible for resistance to anticancer therapy and significant reduction of overall survival. Therefore, based on personalized investigation of each cancer patient including seeking mutant target genes and neoantigens, evaluating immune cytotoxicity in the TME, and recovering immune normalization, precise cellular immunotherapy is highly likely to change cancer treatment into a state of managing chronic disorders and eventually achieve the coexistence *via* normalization of immune surveillance. Due to complex of the TME, precise methodologies used to detect GI cancers at early stage primarily depend on the personalized combination of M2PK, miRNAs, ctDNAs, cancer-produced exosomes, and CTCs with conventional tumor markers and serologically biochemical examinations, in which CTC methodology is far more beneficial in evaluation of treatment efficacy and prognosis. Prior to treatment, a solid tumor is like an onion, in which anticancer mechanism of each layer is highly changeable, thereby, one step-by-step comprehensive treatment plan primarily includes that using BNCT technique efficiently reduces tumor volume and tears the tumor shell, and then applying OVs targeting TAMs, MDSCs, and CSCs with ICIs or dual recognition antibody of TGFβ and PD-1/PDL-1 maximally destroys immunosuppression and amplifies immunotoxicity of infiltrating T cells in the TME; furthermore, alternative infusion of DC-CIKs and allogeneic NK cells significantly eliminates most cancer cells with or without neoantigen expression. Such a therapy plan remarkably shrinks and eradicates the whole onion layer by layer. For CTCs or temporary formation of metastatic microtumors, CAR-T and CAR-NK therapies predominantly contribute to remove them. Surely, through recovering immune normalization in cancer patients and high-risk population, prevention of cancers in the community is far more critical than diagnosis and treatment. Whether precisely selecting the personalized cellular immunotherapy based on the diversity of the TME or rigidly relying on the unspecific chemotherapy, your choice.

AUTHOR CONTRIBUTIONS

HZ made outline, wrote and revised the draft, and finalized the review. XL made outline. All authors contributed to the article and approved the submitted version.

REFERENCES

1. Arnold M, Abnet CC, Neale RE, Vignat J, Giovannucci EL, McGlynn KA, et al. Global Burden of 5 Major Types of Gastrointestinal Cancer. *Gastroenterology* (2020) 159(1):335–49 e15. doi: 10.1053/j.gastro.2020.02.068
2. Wang M, Zhao J, Zhang L, Wei F, Lian Y, Wu Y, et al. Role of Tumor Microenvironment in Tumorigenesis. *J Cancer* (2017) 8(5):761–73. doi: 10.7150/jca.17648
3. Martins D, Schmitt F. Microenvironment in Breast Tumorigenesis: Friend or Foe? *Histol Histopathol* (2019) 34(1):13–24. doi: 10.14670/HH-18-021
4. Xian W, McKeon F. Microenvironment Meets Lineage Complexity in Junctional Tumorigenesis. *Nat Commun* (2019) 10(1):3829. doi: 10.1038/s41467-019-11651-6
5. Tong Q, Wang XL, Li SB, Yang GL, Jin S, Gao ZY, et al. Combined Detection of IL-6 and IL-8 is Beneficial to the Diagnosis of Early Stage Esophageal Squamous Cell Cancer: A Preliminary Study Based on the Screening of Serum Markers Using Protein Chips. *Onco Targets Ther* (2018) 11:5777–87. doi: 10.2147/OTT.S171242
6. Schneider J, Schulze G. Comparison of Tumor M2-pyruvate Kinase (Tumor M2-PK), Carcinoembryonic Antigen (CEA), Carbohydrate Antigens CA 19-9 and CA 72-4 in the Diagnosis of Gastrointestinal Cancer. *Anticancer Res* (2003) 23(6D):5089–93.
7. Li D, Wang G, Mei X. Diagnosis of Cancer at Early Stages Based on the Multiplex Detection of Tumor Markers Using Metal Nanoclusters. *Analyst* (2020) 145(22):7150–61. doi: 10.1039/d0an01538e
8. Killock D. Diagnosis: CancerSEEK and Destroy - a Blood Test for Early Cancer Detection. *Nat Rev Clin Oncol* (2018) 15(3):133. doi: 10.1038/nrclinonc.2018.21
9. Chen X, Gole J, Gore A, He Q, Lu M, Min J, et al. Non-Invasive Early Detection of Cancer Four Years Before Conventional Diagnosis Using a Blood Test. *Nat Commun* (2020) 11(1):3475. doi: 10.1038/s41467-020-17316-z
10. Crosby D, Lyons N, Greenwood E, Harrison S, Hiom S, Moffat J, et al. A Roadmap for the Early Detection and Diagnosis of Cancer. *Lancet Oncol* (2020) 21(11):1397–9. doi: 10.1016/S1470-2045(20)30593-3
11. Schulze G. The Tumor Marker Tumor M2-PK: An Application in the Diagnosis of Gastrointestinal Cancer. *Anticancer Res* (2000) 20(6D):4961–4.
12. Thakkar S, Sharma D, Kalia K, Tekade RK. Tumor Microenvironment Targeted Nanotherapeutics for Cancer Therapy and Diagnosis: A Review. *Acta Biomater* (2020) 101:43–68. doi: 10.1016/j.actbio.2019.09.009

13. Dudley ME, Rosenberg SA. Adoptive-Cell-Transfer Therapy for the Treatment of Patients With Cancer. *Nat Rev Cancer* (2003) 3(9):666–75. doi: 10.1038/nrc1167
14. Marcus A, Eshhar Z. Allogeneic Adoptive Cell Transfer Therapy as a Potent Universal Treatment for Cancer. *Oncotarget* (2011) 2(7):525–6. doi: 10.18632/oncotarget.300
15. Villadangos JA. Antigen-Specific Impairment of Adoptive T-cell Therapy Against Cancer: Players, Mechanisms, Solutions and a Hypothesis. *Immunol Rev* (2016) 272(1):169–82. doi: 10.1111/imr.12433
16. Hinrichs CS, Rosenberg SA. Exploiting the Curative Potential of Adoptive T-cell Therapy for Cancer. *Immunol Rev* (2014) 257(1):56–71. doi: 10.1111/imr.12132
17. Burchett R, Walsh S, Wan Y, Bramson JL. A Rational Relationship: Oncolytic Virus Vaccines as Functional Partners for Adoptive T Cell Therapy. *Cytokine Growth Factor Rev* (2020) 56:149–59. doi: 10.1016/j.cytogfr.2020.07.003
18. Chau I. Clinical Development of PD-1/PD-L1 Immunotherapy for Gastrointestinal Cancers: Facts and Hopes. *Clin Cancer Res* (2017) 23 (20):6002–11. doi: 10.1158/1078-0432.CCR-17-0020
19. Wang D, Lin J, Yang X, Long J, Bai Y, Yang X, et al. Combination Regimens With PD-1/PD-L1 Immune Checkpoint Inhibitors for Gastrointestinal Malignancies. *J Hematol Oncol* (2019) 12(1):42. doi: 10.1186/s13045-019-0730-9
20. Park H, Chen B, Ciorba MA. Progress in PD-1-based Immunotherapy: New Mechanistic Insight may Provide Expanded Hope for Application to Colon and Gastrointestinal Cancers. *Gastroenterology* (2017) 153(4):1162–3. doi: 10.1053/j.gastro.2017.08.050
21. Wang S, Li Y, Xing C, Ding C, Zhang H, Chen L, et al. Tumor Microenvironment in Chemoresistance, Metastasis and Immunotherapy of Pancreatic Cancer. *Am J Cancer Res* (2020) 10(7):1937–53.
22. Zahn LM. Effects of the Tumor Microenvironment. *Science* (2017) 355 (6332):1386–8. doi: 10.1126/science.355.6332.1386-l
23. Dudziak D, Kamphorst AO, Heidkamp GF, Buchholz VR, Trumpfheller C, Yamazaki S, et al. Differential Antigen Processing by Dendritic Cell Subsets In Vivo. *Science* (2007) 315(5808):107–11. doi: 10.1126/science.1136080
24. Steinman RM, Kaplan G, Witmer MD, Cohn ZA. Identification of a Novel Cell Type in Peripheral Lymphoid Organs of Mice. V. Purification of Spleen Dendritic Cells, New Surface Markers, and Maintenance In Vitro. *J Exp Med* (1979) 149(1):1–16. doi: 10.1084/jem.149.1.1
25. Steinman RM, Pack M, Inaba K. Dendritic Cells in the T-cell Areas of Lymphoid Organs. *Immunol Rev* (1997) 156:25–37. doi: 10.1111/j.1600-065x.1997.tb00956.x
26. Gabrilovich D. Mechanisms and Functional Significance of Tumour-Induced Dendritic-Cell Defects. *Nat Rev Immunol* (2004) 4(12):941–52. doi: 10.1038/nri1498
27. Satpathy AT, Kc W, Albring JC, Edelson BT, Kretzer NM, Bhattacharya D, et al. Zbtb46 Expression Distinguishes Classical Dendritic Cells and Their Committed Progenitors From Other Immune Lineages. *J Exp Med* (2012) 209 (6):1135–52. doi: 10.1084/jem.20120030
28. Du H, Yang J, Zhang Y. Cytokine-Induced Killer Cell/Dendritic Cell Combined With Cytokine-Induced Killer Cell Immunotherapy for Treating Advanced Gastrointestinal Cancer. *BMC Cancer* (2020) 20(1):357. doi: 10.1186/s12885-020-06860-y
29. Cai L, Zhang C, Wu J, Zhou W, Chen T. Decreased PD-1 Expression on Circulating CD4(+)T Cell and PD-L1 Expression on Myeloid Dendritic Cell Correlate With Clinical Manifestations in Systemic Juvenile Idiopathic Arthritis. *Joint Bone Spine* (2019) 86(1):61–8. doi: 10.1016/j.jbspin.2018.03.003
30. Jeong Y, Kim GB, Ji Y, Kwak GJ, Nam GH, Hong Y, et al. Dendritic Cell Activation by an E. Coli-Derived Monophosphoryl Lipid A Enhances the Efficacy of PD-1 Blockade. *Cancer Lett* (2020) 472:19–28. doi: 10.1016/j.canlet.2019.12.012
31. Lurje I, Hammerich L, Tacke F. Dendritic Cell and T Cell Crosstalk in Liver Fibrogenesis and Hepatocarcinogenesis: Implications for Prevention and Therapy of Liver Cancer. *Int J Mol Sci* (2020) 21(19):7378. doi: 10.3390/ijms21197378
32. Aloysius MM, Takhar A, Robins A, Eremin O. Dendritic Cell Biology, Dysfunction and Immunotherapy in Gastrointestinal Cancers. *Surgeon* (2006) 4(4):195–210. doi: 10.1016/s1479-666x(06)80061-2
33. Zhu S, Yang N, Wu J, Wang X, Wang W, Liu YJ, et al. Tumor Microenvironment-Related Dendritic Cell Deficiency: A Target to Enhance Tumor Immunotherapy. *Pharmacol Res* (2020) 159:104980. doi: 10.1016/j.phrs.2020.104980
34. Lin JH, Huffman AP, Wattenberg MM, Walter DM, Carpenter EL, Feldser DM, et al. Type 1 Conventional Dendritic Cells are Systemically Dysregulated Early in Pancreatic Carcinogenesis. *J Exp Med* (2020) 217(8):e20190673. doi: 10.1084/jem.20190673
35. Li W, Wang W, Liao P, Song K, Zhu Z, Wang K, et al. High Levels of Tumor-Infiltrating Lymphocytes Showed Better Clinical Outcomes in FOLFOX-treated Gastric Cancer Patients. *Pharmacogenomics* (2020) 21(11):751–9. doi: 10.2217/pgs-2019-0102
36. Okadome K, Baba Y, Yagi T, Kiyozumi Y, Ishimoto T, Iwatsuki M, et al. Prognostic Nutritional Index, Tumor-infiltrating Lymphocytes, and Prognosis in Patients With Esophageal Cancer. *Ann Surg* (2020) 271(4):693–700. doi: 10.1097/SLA.0000000000002985
37. Choi E, Chang MS, Byeon SJ, Jin H, Jung KC, Kim H, et al. Prognostic Perspectives of PD-L1 Combined With Tumor-Infiltrating Lymphocytes, Epstein-Barr Virus, and Microsatellite Instability in Gastric Carcinomas. *Diagn Pathol* (2020) 15(1):69. doi: 10.1186/s13000-020-00979-z
38. Jun SY, Park ES, Lee JJ, Chang HK, Jung ES, Oh YH, et al. Prognostic Significance of Stromal and Intraepithelial Tumor-Infiltrating Lymphocytes in Small Intestinal Adenocarcinoma. *Am J Clin Pathol* (2020) 153(1):105–18. doi: 10.1093/ajcp/aqz136
39. Idos GE, Kwok J, Bonthala N, Kysh L, Gruber SB, Qu C. The Prognostic Implications of Tumor Infiltrating Lymphocytes in Colorectal Cancer: A Systematic Review and Meta-Analysis. *Sci Rep* (2020) 10(1):3360. doi: 10.1038/s41598-020-60255-4
40. Xiao B, Peng J, Wang Y, Deng Y, Ou Q, Wu X, et al. Prognostic Value of Tumor Infiltrating Lymphocytes Combined With PD-L1 Expression for Patients With Solitary Colorectal Cancer Liver Metastasis. *Ann Transl Med* (2020) 8(19):1221. doi: 10.21037/atm-20-2762a
41. Fridman WH, Pages F, Sautes-Fridman C, Galon J. The Immune Contexture in Human Tumours: Impact on Clinical Outcome. *Nat Rev Cancer* (2012) 12 (4):298–306. doi: 10.1038/nrc3245
42. Kawahata K, Misaki Y, Yamauchi M, Tsunekawa S, Setoguchi K, Miyazaki J, et al. Generation of CD4(+)CD25(+) Regulatory T Cells From Autoreactive T Cells Simultaneously With Their Negative Selection in the Thymus and From Nonautoreactive T Cells by Endogenous TCR Expression. *J Immunol* (2002) 168(9):4399–405. doi: 10.4049/jimmunol.168.9.4399
43. Raffin C, Vo LT, Bluestone JA. Treg Cell-Based Therapies: Challenges and Perspectives. *Nat Rev Immunol* (2020) 20(3):158–72. doi: 10.1038/s41577-019-0232-6
44. Hira SK, Rej A, Paladhi A, Singh R, Saha J, Mondal I, et al. Galunisertib Drives Treg Fragility and Promotes Dendritic Cell-Mediated Immunity Against Experimental Lymphoma. *iScience* (2020) 23(10):101623. doi: 10.1016/j.isci.2020.101623
45. Grygorowicz MA, Borycka IS, Nowak E, Paszkiewicz-Kozik E, Rymkiewicz G, Blachnio K, et al. Lenalidomide Potentiates CD4(+)CD25(+)Treg-related Suppression of Lymphoma B-cell Proliferation. *Clin Exp Med* (2017) 17 (2):193–207. doi: 10.1007/s10238-016-0411-8
46. Zhu MX, Wan WL, Tian L, Hu K, Wang J, Wang YF, et al. [Prognostic Significance of Treg/Th17 Cells Imbalance in Patients With Diffuse Large B Cell Lymphoma]. *Zhonghua Xue Ye Xue Za Zhi* (2018) 39(6):507–10. doi: 10.3760/cma.j.issn.0253-2727.2018.06.014
47. Marquez-Medina D, Salla-Fortuny J, Salud-Salvia A. Role of Gamma-Delta T-cells in Cancer: Another Opening Door to Immunotherapy. *Clin Transl Oncol* (2012) 14(12):891–5. doi: 10.1007/s12094-012-0935-7
48. Alam SM, Clark JS, Leech V, Whitford P, George WD, Campbell AM. T Cell Receptor Gamma/Delta Expression on Lymphocyte Populations of Breast Cancer Patients. *Immunol Lett* (1992) 31(3):279–83. doi: 10.1016/0165-2478(92)90127-a
49. Raspollini MR, Castiglione F, Rossi Degl'innocenti D, Amunni G, Villanucci A, Garbini F, et al. Tumour-Infiltrating Gamma/Delta T-lymphocytes are Correlated With a Brief Disease-Free Interval in Advanced Ovarian Serous Carcinoma. *Ann Oncol* (2005) 16(4):590–6. doi: 10.1093/annonc/mdi112
50. Bouet-Toussaint F, Cabillic F, Toutirais O, Le Gallo M, Thomas de la Pintiere C, Daniel P, et al. Vgamma9Vdelta2 T Cell-Mediated Recognition of Human Solid Tumors. Potential for Immunotherapy of Hepatocellular and Colorectal

Carcinomas. *Cancer Immunol Immunother* (2008) 57(4):531–9. doi: 10.1007/s00262-007-0391-3

51. Chitadze G, Oberg HH, Wesch D, Kabelitz D. The Ambiguous Role of Gammadelta T Lymphocytes in Antitumor Immunity. *Trends Immunol* (2017) 38(9):668–78. doi: 10.1016/j.it.2017.06.004
52. Fleming C, Morrissey S, Cai Y, Yan J. Gammadelta T Cells: Unexpected Regulators of Cancer Development and Progression. *Trends Cancer* (2017) 3 (8):561–70. doi: 10.1016/j.trecan.2017.06.003
53. Vivier E, Tomasello E, Baratin M, Walzer T, Ugolini S. Functions of Natural Killer Cells. *Nat Immunol* (2008) 9(5):503–10. doi: 10.1038/ni1582
54. Polidoro MA, Mikulak J, Cazzetta V, Lleo A, Mavilio D, Torzilli G, et al. Tumor Microenvironment in Primary Liver Tumors: A Challenging Role of Natural Killer Cells. *World J Gastroenterol* (2020) 26(33):4900–18. doi: 10.3748/wjg.v26.i33.4900
55. Mugitani H, Suzuki M, Naruki Y, Ohtsuka S, Shinbo T. [Natural Killer Cell Activity in Gastrointestinal Cancer Patients–a Decline in Natural Killer Cell Activity in T Cells and the Action of Interferon on its Increase (Author's Transl)]. *Nihon Gan Chiryo Gakkai Shi* (1981) 16(7):1371–6.
56. Sun C, Xu J, Huang Q, Huang M, Wen H, Zhang C, et al. High NKG2A Expression Contributes to NK Cell Exhaustion and Predicts a Poor Prognosis of Patients With Liver Cancer. *Oncoimmunology* (2017) 6(1):e1264562. doi: 10.1080/2162402X.2016.1264562
57. Lee YE, Ju A, Choi HW, Kim JC, Kim EE, Kim TS, et al. Rationally Designed Redirection of Natural Killer Cells Anchoring a Cytotoxic Ligand for Pancreatic Cancer Treatment. *J Control Release* (2020) 326:310–23. doi: 10.1016/j.jconrel.2020.07.016
58. Park DJ, Sung PS, Kim JH, Lee GW, Jang JW, Jung ES, et al. EpCAM-high Liver Cancer Stem Cells Resist Natural Killer Cell-Mediated Cytotoxicity by Upregulating CEACAM1. *J Immunother Cancer* (2020) 8(1):e000301. doi: 10.1136/jitc-2019-000301
59. Mosser DM, Edwards JP. Exploring the Full Spectrum of Macrophage Activation. *Nat Rev Immunol* (2008) 8(12):958–69. doi: 10.1038/nri2448
60. Mantovani A, Sica A, Allavena P, Garlanda C, Locati M. Tumor-Associated Macrophages and the Related Myeloid-Derived Suppressor Cells as a Paradigm of the Diversity of Macrophage Activation. *Hum Immunol* (2009) 70(5):325–30. doi: 10.1016/j.humimm.2009.02.008
61. Eisinger S, Sarhan D, Boura VF, Ibarlucea-Benitez I, Tyystjarvi S, Oliynyk G, et al. Targeting a Scavenger Receptor on Tumor-Associated Macrophages Activates Tumor Cell Killing by Natural Killer Cells. *Proc Natl Acad Sci USA* (2020) 117(50):32005–16. doi: 10.1073/pnas.2015343117
62. Ojalvo LS, Whittaker CA, Condeelis JS, Pollard JW. Gene Expression Analysis of Macrophages That Facilitate Tumor Invasion Supports a Role for Wnt-signaling in Mediating Their Activity in Primary Mammary Tumors. *J Immunol* (2010) 184(2):702–12. doi: 10.4049/jimmunol.0902360
63. D'Errico G, Alonso-Nocelo M, Vallespinos M, Hermann PC, Alcala S, Garcia CP, et al. Tumor-Associated Macrophage-Secreted 14-3-3zeta Signals Via AXL to Promote Pancreatic Cancer Chemoresistance. *Oncogene* (2019) 38 (27):5469–85. doi: 10.1038/s41388-019-0803-9
64. Kurahara H, Shinchi H, Mataki Y, Maemura K, Noma H, Kubo F, et al. Significance of M2-polarized Tumor-Associated Macrophage in Pancreatic Cancer. *J Surg Res* (2011) 167(2):e211–9. doi: 10.1016/j.jss.2009.05.026
65. Zheng Y, Cai Z, Wang S, Zhang X, Qian J, Hong S, et al. Macrophages are an Abundant Component of Myeloma Microenvironment and Protect Myeloma Cells From Chemotherapy Drug-Induced Apoptosis. *Blood* (2009) 114 (17):3625–8. doi: 10.1182/blood-2009-05-220285
66. Gabrilovich DI, Ostrand-Rosenberg S, Bronte V. Coordinated Regulation of Myeloid Cells by Tumours. *Nat Rev Immunol* (2012) 12(4):253–68. doi: 10.1038/nri3175
67. Yang L, DeBusk LM, Fukuda K, Fingleton B, Green-Jarvis B, Shyr Y, et al. Expansion of Myeloid Immune Suppressor Gr+CD11b+ Cells in Tumor-Bearing Host Directly Promotes Tumor Angiogenesis. *Cancer Cell* (2004) 6 (4):409–21. doi: 10.1016/j.ccr.2004.08.031
68. Nagaraj S, Schrum AG, Cho HI, Celis E, Gabrilovich DI. Mechanism of T Cell Tolerance Induced by Myeloid-Derived Suppressor Cells. *J Immunol* (2010) 184(6):3106–16. doi: 10.4049/jimmunol.0902661
69. Rodriguez PC, Quiceno DG, Zabaleta J, Ortiz B, Zea AH, Piazuelo MB, et al. Arginase I Production in the Tumor Microenvironment by Mature Myeloid Cells Inhibits T-cell Receptor Expression and Antigen-Specific T-cell Responses. *Cancer Res* (2004) 64(16):5839–49. doi: 10.1158/0008-5472.CAN-04-0465
70. Srivastava MK, Sinha P, Clements VK, Rodriguez P, Ostrand-Rosenberg S. Myeloid-Derived Suppressor Cells Inhibit T-cell Activation by Depleting Cystine and Cysteine. *Cancer Res* (2010) 70(1):68–77. doi: 10.1158/0008-5472.CAN-09-2587
71. Molon B, Ugel S, Del Pozzo F, Soldani C, Zilio S, Avella D, et al. Chemokine Nitration Prevents Intratumoral Infiltration of Antigen-Specific T Cells. *J Exp Med* (2011) 208(10):1949–62. doi: 10.1084/jem.20101956
72. Pan PY, Ma G, Weber KJ, Ozao-Choy J, Wang G, Yin B, et al. Immune Stimulatory Receptor CD40 is Required for T-cell Suppression and T Regulatory Cell Activation Mediated by Myeloid-Derived Suppressor Cells in Cancer. *Cancer Res* (2010) 70(1):99–108. doi: 10.1158/0008-5472.CAN-09-1882
73. Serafini P, Mgebroff S, Noonan K, Borrello I. Myeloid-Derived Suppressor Cells Promote Cross-Tolerance in B-cell Lymphoma by Expanding Regulatory T Cells. *Cancer Res* (2008) 68(13):5439–49. doi: 10.1158/0008-5472.CAN-07-6621
74. Cao S, Liu J, Chesi M, Bergsagel PL, Ho IC, Donnelly RP, et al. Differential Regulation of IL-12 and IL-10 Gene Expression in Macrophages by the Basic Leucine Zipper Transcription Factor c-Maf Fibrosarcoma. *J Immunol* (2002) 169(10):5715–25. doi: 10.4049/jimmunol.169.10.5715
75. Murai M, Turovskaya O, Kim G, Madan R, Karp CL, Cheroutre H, et al. Interleukin 10 Acts on Regulatory T Cells to Maintain Expression of the Transcription Factor Foxp3 and Suppressive Function in Mice With Colitis. *Nat Immunol* (2009) 10(11):1178–84. doi: 10.1038/ni.1791
76. DeNardo DG, Barreto JB, Andreu P, Vasquez L, Tawfik D, Kolhatkar N, et al. Cd4(+) T Cells Regulate Pulmonary Metastasis of Mammary Carcinomas by Enhancing Protumor Properties of Macrophages. *Cancer Cell* (2009) 16 (2):91–102. doi: 10.1016/j.ccr.2009.06.018
77. Elkabets M, Ribeiro VS, Dinarello CA, Ostrand-Rosenberg S, Di Santo JP, Apte RN, et al. Il-1beta Regulates a Novel Myeloid-Derived Suppressor Cell Subset That Impairs NK Cell Development and Function. *Eur J Immunol* (2010) 40(12):3347–57. doi: 10.1002/eji.201041037
78. Langowski JL, Zhang X, Wu L, Mattson JD, Chen T, Smith K, et al. Il-23 Promotes Tumour Incidence and Growth. *Nature* (2006) 442(7101):461–5. doi: 10.1038/nature04808
79. Fabian KP, Padget MR, Donahue RN, Solocinski K, Robbins Y, Allen CT, et al. Pd-L1 Targeting High-Affinity NK (t-haNK) Cells Induce Direct Antitumor Effects and Target Suppressive MDSC Populations. *J Immunother Cancer* (2020) 8(1):e000450. doi: 10.1136/jitc-2019-000450
80. Greene S, Robbins Y, Mydlarz WK, Huynh AP, Schmitt NC, Friedman J, et al. Inhibition of MDSC Trafficking With SX-682, a CXCR1/2 Inhibitor, Enhances Nk-Cell Immunotherapy in Head and Neck Cancer Models. *Clin Cancer Res* (2020) 26(6):1420–31. doi: 10.1158/1078-0432.CCR-19-2625
81. Langrish CL, Chen Y, Blumenschein WM, Mattson J, Basham B, Sedgwick JD, et al. Il-23 Drives a Pathogenic T Cell Population That Induces Autoimmune Inflammation. *J Exp Med* (2005) 201(2):233–40. doi: 10.1084/jem.20041257
82. Poschke I, Mao Y, Adamson L, Salazar-Onfray F, Masucci G, Kiessling R. Myeloid-Derived Suppressor Cells Impair the Quality of Dendritic Cell Vaccines. *Cancer Immunol Immunother* (2012) 61(6):827–38. doi: 10.1007/s00262-011-1143-y
83. Zhang J, Li Z, Hu X, Su Q, He C, Liu J, et al. Knockout of P2Y12 Aggravates Experimental Autoimmune Encephalomyelitis in Mice Via Increasing of IL-23 Production and Th17 Cell Differentiation by Dendritic Cells. *Brain Behav Immun* (2017) 62:245–55. doi: 10.1016/j.bbi.2016.12.001
84. Li B, Wang JH. Fibroblasts and Myofibroblasts in Wound Healing: Force Generation and Measurement. *J Tissue Viability* (2011) 20(4):108–20. doi: 10.1016/j.jtv.2009.11.004
85. Rockey DC, Weymouth N, Shi Z. Smooth Muscle Alpha Actin (Acta2) and Myofibroblast Function During Hepatic Wound Healing. *PloS One* (2013) 8 (10):e77166. doi: 10.1371/journal.pone.0077166
86. Sugimoto H, Mundel TM, Kieran MW, Kalluri R. Identification of Fibroblast Heterogeneity in the Tumor Microenvironment. *Cancer Biol Ther* (2006) 5 (12):1640–6. doi: 10.4161/cbt.5.12.3354
87. Dong R, Guo J, Zhang Z, Zhou Y, Hua Y. Polyphyllin I Inhibits Gastric Cancer Cell Proliferation by Downregulating the Expression of Fibroblast Activation Protein Alpha (FAP) and Hepatocyte Growth Factor (HGF) in Cancer-

Associated Fibroblasts. *Biochem Biophys Res Commun* (2018) 497(4):1129–34. doi: 10.1016/j.bbrc.2018.02.193

88. Fukumura D, Xavier R, Sugiura T, Chen Y, Park EC, Lu N, et al. Tumor Induction of VEGF Promoter Activity in Stromal Cells. *Cell* (1998) 94(6):715–25. doi: 10.1016/s0092-8674(00)81731-6
89. Monteran L, Erez N. The Dark Side of Fibroblasts: Cancer-Associated Fibroblasts as Mediators of Immunosuppression in the Tumor Microenvironment. *Front Immunol* (2019) 10:1835. doi: 10.3389/fimmu.2019.01835
90. Fearon DT. The Carcinoma-Associated Fibroblast Expressing Fibroblast Activation Protein and Escape From Immune Surveillance. *Cancer Immunol Res* (2014) 2(3):187–93. doi: 10.1158/2326-6066.Cir-14-0002
91. Feig C, Jones JO, Kraman M, Wells RJ, Deonarine A, Chan DS, et al. Targeting CXCL12 From FAP-expressing Carcinoma-Associated Fibroblasts Synergizes With anti-PD-L1 Immunotherapy in Pancreatic Cancer. *Proc Natl Acad Sci USA* (2013) 110(50):20212–7. doi: 10.1073/pnas.1320318110
92. Jiang H, Hegde S, Knolhoff BL, Zhu Y, Herndon JM, Meyer MA, et al. Targeting Focal Adhesion Kinase Renders Pancreatic Cancers Responsive to Checkpoint Immunotherapy. *Nat Med* (2016) 22(8):851–60. doi: 10.1038/nm.4123
93. Erez N, Truitt M, Olson P, Arron ST, Hanahan D. Cancer-Associated Fibroblasts are Activated in Incipient Neoplasia to Orchestrate Tumor-Promoting Inflammation in an NF-kappaB-Dependent Manner. *Cancer Cell* (2010) 17(2):135–47. doi: 10.1016/j.ccr.2009.12.041
94. Johansson AC, Ansell A, Jerhammar F, Lindh MB, Grenman R, Munck-Wikland E, et al. Cancer-Associated Fibroblasts Induce Matrix Metalloproteinase-Mediated Cetuximab Resistance in Head and Neck Squamous Cell Carcinoma Cells. *Mol Cancer Res* (2012) 10(9):1158–68. doi: 10.1158/1541-7786.MCR-12-0030
95. Yegodayev KM, Novoplansky O, Golden A, Prasad M, Levin L, Jagadeeshan S, et al. Tgf-Beta-Activated Cancer-Associated Fibroblasts Limit Cetuximab Efficacy in Preclinical Models of Head and Neck Cancer. *Cancers (Basel)* (2020) 12(2):339. doi: 10.3390/cancers12020339
96. Katuri V, Tang Y, Marshall B, Rashid A, Jogunoori W, Volpe EA, et al. Inactivation of ELF/TGF-beta Signaling in Human Gastrointestinal Cancer. *Oncogene* (2005) 24(54):8012–24. doi: 10.1038/sj.onc.1208946
97. Principe DR, DeCant B, Mascarinas E, Wayne EA, Diaz AM, Akagi N, et al. Tgfbeta Signaling in the Pancreatic Tumor Microenvironment Promotes Fibrosis and Immune Evasion to Facilitate Tumorigenesis. *Cancer Res* (2016) 76(9):2525–39. doi: 10.1158/0008-5472.CAN-15-1293
98. Lebrun JJ. The Dual Role of TGFbeta in Human Cancer: From Tumor Suppression to Cancer Metastasis. *ISRN Mol Biol* (2012) 2012:381428. doi: 10.5402/2012/381428
99. Massague J. Tgfbeta in Cancer. *Cell* (2008) 134(2):215–30. doi: 10.1016/j.cell.2008.07.001
100. Massague J. Tgfbeta Signalling in Context. *Nat Rev Mol Cell Biol* (2012) 13(10):616–30. doi: 10.1038/nrm3434
101. Bakin AV, Rinehart C, Tomlinson AK, Arteaga CL. p38 Mitogen-Activated Protein Kinase is Required for TGFbeta-mediated Fibroblastic Transdifferentiation and Cell Migration. *J Cell Sci* (2002) 115(Pt 15):3193–206. doi: 10.1242/jcs.115.15.3193
102. Rahimi RA, Leof EB. Tgfbeta Versatility: PI3K as a Critical Mediator of Distinct Cell Type and Context Specific Responses. *Cell Cycle* (2009) 8(12):1813–4. doi: 10.4161/cc.8.12.8828
103. Feng XH, Liang YY, Liang M, Zhai W, Lin X. Direct Interaction of c-Myc With Smad2 and Smad3 to Inhibit TGF-Beta-Mediated Induction of the CDK Inhibitor P15(Ink4B). *Mol Cell* (2016) 63(6):1089. doi: 10.1016/j.molcel.2016.08.027
104. Sanchez-Capelo A. Dual Role for TGF-beta1 in Apoptosis. *Cytokine Growth Factor Rev* (2005) 16(1):15–34. doi: 10.1016/j.cytogfr.2004.11.002
105. Cassar L, Li H, Jiang FX, Liu JP. TGF-Beta Induces Telomerase-Dependent Pancreatic Tumor Cell Cycle Arrest. *Mol Cell Endocrinol* (2010) 320(1-2):97–105. doi: 10.1016/j.mce.2010.02.002
106. Tauriello DVF, Palomo-Ponce S, Stork D, Berenguer-Llergo A, Badia-Ramentol J, Iglesias M, et al. Tgfbeta Drives Immune Evasion in Genetically Reconstituted Colon Cancer Metastasis. *Nature* (2018) 554(7693):538–43. doi: 10.1038/nature25492
107. Mariathasan S, Turley SJ, Nickles D, Castiglioni A, Yuen K, Wang Y, et al. Tgfbeta Attenuates Tumour Response to PD-L1 Blockade by Contributing to Exclusion of T Cells. *Nature* (2018) 554(7693):544–8. doi: 10.1038/nature25501
108. Huang CY, Chung CL, Hu TH, Chen JJ, Liu PF, Chen CL. Recent Progress in TGF-beta Inhibitors for Cancer Therapy. *BioMed Pharmacother* (2021) 134:111046. doi: 10.1016/j.biopha.2020.111046
109. Lind H, Gameiro SR, Jochems C, Donahue RN, Strauss J, Gulley JM, et al. Dual Targeting of TGF-beta and PD-L1 Via a Bifunctional anti-PD-L1/TGF-betaRII Agent: Status of Preclinical and Clinical Advances. *J Immunother Cancer* (2020) 8(1):e000433. doi: 10.1136/jitc-2019-000433
110. Coussens LM, Werb Z. Inflammation and Cancer. *Nature* (2002) 420(6917):860–7. doi: 10.1038/nature01322
111. Dvorakova K, Payne CM, Ramsey L, Holubec H, Sampliner R, Dominguez J, et al. Increased Expression and Secretion of Interleukin-6 in Patients With Barrett's Esophagus. *Clin Cancer Res* (2004) 10(6):2020–8. doi: 10.1158/1078-0432.ccr-0437-03
112. Wang T, Niu G, Kortylewski M, Burdelya L, Shain K, Zhang S, et al. Regulation of the Innate and Adaptive Immune Responses by Stat-3 Signaling in Tumor Cells. *Nat Med* (2004) 10(1):48–54. doi: 10.1038/nm976
113. Huang FL, Yu SJ. Esophageal Cancer: Risk Factors, Genetic Association, and Treatment. *Asian J Surg* (2018) 41(3):210–5. doi: 10.1016/j.asjsur.2016.10.005
114. Tanaka Y, Yoshida K, Suetsugu T, Imai T, Matsuhashi N, Yamaguchi K. Recent Advancements in Esophageal Cancer Treatment in Japan. *Ann Gastroenterol Surg* (2018) 2(4):253–65. doi: 10.1002/ags3.12174
115. Karakasheva TA, Waldron TJ, Eruslanov E, Kim SB, Lee JS, O'Brien S, et al. Cd38-Expressing Myeloid-Derived Suppressor Cells Promote Tumor Growth in a Murine Model of Esophageal Cancer. *Cancer Res* (2015) 75(19):4074–85. doi: 10.1158/0008-5472.CAN-14-3639
116. Pal S, Nandi M, Dey D, Chakraborty BC, Shil A, Ghosh S, et al. Myeloid-Derived Suppressor Cells Induce Regulatory T Cells in Chronically HBV Infected Patients With High Levels of Hepatitis B Surface Antigen and Persist After Antiviral Therapy. *Aliment Pharmacol Ther* (2019) 49(10):1346–59. doi: 10.1111/apt.15226
117. Sohda M, Kuwano H. Current Status and Future Prospects for Esophageal Cancer Treatment. *Ann Thorac Cardiovasc Surg* (2017) 23(1):1–11. doi: 10.5761/atcs.ra.16-00162
118. Miyashita T, Tajima H, Shah FA, Oshima M, Makino I, Nakagawara H, et al. Impact of Inflammation-Metaplasia-Adenocarcinoma Sequence and Inflammatory Microenvironment in Esophageal Carcinogenesis Using Surgical Rat Models. *Ann Surg Oncol* (2014) 21(6):2012–9. doi: 10.1245/s10434-014-3537-5
119. Wang J, Zhang G, Wang J, Wang L, Huang X, Cheng Y. The Role of Cancer-Associated Fibroblasts in Esophageal Cancer. *J Transl Med* (2016) 14:30. doi: 10.1186/s12967-016-0788-x
120. Tomas-Bort E, Kieler M, Sharma S, Candido JB, Loessner D. 3D Approaches to Model the Tumor Microenvironment of Pancreatic Cancer. *Theranostics* (2020) 10(11):5074–89. doi: 10.7150/thno.42441
121. Polk DB, Peek RMJr. Helicobacter Pylori: Gastric Cancer and Beyond. *Nat Rev Cancer* (2010) 10(6):403–14. doi: 10.1038/nrc2857
122. Rasch S, Algul H. A Clinical Perspective on the Role of Chronic Inflammation in Gastrointestinal Cancer. *Clin Exp Gastroenterol* (2014) 7:261–72. doi: 10.2147/CEG.S43457
123. Lee HJ, Park JM, Han YM, Gil HK, Kim J, Chang JY, et al. The Role of Chronic Inflammation in the Development of Gastrointestinal Cancers: Reviewing Cancer Prevention With Natural Anti-Inflammatory Intervention. *Expert Rev Gastroenterol Hepatol* (2016) 10(1):129–39. doi: 10.1586/17474124.2016.1103179
124. Carcas LP. Gastric Cancer Review. *J Carcinog* (2014) 13:14. doi: 10.4103/1477-3163.146506
125. Gyori D, Chessa T, Hawkins PT, Stephens LR. Class (I) Phosphoinositide 3-Kinases in the Tumor Microenvironment. *Cancers (Basel)* (2017) 9(3):24. doi: 10.3390/cancers9030024
126. Zhou H, Liu H, Jiang M, Zhang S, Chen J, Fan X. Targeting MicroRNA-21 Suppresses Gastric Cancer Cell Proliferation and Migration Via PTEN/Akt Signaling Axis. *Cell Transplant* (2019) 28(3):306–17. doi: 10.1177/0963689719825573

127. Wang Z, Ye Y, Liu D, Yang X, Wang F. Hypermethylation of Multiple Wnt Antagonist Genes in Gastric Neoplasia: Is H Pylori Infection Blasting Fuse? *Med (Baltimore)* (2018) 97(52):e13734. doi: 10.1097/MD.0000000000013734
128. Murata-Kamiya N, Kurashima Y, Teishikata Y, Yamahashi Y, Saito Y, Higashi H, et al. Helicobacter Pylori CagA Interacts With E-cadherin and Deregulates the Beta-Catenin Signal That Promotes Intestinal Transdifferentiation in Gastric Epithelial Cells. *Oncogene* (2007) 26 (32):4617–26. doi: 10.1038/sj.onc.1210251
129. Fujii Y, Yoshihashi K, Suzuki H, Tsutsumi S, Mutoh H, Maeda S, et al. CDX1 Confers Intestinal Phenotype on Gastric Epithelial Cells Via Induction of Stemness-Associated Reprogramming Factors SALL4 and KLF5. *Proc Natl Acad Sci USA* (2012) 109(50):20584–9. doi: 10.1073/pnas.1208651109
130. Zhang L, Xu Z, Xu X, Zhang B, Wu H, Wang M, et al. SALL4, a Novel Marker for Human Gastric Carcinogenesis and Metastasis. *Oncogene* (2014) 33(48):5491–500. doi: 10.1038/onc.2013.495
131. Choi YJ, Kim N, Chang H, Lee HS, Park SM, Park JH, et al. Helicobacter Pylori-Induced Epithelial-Mesenchymal Transition, a Potential Role of Gastric Cancer Initiation and an Emergence of Stem Cells. *Carcinogenesis* (2015) 36(5):553–63. doi: 10.1093/carcin/bgv022
132. Terashima M, Kitada K, Ochiai A, Ichikawa W, Kurahashi I, Sakuramoto S, et al. Impact of Expression of Human Epidermal Growth Factor Receptors EGFR and ERBB2 on Survival in Stage II/III Gastric Cancer. *Clin Cancer Res* (2012) 18(21):5992–6000. doi: 10.1158/1078-0432.CCR-12-1318
133. Xu W, Yang Z, Lu N. Molecular Targeted Therapy for the Treatment of Gastric Cancer. *J Exp Clin Cancer Res* (2016) 35:1. doi: 10.1186/s13046-015-0276-9
134. Zhang Z, Li Z, Li Y, Zang A. MicroRNA and Signaling Pathways in Gastric Cancer. *Cancer Gene Ther* (2014) 21(8):305–16. doi: 10.1038/cgt.2014.37
135. Chen X, Gao H, Deng Y, Jin Q, Ji J, Ding D. Supramolecular Aggregation-Induced Emission Nanodots With Programmed Tumor Microenvironment Responsiveness for Image-Guided Orthotopic Pancreatic Cancer Therapy. *ACS Nano* (2020) 14(4):5121–34. doi: 10.1021/acsnano.0c02197
136. Ma L, Hernandez MO, Zhao Y, Mehta M, Tran B, Kelly M, et al. Tumor Cell Biodiversity Drives Microenvironmental Reprogramming in Liver Cancer. *Cancer Cell* (2019) 36(4):418–30 e6. doi: 10.1016/j.ccell.2019.08.007
137. Shen YC, Hsu C, Cheng AL. Molecular Targeted Therapy for Advanced Hepatocellular Carcinoma: Current Status and Future Perspectives. *J Gastroenterol* (2010) 45(8):794–807. doi: 10.1007/s00535-010-0270-0
138. Yoo YG, Oh SH, Park ES, Cho H, Lee N, Park H, et al. Hepatitis B Virus X Protein Enhances Transcriptional Activity of Hypoxia-Inducible factor-1alpha Through Activation of Mitogen-Activated Protein Kinase Pathway. *J Biol Chem* (2003) 278(40):39076–84. doi: 10.1074/jbc.M305101200
139. Thomas H. Liver Cancer: Lenvatinib non-Inferior to Sorafenib for Hepatocellular Carcinoma. *Nat Rev Gastroenterol Hepatol* (2018) 15 (4):190. doi: 10.1038/nrgastro.2018.20
140. Oh SH, Swiderska-Syn M, Jewell ML, Premont RT, Diehl AM. Liver Regeneration Requires Yap1-TGFbeta-dependent Epithelial-Mesenchymal Transition in Hepatocytes. *J Hepatol* (2018) 69(2):359–67. doi: 10.1016/j.jhep.2018.05.008
141. Zhou SJ, Liu FY, Jiang YH, Liang HF. Reply to 'Comment on 'MicroRNA-199b-5p Attenuates TGF-beta1-induced Epithelial-Mesenchymal Transition in Hepatocellular Carcinoma''. *Br J Cancer* (2018) 118(7):1030. doi: 10.1038/s41416-018-0031-z
142. Bi JG, Zheng JF, Li Q, Bao SY, Yu XF, Xu P, et al. MicroRNA-181a-5p Suppresses Cell Proliferation by Targeting Egr1 and Inhibiting Egr1/TGF-beta/Smad Pathway in Hepatocellular Carcinoma. *Int J Biochem Cell Biol* (2019) 106:107–16. doi: 10.1016/j.biocel.2018.11.011
143. Zhou Q, Lui VW, Yeo W. Targeting the PI3K/Akt/mTOR Pathway in Hepatocellular Carcinoma. *Future Oncol* (2011) 7(10):1149–67. doi: 10.2217/fon.11.95
144. Hu TH, Huang CC, Lin PR, Chang HW, Ger LP, Lin YW, et al. Expression and Prognostic Role of Tumor Suppressor Gene PTEN/MMAC1/TEP1 in Hepatocellular Carcinoma. *Cancer* (2003) 97(8):1929–40. doi: 10.1002/cncr.11266
145. Song XZ, Ren XN, Xu XJ, Ruan XX, Wang YL, Yao TT. Lncrna RHPN1-AS1 Promotes Cell Proliferation, Migration and Invasion Through Targeting miR-7-5p and Activating PI3K/AKT/Mtor Pathway in Hepatocellular Carcinoma. *Technol Cancer Res Treat* (2020) 19:1533033820957023. doi: 10.1177/1533033820957023
146. Zhu AX, Abrams TA, Miksad R, Blaszkowsky LS, Meyerhardt JA, Zheng H, et al. Phase 1/2 Study of Everolimus in Advanced Hepatocellular Carcinoma. *Cancer* (2011) 117(22):5094–102. doi: 10.1002/cncr.26165
147. Kirstein MM, Boukouris AE, Pothiraju D, Buitrago-Molina LE, Marhenke S, Schutt J, et al. Activity of the mTOR Inhibitor RAD001, the Dual mTOR and PI3-kinase Inhibitor BEZ235 and the PI3-kinase Inhibitor BKM120 in Hepatocellular Carcinoma. *Liver Int* (2013) 33(5):780–93. doi: 10.1111/liv.12126
148. Wong CM, Fan ST, Ng IO. beta-Catenin Mutation and Overexpression in Hepatocellular Carcinoma: Clinicopathologic and Prognostic Significance. *Cancer* (2001) 92(1):136–45. doi: 10.1002/1097-0142(20010701)92:1<136::aid-cncr1301>3.0.co;2-r
149. Giles RH, van Es JH, Clevers H. Caught Up in a Wnt Storm: Wnt Signaling in Cancer. *Biochim Biophys Acta* (2003) 1653(1):1–24. doi: 10.1016/s0304-419x(03)00005-2
150. Hoshida Y, Nijman SM, Kobayashi M, Chan JA, Brunet JP, Chiang DY, et al. Integrative Transcriptome Analysis Reveals Common Molecular Subclasses of Human Hepatocellular Carcinoma. *Cancer Res* (2009) 69(18):7385–92. doi: 10.1158/0008-5472.CAN-09-1089
151. Tan J, Tong BD, Wu YJ, Xiong W. MicroRNA-29 Mediates TGFbeta1-induced Extracellular Matrix Synthesis by Targeting Wnt/Beta-Catenin Pathway in Human Orbital Fibroblasts. *Int J Clin Exp Pathol* (2014) 7 (11):7571–7.
152. Zhang H, Ye J, Weng X, Liu F, He L, Zhou D, et al. Comparative Transcriptome Analysis Reveals That the Extracellular Matrix Receptor Interaction Contributes to the Venous Metastases of Hepatocellular Carcinoma. *Cancer Genet* (2015) 208(10):482–91. doi: 10.1016/j.cancergen.2015.06.002
153. Carloni V, Luong TV, Rombouts K. Hepatic Stellate Cells and Extracellular Matrix in Hepatocellular Carcinoma: More Complicated Than Ever. *Liver Int* (2014) 34(6):834–43. doi: 10.1111/liv.12465
154. Siegel RL, Miller KD, Jemal A. Cancer Statistics, 2020. *CA Cancer J Clin* (2020) 70(1):7–30. doi: 10.3322/caac.21590
155. Adamska A, Domenichini A, Falasca M. Pancreatic Ductal Adenocarcinoma: Current and Evolving Therapies. *Int J Mol Sci* (2017) 18(7):1338. doi: 10.3390/ijms18071338
156. Paniccia A, Hosokawa P, Henderson W, Schulick RD, Edil BH, McCarter MD, et al. Characteristics of 10-Year Survivors of Pancreatic Ductal Adenocarcinoma. *JAMA Surg* (2015) 150(8):701–10. doi: 10.1001/jamasurg.2015.0668
157. Nakayama H, Ohuchida K, Yoshida M, Miyazaki T, Takesue S, Abe T, et al. Degree of Desmoplasia in Metastatic Lymph Node Lesions is Associated With Lesion Size and Poor Prognosis in Pancreatic Cancer Patients. *Oncol Lett* (2017) 14(3):3141–7. doi: 10.3892/ol.2017.6549
158. Iglesias M, Frontelo P, Gamallo C, Quintanilla M. Blockade of Smad4 in Transformed Keratinocytes Containing a Ras Oncogene Leads to Hyperactivation of the Ras-dependent Erk Signalling Pathway Associated With Progression to Undifferentiated Carcinomas. *Oncogene* (2000) 19 (36):4134–45. doi: 10.1038/sj.onc.1203764
159. Tan Z, Xu J, Zhang B, Shi S, Yu X, Liang C. Hypoxia: A Barricade to Conquer the Pancreatic Cancer. *Cell Mol Life Sci* (2020) 77(16):3077–83. doi: 10.1007/s00018-019-03444-3
160. Samkharadze T, Erkan M, Reiser-Erkan C, Demir IE, Kong B, Ceyhan GO, et al. Pigment Epithelium-Derived Factor Associates With Neuropathy and Fibrosis in Pancreatic Cancer. *Am J Gastroenterol* (2011) 106(5):968–80. doi: 10.1038/ajg.2010.479
161. Kisker O, Onizuka S, Banyard J, Komiyama T, Becker CM, Achilles EG, et al. Generation of Multiple Angiogenesis Inhibitors by Human Pancreatic Cancer. *Cancer Res* (2001) 61(19):7298–304.
162. Xue Y, Beyer G, Mayerle J. Fapalpha in Pancreatic Stellate Cells Upregulated by TGFbeta1: A Novel Insight Into Pancreatic Cancer Progress. *Ann Transl Med* (2020) 8(15):910. doi: 10.21037/atm-20-2559
163. Pothula SP, Pirola RC, Wilson JS, Apte MV. Pancreatic Stellate Cells: Aiding and Abetting Pancreatic Cancer Progression. *Pancreatology* (2020) 20 (3):409–18. doi: 10.1016/j.pan.2020.01.003

164. Mace TA, Ameen Z, Collins A, Wojcik S, Mair M, Young GS, et al. Pancreatic Cancer-Associated Stellate Cells Promote Differentiation of Myeloid-Derived Suppressor Cells in a STAT3-Dependent Manner. *Cancer Res* (2013) 73(10):3007–18. doi: 10.1158/0008-5472.CAN-12-4601
165. Tang D, Yuan Z, Xue X, Lu Z, Zhang Y, Wang H, et al. High Expression of Galectin-1 in Pancreatic Stellate Cells Plays a Role in the Development and Maintenance of an Immunosuppressive Microenvironment in Pancreatic Cancer. *Int J Cancer* (2012) 130(10):2337–48. doi: 10.1002/ijc.26290
166. Zhang Y, Ware MB, Zaidi MY, Ruggieri AN, Olson BM, Komar H, et al. Heat Shock Protein-90 Inhibition Alters Activation of Pancreatic Stellate Cells and Enhances the Efficacy of PD-1 Blockade in Pancreatic Cancer. *Mol Cancer Ther* (2021) 20(1):150–60. doi: 10.1158/1535-7163.MCT-19-0911
167. Masamune A, Kikuta K, Watanabe T, Satoh K, Hirota M, Shimosegawa T. Hypoxia Stimulates Pancreatic Stellate Cells to Induce Fibrosis and Angiogenesis in Pancreatic Cancer. *Am J Physiol Gastrointest Liver Physiol* (2008) 295(4):G709–17. doi: 10.1152/ajpgi.90356.2008
168. Szablowska-Gadomska I, Zayat V, Buzanska L. Influence of Low Oxygen Tensions on Expression of Pluripotency Genes in Stem Cells. *Acta Neurobiol Exp (Wars)* (2011) 71(1):86–93.
169. Hamada S, Masamune A, Takikawa T, Suzuki N, Kikuta K, Hirota M, et al. Pancreatic Stellate Cells Enhance Stem Cell-Like Phenotypes in Pancreatic Cancer Cells. *Biochem Biophys Res Commun* (2012) 421(2):349–54. doi: 10.1016/j.bbrc.2012.04.014
170. Cave DD, Di Guida M, Costa V, Sevillano M, Ferrante L, Heeschen C, et al. TGF-Beta1 Secreted by Pancreatic Stellate Cells Promotes Stemness and Tumourigenicity in Pancreatic Cancer Cells Through L1CAM Downregulation. *Oncogene* (2020) 39(21):4271–85. doi: 10.1038/s41388-020-1289-1
171. Hermann PC, Huber SL, Herrler T, Aicher A, Ellwart JW, Guba M, et al. Distinct Populations of Cancer Stem Cells Determine Tumor Growth and Metastatic Activity in Human Pancreatic Cancer. *Cell Stem Cell* (2007) 1 (3):313–23. doi: 10.1016/j.stem.2007.06.002
172. Quint K, Tonigold M, Di Fazio P, Montalbano R, Lingelbach S, Ruckert F, et al. Pancreatic Cancer Cells Surviving Gemcitabine Treatment Express Markers of Stem Cell Differentiation and Epithelial-Mesenchymal Transition. *Int J Oncol* (2012) 41(6):2093–102. doi: 10.3892/ijo.2012.1648
173. Polireddy K, Chen Q. Cancer of the Pancreas: Molecular Pathways and Current Advancement in Treatment. *J Cancer* (2016) 7(11):1497–514. doi: 10.7150/jca.14922
174. Lonardo E, Hermann PC, Mueller MT, Huber S, Balic A, Miranda-Lorenzo I, et al. Nodal/Activin Signaling Drives Self-Renewal and Tumorigenicity of Pancreatic Cancer Stem Cells and Provides a Target for Combined Drug Therapy. *Cell Stem Cell* (2011) 9(5):433–46. doi: 10.1016/j.stem.2011.10.001
175. Mani SA, Guo W, Liao MJ, Eaton EN, Ayyanan A, Zhou AY, et al. The Epithelial-Mesenchymal Transition Generates Cells With Properties of Stem Cells. *Cell* (2008) 133(4):704–15. doi: 10.1016/j.cell.2008.03.027
176. Lu Y, Lu J, Li X, Zhu H, Fan X, Zhu S, et al. MiR-200a Inhibits Epithelial-Mesenchymal Transition of Pancreatic Cancer Stem Cell. *BMC Cancer* (2014) 14:85. doi: 10.1186/1471-2407-14-85
177. Thompson EW, Newgreen DF, Tarin D. Carcinoma Invasion and Metastasis: A Role for Epithelial-Mesenchymal Transition? *Cancer Res* (2005) 65 (14):5991–5. doi: 10.1158/0008-5472.CAN-05-0616
178. Thiery JP, Sleeman JP. Complex Networks Orchestrate Epithelial-Mesenchymal Transitions. *Nat Rev Mol Cell Biol* (2006) 7(2):131–42. doi: 10.1038/nrm1835
179. Yang MH, Wu MZ, Chiou SH, Chen PM, Chang SY, Liu CJ, et al. Direct Regulation of TWIST by HIF-1alpha Promotes Metastasis. *Nat Cell Biol* (2008) 10(3):295–305. doi: 10.1038/ncb1691
180. Gort EH, van Haaften G, Verlaan I, Groot AJ, Plasterk RH, Shvarts A, et al. The TWIST1 Oncogene is a Direct Target of Hypoxia-Inducible Factor-2alpha. *Oncogene* (2008) 27(11):1501–10. doi: 10.1038/sj.onc.1210795
181. Evans AJ, Russell RC, Roche O, Burry TN, Fish JE, Chow VW, et al. VHL Promotes E2 Box-Dependent E-cadherin Transcription by HIF-mediated Regulation of SIP1 and Snail. *Mol Cell Biol* (2007) 27(1):157–69. doi: 10.1128/MCB.00892-06
182. Joseph JV, Conroy S, Tomar T, Eggens-Meijer E, Bhat K, Copray S, et al. TGF-Beta is an Inducer of ZEB1-dependent Mesenchymal Transdifferentiation in Glioblastoma That is Associated With Tumor Invasion. *Cell Death Dis* (2014) 5:e1443. doi: 10.1038/cddis.2014.395
183. Rhim AD, Mirek ET, Aiello NM, Maitra A, Bailey JM, McAllister F, et al. EMT and Dissemination Precede Pancreatic Tumor Formation. *Cell* (2012) 148(1-2):349–61. doi: 10.1016/j.cell.2011.11.025
184. Li Y, Kong D, Ahmad A, Bao B, Sarkar FH. Pancreatic Cancer Stem Cells: Emerging Target for Designing Novel Therapy. *Cancer Lett* (2013) 338 (1):94–100. doi: 10.1016/j.canlet.2012.03.018
185. Cheung KS, Chen L, Chan EW, Seto WK, Wong ICK, Leung WK. Nonsteroidal Anti-Inflammatory Drugs But Not Aspirin are Associated With a Lower Risk of Post-Colonoscopy Colorectal Cancer. *Aliment Pharmacol Ther* (2020) 51(9):899–908. doi: 10.1111/apt.15693
186. DuBois RN, Giardiello FM, Smalley WE. Nonsteroidal Anti-Inflammatory Drugs, Eicosanoids, and Colorectal Cancer Prevention. *Gastroenterol Clin North Am* (1996) 25(4):773–91. doi: 10.1016/s0889-8553(05)70274-0
187. Liu Y, Borchert GL, Surazynski A, Phang JM. Proline Oxidase, a p53-induced Gene, Targets COX-2/PGE2 Signaling to Induce Apoptosis and Inhibit Tumor Growth in Colorectal Cancers. *Oncogene* (2008) 27(53):6729–37. doi: 10.1038/onc.2008.322
188. Zhu Y, Shi C, Zeng L, Liu G, Jiang W, Zhang X, et al. High COX-2 Expression in Cancer-Associated Fibiroblasts Contributes to Poor Survival and Promotes Migration and Invasiveness in Nasopharyngeal Carcinoma. *Mol Carcinog* (2020) 59(3):265–80. doi: 10.1002/mc.23150
189. Kabir TD, Leigh RJ, Tasena H, Mellone M, Coletta RD, Parkinson EK, et al. A miR-335/COX-2/PTEN Axis Regulates the Secretory Phenotype of Senescent Cancer-Associated Fibroblasts. *Aging (Albany NY)* (2016) 8 (8):1608–35. doi: 10.18632/aging.100987
190. Li T, Yang Y, Hua X, Wang G, Liu W, Jia C, et al. Hepatocellular Carcinoma-Associated Fibroblasts Trigger NK Cell Dysfunction Via PGE2 and IDO. *Cancer Lett* (2012) 318(2):154–61. doi: 10.1016/j.canlet.2011.12.020
191. Erdogan B, Webb DJ. Cancer-Associated Fibroblasts Modulate Growth Factor Signaling and Extracellular Matrix Remodeling to Regulate Tumor Metastasis. *Biochem Soc Trans* (2017) 45(1):229–36. doi: 10.1042/BST20160387
192. Herrera M, Herrera A, Dominguez G, Silva J, Garcia V, Garcia JM, et al. Cancer-Associated Fibroblast and M2 Macrophage Markers Together Predict Outcome in Colorectal Cancer Patients. *Cancer Sci* (2013) 104 (4):437–44. doi: 10.1111/cas.12096
193. Katoh H, Watanabe M. Myeloid-Derived Suppressor Cells and Therapeutic Strategies in Cancer. *Mediators Inflamm* (2015) 2015:159269. doi: 10.1155/2015/159269
194. Pinchuk IV, Beswick EJ, Saada JI, Boya G, Schmitt D, Raju GS, et al. Human Colonic Myofibroblasts Promote Expansion of CD4+ Cd25high Foxp3+ Regulatory T Cells. *Gastroenterology* (2011) 140(7):2019–30. doi: 10.1053/j.gastro.2011.02.059
195. Inoue C, Miki Y, Saito R, Hata S, Abe J, Sato I, et al. Pd-L1 Induction by Cancer-Associated Fibroblast-Derived Factors in Lung Adenocarcinoma Cells. *Cancers (Basel)* (2019) 11(9):1257. doi: 10.3390/cancers11091257
196. Ziani L, Chouaib S, Thiery J. Alteration of the Antitumor Immune Response by Cancer-Associated Fibroblasts. *Front Immunol* (2018) 9:414. doi: 10.3389/fimmu.2018.00414
197. Donnarumma E, Fiore D, Nappa M, Roscigno G, Adamo A, Iaboni M, et al. Cancer-Associated Fibroblasts Release Exosomal microRNAs That Dictate an Aggressive Phenotype in Breast Cancer. *Oncotarget* (2017) 8(12):19592–608. doi: 10.18632/oncotarget.14752
198. Bhome R, Goh RW, Bullock MD, Pillar N, Thirdborough SM, Mellone M, et al. Exosomal microRNAs Derived From Colorectal Cancer-Associated Fibroblasts: Role in Driving Cancer Progression. *Aging (Albany NY)* (2017) 9 (12):2666–94. doi: 10.18632/aging.101355
199. Hu Y, Yan C, Mu L, Huang K, Li X, Tao D, et al. Fibroblast-Derived Exosomes Contribute to Chemoresistance Through Priming Cancer Stem Cells in Colorectal Cancer. *PloS One* (2015) 10(5):e0125625. doi: 10.1371/journal.pone.0125625
200. Lotti F, Jarrar AM, Pai RK, Hitomi M, Lathia J, Mace A, et al. Chemotherapy Activates Cancer-Associated Fibroblasts to Maintain Colorectal Cancer-Initiating Cells by IL-17A. *J Exp Med* (2013) 210(13):2851–72. doi: 10.1084/jem.20131195

201. Neri E, Faggioni L, Cerri F, Turini F, Angeli S, Cini L, et al. CT Colonography Versus Double-Contrast Barium Enema for Screening of Colorectal Cancer: Comparison of Radiation Burden. *Abdom Imaging* (2010) 35(5):596–601. doi: 10.1007/s00261-009-9568-x
202. Brenner H, Chang-Claude J, Jansen L, Knebel P, Stock C, Hoffmeister M. Reduced Risk of Colorectal Cancer Up to 10 Years After Screening, Surveillance, or Diagnostic Colonoscopy. *Gastroenterology* (2014) 146 (3):709–17. doi: 10.1053/j.gastro.2013.09.001
203. Ozguroglu M, Turna H. Do We Really Benefit From Checking Tumor Markers in Detecting Recurrence in Gastrointestinal Cancer? *J BUON* (2004) 9(2):179–82.
204. Duffy MJ. Tumor Markers in Clinical Practice: A Review Focusing on Common Solid Cancers. *Med Princ Pract* (2013) 22(1):4–11. doi: 10.1159/000338393
205. van Veelen CW, Verbiest H, Zulch KJ, van Ketel B, van der Vlist MJ, Vlug AM, et al. [Pyruvate Kinase as a Marker of Human Brain Tumors]. *Ned Tijdschr Geneeskd* (1980) 124(40):1678–85.
206. Mazurek S, Boschek CB, Hugo F, Eigenbrodt E. Pyruvate Kinase Type M2 and its Role in Tumor Growth and Spreading. *Semin Cancer Biol* (2005) 15 (4):300–8. doi: 10.1016/j.semcancer.2005.04.009
207. Eigenbrodt E, Reinacher M, Scheefers-Borchel U, Scheefers H, Friis R. Double Role for Pyruvate Kinase Type M2 in the Expansion of Phosphometabolite Pools Found in Tumor Cells. *Crit Rev Oncog* (1992) 3 (1-2):91–115.
208. Kobierzycki C, Piotrowska A, Latkowski K, Zabel M, Nowak-Markwitz E, Spaczynski M, et al. Correlation of Pyruvate Kinase M2 Expression With Clinicopathological Data in Ovarian Cancer. *Anticancer Res* (2018) 38 (1):295–300. doi: 10.21873/anticanres.12221
209. Liu B, Song M, Qin H, Zhang B, Liu Y, Sun Y, et al. Phosphoribosyl Pyrophosphate Amidotransferase Promotes the Progression of Thyroid Cancer Via Regulating Pyruvate Kinase M2. *Onco Targets Ther* (2020) 13:7629–39. doi: 10.2147/OTT.S253137
210. Yang Y, Wu K, Liu Y, Shi L, Tao K, Wang G. Prognostic Significance of Metabolic Enzyme Pyruvate Kinase M2 in Breast Cancer: A Meta-Analysis. *Med (Baltimore)* (2017) 96(46):e8690. doi: 10.1097/MD.0000000000008690
211. Zhu Q, Hong B, Zhang L, Wang J. Pyruvate Kinase M2 Inhibits the Progression of Bladder Cancer by Targeting MAKP Pathway. *J Cancer Res Ther* (2018) 14(Supplement):S616–S21. doi: 10.4103/0973-1482.187302
212. Guo W, Zhang Z, Li G, Lai X, Gu R, Xu W, et al. Pyruvate Kinase M2 Promotes Prostate Cancer Metastasis Through Regulating ERK1/2-COX-2 Signaling. *Front Oncol* (2020) 10:544288. doi: 10.3389/fonc.2020.544288
213. Wang C, Zhang S, Liu J, Tian Y, Ma B, Xu S, et al. Secreted Pyruvate Kinase M2 Promotes Lung Cancer Metastasis Through Activating the Integrin Beta1/Fak Signaling Pathway. *Cell Rep* (2020) 30(6):1780–97.e6. doi: 10.1016/j.celrep.2020.01.037
214. Landt S, Jeschke S, Koeninger A, Thomas A, Heusner T, Korlach S, et al. Tumor-Specific Correlation of Tumor M2 Pyruvate Kinase in Pre-Invasive, Invasive and Recurrent Cervical Cancer. *Anticancer Res* (2010) 30(2):375–81.
215. Wechsel HW, Petri E, Bichler KH, Feil G. Marker for Renal Cell Carcinoma (RCC): The Dimeric Form of Pyruvate Kinase Type M2 (Tu M2-Pk). *Anticancer Res* (1999) 19(4A):2583–90.
216. Kumar Y, Tapuria N, Kirmani N, Davidson BR. Tumour M2-pyruvate Kinase: A Gastrointestinal Cancer Marker. *Eur J Gastroenterol Hepatol* (2007) 19(3):265–76. doi: 10.1097/MEG.0b013e3280102f78
217. Hardt PD, Ewald N. Tumor M2 Pyruvate Kinase: A Tumor Marker and its Clinical Application in Gastrointestinal Malignancy. *Expert Rev Mol Diagn* (2008) 8(5):579–85. doi: 10.1586/14737159.8.5.579
218. Pantel K, Speicher MR. The Biology of Circulating Tumor Cells. *Oncogene* (2016) 35(10):1216–24. doi: 10.1038/onc.2015.192
219. Toyoshima K, Hayashi A, Kashiwagi M, Hayashi N, Iwatsuki M, Ishimoto T, et al. Analysis of Circulating Tumor Cells Derived From Advanced Gastric Cancer. *Int J Cancer* (2015) 137(4):991–8. doi: 10.1002/ijc.29455
220. Witzig TE, Bossy B, Kimlinger T, Roche PC, Ingle JN, Grant C, et al. Detection of Circulating Cytokeratin-Positive Cells in the Blood of Breast Cancer Patients Using Immunomagnetic Enrichment and Digital Microscopy. *Clin Cancer Res* (2002) 8(5):1085–91.
221. Baccelli I, Schneeweiss A, Riethdorf S, Stenzinger A, Schillert A, Vogel V, et al. Identification of a Population of Blood Circulating Tumor Cells From Breast Cancer Patients That Initiates Metastasis in a Xenograft Assay. *Nat Biotechnol* (2013) 31(6):539–44. doi: 10.1038/nbt.2576
222. Uenosono Y, Arigami T, Kozono T, Yanagita S, Hagihara T, Haraguchi N, et al. Clinical Significance of Circulating Tumor Cells in Peripheral Blood From Patients With Gastric Cancer. *Cancer* (2013) 119(22):3984–91. doi: 10.1002/cncr.28309
223. Tang L, Zhao S, Liu W, Parchim NF, Huang J, Tang Y, et al. Diagnostic Accuracy of Circulating Tumor Cells Detection in Gastric Cancer: Systematic Review and Meta-Analysis. *BMC Cancer* (2013) 13:314. doi: 10.1186/1471-2407-13-314
224. Chen CJ, Sung WW, Chen HC, Chern YJ, Hsu HT, Lin YM, et al. Early Assessment of Colorectal Cancer by Quantifying Circulating Tumor Cells in Peripheral Blood: ECT2 in Diagnosis of Colorectal Cancer. *Int J Mol Sci* (2017) 18(4):743. doi: 10.3390/ijms18040743
225. Yang C, Shi D, Wang S, Wei C, Zhang C, Xiong B. Prognostic Value of Pre- and Post-Operative Circulating Tumor Cells Detection in Colorectal Cancer Patients Treated With Curative Resection: A Prospective Cohort Study Based on ISET Device. *Cancer Manag Res* (2018) 10:4135–44. doi: 10.2147/CMAR.S176575
226. Kahlert C, Melo SA, Protopopov A, Tang J, Seth S, Koch M, et al. Identification of Double-Stranded Genomic DNA Spanning All Chromosomes With Mutated KRAS and P53 DNA in the Serum Exosomes of Patients With Pancreatic Cancer. *J Biol Chem* (2014) 289 (7):3869–75. doi: 10.1074/jbc.C113.532267
227. Wan JCM, Massie C, Garcia-Corbacho J, Mouliere F, Brenton JD, Caldas C, et al. Liquid Biopsies Come of Age: Towards Implementation of Circulating Tumour DNA. *Nat Rev Cancer* (2017) 17(4):223–38. doi: 10.1038/nrc.2017.7
228. Sumbal S, Javed A, Afroze B, Zulfiqar HF, Javed F, Noreen S, et al. Circulating Tumor DNA in Blood: Future Genomic Biomarkers for Cancer Detection. *Exp Hematol* (2018) 65:17–28. doi: 10.1016/j.exphem.2018.06.003
229. Newman AM, Lovejoy AF, Klass DM, Kurtz DM, Chabon JJ, Scherer F, et al. Integrated Digital Error Suppression for Improved Detection of Circulating Tumor DNA. *Nat Biotechnol* (2016) 34(5):547–55. doi: 10.1038/nbt.3520
230. Leary RJ, Sausen M, Kinde I, Papadopoulos N, Carpten JD, Craig D, et al. Detection of Chromosomal Alterations in the Circulation of Cancer Patients With Whole-Genome Sequencing. *Sci Transl Med* (2012) 4(162):162ra54. doi: 10.1126/scitranslmed.3004742
231. Haber DA, Velculescu VE. Blood-Based Analyses of Cancer: Circulating Tumor Cells and Circulating Tumor DNA. *Cancer Discov* (2014) 4(6):650–61. doi: 10.1158/2159-8290.CD-13-1014
232. Kidess E, Jeffrey SS. Circulating Tumor Cells Versus Tumor-Derived Cell-Free DNA: Rivals or Partners in Cancer Care in the Era of Single-Cell Analysis? *Genome Med* (2013) 5(8):70. doi: 10.1186/gm474
233. Fiala C, Diamandis EP. Utility of Circulating Tumor DNA in Cancer Diagnostics With Emphasis on Early Detection. *BMC Med* (2018) 16 (1):166. doi: 10.1186/s12916-018-1157-9
234. Wang HQ, Yang CY, Wang SY, Wang T, Han JL, Wei K, et al. Cell-Free Plasma Hypermethylated CASZ1, CDH13 and ING2 are Promising Biomarkers of Esophageal Cancer. *J BioMed Res* (2018) 32(5):424–33. doi: 10.7555/JBR.32.20170065
235. Tian X, Sun B, Chen C, Gao C, Zhang J, Lu X, et al. Circulating Tumor DNA 5-Hydroxymethylcytosine as a Novel Diagnostic Biomarker for Esophageal Cancer. *Cell Res* (2018) 28(5):597–600. doi: 10.1038/s41422-018-0014-x
236. Qian C, Ju S, Qi J, Zhao J, Shen X, Jing R, et al. Alu-Based Cell-Free DNA: A Novel Biomarker for Screening of Gastric Cancer. *Oncotarget* (2017) 8 (33):54037–45. doi: 10.18632/oncotarget.11079
237. Gao Y, Zhang K, Xi H, Cai A, Wu X, Cui J, et al. Diagnostic and Prognostic Value of Circulating Tumor DNA in Gastric Cancer: A Meta-Analysis. *Oncotarget* (2017) 8(4):6330–40. doi: 10.18632/oncotarget.14064
238. Xu RH, Wei W, Krawczyk M, Wang W, Luo H, Flagg K, et al. Circulating Tumour DNA Methylation Markers for Diagnosis and Prognosis of Hepatocellular Carcinoma. *Nat Mater* (2017) 16(11):1155–61. doi: 10.1038/nmat4997
239. Tao K, Bian Z, Zhang Q, Guo X, Yin C, Wang Y, et al. Machine Learning-Based Genome-Wide Interrogation of Somatic Copy Number Aberrations in Circulating Tumor DNA for Early Detection of Hepatocellular Carcinoma. *EBioMedicine* (2020) 56:102811. doi: 10.1016/j.ebiom.2020.102811

240. Jaworski JJ, Morgan RD, Sivakumar S. Circulating Cell-Free Tumour DNA for Early Detection of Pancreatic Cancer. *Cancers (Basel)* (2020) 12(12):3704. doi: 10.3390/cancers12123704
241. Grunvald MW, Jacobson RA, Kuzel TM, Pappas SG, Masood A. Current Status of Circulating Tumor DNA Liquid Biopsy in Pancreatic Cancer. *Int J Mol Sci* (2020) 21(20):7651. doi: 10.3390/ijms21207651
242. Liggett T, Melnikov A, Yi QL, Replogle C, Brand R, Kaul K, et al. Differential Methylation of Cell-Free Circulating DNA Among Patients With Pancreatic Cancer Versus Chronic Pancreatitis. *Cancer* (2010) 116(7):1674–80. doi: 10.1002/cncr.24893
243. Eissa MAL, Lerner L, Abdelfatah E, Shankar N, Canner JK, Hasan NM, et al. Promoter Methylation of ADAMTS1 and BNC1 as Potential Biomarkers for Early Detection of Pancreatic Cancer in Blood. *Clin Epigenet* (2019) 11(1):59. doi: 10.1186/s13148-019-0650-0
244. Cohen JD, Javed AA, Thoburn C, Wong F, Tie J, Gibbs P, et al. Combined Circulating Tumor DNA and Protein Biomarker-Based Liquid Biopsy for the Earlier Detection of Pancreatic Cancers. *Proc Natl Acad Sci USA* (2017) 114 (38):10202–7. doi: 10.1073/pnas.1704961114
245. Bedin C, Enzo MV, Del Bianco P, Pucciarelli S, Nitti D, Agostini M. Diagnostic and Prognostic Role of Cell-Free DNA Testing for Colorectal Cancer Patients. *Int J Cancer* (2017) 140(8):1888–98. doi: 10.1002/ijc.30565
246. Nagai Y, Sunami E, Yamamoto Y, Hata K, Okada S, Murono K, et al. LINE-1 Hypomethylation Status of Circulating Cell-Free DNA in Plasma as a Biomarker for Colorectal Cancer. *Oncotarget* (2017) 8(7):11906–16. doi: 10.18632/oncotarget.14439
247. Brennecke J, Stark A, Russell RB, Cohen SM. Principles of microRNA-target Recognition. *PloS Biol* (2005) 3(3):e85. doi: 10.1371/journal.pbio.0030085
248. Weber JA, Baxter DH, Zhang S, Huang DY, Huang KH, Lee MJ, et al. The microRNA Spectrum in 12 Body Fluids. *Clin Chem* (2010) 56(11):1733–41. doi: 10.1373/clinchem.2010.147405
249. Calin GA, Dumitru CD, Shimizu M, Bichi R, Zupo S, Noch E, et al. Frequent Deletions and Down-Regulation of Micro- RNA Genes miR15 and miR16 at 13q14 in Chronic Lymphocytic Leukemia. *Proc Natl Acad Sci USA* (2002) 99 (24):15524–9. doi: 10.1073/pnas.242606799
250. Shen Y, Ding Y, Ma Q, Zhao L, Guo X, Shao Y, et al. Identification of Novel Circulating Mirna Biomarkers for the Diagnosis of Esophageal Squamous Cell Carcinoma and Squamous Dysplasia. *Cancer Epidemiol Biomarkers Prev* (2019) 28(7):1212–20. doi: 10.1158/1055-9965.EPI-18-1199
251. Yang M, Liu R, Sheng J, Liao J, Wang Y, Pan E, et al. Differential Expression Profiles of microRNAs as Potential Biomarkers for the Early Diagnosis of Esophageal Squamous Cell Carcinoma. *Oncol Rep* (2013) 29(1):169–76. doi: 10.3892/or.2012.2105
252. So JBY, Kapoor R, Zhu F, Koh C, Zhou L, Zou R, et al. Development and Validation of a Serum microRNA Biomarker Panel for Detecting Gastric Cancer in a High-Risk Population. *Gut* (2020) 70(5):829–37. doi: 10.1136/gutjnl-2020-322065
253. Shen S, Lin Y, Yuan X, Shen L, Chen J, Chen L, et al. Biomarker MicroRNAs for Diagnosis, Prognosis and Treatment of Hepatocellular Carcinoma: A Functional Survey and Comparison. *Sci Rep* (2016) 6:38311. doi: 10.1038/srep38311
254. Shams R, Saberi S, Zali M, Sadeghi A, Ghafouri-Fard S, Aghdaei HA. Identification of Potential microRNA Panels for Pancreatic Cancer Diagnosis Using Microarray Datasets and Bioinformatics Methods. *Sci Rep* (2020) 10(1):7559. doi: 10.1038/s41598-020-64569-1
255. Eslamizadeh S, Heidari M, Agah S, Faghihloo E, Ghazi H, Mirzaei A, et al. The Role of MicroRNA Signature as Diagnostic Biomarkers in Different Clinical Stages of Colorectal Cancer. *Cell J* (2018) 20(2):220–30. doi: 10.22074/cellj.2018.5366
256. Li G, Shen Q, Li C, Li D, Chen J, He M. Identification of Circulating MicroRNAs as Novel Potential Biomarkers for Hepatocellular Carcinoma Detection: A Systematic Review and Meta-Analysis. *Clin Transl Oncol* (2015) 17(9):684–93. doi: 10.1007/s12094-015-1294-y
257. Pan C, Yan X, Li H, Huang L, Yin M, Yang Y, et al. Systematic Literature Review and Clinical Validation of Circulating microRNAs as Diagnostic Biomarkers for Colorectal Cancer. *Oncotarget* (2017) 8(40):68317–28. doi: 10.18632/oncotarget.19344
258. Nedaeinia R, Manian M, Jazayeri MH, Ranjbar M, Salehi R, Sharifi M, et al. Circulating Exosomes and Exosomal microRNAs as Biomarkers in Gastrointestinal Cancer. *Cancer Gene Ther* (2017) 24(2):48–56. doi: 10.1038/cgt.2016.77
259. Wang R, Wen H, Xu Y, Chen Q, Luo Y, Lin Y, et al. Circulating microRNAs as a Novel Class of Diagnostic Biomarkers in Gastrointestinal Tumors Detection: A Meta-Analysis Based on 42 Articles. *PloS One* (2014) 9(11): e113401. doi: 10.1371/journal.pone.0113401
260. Salzman J. Circular RNA Expression: Its Potential Regulation and Function. *Trends Genet* (2016) 32(5):309–16. doi: 10.1016/j.tig.2016.03.002
261. Wang S, Zhang K, Tan S, Xin J, Yuan Q, Xu H, et al. Circular RNAs in Body Fluids as Cancer Biomarkers: The New Frontier of Liquid Biopsies. *Mol Cancer* (2021) 20(1):13. doi: 10.1186/s12943-020-01298-z
262. Liu X, Abraham JM, Cheng Y, Wang Z, Wang Z, Zhang G, et al. Synthetic Circular Rna Functions as a Mir-21 Sponge to Suppress Gastric Carcinoma Cell Proliferation. *Mol Ther Nucleic Acids* (2018) 13:312–21. doi: 10.1016/j.omtn.2018.09.010
263. Niu C, Zhao L, Guo X, Shen Y, Shao Y, Liu F. Diagnostic Accuracy of circRNAs in Esophageal Cancer: A Meta-Analysis. *Dis Markers* (2019) 2019:9673129. doi: 10.1155/2019/9673129
264. Li T, Shao Y, Fu L, Xie Y, Zhu L, Sun W, et al. Plasma Circular RNA Profiling of Patients With Gastric Cancer and Their Droplet Digital RT-PCR Detection. *J Mol Med (Berl)* (2018) 96(1):85–96. doi: 10.1007/s00109-017-1600-y
265. Zhao Q, Chen S, Li T, Xiao B, Zhang X. Clinical Values of Circular RNA 0000181 in the Screening of Gastric Cancer. *J Clin Lab Anal* (2018) 32(4): e22333. doi: 10.1002/jcla.22333
266. Sun XH, Wang YT, Li GF, Zhang N, Fan L. Serum-Derived three-circRNA Signature as a Diagnostic Biomarker for Hepatocellular Carcinoma. *Cancer Cell Int* (2020) 20:226. doi: 10.1186/s12935-020-01302-y
267. Yang F, Liu DY, Guo JT, Ge N, Zhu P, Liu X, et al. Circular RNA circ-LDLRAD3 as a Biomarker in Diagnosis of Pancreatic Cancer. *World J Gastroenterol* (2017) 23(47):8345–54. doi: 10.3748/wjg.v23.i47.8345
268. Yao J, Zhang C, Chen Y, Gao S. Downregulation of Circular RNA circ-LDLRAD3 Suppresses Pancreatic Cancer Progression Through miR-137-3p/PTN Axis. *Life Sci* (2019) 239:116871. doi: 10.1016/j.lfs.2019.116871
269. Lin J, Cai D, Li W, Yu T, Mao H, Jiang S, et al. Plasma Circular RNA Panel Acts as a Novel Diagnostic Biomarker for Colorectal Cancer. *Clin Biochem* (2019) 74:60–8. doi: 10.1016/j.clinbiochem.2019.10.012
270. Li J, Song Y, Wang J, Huang J. Plasma Circular RNA Panel Acts as a Novel Diagnostic Biomarker for Colorectal Cancer Detection. *Am J Transl Res* (2020) 12(11):7395–403.
271. Tao Z, Li S, Ichim TE, Yang J, Riordan N, Yenugonda V, et al. Cellular Immunotherapy of Cancer: An Overview and Future Directions. *Immunotherapy* (2017) 9(7):589–606. doi: 10.2217/imt-2016-0086
272. Rodriguez Perez A, Campillo-Davo D, Van Tendeloo VFI, Benitez-Ribas D. Cellular Immunotherapy: A Clinical State-of-the-Art of a New Paradigm for Cancer Treatment. *Clin Transl Oncol* (2020) 22(11):1923–37. doi: 10.1007/s12094-020-02344-4
273. Krzyszczyk P, Acevedo A, Davidoff EJ, Timmins LM, Marrero-Berrios I, Patel M, et al. The Growing Role of Precision and Personalized Medicine for Cancer Treatment. *Technol (Singap World Sci)* (2018) 6(3-4):79–100. doi: 10.1142/S2339547818300020
274. Dumbrava EI, Meric-Bernstam F. Personalized Cancer Therapy-Leveraging a Knowledge Base for Clinical Decision-Making. *Cold Spring Harb Mol Case Stud* (2018) 4(2):a001578. doi: 10.1101/mcs.a001578
275. McCarthy EF. The Toxins of William B. Coley and the Treatment of Bone and Soft-Tissue Sarcomas. *Iowa Orthop J* (2006) 26:154–8. doi: 10.1177/104990919100800102
276. Rasmussen L, Arvin A. Chemotherapy-Induced Immunosuppression. *Environ Health Perspect* (1982) 43:21–5. doi: 10.1289/ehp.824321
277. Steele TA. Chemotherapy-Induced Immunosuppression and Reconstitution of Immune Function. *Leuk Res* (2002) 26(4):411–4. doi: 10.1016/s0145-2126(01)00138-2
278. Peng J, Hamanishi J, Matsumura N, Abiko K, Murat K, Baba T, et al. Chemotherapy Induces Programmed Cell Death-Ligand 1 Overexpression Via the Nuclear Factor-Kappab to Foster an Immunosuppressive Tumor Microenvironment in Ovarian Cancer. *Cancer Res* (2015) 75(23):5034–45. doi: 10.1158/0008-5472.CAN-14-3098

279. Daenen LG, Roodhart JM, van Amersfoort M, Dehnad M, Roessingh W, Ulfman LH, et al. Chemotherapy Enhances Metastasis Formation Via VEGFR-1-expressing Endothelial Cells. *Cancer Res* (2011) 71(22):6976–85. doi: 10.1158/0008-5472.CAN-11-0627
280. Palmieri LJ, Dubreuil O, Bachet JB, Trouilloud I, Locher C, Coriat R, et al. Reasons for Chemotherapy Discontinuation and End-of-Life in Patients With Gastrointestinal Cancer: A Multicenter Prospective AGEO Study. *Clin Res Hepatol Gastroenterol* (2021) 45(1):101431. doi: 10.1016/j.clinre.2020.03.029
281. Park SE, Lee SH, Ahn JS, Ahn MJ, Park K, Sun JM. Increased Response Rates to Salvage Chemotherapy Administered After PD-1/PD-L1 Inhibitors in Patients With Non-Small Cell Lung Cancer. *J Thorac Oncol* (2018) 13 (1):106–11. doi: 10.1016/j.jtho.2017.10.011
282. Jiang J, Xu N, Wu C, Deng H, Lu M, Li M, et al. Treatment of Advanced Gastric Cancer by Chemotherapy Combined With Autologous Cytokine-Induced Killer Cells. *Anticancer Res* (2006) 26(3B):2237–42.
283. Hirsch HA, Iliopoulos D, Tsichlis PN, Struhl K. Metformin Selectively Targets Cancer Stem Cells, and Acts Together With Chemotherapy to Block Tumor Growth and Prolong Remission. *Cancer Res* (2009) 69 (19):7507–11. doi: 10.1158/0008-5472.CAN-09-2994
284. Helleday T. Making Immunotherapy 'Cold' Tumours 'Hot' by Chemotherapy-Induced Mutations-a Misconception. *Ann Oncol* (2019) 30 (3):360–1. doi: 10.1093/annonc/mdz013
285. Spiegel S, Milstien S, Grant S. Endogenous Modulators and Pharmacological Inhibitors of Histone Deacetylases in Cancer Therapy. *Oncogene* (2012) 31 (5):537–51. doi: 10.1038/onc.2011.267
286. Li G, Tian Y, Zhu WG. The Roles of Histone Deacetylases and Their Inhibitors in Cancer Therapy. *Front Cell Dev Biol* (2020) 8:576946. doi: 10.3389/fcell.2020.576946
287. Masunaga SI, Sanada Y, Tano K, Sakurai Y, Tanaka H, Takata T, et al. An Attempt to Improve the Therapeutic Effect of Boron Neutron Capture Therapy Using Commonly Employed 10B-Carriers Based on Analytical Studies on the Correlation Among Quiescent Tumor Cell Characteristics, Tumor Heterogeneity and Cancer Stemness. *J Radiat Res* (2020) 61(6):876–85. doi: 10.1093/jrr/rraa048
288. Hatanaka H, Amano K, Kamano S, Fankhauser H, Hanamura T, Sano K. Boron-Neutron Capture Therapy in Relation to Immunotherapy. *Acta Neurochir (Wien)* (1978) 42(1-2):57–72. doi: 10.1007/BF01406631
289. Rosenberg SA, Spiess P, Lafreniere R. A New Approach to the Adoptive Immunotherapy of Cancer With Tumor-Infiltrating Lymphocytes. *Science* (1986) 233(4770):1318–21. doi: 10.1126/science.3489291
290. Lin B, Du L, Li H, Zhu X, Cui L, Li X. Tumor-Infiltrating Lymphocytes: Warriors Fight Against Tumors Powerfully. *BioMed Pharmacother* (2020) 132:110873. doi: 10.1016/j.biopha.2020.110873
291. D'Andrea MA, Reddy GK. Systemic Effects of Radiation Therapy-Induced Abscopal Responses in Patients With Advanced Lung Cancer. *Oncology* (2021) 99(1):1–14. doi: 10.1159/000510287
292. Yang C, Li Y, Yang Y, Chen Z. Overview of Strategies to Improve Therapy Against Tumors Using Natural Killer Cell. *J Immunol Res* (2020) 2020:8459496. doi: 10.1155/2020/8459496
293. Xie G, Dong H, Liang Y, Ham JD, Rizwan R, Chen J. Car-NK Cells: A Promising Cellular Immunotherapy for Cancer. *EBioMedicine* (2020) 59:102975. doi: 10.1016/j.ebiom.2020.102975
294. Marangon M, Visco C, Barbui AM, Chiappella A, Fabbri A, Ferrero S, et al. Allogeneic Stem Cell Transplantation in Mantle Cell Lymphoma in the Era of New Drugs and CAR-T Cell Therapy. *Cancers (Basel)* (2021) 13(2):291. doi: 10.3390/cancers13020291
295. Zhao YJ, Jiang N, Song QK, Wu JP, Song YG, Zhang HM, et al. Continuous DC-CIK Infusions Restore CD8+ Cellular Immunity, Physical Activity and Improve Clinical Efficacy in Advanced Cancer Patients Unresponsive to Conventional Treatments. *Asian Pac J Cancer Prev* (2015) 16(6):2419–23. doi: 10.7314/apjcp.2015.16.6.2419
296. Zhang L, Mu Y, Zhang A, Xie J, Chen S, Xu F, et al. Cytokine-Induced Killer Cells/Dendritic Cells-Cytokine Induced Killer Cells Immunotherapy Combined With Chemotherapy for Treatment of Colorectal Cancer in China: A Meta-Analysis of 29 Trials Involving 2,610 Patients. *Oncotarget* (2017) 8(28):45164–77. doi: 10.18632/oncotarget.16665
297. Mu Y, Zhou CH, Chen SF, Ding J, Zhang YX, Yang YP, et al. Effectiveness and Safety of Chemotherapy Combined With Cytokine-Induced Killer Cell /Dendritic Cell-Cytokine-Induced Killer Cell Therapy for Treatment of Gastric Cancer in China: A Systematic Review and Meta-Analysis. *Cytotherapy* (2016) 18(9):1162–77. doi: 10.1016/j.jcyt.2016.05.015
298. Jiang N, Qiao G, Wang X, Morse MA, Gwin WR, Zhou L, et al. Dendritic Cell/Cytokine-Induced Killer Cell Immunotherapy Combined With S-1 in Patients With Advanced Pancreatic Cancer: A Prospective Study. *Clin Cancer Res* (2017) 23(17):5066–73. doi: 10.1158/1078-0432.CCR-17-0492
299. Cao J, Kong FH, Liu X, Wang XB. Immunotherapy With Dendritic Cells and Cytokine-Induced Killer Cells for Hepatocellular Carcinoma: A Meta-Analysis. *World J Gastroenterol* (2019) 25(27):3649–63. doi: 10.3748/wjg.v25.i27.3649
300. Merker M, Salzmann-Manrique E, Katzki V, Huenecke S, Bremm M, Bakhtiar S, et al. Clearance of Hematologic Malignancies by Allogeneic Cytokine-Induced Killer Cell or Donor Lymphocyte Infusions. *Biol Blood Marrow Transplant* (2019) 25(7):1281–92. doi: 10.1016/j.bbmt.2019.03.004
301. Liang S, Xu K, Niu L, Wang X, Liang Y, Zhang M, et al. Comparison of Autogeneic and Allogeneic Natural Killer Cells Immunotherapy on the Clinical Outcome of Recurrent Breast Cancer. *Onco Targets Ther* (2017) 10:4273–81. doi: 10.2147/OTT.S139986
302. Wang F, Lau JKC, Yu J. The Role of Natural Killer Cell in Gastrointestinal Cancer: Killer or Helper. *Oncogene* (2020) 40(4):717–30. doi: 10.1038/s41388-020-01561-z
303. Lin M, Liang S, Wang X, Liang Y, Zhang M, Chen J, et al. Percutaneous Irreversible Electroporation Combined With Allogeneic Natural Killer Cell Immunotherapy for Patients With Unresectable (Stage III/IV) Pancreatic Cancer: A Promising Treatment. *J Cancer Res Clin Oncol* (2017) 143 (12):2607–18. doi: 10.1007/s00432-017-2513-4
304. Yang Y, Qin Z, Du D, Wu Y, Qiu S, Mu F, et al. Safety and Short-Term Efficacy of Irreversible Electroporation and Allogenic Natural Killer Cell Immunotherapy Combination in the Treatment of Patients With Unresectable Primary Liver Cancer. *Cardiovasc Intervent Radiol* (2019) 42 (1):48–59. doi: 10.1007/s00270-018-2069-y
305. Lim TS, Chew V, Sieow JL, Goh S, Yeong JP, Soon AL, et al. PD-1 Expression on Dendritic Cells Suppresses CD8(+) T Cell Function and Antitumor Immunity. *Oncoimmunology* (2016) 5(3):e1085146. doi: 10.1080/2162402X.2015.1085146
306. Peng Q, Qiu X, Zhang Z, Zhang S, Zhang Y, Liang Y, et al. Pd-L1 on Dendritic Cells Attenuates T Cell Activation and Regulates Response to Immune Checkpoint Blockade. *Nat Commun* (2020) 11(1):4835. doi: 10.1038/s41467-020-18570-x
307. Vari F, Arpon D, Keane C, Hertzberg MS, Talaulikar D, Jain S, et al. Immune Evasion Via PD-1/PD-L1 on NK Cells and Monocyte/Macrophages is More Prominent in Hodgkin Lymphoma Than DLBCL. *Blood* (2018) 131 (16):1809–19. doi: 10.1182/blood-2017-07-796342
308. Norris S, Coleman A, Kuri-Cervantes L, Bower M, Nelson M, Goodier MR. PD-1 Expression on Natural Killer Cells and CD8(+) T Cells During Chronic HIV-1 Infection. *Viral Immunol* (2012) 25(4):329–32. doi: 10.1089/vim.2011.0096
309. Mariotti FR, Petrini S, Ingegnere T, Tumino N, Besi F, Scordamaglia F, et al. PD-1 in Human NK Cells: Evidence of Cytoplasmic mRNA and Protein Expression. *Oncoimmunology* (2019) 8(3):1557030. doi: 10.1080/2162402X.2018.1557030
310. Beldi-Ferchiou A, Lambert M, Dogniaux S, Vely F, Vivier E, Olive D, et al. PD-1 Mediates Functional Exhaustion of Activated NK Cells in Patients With Kaposi Sarcoma. *Oncotarget* (2016) 7(45):72961–77. doi: 10.18632/oncotarget.12150
311. Niu C, Li M, Zhu S, Chen Y, Zhou L, Xu D, et al. PD-1-Positive Natural Killer Cells Have a Weaker Antitumor Function Than That of PD-1-negative Natural Killer Cells in Lung Cancer. *Int J Med Sci* (2020) 17(13):1964–73. doi: 10.7150/ijms.47701
312. Concha-Benavente F, Kansy B, Moskovitz J, Moy J, Chandran U, Ferris RL. Pd-L1 Mediates Dysfunction in Activated Pd-1(+) NK Cells in Head and Neck Cancer Patients. *Cancer Immunol Res* (2018) 6(12):1548–60. doi: 10.1158/2326-6066.CIR-18-0062
313. Giuliani M, Janji B, Berchem G. Activation of NK Cells and Disruption of PD-L1/PD-1 Axis: Two Different Ways for Lenalidomide to Block Myeloma

Progression. *Oncotarget* (2017) 8(14):24031–44. doi: 10.18632/oncotarget.15234

314. Zhang W, Song Z, Xiao J, Liu X, Luo Y, Yang Z, et al. Blocking the PD-1/PD-L1 Axis in Dendritic Cell-Stimulated Cytokine-Induced Killer Cells With Pembrolizumab Enhances Their Therapeutic Effects Against Hepatocellular Carcinoma. *J Cancer* (2019) 10(11):2578–87. doi: 10.7150/jca.26961
315. Oyer JL, Gitto SB, Altomare DA, Copik AJ. Pd-L1 Blockade Enhances Anti-Tumor Efficacy of NK Cells. *Oncoimmunology* (2018) 7(11):e1509819. doi: 10.1080/2162402X.2018.1509819
316. Itzhaki O, Jacoby E, Nissani A, Levi M, Nagler A, Kubi A, et al. Head-to-Head Comparison of in-House Produced CD19 CAR-T Cell in ALL and NHL Patients. *J Immunother Cancer* (2020) 8(1):e000148. doi: 10.1136/jitc-2019-000148
317. Li J, Li W, Huang K, Zhang Y, Kupfer G, Zhao Q. Chimeric Antigen Receptor T Cell (CAR-T) Immunotherapy for Solid Tumors: Lessons Learned and Strategies for Moving Forward. *J Hematol Oncol* (2018) 11(1):22. doi: 10.1186/s13045-018-0568-6
318. Parkhurst MR, Yang JC, Langan RC, Dudley ME, Nathan DA, Feldman SA, et al. T Cells Targeting Carcinoembryonic Antigen can Mediate Regression of Metastatic Colorectal Cancer But Induce Severe Transient Colitis. *Mol Ther* (2011) 19(3):620–6. doi: 10.1038/mt.2010.272
319. Sanmamed MF, Chen L. A Paradigm Shift in Cancer Immunotherapy: From Enhancement to Normalization. *Cell* (2019) 176(3):677. doi: 10.1016/j.cell.2019.01.008
320. Tang X, Yang L, Li Z, Nalin AP, Dai H, Xu T, et al. First-in-Man Clinical Trial of CAR Nk-92 Cells: Safety Test of CD33-CAR Nk-92 Cells in Patients With Relapsed and Refractory Acute Myeloid Leukemia. *Am J Cancer Res* (2018) 8(6):1083–9.
321. Hollingsworth RE, Jansen K. Turning the Corner on Therapeutic Cancer Vaccines. *NPJ Vaccines* (2019) 4:7. doi: 10.1038/s41541-019-0103-y
322. Leitner WW, Ying H, Restifo NP. DNA and RNA-based Vaccines: Principles, Progress and Prospects. *Vaccine* (1999) 18(9-10):765–77. doi: 10.1016/s0264-410x(99)00271-6
323. Trimble CL, Morrow MP, Kraynyak KA, Shen X, Dallas M, Yan J, et al. Safety, Efficacy, and Immunogenicity of VGX-3100, a Therapeutic Synthetic DNA Vaccine Targeting Human Papillomavirus 16 and 18 E6 and E7 Proteins for Cervical Intraepithelial Neoplasia 2/3: A Randomised, Double-Blind, Placebo-Controlled Phase 2b Trial. *Lancet* (2015) 386(10008):2078–88. doi: 10.1016/S0140-6736(15)00239-1
324. Norell H, Poschke I, Charo J, Wei WZ, Erskine C, Piechocki MP, et al. Vaccination With a Plasmid DNA Encoding HER-2/neu Together With Low Doses of GM-CSF and IL-2 in Patients With Metastatic Breast Carcinoma: A Pilot Clinical Trial. *J Transl Med* (2010) 8:53. doi: 10.1186/1479-5876-8-53
325. Staff C, Mozaffari F, Haller BK, Wahren B, Liljefors M. A Phase I Safety Study of Plasmid DNA Immunization Targeting Carcinoembryonic Antigen in Colorectal Cancer Patients. *Vaccine* (2011) 29(39):6817–22. doi: 10.1016/j.vaccine.2010.12.063
326. Chudley L, McCann K, Mander A, Tjelle T, Campos-Perez J, Godeseth R, et al. DNA Fusion-Gene Vaccination in Patients With Prostate Cancer Induces High-Frequency CD8(+) T-Cell Responses and Increases PSA Doubling Time. *Cancer Immunol Immunother* (2012) 61(11):2161–70. doi: 10.1007/s00262-012-1270-0
327. Ginsberg BA, Gallardo HF, Rasalan TS, Adamow M, Mu Z, Tandon S, et al. Immunologic Response to Xenogeneic Gp100 DNA in Melanoma Patients: Comparison of Particle-Mediated Epidermal Delivery With Intramuscular Injection. *Clin Cancer Res* (2010) 16(15):4057–65. doi: 10.1158/1078-0432.CCR-10-1093
328. Cafri G, Gartner JJ, Zaks T, Hopson K, Levin N, Paria BC, et al. mRNA Vaccine-Induced Neoantigen-Specific T Cell Immunity in Patients With Gastrointestinal Cancer. *J Clin Invest* (2020) 130(11):5976–88. doi: 10.1172/JCI134915
329. Sadanaga N, Nagashima H, Mashino K, Tahara K, Yamaguchi H, Ohta M, et al. Dendritic Cell Vaccination With MAGE Peptide is a Novel Therapeutic Approach for Gastrointestinal Carcinomas. *Clin Cancer Res* (2001) 7 (8):2277–84.
330. Lion E, Smits EL, Berneman ZN, Van Tendeloo VF. NK Cells: Key to Success of DC-based Cancer Vaccines? *Oncologist* (2012) 17(10):1256–70. doi: 10.1634/theoncologist.2011-0122
331. Hammerich L, Binder A, Brody JD. *In Situ* Vaccination: Cancer Immunotherapy Both Personalized and Off-the-Shelf. *Mol Oncol* (2015) 9 (10):1966–81. doi: 10.1016/j.molonc.2015.10.016
332. Sheen MR, Fiering S. In Situ Vaccination: Harvesting Low Hanging Fruit on the Cancer Immunotherapy Tree. *Wiley Interdiscip Rev Nanomed Nanobiotechnol* (2019) 11(1):e1524. doi: 10.1002/wnan.1524
333. Cebon J. Perspective: Cancer Vaccines in the Era of Immune Checkpoint Blockade. *Mamm Genome* (2018) 29(11-12):703–13. doi: 10.1007/s00335-018-9786-z
334. Mougel A, Terme M, Tanchot C. Therapeutic Cancer Vaccine and Combinations With Antiangiogenic Therapies and Immune Checkpoint Blockade. *Front Immunol* (2019) 10:467. doi: 10.3389/fimmu.2019.00467
335. Stojdl DF, Lichty B, Knowles S, Marius R, Atkins H, Sonenberg N, et al. Exploiting Tumor-Specific Defects in the Interferon Pathway With a Previously Unknown Oncolytic Virus. *Nat Med* (2000) 6(7):821–5. doi: 10.1038/77558
336. Coffey MC, Strong JE, Forsyth PA, Lee PW. Reovirus Therapy of Tumors With Activated Ras Pathway. *Science* (1998) 282(5392):1332–4. doi: 10.1126/science.282.5392.1332
337. Yokoda RT, Nagalo BM, Borad MJ. Oncolytic Adenoviruses in Gastrointestinal Cancers. *Biomedicines* (2018) 6(1):33. doi: 10.3390/biomedicines6010033
338. Rahman MM, McFadden G. Oncolytic Virotherapy With Myxoma Virus. *J Clin Med* (2020) 9(1):171. doi: 10.3390/jcm9010171
339. Abate-Daga D, Andreu N, Camacho-Sanchez J, Alemany R, Herance R, Millan O, et al. Oncolytic Adenoviruses Armed With Thymidine Kinase can be Traced by PET Imaging and Show Potent Antitumoural Effects by Ganciclovir Dosing. *PloS One* (2011) 6(10):e26142. doi: 10.1371/journal.pone.0026142
340. Galanis E, Atherton PJ, Maurer MJ, Knutson KL, Dowdy SC, Cliby WA, et al. Oncolytic Measles Virus Expressing the Sodium Iodide Symporter to Treat Drug-Resistant Ovarian Cancer. *Cancer Res* (2015) 75(1):22–30. doi: 10.1158/0008-5472.CAN-14-2533
341. McCart JA, Mehta N, Scollard D, Reilly RM, Carrasquillo JA, Tang N, et al. Oncolytic Vaccinia Virus Expressing the Human Somatostatin Receptor SSTR2: Molecular Imaging After Systemic Delivery Using 111In-Pentetreotide. *Mol Ther* (2004) 10(3):553–61. doi: 10.1016/j.ymthe.2004.06.158
342. Barton KN, Stricker H, Brown SL, Elshaikh M, Aref I, Lu M, et al. Phase I Study of Noninvasive Imaging of Adenovirus-Mediated Gene Expression in the Human Prostate. *Mol Ther* (2008) 16(10):1761–9. doi: 10.1038/mt.2008.172
343. Jacobs A, Tjuvajev JG, Dubrovin M, Akhurst T, Balatoni J, Beattie B, et al. Positron Emission Tomography-Based Imaging of Transgene Expression Mediated by Replication-Conditional, Oncolytic Herpes Simplex Virus Type 1 Mutant Vectors In Vivo. *Cancer Res* (2001) 61(7):2983–95.
344. Zellmer VR, Zhang S. Evolving Concepts of Tumor Heterogeneity. *Cell Biosci* (2014) 4:69. doi: 10.1186/2045-3701-4-69
345. McGranahan N, Swanton C. Clonal Heterogeneity and Tumor Evolution: Past, Present, and the Future. *Cell* (2017) 168(4):613–28. doi: 10.1016/j.cell.2017.01.018
346. Parikh AR, Leshchiner I, Elagina L, Goyal L, Levovitz C, Siravegna G, et al. Liquid Versus Tissue Biopsy for Detecting Acquired Resistance and Tumor Heterogeneity in Gastrointestinal Cancers. *Nat Med* (2019) 25(9):1415–21. doi: 10.1038/s41591-019-0561-9
347. Aravanis AM, Lee M, Klausner RD. Next-Generation Sequencing of Circulating Tumor DNA for Early Cancer Detection. *Cell* (2017) 168 (4):571–4. doi: 10.1016/j.cell.2017.01.030
348. Hass R, von der Ohe J, Ungefroren H. Impact of the Tumor Microenvironment on Tumor Heterogeneity and Consequences for Cancer Cell Plasticity and Stemness. *Cancers (Basel)* (2020) 12(12):3716. doi: 10.3390/cancers12123716
349. Yuan Y. Spatial Heterogeneity in the Tumor Microenvironment. *Cold Spring Harb Perspect Med* (2016) 6(8):a026583. doi: 10.1101/cshperspect.a026583
350. Cell Editorial T. Cancer: The Road Ahead. *Cell* (2017) 168(4):545–6. doi: 10.1016/j.cell.2017.01.036
351. El-Deiry WS, Taylor B, Neal JW. Tumor Evolution, Heterogeneity, and Therapy for Our Patients With Advanced Cancer: How Far Have We Come? *Am Soc Clin Oncol Educ Book* (2017) 37:e8–15. doi: 10.14694/EDBK_175524

4

siRNAs Targeting Mouse-Specific lncRNA AA388235 Induce Human Tumor Cell Pyroptosis/Apoptosis

Yan-Ru Chen[1,2†], Wan-Ying Feng[1†], Yuan-Xiong Cheng[3], Hao Zhu[4], Hong-Juan Liu ,
Yi Gao[5] and Wei-Jie Zhou[1,3,5,6,7*]

[1] State Key Laboratory of Organ Failure Research, Guangdong Province Key Laboratory of Molecular Tumor Pathology, Department of Pathology, Nanfang Hospital, School of Basic Medical Sciences, Southern Medical University, Guangzhou, China, [2] Department of Research and Teaching, Huizhou Municipal Central Hospital, Huizhou, China, [3] Department of Respiratory and Critical Care Medicine, The Third Affiliated Hospital, Southern Medical University, Guangzhou, China, [4] Department of Bioinformation, School of Basic Medical Sciences, Southern Medical University, Guangzhou, China, [5] General Surgery Center, Department of Hepatobiliary Surgery II, Guangdong Provincial, Research Center for Artificial Organ and Tissue Engineering, Guangzhou Clinical Research and Transformation Center for Artificial Liver, Institute of Regenerative Medicine, Zhujiang Hospital, Southern Medical University, Guangzhou, China, [6] Microbiome Medicine Center, Zhujiang Hospital, Southern Medical University, Guangzhou, China, [7] Bioland Laboratory (Guangzhou Regenerative Medicine and Health Guangdong Laboratory), Guangzhou, China

***Correspondence:**
Wei-Jie Zhou
weijiezhouum@163.com

†These authors have contributed equally to this work and share first authorship

Species-specific lncRNAs significantly determine species-specific functions through various ways, such as epigenetic regulation. However, there has been no study focusing on the role of species-specific lncRNAs in other species yet. Here, we found that siRNAs targeting mouse-specific lncRNA AA388235 could significantly induce death of human tumor cells, although it has no effect on mouse tumor cells and normal human cells. The mechanism studies showed that these siRNAs could activate the response of human tumor cells to exogenous nucleic acids, induce pyroptosis and apoptosis in the presence of GSDME, but induce apoptosis in the absence of GSDME. They also significantly inhibited the growth of human tumor cells *in vivo*. 17 siRNAs were designed for seven more mouse-specific lncRNAs selected randomly, among which 12 siRNAs targeting five lncRNAs induced death in human tumor cell. Our study not only demonstrates that the siRNAs designed for knocking down mouse-specific lncRNA AA388235 can be potential tumor therapeutic drugs, but also suggests that non-human species-specific lncRNAs are a huge potential library that can be used to design siRNAs for tumor treatment. Large-scale screening based on this is promising.

Keywords: siRNAs, lncRNAs, pyroptosis, apoptosis, tumor

INTRODUCTION

The sequencing of the human genome has revealed that only ~1.2% of the human genome encodes for protein-coding genes, yet the large majority of the human genome is transcribed into non-protein-coding RNAs (ncRNAs) (1, 2). Long non-coding RNAs (lncRNAs) represent the largest group of non-coding RNAs produced from the genome. In the most recent GENCODE V30 release, there are 16,193 annotated lncRNAs in the human genome (3). lncRNAs are defined as transcripts longer than 200 nucleotides that are not translated into proteins, although some transcripts annotated as lncRNAs in fact encode for small proteins (4, 5). They comprise intergenic transcripts (lincRNAs), enhancer RNAs (eRNAs), and sense or antisense transcripts of protein-coding genes (3–6). lncRNAs are reported to have diverse functions, including organization of nuclear architecture, transcription regulation in cis or trans, modulation of mRNA stability, translation and post-translational modification (7, 8).

Compared with highly conserved protein-coding RNAs, lncRNAs generally are poorly conserved and many lncRNA genes are clade- and species-specific (3–9). A recent study reports that lncRNAs evolve rapidly, with >70% of lncRNAs having no sequence-similar orthologs in species separated by >50 million years of evolutionary divergence (8). Increasing reports show that species-specific lncRNAs significantly determine species-specific epigenetic regulation (10–12). However, no studies paid attention to the roles of species-specific lncRNAs in other species.

AA388235 is a mouse-specific lncRNA with a length of 3,867 bp, located in chr17:33981491–33985358, mainly expressed in the testis and heart (13). So far, there is no report focusing on its function. First of all, we randomly designed six siRNAs to knock down lncRNA AA388235. Unexpectedly, although these siRNAs had no effect on the death of mouse tumor cells and normal human cells, they caused death of human colorectal tumor cells and breast tumor cells. These siRNAs increased the response of human tumor cells to exogenous nucleic acids, induced pyroptosis and apoptosis in the presence of GSDME (Gasdermin E), but induced apoptosis in the absence of GSDME. In addition, we randomly designed 17 siRNAs for seven more mouse-specific lncRNAs. 12 of the 17 siRNAs (targeting five different lncRNAs) induced death of human colorectal tumor cells, suggesting that species-specific lncRNAs other than human can be used as targets for designing siRNAs for tumor therapy.

MATERIALS AND METHODS

Antibodies and Reagents

The antibodies to detect P-PKR (ab81303, 1:1,000), GSDME (ab215191, 1:1,000), GSDMA (ab230768, 1:500), and GSDMB (ab215729, 1:500) were obtained from Abcam. Antibodies against caspase-3 (9662S, 1:1,000), cleaved-caspase-3 (9664T, 1:500), PARP (9532T, 1:1,000), MAVS (3993T, 1:1,000), and MDA5 (5321T, 1:1,000) were purchased from Cell Signaling Technologies. Antibodies targeting GSDMD (20770-1-AP, 1:1,000), GSDMC (27630-1-AP, 1:1,000), and caspase9 (10380-1-AP, 1:1,000) were obtained from Proteintech. Anti-RIGI (sc-376845, 1:200) and Anti-TLR3 (sc-32232, 1:200) were obtained from Santa Cruz Biotechnology. Anti-a-tubulin (RM2007, 1:10,000) was obtained from Ray. Caspase-3 inhibitors Z-DEVD-FMK (S7312, 40 μM) were purchased from Selleck.

Cell Culture

Mouse colorectal tumor cell lines MC38 and CT26 were kindly provided by Professor Wei Yang of the Southern Medical University. Human normal intestinal epithelial cells NCM460 were kindly provided by Professor Side Liu of Nanfang Hospital. Human colorectal tumor cell lines HCT116 and DLD1, mouse breast tumor lines 4T1, human breast tumor cell lines MDA-MB-453, and human normal intestinal epithelial cells FHC were obtained from the American Type Culture Collection (ATCC, Philadelphia, PA, USA). MC38, CT26, and MDA-MB-453 cells were cultured in DMEM (GIBCO) supplemented with 10% fetal bovine serum (FBS). FHCs were cultured in DMEM (GIBCO) supplemented with 20% fetal bovine serum (FBS). HCT116, DLD1, NCM460, and 4T1 cells were cultured in RPMI 1640 (GIBCO) supplemented with 10% fetal bovine serum (FBS). All cells were cultured at 37°C in a humidified 5% CO_2 incubator.

Plasmids, siRNAs and Transfection

Penter-human-GSDME-FLAG, PCDNA3.1-mouse-Gsdme-FLAG, PCDNA3.1-mouse-AA388235, and relative negative control plasmids were purchased from Vigene (Shan Dong, China). shNC, shAA388235-2 and shAA388235-6 were purchased from Gene (Shang Hai, China). DsDNAs and siRNAs including ssRNA and dsRNA were synthesized from RiboBio (Guangzhou, China), and all the sequences are listed in **Supplementary Table S1**. For siRNA transfection, cells were plated with 40% confluence in six-well plates, and 50 nM siRNA mixed with 5 μl Lipofectamine 3000 (Invitrogen) was added into the cells after 24 h according to the protocol offered by the manufacturer. For siRNA co-transfection with plasmid, cells were plated with 40% confluence in six-well plates; 50 nM siRNA and 2 μg plasmids mixed with the mixture of 5 μl Lipofectamine 3000 and 10 μl P3000 (Invitrogen) were added into the cells after 24 h. For Z-DEVD treatment, after transfection of the siRNA mixture, 40 μM Z-DEVD was added immediately.

Microscopy Images

Cells were seeded in the six-well plate format (NEST, China) and treated as indicated. Then static bright-field cell images were captured using an Olympus CKX31 microscope at room temperature. The pictures shown in the figures were processed using ImageJ software. Then the dead cells were washed off with PBS, and the living cells were captured to measure the area percentage of survival cells using Image J software from five independent perspectives.

SiAA388235-2/4/5/6 Off-Target Prediction

The prediction of siAA388235-2/4/5/6 off-target gene was mainly based on the complementary pairing of siAA388235-2/4/5/6 and the gene, which referred to miRNA. Different software had different algorithms for predicting target genes, and we mainly predicted the off-target gene of siAA388235-2/4/5/6 through four databases: TargetScan, miRanda, RNAhybrid, and pita. We further screened and sorted out the prediction results of the four databases or the random three databases, and the same target genes presented in four or three online databases were considered as potential targets of siAA388235-2/4/5/6.

RNA Extraction and Quantitative Real-Time PCR

For the Quantitative Real-Time PCR assay, total RNA from cell lines was extracted by Trizol (Takara, Japan) and then reverse-transcribed into cDNA using M-MLV reverse transcriptase (Takara, Japan). qRT–PCR analysis was performed on Applied Biosystems 7500 Fast Real-Time PCR System with the SYBR Premix Ex Taq (Takara, Japan). Primers used for qRT–PCR analysis are listed in **Supplementary Table S2**. All data were using endogenous GAPDH as an internal control.

Western Blot

Cells were lysed in lysis solution (P0013, Beyotime, China) buffer supplemented with PMSF and under ultrasonic treatment before being boiled in 5× SDS loading buffer (WB-0091, Dingguo, China). Equal amounts of proteins were separated in 10% gradient SDS-PAGE and then electroblotted onto polyvinylidene fluoride (PVDF) membranes, which were then blocked with 5% milk in 0.1% TBST buffer for 1 h before incubation with primary antibodies at 4°C overnight. After washing with TBST 5 min each time for five times, the polyvinylidene fluoride membrane was incubated with appropriate secondary antibody for 1 h at room temperature. The bands were detected using the enhanced chemiluminescence detection system (Amersham Biosciences Europe, Freiberg, Germany).

LDH Release Assay

Culture supernatants were collected and centrifuged at 250×g for 5 min after treatments. The LDH concentration was measured with the CytoTox 96 cytotoxicity assay (G1780, Promega, USA) at 490 nm according to the protocol offered by the manufacturer. The percentage of LDH release was calculated as follows: (Sample − Background)/(Maximum − Background) × 100%. Each subject was repeated at least three times.

ATP Cell Viability

To evaluate the overall cell death, we used the CellTiter-Glo kit (G7570, Promega, USA) to assess cell viability by measuring ATP level. The substrate luciferin and the enzyme luciferase were added into lysed cells to attach to the ATP; the ATP level of treated cells was normalized to the control cells.

FACS Analysis

Dead and living cells were collected, washed with cold PBS twice, and stained with the FITC-labeled Annexin V and PI (propidium iodide) according to the manufacturer's recommendation (KGA107, KeyGEN BioTECH, China). After staining, data would be collected by BD FACSCanto II (BD Biosciences) and analyzed by FlowJo V.10 (TreeStar) software. Cell death was assessed by counting Annexin V positive cells. The percentage of Annexin$^+$ cells is the sum of PI$^+$/Annexin V$^+$ and PI$^-$/Annexin V$^+$ cells.

Xenograft Mouse Model

Female BALB/c nude mice (4 weeks old) were purchased from the Animal Center of Southern Medical University, Guangzhou, China (NO: 2019038). All the mice used in this study were housed under the specific pathogen-free environment, and animal experiments were conducted in accordance with standard procedures and approved by the Institutional Use Committee for Animal Care. All mice were maintained in a sterile environment. Cells HCT116-shNC (1×10^6), HCT116-shAA388235-2 (1×10^6), and HCT116-shAA388235-6 (1×10^6) were injected into the right flank of the nude mice. Measurement of tumors started 4 days after injection with one measurement every three days. 40 days after injection, the mice were sacrificed; the tumors were excised, weighed, and photographed.

Statistical Analysis

Data were calculated using SPSS 21.0 (SPSS Inc., Chicago, IL, USA) and GraphPad Prism 6.0 (GraphPad Software Inc., San Diego, CA, USA) then were statistically analyzed by Student's t-test or analysis of variance (ANOVA). In all cases, data from at least three independent experiments are represented as the mean ± standard error of the mean (SEM). P <0.05 was considered to be statistically significant.

RESULTS

siRNAs Targeting Mouse-Specific lncRNA AA388235 Induce Human Tumor Cells Death

LncRNA AA388235 is low conserved among species and expressed in mouse but not human (**Figure 1A**). So far, no studies have explored the function of lncRNA AA388235. We first randomly designed six siRNAs targeting mouse lncRNA AA388235. Then, we found that these siRNAs could knocked down the expression of lncRNA AA388235 in mouse colorectal tumor cell lines MC38 and CT26 cells (**Figures 1B, C**). However, they had no effect on the death of MC38 and CT26 cells (**Figures 1D–G**). Neither did they have any effect on the death of mouse breast tumor cells 4T1 (**Supplementary Figures S1A, B**). Surprisingly, four of the six siRNAs targeting mouse lncRNA AA388235 (siAA388235-2, siAA388235-4, siAA388235-5, and siAA388235-6) induced death in human colorectal tumor cell line HCT116 and DLD1; siAA388235-1 had no effect on HCT116 but seemed to inhibit the growth of DLD1 due to fewer survival cells without shedding cells in the phenotype, and siAA388235-3 also seemed to inhibit the growth of HCT116 and DLD1 cells due to fewer survival cells without shedding cells in the phenotype (**Figures 1H–K** and **Supplementary Figures S1C–F**).SiAA388235-2, siAA388235-4, siAA388235-5, and siAA388235-6 also showed death activity in human breast tumor cell line MDA-MB-453 (**Supplementary Figures S1G, H**). However, siAA388235-1/2/3/4/5/6 did not induce death in FHC (human normal intestinal epithelial cells), MCF12A (human normal breast epithelial cells), and HEK293 (human embryonic kidney epithelial cells). In addition, some siRNAs increased the growth of MCF12A and HEK293 cells for unknown reasons (**Supplementary Figures S1I–N**). No death was also observed with the transfection of siAA388235-1/3/4/5/6 into NCM460 (human normal intestinal epithelial cells) except the

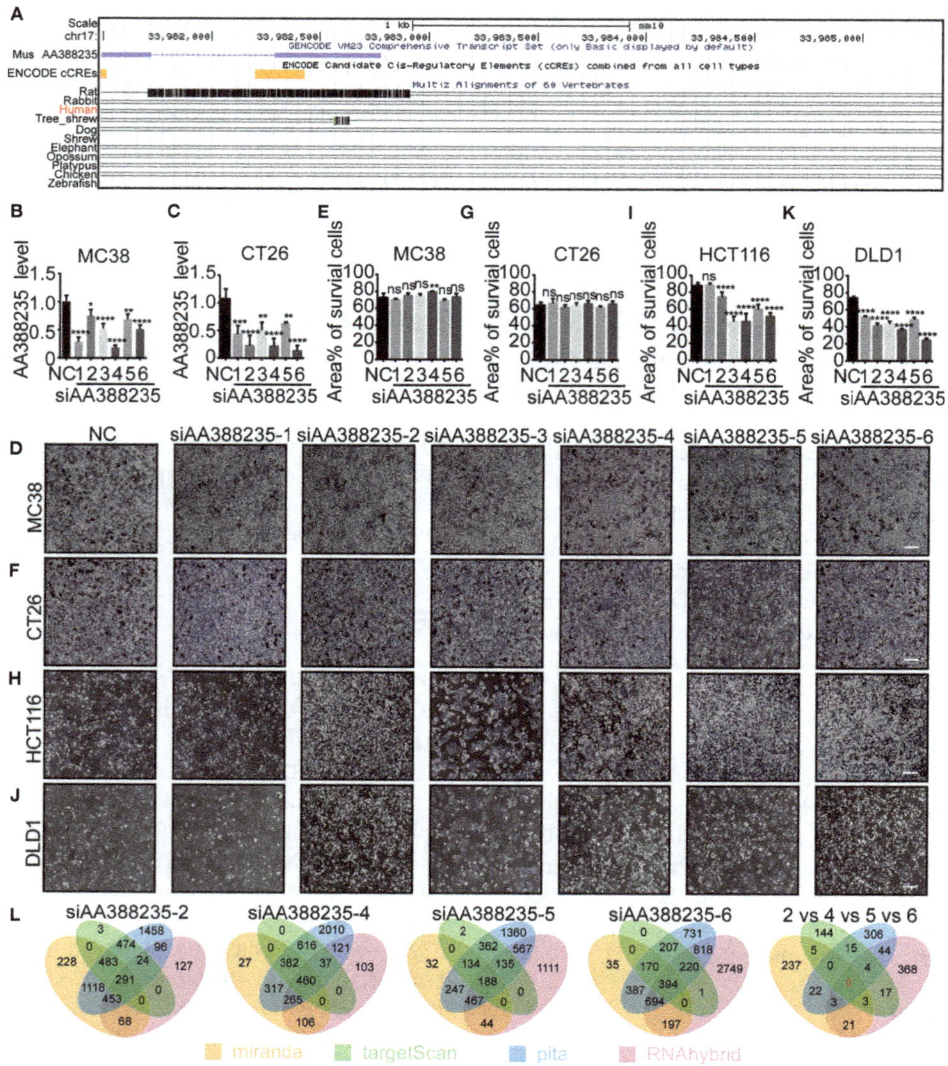

FIGURE 1 | siRNAs targeting mouse-specific lncRNA AA388235 induce human colorectal tumor cells death. **(A)** Graphical views showing multiple-species conversation comparisons with mouse LncRNA AA388235 using UCSC genome browser. The conservation scores were indicated by the gray peaks. **(B, C)** "NC" was a random arrangement and meaningless 19 bp siRNA, which was desired by RiboBio to act as the negative control."siAA388235-1/2/3/4/5/6"meant six 19 bp siRNAs targeting six different regions of mouse LncRNA AA388235. The AA388235 level in MC38 and CT26 cells transfected with siRNAs as indicated. *P* value was calculated by one-way ANOVA. **(D–G)** MC38 and CT26 were seeded and treated as indicated. After 48 h, the static bright-field cell images were captured **(D, F)**. Then the dead cells were washed off with PBS, and the living cells were captured to measure the area percentage of survival cells using Image J software from five independent perspectives **(E, G)**. Scale bar, 200μm. *P* value was calculated by one-way ANOVA. **(H–K)** HCT116 and DLD1 were seeded and treated as indicated. After 48 h, the static bright-field cell images were captured **(H, J)**. Then the dead cells were washed off with PBS, and the living cells were captured to measure the area percentage of survival cells using Image J software from five independent perspectives **(I, K)**. Scale bar, 200μm. *P* value was calculated by one-way ANOVA. **(L)** Prediction of off-target genes of siAA388235 using database: miranda, targetScan, pita, and RNAhybrid. "2 *vs* 4 *vs* 5 *vs* 6" meant the prediction of common off-target genes between the siAA388235-2,4,5, and 6. There were no common off-target genes between the siAA388235-2,4,5, and 6 in four databases and ten off-target genes in random three databases including AHRR, C3ORF14, SLC15A2, COQ8A, FAM46C, GOLGA8H, TNRC6C, TLK2,PAGR1, PGS1. Mean ± SEM, $^{*}P < 0.05$, $^{**}P < 0.01$, $^{***}P < 0.001$, $^{****}P < 0.0001$, "ns" indicates no significance.

siAA388235-2 which induced slight death (**Supplementary Figures S1O, P**).

Since lncRNA AA388235 is absent in human cells, we first suspected that the cell death was due to off-target effects of these siRNAs. Miranda, targetscan, pita, and rnahybrid databases were applied to predict the off-target genes of these siRNAs.The results showed that there was no common target gene recognized by four databases among siAA388235-2, siAA388235-4, siAA388235-5, and siAA388235-6, and that 10 genes were recognized by three random databases including AHRR, C3orf14, SLC15A2, COQ8A,

FAM46C, GOLGA8H, TNRC6C, TLK2, PAGR1, PGS1 (**Figure 1L**). However, using qPCR assay, we found that there was no correlation between the mRNA level of these ten genes and the four siRNAs targeting mouse lncRNA AA388235 (siAA388235-2, siAA388235-4, siAA388235-5, and siAA388235-6), which further indicated that the death activity caused by siRNAs targeting mouse lncRNA AA388235 was not because they happened to target one common human gene (**Supplementary Figure S2**).

siRNAs Targeting Mouse-Specific lncRNA AA388235 Induce Human Tumor Cells Pyroptosis or Apoptosis

Next, we explored the mechanism how siRNAs targeting mouse-specific lncRNA AA388235 induce human colorectal tumor cells' death. siRNAs No. 2 (siAA388235-2) and No. 6 (siAA388235-6) of the six siRNAs were used for the following experiments. We found that the dying HCT116 cells showed evident swelling with characteristic large bubbles from the plasma membrane indicating pyroptosis and shrank and agglomerated indicating apoptosis (**Figure 2A**). Whereas the dying DLD1 cells shrank and agglomerated indicating apoptosis (**Figure 2B**). Recently, Gasdermin E (GSDME) was reported to be cleaved and activated by caspase-3 to cause pyroptosis; therefore it's expression determined the form of death in caspase-3-activated cells (14, 15). In this study, we found that GSDME was expressed in HCT116 cells and was cleaved upon siRNAs targeting mouse-specific lncRNA AA388235 stimulation (**Figure 2C**), whereas DLD1 cells did not express GSDME with or without siRNA treatment (**Figure 2D**). The other gasdermins (GSDMA, GSDMB, GSDMC, GSDMD) were not expressed or cleaved in DLD1 cells either (**Figure 2E**). The nature of cell death was further confirmed by a lactate dehydrogenase (LDH)-release assay (**Figures 2F, G**). Moreover, overexpression of GSDME in DLD1 cells caused an apoptosis-to-pyroptosis switch upon siAA388235-2 and siAA388235-6 stimulation (**Figures 2H–J**). Similarly, human breast tumor cell line MDA-MB-453, which expressed a high level of GSDME, processed pyroptosis and apoptosis (**Supplementary Figures S3A–C**). However, siAA388235-2 and siAA388235-6 failed to induce pyroptosis or apoptosis in normal human cell lines FHC, MCF12A, and HEK293, regardless of whether the cells expressed GSDME or not (**Supplementary Figures S3D–I**). siAA388235-2 induced slight pyroptosis/apoptosis and the cleavage of GSDME/caspase-3 in NCM460, but siAA388235-6 had no such effect (**Supplementary Figures S3J, K**).

Meanwhile, pyroptosis/apoptosis induced by siAA388235-2 or siAA388235-6 was not observed in mouse colorectal tumor cell lines MC38 and CT26, regardless of whether the cells expressed Gsdme or not (**Supplementary Figures S4A–D**). Overexpression of Gsdme induced MC38 cells pyroptosis, but the cells did not respond to siAA388235-2 and siAA388235-6 (**Supplementary Figures S4E–G**). These results demonstrated that siRNAs targeting mouse-specific lncRNA AA388235 induced human tumor cell pyroptosis and apoptosis in the presence of GSDME, whereas induced human tumor cell apoptosis in the absence of GSDME.

Caspase-3 Activation Is Necessary for siRNAs Targeting Mouse-Specific lncRNA AA388235 to Induce Human Tumor Cells Pyroptosis or Apoptosis

Caspase-3 has long been regarded as the hallmark of apoptosis. Recent studies have shown that GSDME is cleaved and activated by caspase-3, which causes pyroptosis (14, 15). To explore whether caspase-3 activation is necessary for cell pyroptosis or apoptosis induced by siRNAs targeting mouse-specific lncRNA AA388235, caspase-3 inhibitor Z-DEVD was employed. Then, the result showed that caspase-3 cleavage induced by siAA388235-2 and siAA388235-6 was inhibited by Z-DEVD both in HCT116 cells and DLD1 cells (**Figures 3A, B**). Furthermore, both pyroptosis and apoptosis of HCT116 cells and apoptosis of DLD1 cells were inhibited by Z-DEVD (**Figures 3C, D**). These fundings support that caspase-3 activation is necessary for siRNAs targeting mouse-specific lncRNA AA388235 to trigger pyroptosis and apoptosis in human tumor cell.

siRNAs Targeting Mouse-Specific lncRNA AA388235 Increase RNA Sensor

As siRNAs targeting mouse-specific lncRNA AA388235 are exogenous nucleic acids to human cells, we explored whether they activated host defense pathways. The result showed that the cytosolic double-stranded RNA (dsRNA) sensor RIG-I, MDA5, and MAVS (16, 17) were upregulated upon siAA388235-2 and siAA388235-6 stimulation, whereas the levels of TLR3 (18) and P-PKR did not change (**Figure 3E**). Caspase-9, as the initiator caspase of the intrinsic apoptosis pathway (19), was also activated with the treatment of siAA388235-2 and siAA388235-6 (**Figure 3F**).

The Form of dsRNA Is Necessary for siRNAs Targeting Mouse-Specific lncRNA AA388235 to Induce Human Tumor Cells Pyroptosis or Apoptosis

As a double-strand RNA (dsRNA), siRNA consists of two complementary pairs of strands: the strand that determines the specificity of the targeting mRNA serves as the guide RNA, and the other one is a passenger RNA. To test whether the form of dsRNA is necessary for siRNAs targeting mouse-specific lncRNA AA388235 to induce human tumor cells' pyroptosis or apoptosis, we designed the following experiments. HCT116 cells and DLD1 cells were transfected with dsRNA, single-anti-sense-strand of siRNA (guide), single-sense-strand of siRNA (passenger), single-anti-sense-strand of siRNA plus single-sense-strand of siRNA (guide + passenger) and double-strand DNA (dsDNA), respectively. We found that only dsRNA induced human tumor cells' pyroptosis and apoptosis (**Figure 4A**) or apoptosis only (**Figure 4B**). Consistently, cleavage of GSDME, caspase-3 and poly ADP-ribose polymerase (PARP) was observed only in HCT116 cells transfected with dsRNA (**Figure 4C**), and cleavage of caspase-3 and PARP was observed only in DLD1 cells transfected with dsRNA (**Figure 4D**). Furthermore, short hairpin RNAs (shRNAs) targeting mouse-specific lncRNA

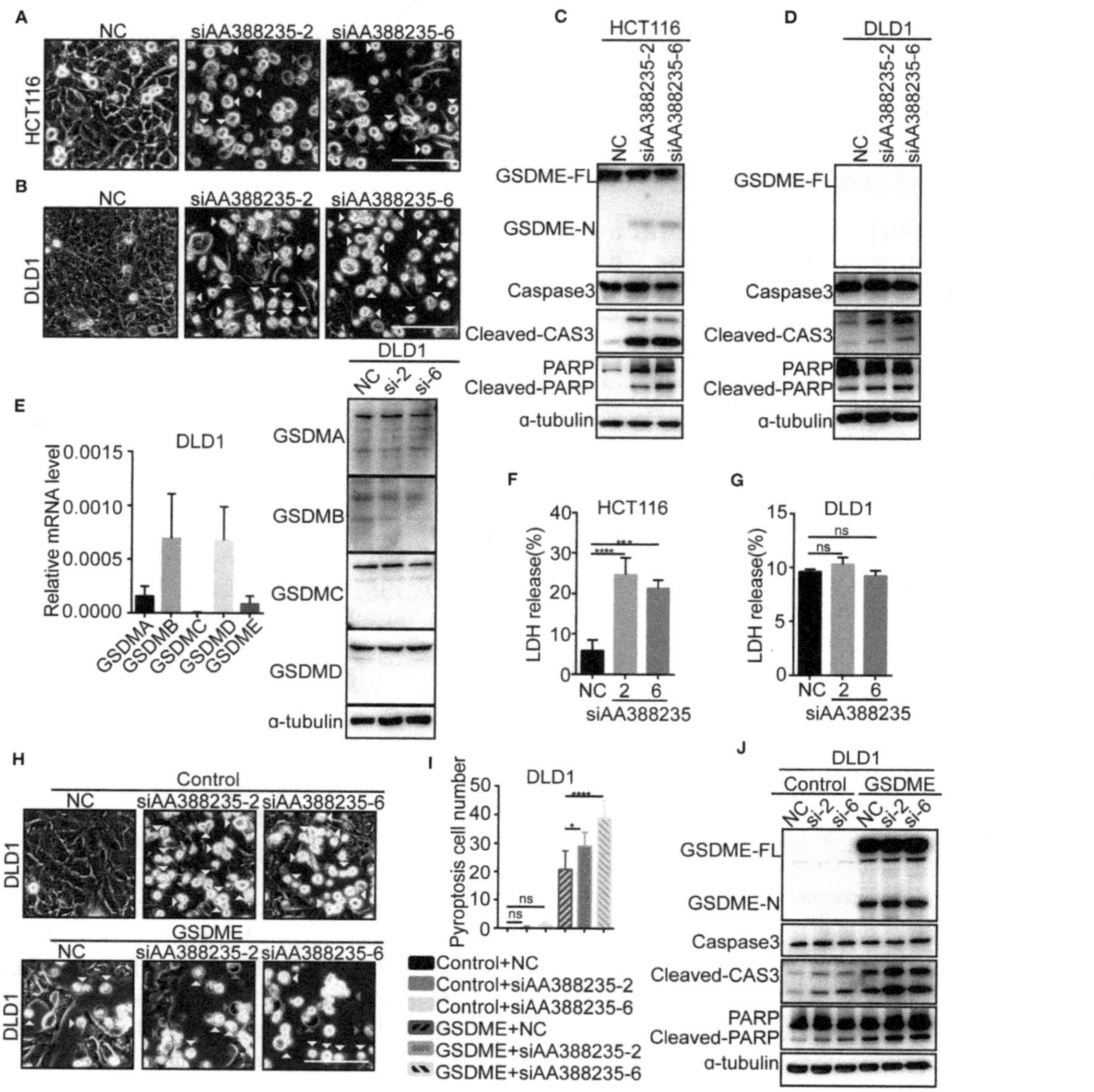

FIGURE 2 | siRNAs targeting mouse-specific lncRNA AA388235 induce human colorectal tumor cells pyroptosis or apoptosis. **(A, B)** Microscopic images of HCT116 and DLD1 cells transfected with siRNAs as indicated. Red arrowheads indicated the pyroptotic cells, and yellow arrowheads indicated the apoptosis cells. Scale bar, 100 μm. **(C, D)** Immunoblotting assay of HCT116 and DLD1 cells transfected as indicated. GSDME-FL, full-length of GSDME; GSDME-N, the N-terminal cleavage of GSDME; Cleaved-CAS3, the cleavage of caspase-3 p19/p17; cleaved-PARP, the cleavage of PARP. **(E)** The mRNA level of GSDM families in wild-type DLD1 cells and the protein level of GSDM families in DLD1 cells transfected with siRNA as indicated. si-2, siAA388235-2; si-6, siAA388235-6. **(F, G)** Comparison of LDH release-based cell death in HCT116 and DLD1 cells transfected with the siRNAs as indicated. *P* value was calculated by one-way ANOVA. **(H)** Microscopic images of DLD1 cells co-transfected with GSDME and siRNA as indicated. Red arrowheads indicate the pyroptotic cells, and yellow arrowheads indicate the apoptosis cells. Scale bar, 100 μm. **(I)** The numbers of the pyroptotic cells of DLD1 co-transfected with GSDME and siRNAs as indicated were calculated in randomly select five fields of view (×200). *P* value was calculated by one-way ANOVA. **(J)** Immunoblotting assay of DLD1 cells co-transfected with GSDME and siRNAs as indicated. GSDME-FL, full-length of GSDME; GSDME-N, the N-terminal cleavage of GSDME; Cleaved-CAS3, the cleavage of Caspase3 p19/p17; Cleaved-PARP, the cleavage of PARP. *P* value was calculated by one-way ANOVA. si-2, siAA388235-2; si-6, siAA388235-6. Mean ± SEM, **P* < 0.05, ****P* < 0.001, *****P* < 0.0001, "ns" indicates no significance.

AA388235 also induced pyroptosis and apoptosis in HCT116 cells and apoptosis in DLD1 cells successfully (**Figures 4E–H**). The primary transcript of shRNA contains a hairpin like stem-loop structure, which is transported to the cytoplasm where the loop of the hairpin is processed off to form a double-stranded siRNA (20). These results suggest that the form of dsRNA is necessary for siRNAs targeting mouse-specific lncRNA AA388235 to induce human tumor cells' pyroptosis or apoptosis.

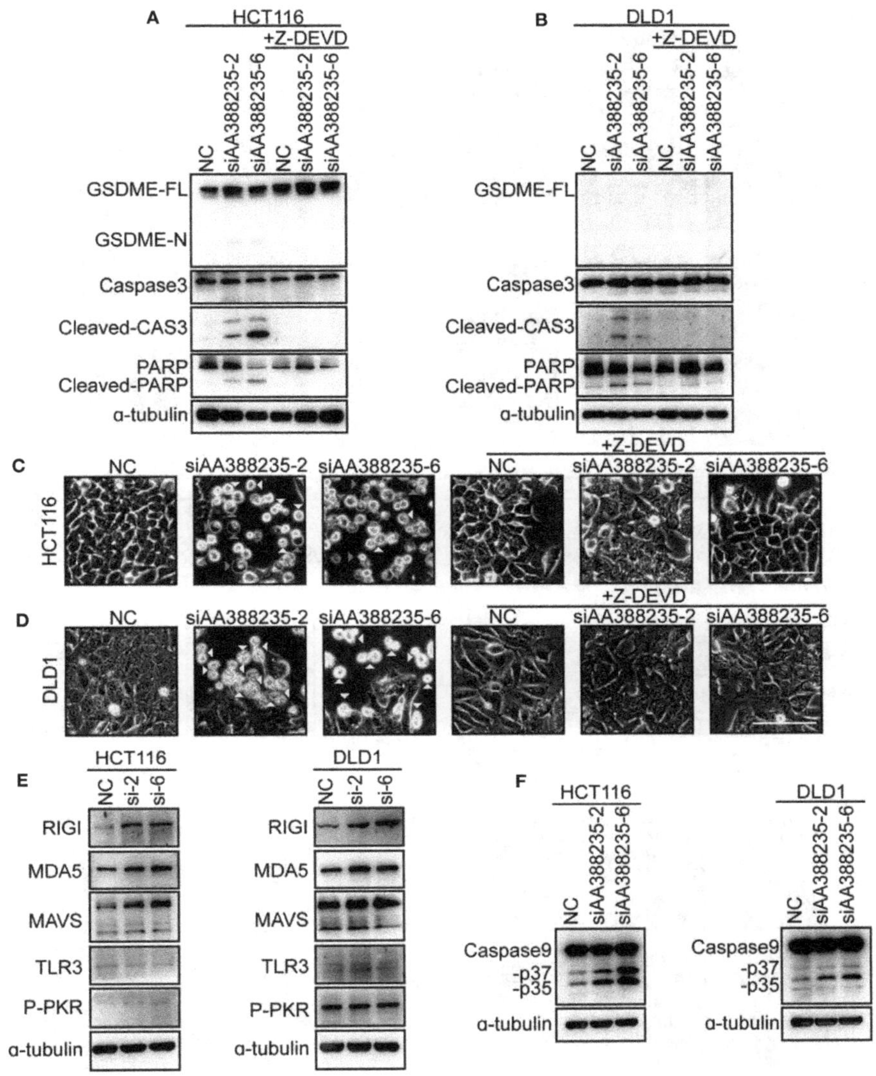

FIGURE 3 | siRNAs targeting mouse-specific lncRNA AA388235 activate caspase-3 and increase RNA sensor. **(A, B)** Effects of Z-DEVD on the cleavage of GSDME and caspase-3 in HCT116 and DLD1 cells transfected with siRNAs as indicated and treated with caspase-3 inhibitor Z-DEVD. GSDME-FL, full-length of GSDME; GSDME-N, the N-terminal cleavage of GSDME; Cleaved-CAS3, the cleavage of caspase-3 p19/p17; cleaved-PARP, the cleavage of PARP. **(C, D)** Effects of Z-DEVD on siRNAs targeting AA388235-induced pyroptosis, and apoptosis in HCT116 and DLD1 cells. Red arrowheads indicated the pyroptotic cells and yellow arrowheads indicated the apoptosis cells. Scale bar, 100 μm. **(E)** Immunoblots of MAVS, RIGI, MDA5, TLR3, and P-PKR (phosphor T451) in HCT116 and DLD1 cells transfected with siRNAs as indicated. si-2, siAA388235-2; si-6, siAA388235-6. **(F)** Immunoblots of caspase-9 in HCT116 and DLD1 cells transfected with siRNAs as indicated. -p37, the cleavage of caspase-9 p37; -p35, the cleavage of caspase-9 p35.

shRNAs Targeting Mouse-Specific lncRNA AA388235 Inhibit the Growth of Human Tumor Cells *In Vivo*

To investigate whether the shRNAs targeting mouse-specific lncRNA AA388235 inhibited the growth of human tumor cells *in vivo*, HCT116 cells transfected with control shRNA, shAA388235-2, or shAA388235-6 were subcutaneously inoculated into BALB/c nude mice. The tumor incidence and tumor size were dramatically reduced by shAA388235-2 or shAA388235-6 (**Figures 5A–C**).

Multiple siRNAs Targeting Different Mouse-Specific lncRNAs Induce Human Tumor Cells Pyroptosis or Apoptosis

There are thousands of mouse-specific lncRNAs. Seven more mouse-specific lncRNAs (GM11815, BC026762, GM15298, GM19792, GM14951, GM11851, and GM15758) were randomly selected. Conservation comparisons using UC Santa Cruz (UCSC) genome browse showed that these seven lncRNAs were not found in humans (**Supplementary Figures S5**). In total, 17 siRNAs were designed for these seven mouse-specific lncRNAs.

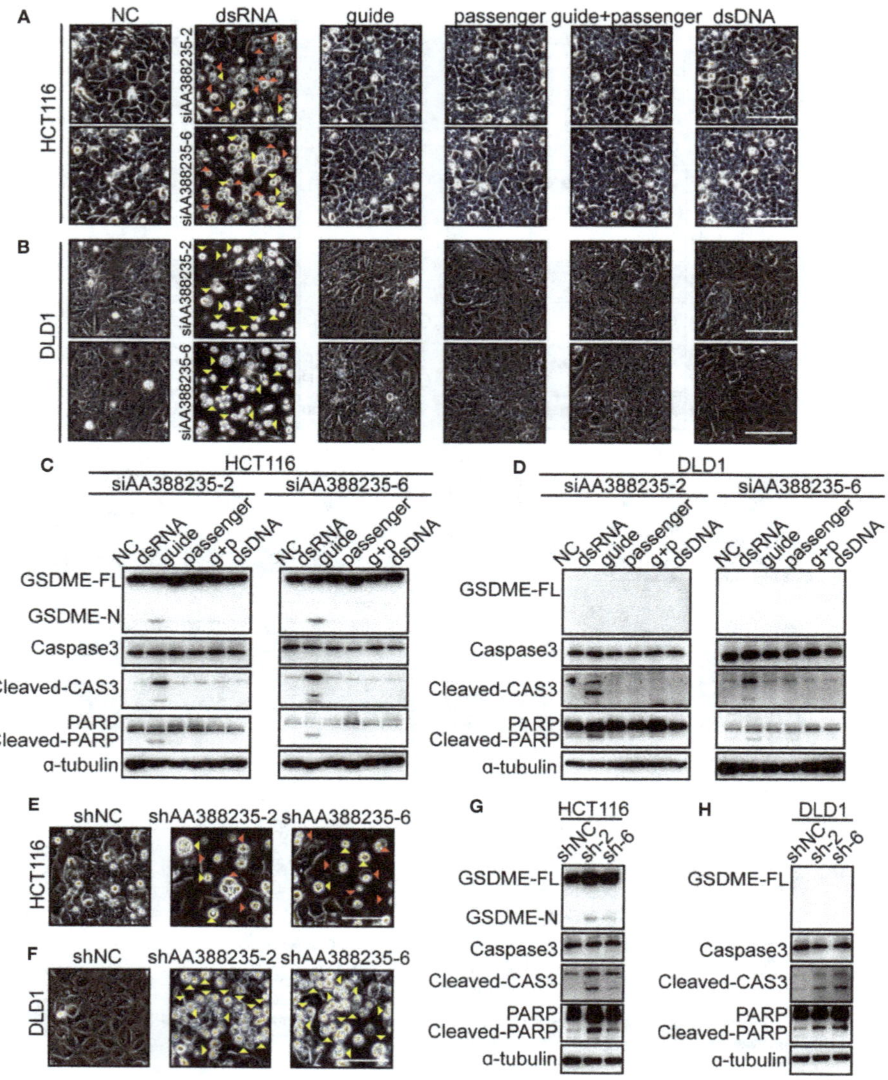

FIGURE 4 | DsRNA is necessary for siRNAs targeting mouse-specific lncRNA AA388235 to induce human tumor cell pyroptosis/apoptosis. **(A, B)** Microscopic images of HCT116 and DLD1 cells transfected as indicated. dsRNA, double-stranded siRNA; guide, single-stranded-anti-sense of siRNA; passenger, single-stranded sense of siRNA; guide + passenger, single-stranded-anti-sense of siRNA and single-stranded-sense of siRNA; dsDNA, double-stranded DNA which has the same sequence as siRNA. Red arrowheads indicated the pyroptotic cells, and yellow arrowheads indicated the apoptosis cells. Scale bar, 100 μm. **(C, D)** Immunoblotting assay of HCT116 and DLD1 cells transfected as indicated. g + p, guide + passenger, single-stranded-anti-sense of siRNA and single-stranded-sense of siRNA. GSDME-FL, full-length of GSDME; GSDME-N, the N-terminal cleavage of GSDME; Cleaved-CAS3, the cleavage of caspase-3 p19/p17; cleaved-PARP, the cleavage of PARP. **(E, F)** Microscopic images of HCT116 and DLD1 cells transfected with shRNA plasmids as indicated. Red arrowheads indicated the pyroptotic cells, and yellow arrowheads indicated the apoptosis cells. Scale bar,100μm. **(G, H)** Immunoblotting assay of HCT116 and DLD1 cells transfected with shRNA plasmids as indicated. sh-2, shAA388235-2; sh-6, shAA388235-6; GSDME-FL, full-length of GSDME; GSDME-N, the N-terminal cleavage of GSDME; Cleaved-CAS3, the cleavage of caspase-3 p19/p17; cleaved-PARP, the cleavage of PARP.

Next, we found that 12 siRNAs (targeting five different lncRNAs: GM11815, BC026762, GM15298, GM19792, and GM14951) induced HCT116 cells' pyroptosis and apoptosis (**Figures 6A–F**). Consistently, these 12 siRNAs induced cleavage of GSDME, caspase-3, and PARP (**Supplementary Figures S6A–F**). Eight siRNAs (targeting three different lncRNAs: GM11815, BC026762, and GM14951) induced DLD1 cells' apoptosis (**Figures 6G–L**). Consistently, these eight siRNAs induced cleavage of caspase-3 and PARP (**Supplementary Figures S6G–L**). Among these siRNAs, siRNAs targeting GM11815, BC026762, and GM14951 had similar functions to those targeting AA388235, which induced pyroptosis and apoptosis in HCT116 cells (**Figures 6A, B, E**) and induced apoptosis in DLD1 cells (**Figures 6G, H, K**). Whereas siRNAs targeting GM15298 induced HCT116 cells' pyroptosis and apoptosis (**Figure 6C**), inhibited DLD1 cells' growth rather than induced apoptosis (**Figure 6I**). SiRNAs targeting GM19792

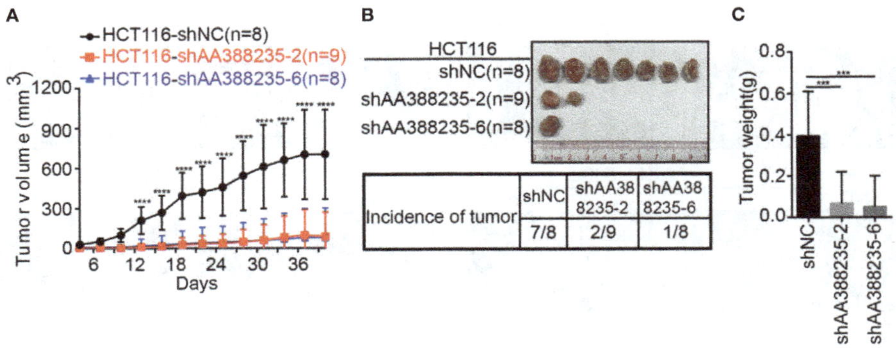

FIGURE 5 | shRNAs targeting mouse-specific lncRNA AA388235 inhibit the growth of human tumor cells *in vivo*. **(A)** Xenograft model in BALB/c nude mice, 1 × 10^6 cells as indicated were injected to the right flank of nude mice. Measurement of tumor started 4 days after injection and ended 40 days after injection. **(B)** Representative tumor samples from each injected mouse. Only 7/8 mice in the HCT116-shNC group, 2/9 mice in the HCT116-shAA388235-2 group, and 1/8 mice in the HCT116-shAA388235-6 group developed tumors 40 days after injection. **(C)** The weights (g) of tumors in each group as indicated. *P* value was calculated by one-way ANOVA. Mean ± SEM, $^{***}P < 0.001$, $^{****}P < 0.0001$.

induced HCT116 cells' pyroptosis and apoptosis (**Figure 6D**) and had no effect on DLD1 cells (**Figure 6J**). Meanwhile, siRNAs targeting GM11851 and GM15758 had no effect on HCT116 cells and DLD1 cells (**Figures 6F, L**). These results indicate that siRNAs targeting mouse-specific lncRNAs have cytotoxicity to human tumor cells, which is a broad-spectrum phenomenon.

lncRNA AA388235 Induces Pyroptosis or Apoptosis of Human Tumor Cells Rather Than Mouse Tumor Cells

We next examined whether lncRNA AA388235 itself affects human tumor cells. Similar to siRNAs targeting lncRNA AA388235, overexpression of lncRNA AA388235 (**Supplementary Figures S7A, B**) induced pyroptosis and apoptosis in HCT116 cells (**Figure 7A**) and apoptosis in DLD1 cells (**Figure 7B**). Consistently, cleavage of GSDME, caspase-3, and PARP was observed in HCT116 cells transfected with AA388235 (**Figure 7C**), whereas only cleavage of caspase-3 and PARP was observed in DLD1 cells transfected with AA388235 (**Figure 7D**). However, overexpression of lncRNA AA388235 (**Supplementary Figures S7C, D**) had no effect on mouse tumor cell lines MC38 and CT26 cells (**Figures 7E–H**). Furthermore, the combination of lncRNA AA388235 and siRNAs targeting lncRNA AA388235 increased cell death compared with siRNAs targeting lncRNA AA388235 alone (**Figures 7I–N** and **Supplementary Figures S7E, F**), which was probably because more fragments were produced during the degradation of AA388235 by siRNAs.

DISCUSSION

In recent decades, scientists have been searching for reliable targets for tumor treatment from various perspectives. One of the most common research strategies is to target some mutated genes or abnormal signaling pathways. As more cancer genomes are sequenced, a large number of cancer genes were identified which is critical for the development of target-based cancer therapeutics. Therefore, it is of great significance to search for new sources of tumor therapeutic targets. We suggest that species-specific lncRNAs can be used to construct new screening libraries, which was supported by our discoveries from this study. We randomly selected eight mouse-specific lncRNAs (absent in human) and designed 23 siRNAs targeting these eight lncRNAs. Among them, around 12–16 siRNAs (targeting six different mouse-specific lncRNAs) induced human tumor cells' pyroptosis or apoptosis. Among them, the mouse-specific lncRNA AA388235 was used to study the underlying mechanism. We next randomly designed six siRNAs targeting AA388235, four of which caused the death of human tumor cell. It was found that siRNAs targeting AA388235 activated the response of human tumor cells to exogenous nucleic acids then induced pyroptosis and apoptosis in the presence of GSDME, but only apoptosis in the absence of GSDME. By sequence analysis and qPCR, we ruled out the possibility that these siRNAs were targeting a common gene that could cause cell death. The reasonable explanation of these findings is that these siRNAs induce cell death by activating the host cell response to exogenous nucleic acids. Further experiments were performed to verify this explanation, with results showing that RNA sensors RIG-I, MDA5, and MAVS are increased.

Numerous metazoan lncRNAs have been discovered from cDNA libraries and RNA-seq data by high-throughput transcriptome projects. Among them, only a handful of lncRNAs have been functionally characterized. Meanwhile, many lncRNAs do not show the same pattern of high interspecies conservation as protein-coding genes. The lack of functional studies and poor evolutionary conservation have raised concerns of whether non-coding RNAs represent "transcriptional noise" or truly functional biomolecules (20–22). At present, the understanding of the function of lncRNA is only

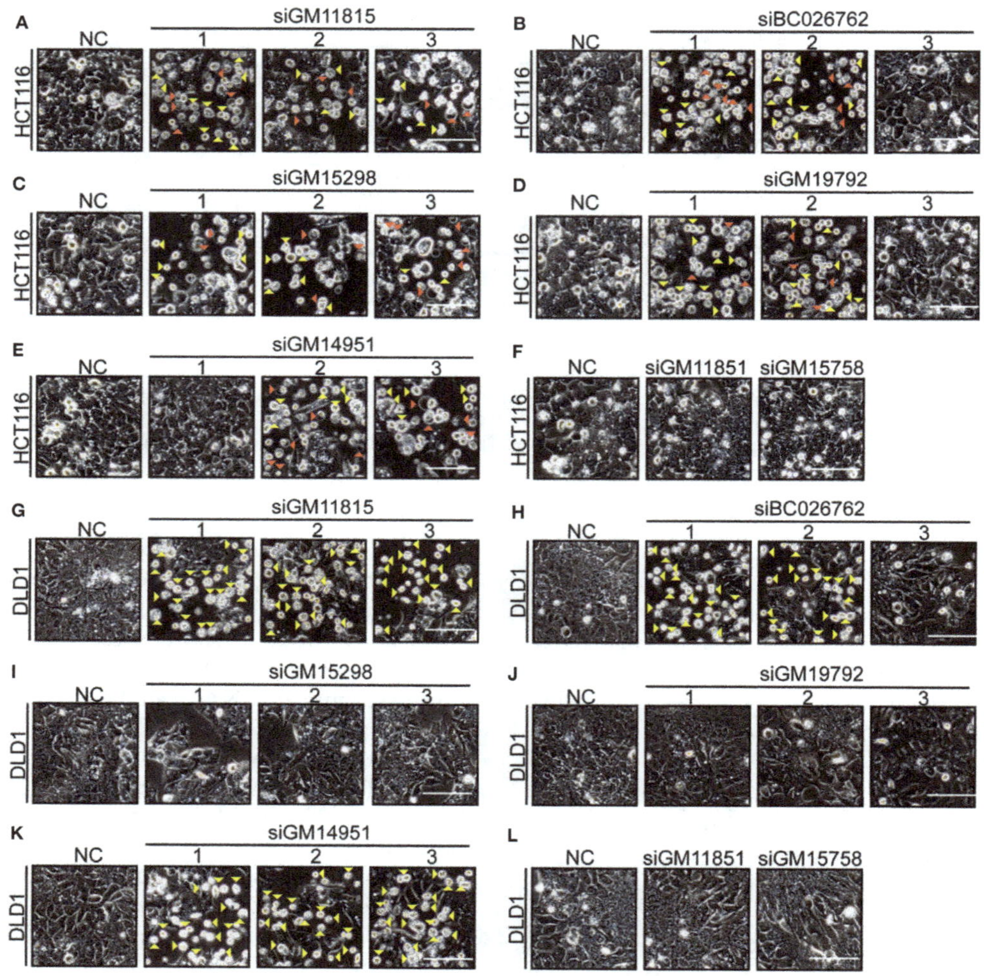

FIGURE 6 | Multiple siRNAs targeting different mouse-specific lncRNAs induce human colorectal tumor cells pyroptosis or apoptosis. Microscopic images of HCT116 and DLD1 cells transfected with siRNAs as indicated. Red arrowheads indicated the pyroptotic cells, and yellow arrowheads indicated the apoptosis cells. Scale bar, 100 μm. **(A)** Transfection with si-GM11815-1/2/3 induced HCT116 cells' pyroptosis and apoptosis. **(B)** Transfection with si-BC026762-1/2 induced HCT116 cells' pyroptosis and apoptosis, and transfection with si-BC026762-3 had no effect on HCT116 cells. **(C)** Transfection with si-GM15298-1/2/3 induced HCT116 cells' pyroptosis and apoptosis. **(D)** Transfection with si-GM19792-1/2 induced HCT116 cells' pyroptosis and apoptosis, and transfection with si-GM19792-3 had no effect on HCT116 cells. **(E)** Transfection with si-GM14951-1 had no effect on HCT116 cells, and transfection with si-GM14951-2/3 induced HCT116 cells' pyroptosis and apoptosis. **(F)** Transfection with si-GM11851 and si-GM15758 had no effect on HCT116 cells. **(G)** Transfection with si-GM11815-1/2/3 induced DLD1 cells apoptosis. **(H)** Transfection with si-BC026762-1/2 induced DLD1 cells apoptosis and transfection with si-BC026762-3 had no effect on DLD1 cells. **(I)** Transfection with si-GM15298-1/2/3 inhibited the growth of DLD1 cells. **(J)** Transfection with si-GM19792-1/2/3 had no effect on DLD1 cells. **(K)** Transfection with si-GM14951-1/2/3 induced DLD1 cells apoptosis. **(L)** Transfection with si-GM11851 and si-GM15758 had no effect on DLD1 cells. Scale bar, 100 μm.

achieved from detailed studies on a case-by-case basis, which only focus on lncRNA function in its expression site. No attention has been paid to the fact that non-conserved lncRNAs may serve as species-specific features, and the possibility that species-specific lncRNAs can be recognized as exogenous nucleic acids by the host. For the first time, our studies showed that mouse-specific lncRNA AA388235 induces human tumor cells' pyroptosis or apoptosis, although it has no effect on mouse tumor cells. More interestingly, siRNAs targeting lncRNA AA388235 have the same effect as lncRNA AA388235. In addition to AA388235, siRNAs targeting seven other mouse-specific lncRNAs were randomly designed, and multiple siRNAs also induced death in human tumor cell. We hypothesized that the effect of such species-specific lncRNAs might be universal and unveiled a new source of target libraries. As there are abundant lncRNAs specific to other mammals, with many of which having similar functions, a lot of siRNAs targeting these lncRNAs can be designed to build a siRNA library. And we are trying to build an extensive screening siRNA library to find out new anti-tumor drugs.

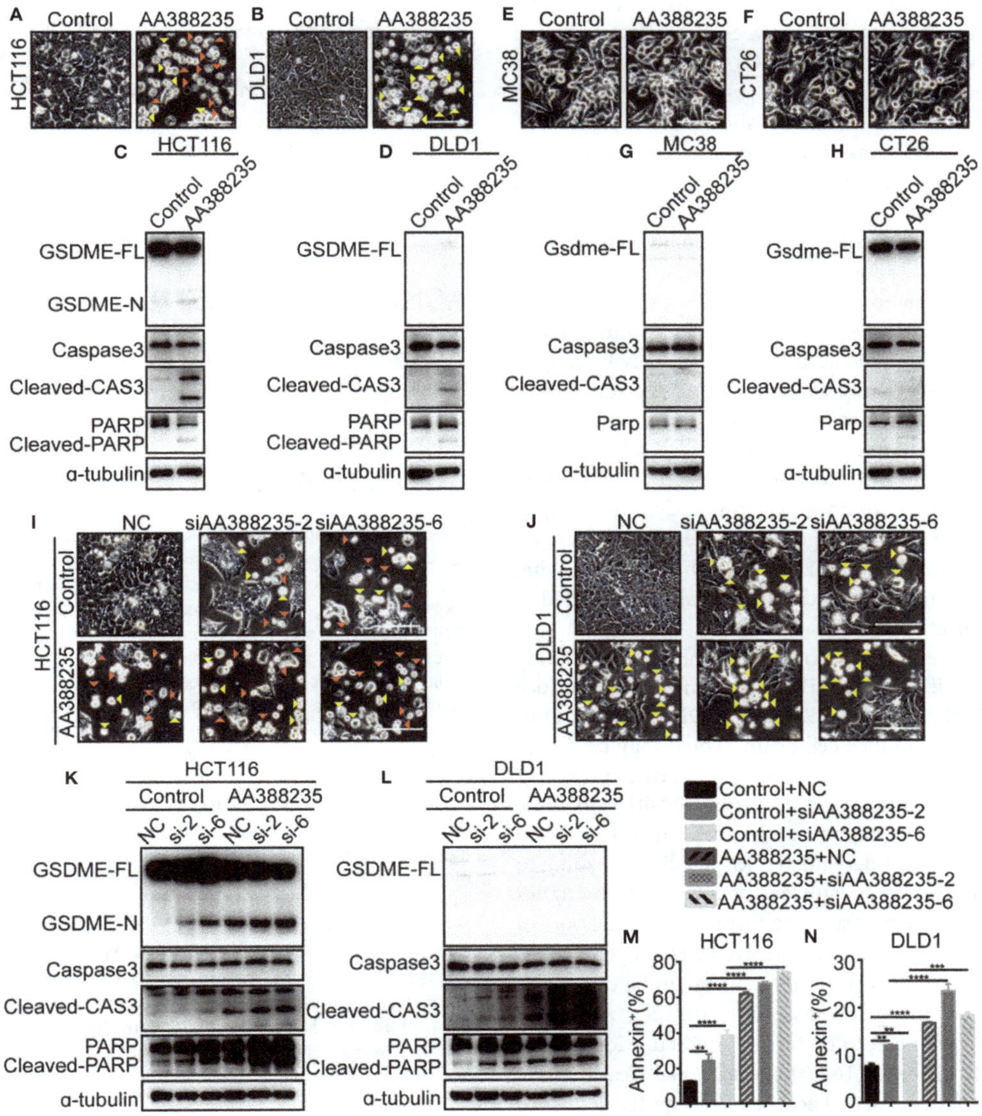

FIGURE 7 | lncRNA AA388235 induces pyroptosis or apoptosis of human tumor cells rather than mouse tumor cells. **(A, B)** Microscopic images of HCT116 and DLD1 cells transfected with plasmids as indicated. Red arrowheads indicated the pyroptotic cells, and yellow arrowheads indicated the apoptosis cells. Scale bar, 100 μm. **(C, D)** Immunoblotting assay of HCT116 and DLD1 cells transfected with plasmids as indicated. GSDME-FL, full-length of GSDME; GSDME-N, the N-terminal cleavage of GSDME; cleaved-CAS3, the cleavage of caspase-3 p19/p17; cleaved-PARP, the cleavage of PARP **(E, F)** Microscopic images of MC38 and CT26 cells transfected with plasmids as indicated. Scale bar, 100 μm. **(G, H)** Immunoblotting assay of MC38 and CT26 cells transfected with plasmid as indicated. Gsdme-FL, full-length of Gsdme; Cleaved-CAS3, the cleavage of caspase-3 p19/p17. **(I, J)** Microscopic images of HCT116 and DLD1 cells co-transfected with control or AA388235 plasmids and siRNAs as indicated. Red arrowheads indicated the pyroptotic cells, and yellow arrowheads indicated the apoptosis cells. Scale bar, 100 μm. **(K, L)** Immunoblotting assay of HCT116 and DLD1 cells co-transfected with control or AA388235 plasmid and siRNA as indicated. si-2, siAA388235-2; si-6, siAA388235-6. GSDME-FL, full-length of GSDME; GSDME-N, the N-terminal cleavage of GSDME; Cleaved-CAS3, the cleavage of caspase-3 p19/p17; cleaved-PARP, the cleavage of PARP. **(M, N)** Flow cytometry of PI (propidium iodide) and Annexin V-fluorescein isothiocyanate (FITC)-stained cells. The percentage of Annexin$^+$ cells is the sum of PI$^+$/Annexin V$^+$ and PI$^-$/Annexin V$^+$ cells. *P* value was calculated by one-way ANOVA. Mean ± SEM, $^{**}P < 0.01$, $^{***}P < 0.001$, $^{****}P < 0.0001$.

The discovery of RNA interference (RNAi) is a seminal work (23). Currently, siRNAs have been used as useful tools in biological research to suppress any gene achieved conveniently by a base sequence alone (24, 25). At the same time, siRNAs can be easily chemically synthesized and have the prospect to inhibit the genes encoding proteins that are "undruggable" by classical small molecules (26, 27). This has led many companies to develop the therapeutic potential of siRNAs. However, the clinical trials have shown non-specific toxicity and insufficient efficacy (28–30). Non-specific toxicity causes severe side effects in the development of siRNA therapy, including immunogenic reactions to dsRNA, unintended RNAi activity caused by unintended seed region matches between guide strands and non-targeted mRNAs, and on-target RNAi activity by siRNA drugs that accumulated in non-target tissues (30–32). These challenges make it difficult to utilize siRNA in clinical trial. However, siRNAs targeting non-human species-specific lncRNAs offer new opportunities to overcome these challenges. First, these siRNAs induce human tumor cells death by activating cell responses to exogenous nucleic acids, but do not activate toll-like receptors (TLRs) that activate immune system cells. Second, siRNAs that may activate host immune reactions or are toxic to human normal cells can be excluded by pre-screening. Thus, unintended RNAi activities and accumulation of siRNAs in non-target tissues can be effectively avoided. The large number of species-specific lncRNAs allows many siRNAs to be designed upon their sequences. After pre-screening siRNAs causing immune reactions and toxicity to normal cells, lots of siRNAs may still remain as candidate drugs. In this study, for example, we found that multiple siRNAs targeting mouse-specific lncRNA AA388235 induced human tumor cells death without having toxicity to human normal cells. And clinical trials are expected to test their anti-tumor effect.

More studies are needed to explore the mechanism. Our study shows that both double stranded siRNA and shRNA can induce cell death, while single stranded siRNA or dsDNA cannot. Full-length lncRNA can also induce cell death, which may be due to the formation of special secondary structures. Furthermore, it is unknown why human tumor cells are more sensitive to these siRNA induced death than human normal cells. It was reported that many oncogenic insults deregulated RNA splicing leading to hypersensitivity of tumors to spliceosome targeted therapies (STTs) which caused widespread cytoplasmic accumulation of dsRNA to trigger antiviral signaling and extrinsic apoptosis (33), suggesting that the sensitivity of tumor cells might be due to the abnormally activated oncogenic gene. The detailed molecules and signaling pathways need to be further studied. Moreover, a large proportion of siRNAs (16/23) induced cell death, while some other siRNAs failed, partly because of the special sequence characteristics of these siRNAs. High throughput screening and sequence analysis are considered to help address these issues.

In conclusion, we found that siRNAs targeting mouse-specific lncRNA AA388235 could induce pyroptosis or apoptosis in human tumor cells without toxicity to human normal cells. Through the functional verification of 17 siRNAs designed for the seven other mouse-specific lncRNAs, we propose that species-specific lncRNAs can be used as sequence targets to design siRNAs for tumor treatment, which highlights a novel approach to tumor drug design.

ETHICS STATEMENT

The animal study was reviewed and approved by Ethics Committee of Southern Medical University, Guangzhou, China (NO:2019038).

AUTHOR CONTRIBUTIONS

The project was conceived by W-JZ. The experiments were designed by W-JZ and Y-RC. The cell biology function experiments and animal experiments were performed by Y-RC and W-YF. The statistical analysis was completed by Y-RC, HZ and H-JL. Data were analyzed by W-JZ, Y-RC, YC and YG. The manuscript was written by W-JZ. All authors contributed to the article and approved the submitted version.

ACKNOWLEDGMENTS

We thank Central Laboratory, Southern Medical University for providing facilities and technical support.

SUPPLEMENTARY MATERIAL

Supplementary Figure 1 | siRNAs targeting mouse-specific lncRNA AA388235 have no/little effect on 4T1 and human normal cells but induce human tumor cells death. **(A, B)** 4T1 cells were seeded and treated as indicated. After 48 h, the static bright-field cell images were captured **(A)**. Then the dead cells were washed off with PBS, and the living cells were captured to measure the area percentage of survival cells using Image J software from five independent perspectives **(B)**.Scale bar, 200μm. *P* value was calculated by one-way ANOVA. **(C, D)** Comparison of ATP cell viability in HCT116 and DLD1 cells transfected with the siRNAs as indicated. *P* value was calculated by one-way ANOVA. **(E, F)** Flow cytometry of PI (propidium iodide) and Annexin V-fluorescein isothiocyanate (FITC)-stained cells. The percentage of $Annexin^+$ cells is the sum of PI^+/Annexin V^+ and PI^-/Annexin V^+ cells. *P* value was calculated by one-way ANOVA. **(G, H)** MDA-MB-453 cells were seeded and treated as indicated. After 48 h, the static bright-field cell images were captured **(G)**. Then the dead cells were washed off with PBS, and the living cells were captured to measure the area percentage of survival cells using Image J software from five independent perspectives **(H)**.Scale bar, 200μm. *P* value was calculated by one-way ANOVA. **(I–P)** Cells were seeded and treated as indicated. After 48 h, the static bright-field cell images were captured **(I, K, M, O)**. Then the dead cells were washed off with PBS, and the living cells were captured to measure the area percentage of survival cells using Image J software from five independent perspectives **(J, L, N, P)**. Scale bar, 200μm. *P* value was calculated by one-way ANOVA. Mean ± SEM, *$P < 0.05$, **$P < 0.01$, ***$P < 0.001$, ****$P < 0.0001$, "ns" indicates no significance.

Supplementary Figure 2 | siRNAs targeting mouse-specific lncRNA AA388235 do not target one common human gene. **(A, B)** The detection of predicted common off-target gene between the siAA388235-2,4,5, and 6 recognized by random 3 databases by qPCR in HCT116 and DLD1 cells transfected with siRNAs as indicated.

Supplementary Figure 3 | The detection of GSDME/caspase-3 in MDA-MB-453 and normal human cells treated with siRNA targeting lncRNA AA388235. **(A)** Microscopic images of MDA-MB-453 cells transfected with siRNA as indicated. Red arrowheads indicated the pyroptotic cells and yellow arrowheads indicated the apoptosis cells. Scale bar, 100μm. **(B)** Immunoblotting assay of MDA-MB-453 cells transfected with siRNA as indicated. GSDME-FL, full-length of GSDME; GSDME-N, the N-terminal cleavage of GSDME; Cleaved-CAS3, the cleavage of Caspase3 p19/p17; Cleaved-PARP, the cleavage of PARP. **(C)** Comparison of LDH release-based cell death in MDA-MB-453 cells transfected with the siRNA as indicated. *P* value was calculated by one-way ANOVA. Mean ± SEM, ***$P < 0.001$, ****$P < 0.0001$. **(D, F, H, J)** Microscopic images of FHC, MCF12A, HEK293, and NCM460 cells transfected with siRNA as indicated. Red arrowheads indicated the pyroptotic cells, and yellow arrowheads indicated the apoptosis cells. Scale bar, 100μm. **(E, G, I, K)** Immunoblotting assay of FHC, MCF12A, HEK293, and NCM460 cells transfected with siRNA as indicated. si-2, siAA388235-2; si-6, siAA388235-6. GSDME-FL, full-length of GSDME; GSDME-N, the N-terminal cleavage of GSDME; Cleaved-CAS3, the cleavage of caspase-3 p19/p17; cleaved-PARP, the cleavage of PARP.

Supplementary Figure 4 | siRNAs targeting mouse-specific lncRNA AA388235 have no effect on the death of mouse colorectal cancer cells. **(A, B)** Microscopic images of MC38 and CT26 cells transfected with siRNA as indicated. Scale bar, 100 µm. **(C, D)** Immunoblotting assay of MC38 and CT26 cells transfected with siRNA as indicated. Gsdme-FL, full-length of Gsdme; Cleaved-CAS3, the cleavage of caspase-3 p19/p17; cleaved-Parp, the cleavage of Parp. **(E)** Microscopic images of MC38 co-transfected with plasmid and siRNA as indicated. Red arrowheads indicated the pyroptotic cells. Scale bar, 100 µm. **(F)** The numbers of the pyroptotic cells of MC38 co-transfected with Gsdme and siRNA as indicated were calculated in randomly select five fields of view (×200). *P* value was calculated by one-way ANOVA. **(G)** Immunoblotting assay of MC38 co-transfected with Gsdme and siRNA as indicated. Gsdme-FL, full-length of Gsdme; Gsdme-N, the N-terminal cleavage products of Gsdme; Cleaved-CAS3, the cleavage of caspase-3 p19/p17; cleaved-Parp, the cleavage of Parp. Mean ± SEM, "ns" indicates no significance.

Supplementary Figure 5 | Multiple-species conversation comparisons with mouse specific LncRNAs. **(A–G)** Graphical views showing multiple-species conversation comparisons with mouse specific LncRNAs using UCSC genome browser. The conservation scores were indicated by the gray peaks. This result showed that the seven randomly selected mouse LncRNA including GM11815 **(A)**, BC026762 **(B)**, GM15298 **(C)**, GM19792 **(D)**, GM14951 **(E)**, GM11851 **(F)** and GM15758 **(G)** only express in mouse.

Supplementary Figure 6 | Multiple siRNAs targeting different mouse-specific lncRNAs induce cleavage of GSDME, caspase-3 and PARP. Immunoblotting assay of HCT116 and DLD1 cells transfected with siRNA as indicated. GSDME-FL, full-length of GSDME; GSDME-N, the N-terminal cleavage of GSDME; Cleaved-CAS3, the cleavage of caspase-3 p19/p17; cleaved-PARP, the cleavage of PARP. **(A)** Transfection with si-GM11815-1/2/3 induced the cleavage of GSDME, caspase-3 and PARP in HCT116. **(B)** Transfection with si-BC026762-1/2 induced the cleavage of GSDME, caspase-3 and PARP, and si-BC026762-3 had no effect in HCT116. **(C)** Transfection with si-GM15298-1/2/3 induced the cleavage of GSDME, caspase-3 and PARP in HCT116. **(D)** Transfection with si-GM19792-1/2 induced the cleavage of GSDME, caspase-3, and PARP, and si-GM19792-3 had no effect. **(E)** Transfection with si-GM14951-1 had no effect, and si-GM14951-2/3 induced the cleavage of GSDME, caspase-3 and PARP in HCT116. **(F)** Transfection with si-GM11851 and si-GM15758 had no effect on the cleavage of GSDME, caspase-3 and PARP in HCT116. **(G)** Transfection with si-GM11815-1/2/3 induced the cleavage of caspase-3 and PARP in DLD1. **(H)** Transfection with si-BC026762-1/2 induced the cleavage of caspase-3 and PARP in DLD1, and si-BC026762-3 had no effect. **(I)** Transfection with si-GM15298-1/2/3 had no effect on the cleavage of caspase-3 and PARP in DLD1. **(J)** Transfection with si-GM19792-1/2/3 had no effect on the cleavage of caspase-3 and PARP in DLD1. **(K)** Transfection with si-GM14951-1/2/3 induced the cleavage of caspase-3 and PARP in DLD1. **(L)** Transfection with si-GM11851 and si-GM15758 had no effect on the cleavage of caspase-3 and PARP in DLD1.

Supplementary Figure 7 | The detection of AA388235 level by qPCR in different transfection as indicated. **(A, B)** The level of AA388235 in HCT116 and DLD1 cells transfected with plasmid as indicated. *P* value was calculated by Student's t test. **(C, D)** The level of AA388235 in MC38 and CT26 cells transfected with plasmid as indicated. *P* value was calculated by Student's t test. **(E, F)** The level of AA388235 in HCT116 and DLD1 cells co-transfected with plasmid and siRNA as indicated. *P* value was calculated by two-way ANOVA. Mean ± SEM, $^{**}P < 0.01$, $^{***}P < 0.001$, $^{****}P < 0.0001$.

REFERENCES

1. International Human Genome Sequencing C. Finishing the Euchromatic Sequence of the Human Genome. *Nature* (2004) 431(7011):931–45. doi: 10.1038/nature03001
2. Djebali S, Davis CA, Merkel A, Dobin A, Lassmann T, Mortazavi A, et al. Landscape of Transcription in Human Cells. *Nature* (2012) 489(7414):101–8. doi: 10.1038/nature11233
3. Derrien T, Johnson R, Bussotti G, Tanzer A, Djebali S, Tilgner H, et al. The Gencode V7 Catalog of Human Long Noncoding RNAs: Analysis of Their Gene Structure, Evolution, and Expression. *Genome Res* (2012) 22(9):1775–89. doi: 10.1101/gr.132159.111
4. Anderson DM, Anderson KM, Chang CL, Makarewich CA, Nelson BR, McAnally JR, et al. A Micropeptide Encoded by a Putative Long Noncoding Rna Regulates Muscle Performance. *Cell* (2015) 160(4):595–606. doi: 10.1016/j.cell.2015.01.009
5. Matsumoto A, Pasut A, Matsumoto M, Yamashita R, Fung J, Monteleone E, et al. MTORC1 and Muscle Regeneration Are Regulated by the LINC00961-Encoded Spar Polypeptide. *Nature* (2017) 541(7636):228–32. doi: 10.1038/nature21034
6. Ulitsky I, Bartel DP. LincRNAs: Genomics, Evolution, and Mechanisms. *Cell* (2013) 154(1):26–46. doi: 10.1016/j.cell.2013.06.020
7. Kopp F, Mendell JT. Functional Classification and Experimental Dissection of Long Noncoding RNAs. *Cell* (2018) 172(3):393–407. doi: 10.1016/j.cell.2018.01.011
8. Hezroni H, Koppstein D, Schwartz MG, Avrutin A, Bartel DP, Ulitsky I. Principles of Long Noncoding RNA Evolution Derived From Direct Comparison of Transcriptomes in 17 Species. *Cell Rep* (2015) 11(7):1110–22. doi: 10.1016/j.celrep.2015.04.023
9. Wang J, Zhang JG, Zheng HK, Li J, Liu DY, Li H, et al. Mouse Transcriptome: Neutral Evolution of 'Non-Coding' Complementary DNAs. *Nature* (2004) 431(7010):757. doi: 10.1038/nature03016
10. Hernando Herraez I, Garcia Perez R, Sharp A J, Marques Bonet T. DNA Methylation: Insights Into Human Evolution. *PloS Genet* (2015) 11(12): e1005661–e. doi: 10.1371/journal.pgen.1005661
11. Sarropoulos I, Marin R, Cardoso Moreira M, Kaessmann H. Developmental Dynamics of LncRNAs Across Mammalian Organs and Species. *Nature* (2019) 571(7766):510–4. doi: 10.1038/s41586-019-1341-x
12. Hodge RD, Bakken TE, Miller JA, Smith KA, Barkan ER, Graybuck LT, et al. Conserved Cell Types With Divergent Features in Human Versus Mouse Cortex. *Nature* (2019) 573(7772):61–8. doi: 10.1038/s41586-019-1506-7
13. Brawand D, Soumillon M, Necsulea A, Julien P, Csárdi G, Harrigan P, et al. The Evolution of Gene Expression Levels in Mammalian Organs. *Nature* (2011) 478(7369):343–8. doi: 10.1038/nature10532
14. Rogers C, Fernandes Alnemri T, Mayes L, Alnemri D, Cingolani G, Alnemri ES. Cleavage of DFNA5 by Caspase-3 During Apoptosis Mediates Progression to Secondary Necrotic/Pyroptotic Cell Death. *Nat Commun* (2017) 8:14128. doi: 10.1038/ncomms14128
15. Wang Y, Gao W, Shi X, Ding J, Liu W, He H, et al. Chemotherapy Drugs Induce Pyroptosis Through Caspase-3 Cleavage of a Gasdermin. *Nature* (2017) 547(7661):99–103. doi: 10.1038/nature22393
16. Yu CY, Chiang RL, Chang TH, Liao CL, Lin YL. The Interferon Stimulator Mitochondrial Antiviral Signaling Protein Facilitates Cell Death by Disrupting the Mitochondrial Membrane Potential and by Activating Caspases. *J Virol* (2010) 84(5):2421–31. doi: 10.1128/JVI.02174-09
17. Blander JM. A Long-Awaited Merger of the Pathways Mediating Host Defence and Programmed Cell Death. *Nat Rev Immunol* (2014) 14(9):601–18. doi: 10.1038/nri3720
18. Meylan E, Tschopp J. Toll-Like Receptors and RNA Helicases: Two Parallel Ways to Trigger Antiviral Responses. *Mol Cell* (2006) 22(5):561–9. doi: 10.1016/j.molcel.2006.05.012

19. Li P, Zhou L, Zhao T, Liu X, Zhang P, Liu Y, et al. Caspase-9: Structure, Mechanisms and Clinical Application. *Oncotarget* (2017) 8(14):23996–4008. doi: 10.18632/oncotarget.15098
20. Rao DD, Vorhies JS, Senzer N, Nemunaitis J. SiRNA *vs.* ShRNA: Similarities and Differences. *Adv Drug Delivery Rev* (2009) 61(9):746–59. doi: 10.1016/j.addr.2009.04.004
21. Guttman M, Amit I, Garber M, French C, Lin MF, Feldser D, et al. Chromatin Signature Reveals Over a Thousand Highly Conserved Large Non-Coding RNAs in Mammals. *Nature* (2009) 458(7235):223–7. doi: 10.1038/nature07672
22. Struhl K. Transcriptional Noise and the Fidelity of Initiation by RNA Polymerase II. *Nat Struct Mol Biol* (2007) 14(2):103–5. doi: 10.1038/nsmb0207-103
23. Fire A, Xu S, Montgomery MK, Kostas SA, Driver SE, Mello CC. Potent and Specific Genetic Interference by Double-Stranded RNA in Caenorhabditis Elegans. *Nature* (1998) 391(6669):806–11. doi: 10.1038/35888
24. Elbashir SM, Harborth J, Lendeckel W, Yalcin A, Weber K, Tuschl T. Duplexes of 21-Nucleotide RNAs Mediate RNA Interference in Cultured Mammalian Cells. *Nature* (2001) 411(6836):494–8. doi: 10.1038/35078107
25. Caplen NJ, Parrish S, Imani F, Fire A, Morgan RA. Specific Inhibition of Gene Expression by Small Double-Stranded RNAs in Invertebrate and Vertebrate Systems. *Proc Natl Acad Sci USA* (2001) 98(17):9742–7. doi: 10.1073/pnas.171251798
26. Hopkins A L, Groom CR. The Druggable Genome. *Nat Rev Drug Discov* (2002) 1(9):727–30. doi: 10.1038/nrd892
27. Wu SY, Lopez Berestein G, Calin GA, Sood AK. Rnai Therapies: Drugging the Undruggable. *Sci Transl Med* (2014) 6(240):240ps7–ps7. doi: 10.1126/scitranslmed.3008362
28. DeVincenzo J, Lambkin-Williams R, Wilkinson T, Cehelsky J, Nochur S, Walsh E, et al. A Randomized, Double-Blind, Placebo-Controlled Study of An RNAi-Based Therapy Directed Against Respiratory Syncytial Virus. *Proc Natl Acad Sci USA* (2010) 107(19):8800–5. doi: 10.1073/pnas.0912186107
29. Davis ME, Zuckerman JE, Choi CHJ, Seligson D, Tolcher A, Alabi CA, et al. Evidence of RNAi in Humans From Systemically Administered siRNA *Via* Targeted Nanoparticles. *Nature* (2010) 464(7291):1067–70. doi: 10.1038/nature08956
30. Kleinman ME, Yamada K, Takeda A, Chandrasekaran V, Nozaki M, Baffi JZ, et al. Sequence- and Target-Independent Angiogenesis Suppression by sirRNA *Via* TLR3. *Nature* (2008) 452(7187):591–7. doi: 10.1038/nature06765
31. Janas MM, Schlegel MK, Harbison CE, Yilmaz VO, Jiang Y, Parmar R, et al. Selection of Galnac-Conjugated Sirnas With Limited Off-Target-Driven Rat Hepatotoxicity. *Nat Commun* (2018) 9(1):723. doi: 10.1038/s41467-018-02989-4
32. Setten RL, Rossi JJ, Han SP. The Current State and Future Directions of RNAi-Based Therapeutics. *Nat Rev Drug Discov* (2019) 18(6):421–46. doi: 10.1038/s41573-019-0017-4
33. Bowling EA, Wang JH, Gong F, Wu W, Neill NJ, Kim IS, et al. Spliceosome-Targeted Therapies Trigger an Antiviral Immune Response in Triple-Negative Breast Cancer. *Cell* (2021) 184(2):384–403.e21. doi: 10.1016/j.cell.2020.12.031

5

Gankyrin as Potential Biomarker for Colorectal Cancer With Occult Liver Metastases

Chengxing Wang[1†], Xiaoping Li[1†], Liangliang Ren[2], Changyi Ma[3], Meimei Wu[2], Weijun Liang[1], Jinglin Zhao[1], Shangren Li[1], Qunying Tan[1], Yuehua Liao[4], Lixia Sun[4], Xin Zhang[2] and Yaoming He[1]*

[1] Department of Gastrointestinal Surgery, Jiangmen Central Hospital, Affiliated Jiangmen Hospital of Sun Yat-sen University, Jiangmen, China, [2] Clinical Experimental Center, Jiangmen Key Laboratory of Clinical Biobanks and Translational Research, Jiangmen Central Hospital, Affiliated Jiangmen Hospital of Sun Yat-sen University, Jiangmen, China, [3] Department of Radiology, Jiangmen Central Hospital, Affiliated Jiangmen Hospital of Sun Yat-sen University, Jiangmen, China, [4] Department of Pathology, Jiangmen Central Hospital, Affiliated Jiangmen Hospital of Sun Yat-sen University, Jiangmen, China

***Correspondence:**
Yaoming He
heyaoming1981@sina.com*

The majority of occult liver metastases cannot be detected by computed tomography (CT), magnetic resonance imaging (MRI) or other traditionally morphological imaging approaches since the lesions are too small or they have not yet formed cancer nodules. Gankyrin is a small molecular protein composed of seven ankyrin domains. In this study, the expression of Gankyrin in colorectal cancer (CRC) patients with liver metastases was investigated to determine its prognosis value. Gankyrin expression in CRC patients was initially analyzed using data from The Cancer Genome Atlas (TCGA) database and bioinformatics tools. RT-qPCR, western blotting, immunohistochemistry (IHC) and transwell migration and invasion assays were then performed to verify the expression and function of Gankyrin in CRC cell line, CRC tissues and matched non-tumor tissues of clinical patients. General clinicopathological information including TNM stage as well as preoperative and postoperative imaging results were collected. The main outcome indicator was overall survival (OS), referring to the length of time from surgery to either death or the last visit. Statistical analyses included chi-squared tests, Cox analyses, progression free survival (PFS) rates and OS rates. Elevated Gankyrin expression was confirmed in CRC patients. The upregulated Gankyrin expression was positively correlated with the progression of disease and liver metastasis in CRC patients. OS analysis revealed that prognosis was worse in CRC patients with high Gankyrin expression compared to those with low expression. CRC patients with higher Gankyrin expression also had a higher risk of occult liver metastases and a lower PFS rate. Therefore, Gankyrin can be used as a potential biomarker for early diagnosis of CRC with occult liver metastasis.

Keywords: Gankyrin, colorectal cancer, occult, liver metastasis, biomarker

INTRODUCTION

Metastasis is a biological characteristics of malignant tumors, and poses a challenge in clinical practice (1). In recent years, considerable progress has been made regarding the diagnosis and treatment of tumors, but tumor metastases are still responsible for 90% of cancer-related deaths. For colorectal cancer (CRC) patients, liver metastasis is the leading cause of mortality. It has been reported that 70% of patients who died of CRC had metastatic liver disease (2). The early diagnosis of liver metastasis in CRC strongly influences the choice of treatment and prognosis. However, most occult liver metastases cannot be detected by computed tomography (CT), magnetic resonance imaging (MRI) or other traditional morphological imaging techniques since the lesions can be very small or may not have yet formed cancer nodules (3). Therefore, a simple technique for early detection of occult liver metastases in CRC patients is an important measure to investigate to improve overall survival (OS) rates and quality of life.

Gankyrin, encoded by the *PSMD10* gene, is a small molecular protein composed of seven ankyrin domains, is involved in the formation of the 26S proteasome, and is related to the cell cycle and apoptotic processes in tumor cells (4, 5). Moreover, several studies have shown that Gankyrin mRNA or protein expression was upregulated in many types of cancer to varying degrees (6–8). The biological function and clinical significance of Gankyrin (*PSMD10*) in occult liver metastasis of CRC have not yet been thoroughly explored.

In this study, the elevated expression of Gankyrin and its positive correlation with disease progression as well as liver metastases in CRC patients were investigated. Gankyrin overexpression was shown to be an independent risk factor for the poor prognosis of CRC patients. Furthermore, CRC patients who did not have detectable liver metastases by conventional imaging examinations before their operation were followed up. It was discovered that patients with higher Gankyrin expression had a higher risk of liver metastasis and lower progression free survival (PFS) rates. Collectively, these data suggest that Gankyrin has the potential to serve as a biomarker for early detection of occult liver metastasis in CRC.

MATERIALS AND METHODS

Bioinformatics Analysis

The Cancer Genome Atlas (TCGA) database of Gene Expression Profiling Interactive Analysis (GEPIA) platform (gepia.cancer-pku.cn) was used to analyze the PSMD10 mRNA levels in human CRC samples. The keywords "colorectal cancer" and "human" were input into the Gene Expression Omnibus (GEO) (www.ncbi.nlm.nih.gov/geo) search, and GEO series (GSE) was selected for data set analysis. Meta-analysis was performed on one group of microarray data through the ONCOMINE databases (www.oncomine.org). The data type was set to mRNA and filtered by "colorectal cancer", "normal tissues" and "PSMD10". Then, five data sets were selected for meta-analysis to compare the expression of Gankyrin in CRC and in matched normal colorectal tissues.

Subjects and Specimens

One hundred and fifty patients with a pathologically confirmed CRC diagnosis from 2014 to 2016 at Jiangmen Central Hospital (Affiliated Jiangmen Hospital of Sun Yat-sen University) were enrolled in this study. Colorectal tissues were collected by colonoscopy or surgery and stored at the Clinical Experimental Center of Jiangmen Central Hospital. Among them, 65 were male and 85 were female. Ages ranged from 22 to 81, with an average age of 63 ± 12 years. The end time point of follow-up was February 2021 or the time of patient death. The death of a patient that was not tumor-related was classified as a loss of visit. The main outcome indicator was OS, which refers to the follow-up time from surgery to either death or the last visit. PFS, which was the period of time from the start of treatment to either worsening of the disease or patient death, was also recorded. This study was approved and supervised by the ethics committee of Jiangmen Central Hospital (decision no. JXY201839). Patients and volunteers all provided signed informed consent.

Reverse Transcription Quantitative Polymerase Chain Reaction (RT-qPCR)

Total RNA from CRC tissues and paired non-tumor tissues was extracted using Minibest universal RNA Extraction Kit (Takara company, Japan), and RNA concentrations were quantified using a Nanodrop (Thermo company, Japan). mRNA was reverse transcribed using PrimeScript^{TM} II (TaKaRaBio, Dalian, China) and the synthesized cDNA was subjected to RT-qPCR using the Golden SYBR Green Mix (2×) kit (Toneker Biotech, Shanghai, China) according to manufacturer's instructions. Glyceraldehyde 3-phosphate dehydrogenase (GAPDH) was used as the internal control. Primer sequences used were: PSMD10-forward, 5′-AACTGACCAGGACAGCAGAACT-3′; PSMD10-reverse, 5′-ACAGCATTCACTTGAGCACCTT-3′; GAPDH-forward, 5′-TGAACGGGAAGCTCACTGG-3′; and GAPDH-reverse, 5′-TCCACCACCCTGTTGCTGTA-3′. The melting curves and $E = 2^{-\triangle\triangle Ct}$ algorithm was analyzed using LightCycler software (Roche Diagnostics). The cycling conditions were as follows: initial denaturation at 95°C for 10 min, followed by 40 cycles of denaturation at 95°C for 1 min and annealing/extension at 56°C for 1 min. All samples were run in triplicate and normalized to internal controls. The fold-changes or relative PSMD10 expression levels were calculated based on the $2^{-\triangle\triangle Ct}$ method.

Western Blot

Western blotting was performed according to our previous publication (9, 10). The antibodies used included rabbit anti-Gankyrin monoclonal antibody (1:1000; Abcam, USA), rabbit anti-GAPDH monoclonal antibody (1:1000; Abcam, USA) and

---

Abbreviations: CEA, Carcinoembryonic Antigen; CT, Computed Tomography; CRC, Colorectal Cancer; EMT, Epithelial-mesenchymal transition; GEPIA, Gene Expression Profiling Interactive Analysis; GEO, Gene Expression Omnibus; IHC, Immunohistochemistry; MRI, Magnetic Resonance Imaging; OS, Overall Survival; PFS, Progression Free Survival; Rb, Retinoblastoma; TCGA, The Cancer Genome Atlas.

goat anti-rabbit IgG-horse radish peroxidase (HRP)-linked secondary antibody (1:1500; Thermo Fisher Scientific, Inc. USA). Briefly, after blocking with 5% non-fat milk dissolved in Tris-buffered saline containing Tween-20 (TBST) at 37°C for 1 hour, the membranes were incubated with the anti-Gankyrin or anti-GAPDH primary antibody at 4°C overnight. The following day, the membranes were incubated with the secondary antibody at room temperature for 1 hour. The specific bands were developed using an enhanced chemiluminescence reagent in a gel imaging system, and the bands were analyzed using Image J software. A total of three independent experiments were performed.

Immunohistochemistry (IHC)

The experimental operation was based on our previous publication (11). Paraffin embedded sections of CRC tissues were deparaffinized and rehydrated. Antigen retrieval was performed by immersion in citrate buffer (pH 6.0) for 15 min at 95°C prior to incubation with 0.3% hydrogen peroxide for 15 min at room temperature to block endogenous peroxidase activity. After rinsing with phosphate-buffered saline (PBS) and blocking with 5% normal goat serum (Thermo Fisher Scientific, Inc. USA) for 30 minutes at room temperature, primary anti-Gankyrin antibody (1:50;, Abcam, USA) was added to sections and incubated overnight at 4°C. The peroxidase-anti-peroxidase detection method was used for all sections, which were subsequently counterstained, dehydrated and mounted with a coverslip at room temperature. Yellow particles in the cytoplasm and/or nucleus were used to estimate the proportion of positive colorectal cells, and the intensity of staining was scored as negative (–), weak positive (+), medium positive (++) or strong positive (+++). The H-score was then calculated from multiplying the intensity score (from 0-3) by the percentage of positive cells (range 0-300) (12). Two experienced pathologists calculated the H-score according to a double-blind procedure.

Transwell Migration and Invasion Assays

SW480 cells were transfected with lenti-virus expressing Gankyrin (Lenti-Gankyrin) or empty lentiviral vector (Lenti-vector). SW480-vector cells and SW480-Gankyrin cells were added to the upper chamber of the polycarbonate Transwell filter (pre-coated with Matrigel) in the BioCoatTM Invasion Chambers (BD Biosciences, San Jose, CA) respectively. RPMI1600 medium with 10% FBS was added to the lower chamber. The cells were allowed to migrate for 12 h at 37°C. After removing cells on the upper side of the transwell, the invading cells on the underside were fixed and stained with Giemsa solution. The stained invasive cells were photographed under a microscope. Three independent experiments were performed and the data are presented as the mean ± standard deviation (SD).

Statistical Analysis

Statistical analysis was performed with Prism 8 (GraphPad Software Inc., San Diego, CA, USA) and SPSS 22.0 software (SPSS Inc., Chicago, IL, USA). Numerical data were expressed as the mean ± SD. The relationship between Gankyrin expression and the clinicopathological features was analyzed using the χ^2 test. Survival analysis were performed using the Kaplan-Meier method and compared *via* the log-rank test. Variables were analyzed using univariate and multivariate Cox regression. A p value < 0.05 was considered statistically significant.

RESULTS

Gankyrin Was Overexpressed in CRC

The analysis using the TCGA, ONCOMINE and GEO databases showed that Gankyrin had higher mRNA expression in CRC tissues compared to matched non-tumor colorectal tissues (**Figures 1A–C**). To verify this finding, RT-qPCR and western blotting were used to measure the expression of Gankyrin. The RT-qPCR results revealed that the expression of Gankyrin mRNA in most CRC tissues was higher compared to non-tumor tissues (36/40; **Figure 2A**). Consistently, western blot analysis also showed that the expression of Gankyrin was increased in most CRC tissues (T) compared to matched non-tumor colorectal tissues (N; **Figure 2B**). In addition, the expression of Gankyrin was detected by IHC in all tissue specimens of CRC patients (n = 150). In most cases (146/150), the H-score of Gankyrin was higher in CRC tissues compared to matched non-tumor colorectal tissues (**Figure 2C**), which was in line with both the RT-qPCR and western blot data.

The Overexpression of Gankyrin Was Positively Correlated With Liver Metastasis

The expression of Gankyrin in paired non-tumor tissues and CRC tissues with or without liver metastasis were compared. Both the results of RT-qPCR and western blot revealed that the expression of Gankyrin was lower in non-tumor colorectal mucosa compared to paired CRC tissues ($p < 0.05$). In addition, the expression of Gankyrin in CRC tissues with liver metastasis was higher than in CRC tissues without liver metastasis ($p < 0.05$; **Figures 3A, B**). Similarly, a significant difference was verified by IHC ($p < 0.05$; **Figure 3C**). Furthermore, we found that epithelial markers of E-cadherin was drastically downregulated, but N-cadherin was dramatically upregulated in Gankyrin-transduced cells (SW480-Gankyrin) (**Figure 3D**). Moreover, the transwell matrix penetration assay showed that Gankyrin-overexpressing CRC cells enhanced the migration and invasion capacity (**Figure 3E**).These results collectively indicated that the elevated Gankyrin expression was positively correlated with liver metastasis of CRC, and it may promote CRC liver metastasis by inducing EMT.

Elevated Expression of Gankyrin Suggested Poorer Outcomes for CRC Patients

First, the relationship between high Gankyrin expression and the clinicopathological characteristics of 150 CRC patients were analyzed by univariate analysis. The results showed that the high Gankyrin expression was positively related to CEA level

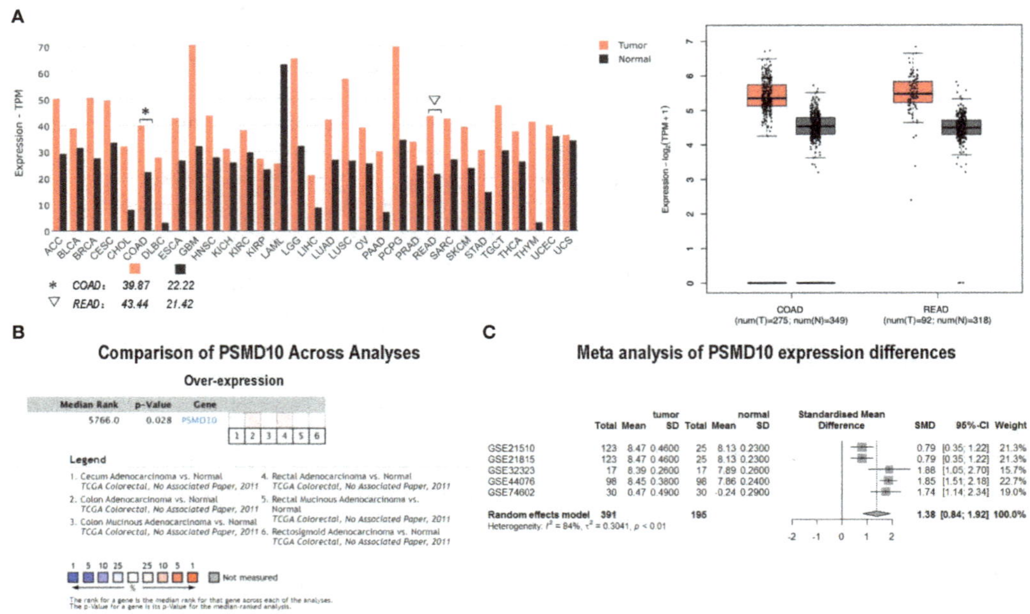

FIGURE 1 | Bioinformatic analyses suggested that Gankyrin was upregulated in colorectal cancer (CRC). **(A)** The expression of Gankyrin (PSMD10) in human CRC tissues and matched non-tumor colorectal tissues was analyzed using The Cancer Genome Atlas (TCGA) database (COAD [colorectal adenocarcinoma] and READ [rectum adenocarcinoma])-based Gene Expression Profiling Interactive Analysis (GEPIA) platform. Box plot graph presented statistical results. **(B)** Using six independent studies from ONCOMINE database, comparison of the relative mRNA expression of Gankyrin in CRC with that in non-tumor colorectal tissue. **(C)** A meta-analysis of Gankyrin using five data sets is represented by forest plot.

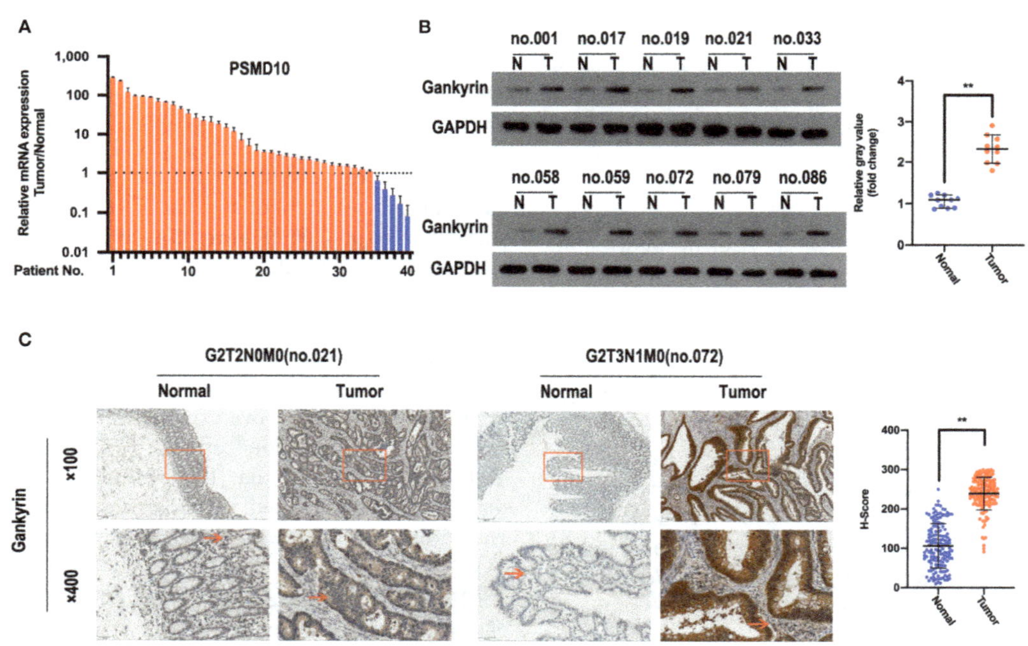

FIGURE 2 | Gankyrin was overexpressed in colorectal cancer (CRC) tissues. **(A)** Gankyrin expression in CRC and matched non-tumor colorectal tissues were measured by RT-qPCR (n = 40), and values were presented as mean ± standard deviation (SD). **(B)** The expression of Gankyrin in CRC and matched non-tumor colorectal tissues was detected by western blot (n = 10), and numerical values were expressed as mean ± SD. Scatter plot displayed the difference of Gankyrin expression level. **(C)** Immunohistochemistry (IHC) staining of Gankyrin in CRC and matched non-tumor colorectal tissues (n = 150; scale bars, 50 μm and 200 μm), numerical values were expressed as mean ± SD. Scatter plot indicated the H-score of Gankyrin staining intensity. **$p < 0.01$.

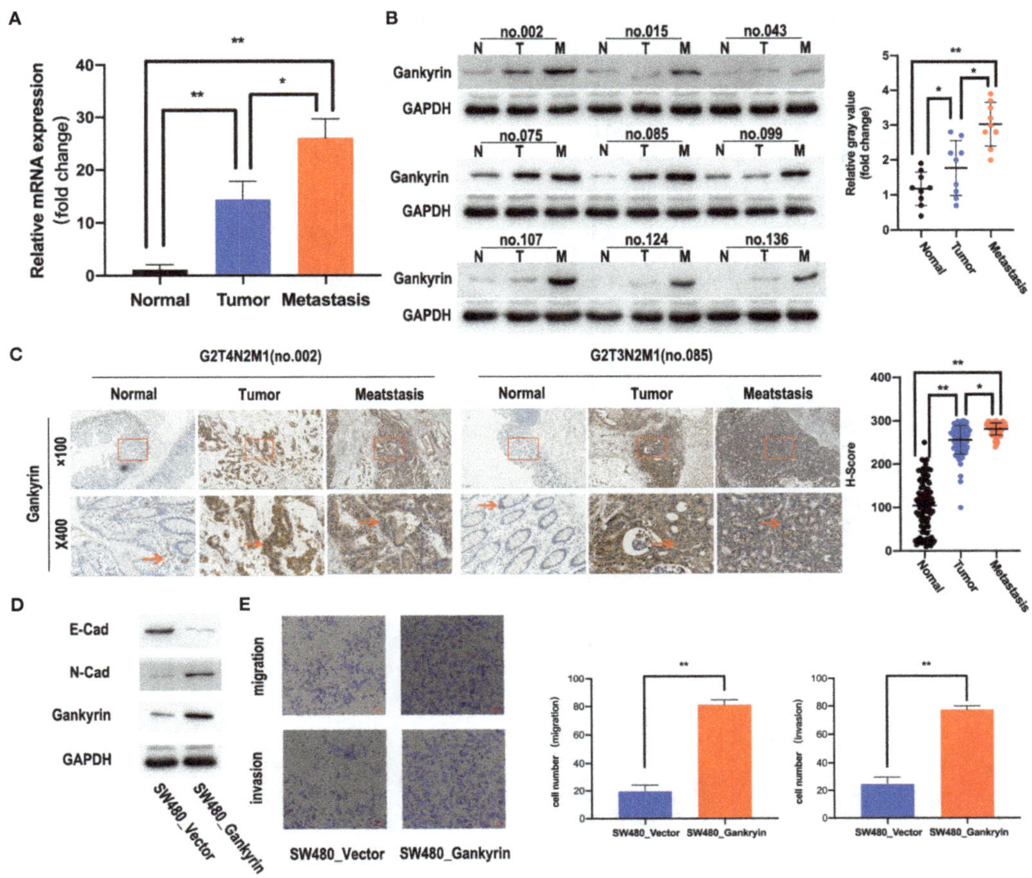

FIGURE 3 | High Gankyrin expression was associated with liver metastasis of CRC. **(A)** Detection of Gankyrin expression in non-tumor colorectal tissues and matched CRC with or without liver metastasis tissues by RT-qPCR (n = 20). **(B)** The expression of Gankyrin in non-tumor colorectal tissues and matched CRC with or without liver metastasis tissues were detected by western blot (n = 9). Scatter plot showed the difference of Gankyrin expression level. **(C)** Immunohistochemistry (IHC) staining of Gankyrin in non-tumor colorectal tissues and matched CRC with or without liver metastasis tissues sections (n = 60; scale bars, 50 μm and 200 μm). Scatter plot indicated the H-score of Gankyrin IHC staining intensity. **(D)** SW480 cells were transfected with lenti-virus overexpressing Gankyrin (SW480-Gankyrin) or empty lentiviral vector (SW480-vector). 48 hours after transfection, total protein extracts were analyzed on Western blot for E-cadherin, N-cadherin and Gankyrin. **(E)** Matrigel invasion assay was used to measure CRC invasive ability, after 48 hours incubation, invaded cells were stained by hematoxylin and counted under a light microscope. The data represent the means of three independent experiments with SEM bars. In this series of statistical analysis, numerical value was expressed as the mean ± standard deviation (SD). *p < 0.05, **p < 0.01.

($p < 0.001$), advanced TNM stage ($p < 0.001$), liver metastasis ($p < 0.001$) and lymph node metastasis ($p < 0.001$) in CRC patients (**Table 1**). Next, the risk factors for OS of 150 CRC patients were analyzed by univariate and multivariate Cox regression analyses. Multivariate Cox regression analysis showed that liver metastasis ($p = 0.041$) and a higher expression of Gankyrin ($p < 0.001$) were the risk factors associated with a poor prognosis in CRC patients (**Table 2**). Second, IHC was applied to examine the tissue expression of Gankyrin in the CRC patients (n=150), and Gankyrin expression was determined by the H-score. The optimal cut-off values for dividing patients into the low and high Gankyrin expression groups were determined by X-tile analysis, which indicated that the best cut-off value was 226 (H-score) using 5-year overall survival as the end point in the cohort (**Figure 4A**). In addition, Kaplan-Meier survival curves combined with the log rank test showed that the prognosis of CRC patients with high expression of Gankyrin was poor, and that the five-year survival rate was significantly reduced ($p < 0.001$; **Figure 4B**). In the localized group (stages I + II), the five-year survival rate of patients with high expression of Gankyrin was also lower compared to patients with low Gankyrin expression ($p < 0.001$; **Figure 4B**), but a comparison of the five-year survival rates in the advanced group (stages III + IV), the expression level of Gankyrin did not reflect a difference in survival ($p = 0.056$; **Figure 4C**).

Overexpression of Gankyrin Suggested a High Risk of Liver Metastasis in CRC

The multivariate Cox regression analysis showed that high expression of Gankyrin was an independent risk factor for liver metastasis in CRC patients ($p = 0.010$; **Table 3**). During the follow-up of 60 CRC patients without liver metastasis before

TABLE 1 | The relationship between Gankyrin expression and the clinicopathological features of 150 colorectal cancer (CRC) patients.

Characteristic	Sum	Number of Patients (%)		χ^2 value	p value
		Gankyrin (High)	Gankyrin (Low)		
Age				0.018	0.895
≥ 55 years	65	46 (70.8)	19 (29.2)		
< 55 years	85	61 (71.8)	24 (28.2)		
Gender				0.350	0.555
Male	65	48 (73.8)	17 (26.2)		
Female	85	59 (69.4)	26 (30.6)		
Smoke				0.006	.0941
Yes	67	48 (71.6)	19 (28.4)		
No	83	59 (71.1)	24 (28.9)		
Drink				0.510	0.822
Yes	81	57 (70.4)	24 (29.6)		
No	69	50 (72.5)	19 (27.5)		
CEA				155.660	< 0.001
≥ 5 ng/mL	103	96 (93.2)	7 (6.8)		
< 5 ng/mL	47	11 (23.4)	36 (76.6)		
Tumor size				0.032	0.858
≥ 5 cm	75	53 (70.7)	22 (29.3)		
< 5 cm	75	54 (72.0)	21 (28.0)		
Tumor location				2.169	0.143
Colon	80	53 (66.3)	27 (33.7)		
Rectum	70	54 (77.1)	16 (22.9)		
TNM stage				62.071	< 0.001
I + II	41	14 (34.1)	27 (65.9)		
III + IV	109	93 (85.3)	16 (14.7)		
Family history				0.001	0.992
Yes	21	15 (71.4)	6 (28.6)		
No	129	92 (72.1)	37 (27.9)		
Liver metastasis				186.071	< 0.001
Positive	90	89 (98.9)	1 (1.1)		
Negative	60	18 (30.0)	42 (70.0)		
Lymph node metastasis				106.938	< 0.001
Positive	112	99 (88.4)	13 (11.6)		
Negative	38	8 (21.1)	30 (78.9)		
Total	150	107	43		

CEA, carcinoembryonic antigen. TNM, tumor node metastasis.

the operation, it was found that Gankyrin was strongly expressed in nine patients with CRC who did not show liver metastasis by preoperative CT or MRI (**Figure 5**). However, all nine of these patients developed detectable liver metastases within six months following the operation. The PFS of patients with strong Gankyrin expression was significantly shorter than that of patients with weak or no expression of Gankyrin ($p < 0.001$; **Figure 6**).

TABLE 2 | Cox regression analysis of five years overall survival in 150 colorectal cancer (CRC) patients.

Predictor variables	Hazard Ratio	95% CI	p value
Age (≥ 55 years *vs* < 55 years)	0.880	0.628-1.232	0.456
Gender (Male *vs* Female)	0.829	0.592-1.161	0.275
Smoke (Yes *vs* No)	0.737	0.528-1.030	0.074
Drink (Yes *vs* No)	1.189	0.850-1.662	0.312
CEA (≥ 5 ng/mL *vs* < 5 ng/mL)	0.146	0.091-0.234	< 0.001
Tumor size (≥ 5 cm *vs* < 5 cm)	1.126	0.807-1.573	0.484
Tumor location (Colon *vs* Rectum)	1.243	0.889-1.737	0.203
TNM stage (III + IV *vs* I + II)	0.219	0.145-0.330	< 0.001
Family history (Yes *vs* No)	0.733	0.460-1.168	0.191
Lymph node metastasis (Positive *vs* Negative)	0.190	0.122-0.298	< 0.001
Liver metastasis (Positive *vs* Negative)	0.114	0.070-0.188	< 0.001
Gankyrin expression (High *vs* Low)	0.117	0.068-0.203	< 0.001
Multivariable model			
Liver metastasis (Positive *vs* Negative)	2.128	1.031-4.392	0.041
Gankyrin expression (High *vs* Low)	0.276	0.125-0.610	0.001

CI, confidence interval; CEA, carcinoembryonic antigen; TNM, tumor node metastasis.

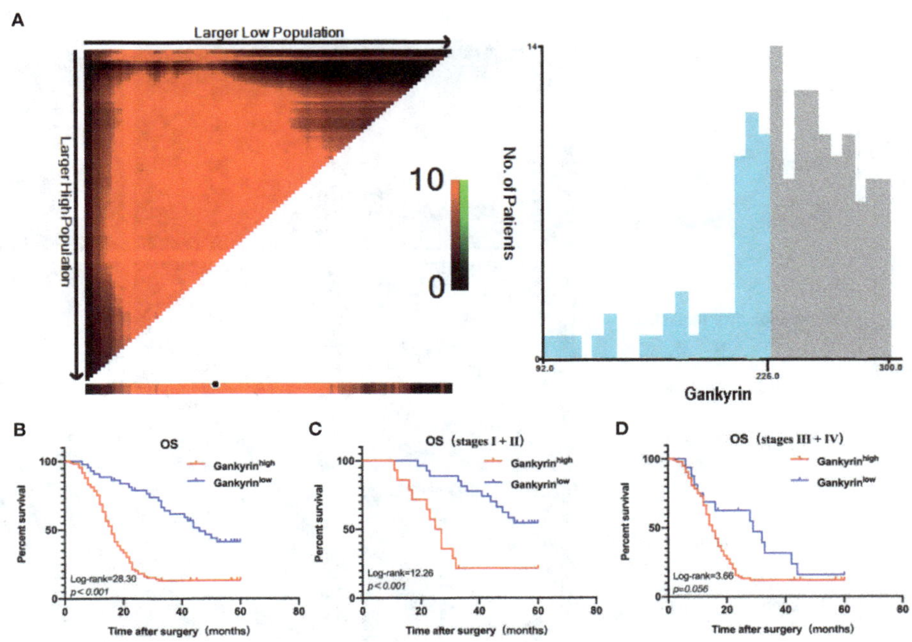

FIGURE 4 | X-tile analysis of survival data. **(A)** The optimum cut-off points for Gankyrin was 226 (H-score) according to the X-tile program. **(B)** Kaplan-Meier overall survival (OS) analysis of colorectal cancer (CRC) patients with high and low expression levels of Gankyrin. **(C)** OS analysis of CRC patients with localized disease (stages I + II). **(D)** OS analysis of CRC patients with advanced disease (stages III + IV).

DISCUSSION

At present, an early diagnosis of occult liver metastasis from CRC and an accurate judgement of prognosis remains clinically challenging (2, 13). To achieve individualized treatment for patients with different levels of risk, researchers are trying to find potential biomarkers that can accurately predict the outcome of CRC patients with liver metastasis. Gankyrin overexpression has been reported to be associated with the occurrence and progression of various cancers, including liver, pancreatic, kidney, endometrial, breast, and CRC (14–19).

TABLE 3 | Cox regression analysis of liver metastasis risk factors in colorectal cancer (CRC) patients.

Univariate Cox regression analysis	**Overall survival**		
	Hazard Ratio	**95% CI**	**p value**
Age (≥ 55 years *vs* < 55 years)	1.016	0.670-1.542	0.940
Gender (Male *vs* Female)	0.820	0.541-1.242	0.349
Smoke (Yes *vs* No)	0.674	0.447-1.023	0.064
Drink (Yes *vs* No)	1.123	0.740-1.704	0.585
CEA (≥ 5 ng/ml *vs* < 5 ng/ml)	0.013	0.002-0.074	< 0.001
Tumor size (≥ 5 cm *vs* < 5 cm)	0.948	0.627-1.433	0.800
Tumor location (Colon *vs* Rectum)	1.338	0.883-2.026	0.169
TNM stage (III + IV *vs* I + II)	0.015	0.003-0.089	< 0.001
Family history (Yes *vs* No)	0.670	0.384-1.168	0.158
Lymph node metastasis (Positive *vs* Negative)	0.018	0.003-0.110	< 0.001
Gankyrin expression (High *vs* Low)	0.012	0.002-0.090	< 0.001
Multivariate Cox regression analysis*	**Overall survival**		
	Hazard Ratio	**95% CI**	**p value**
Gankyrin expression (High *vs* Low)	13.573	1.854-99.384	0.010

CI, confidence interval; CEA, carcinoembryonic antigen; TNM, tumor node metastasis.

**Adjusted for variables from the above predictor variables using a backward stepwise cox proportional hazards model with a stay criterion of 0.10. p < 0.05 represents statistical significance.*

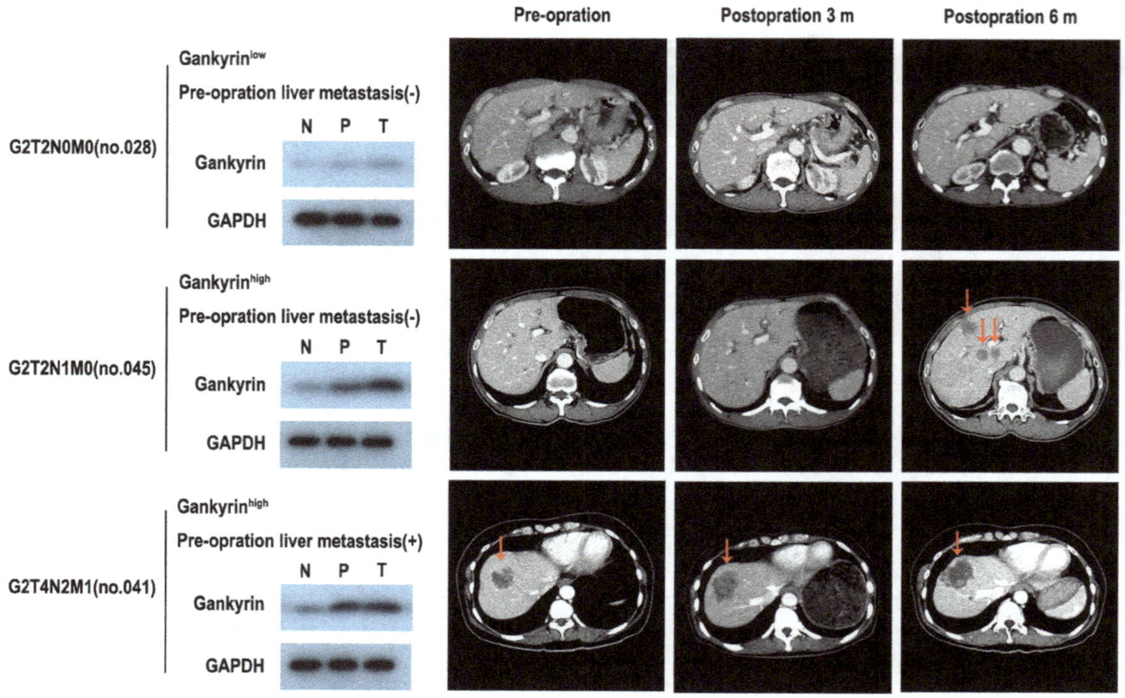

FIGURE 5 | The expression of Gankyrin association with occult liver metastasis. Through the comparison of gankyin in non-tumor tissues, paracancerous tissues and cancerous tissues of colorectal cancer (CRC) patients, it is revealed that partial patients with high expression of Gankyrin are more likely to be in the state of occult liver metastasis, and then develop into CRC liver metastasis.

Gankyrin can reduce the stability of the retinoblastoma (Rb) protein, causing dephosphorylation and inactivation of Rb, which activates E2 factor (E2F) transcription factors that induce the expression of genes related to cell cycle progression from G1 to S phase, and ultimately promotes cell division and growth that can lead to tumorigenesis (20). Gankyrin also interacts with cyclin-dependent kinase 4 (CDK4) to regulate the cell cycle and proliferation (21). In addition, Gankyrin can degrade tumor protein p53 (p53) through the ubiquitination pathway, resulting in decreased activity of this important tumor suppressor protein (22).

More importantly, many studies have shown that Gankyrin is expected to be a promising target for the treatment of a wide range of cancers involving metastasis in the future. Jin et al. found that Gankyrin was closely related to Ras-induced transformation (23). The study conducted by Man and colleagues revealed that Gankyrin is highly expressed in lung cancer cell lines and lung cancer tissues, and mediates phosphatase and tensin homolog (PTEN) degradation through an interaction with Rho GDP-dissociation inhibitor (RhoGDI). This in turn regulates the activation of phosphoinositide 3-kinase (PI3K)/Akt signaling to promote the occurrence of lung cancer (24). Bai et al. reported that Gankyrin is highly expressed in human CRC cell lines and tissues and can promote the migration of CRC cells by upregulating IL-8 signaling (25). Liu and colleagues have suggested that Gankyrin promotes tumor occurrence, metastasis and drug resistance by activating the β-catenin/c-myc signaling pathway in human hepatocellular carcinoma cell lines (26). Recently, He and colleagues found that Gankyrin promotes the invasion and progression of CRC by maintaining PI3K/GSK-3β/β-catenin signal activation (27). Taken together, these data indicate that the application of biomarkers for the early diagnosis of occult liver metastases from CRC is still in preliminary stages, and finding a suitable biomarker is important for current research.

In the present study, from analyses using the GEPIA platform of TCGA database, as well as the ONCOMIE and GEO databases, we found that Gankyrin mRNA expression was significantly upregulated in CRC tissues but not in matched non-tumor tissues. To verify these bioinformatics results, used RT-qPCR, western blotting, IHC and transwell migration and invasion assays were used to detect the expression and function of Gankyrin in CRC cell line, CRC tissues and matched non-tumor tissues. Additionally, Gankyrin was found to be highly expressed in CRC tissues experimentally and was even higher in CRC tissues from patients with known liver metastases. Therefore, we concluded that the expression of Gankyrin is positively correlated with liver metastasis, and it may promote CRC liver metastasis by inducing EMT. In addition, correlation analysis showed that high expression of Gankyrin and TNM staging were independent risk factors for CRC, and the high expression of Gankyrin may be related to liver metastasis of

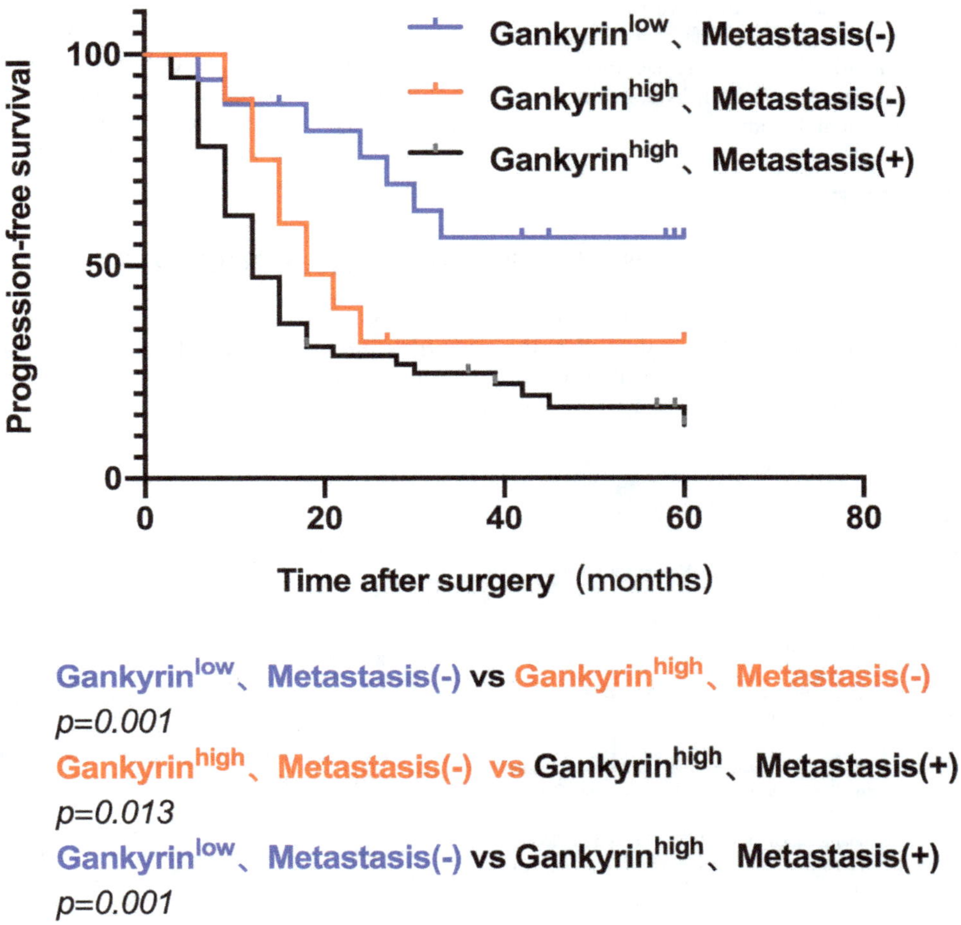

FIGURE 6 | The progression free survival (PFS) of colorectal cancer (CRC) patients. The PFS was compared according to the expression of Gankyrin and the presence of liver metastasis, which characterized three groups: low Gankyrin expression without liver metastasis; high Gankyrin expression without liver metastasis; and high Gankyrin expression with liver metastasis.

CRC. The OS analysis suggested that patients with high Gankyrin expression had shorter survival times and worse prognoses. Moreover, in CRC patients without detectable liver metastasis by preoperative CT and/or MRI, those patients with stronger Gankyrin expression were found to have a higher risk of developing detectable liver metastasis and had shorter PFS rates at follow up. At the first visit, some patients with CRC have a higher risk of liver metastasis or already have occult metastases that cannot be found by conventional imaging examinations such as CT and MRI. Since the routine preoperative evaluation cannot detect this state, there will be no additional examinations (that are typically more sensitive but also more costly) in the process of diagnosis and treatment, which leads to an incorrect evaluation of the disease staging in patients. We hope that we can take advantage of Gankyrin to evaluate patients with a higher risk of occult liver metastasis or identify patients who already have occult liver metastasis at their first visit, which can better guide the choice of treatment and the frequency of postoperative follow-ups. Taken together, our results suggest that Gankyrin is a promising biomarker to indicate occult liver metastasis in CRC patients when it is difficult to detect through imaging examinations.

Our study has some limitations. Firstly, this single center study only included a small cohort. We plan to further investigate the role of Gankyrin in the diagnosis of CRC with occult liver metastases through a multicenter study. Secondly, we need further research to explore the correlation between Gankyrin expression in CRC tumor tissue and peripheral blood to improve the clinical feasibility for its use as a biomarker. Finally, the Gankyrin signaling pathway in liver metastases stemming from CRC has not been fully elucidated. As such, further *in vivo* and *in vitro* experiments are required.

In conclusion, Gankyrin can be used as a biomarker to predict the progression and prognosis of CRC in patients, and has the potential to allow for early diagnosis of CRC occult liver metastasis. The measurement of Gankyrin expression, combined with carcinoembryonic antigen (CEA) detection and other clinical indicators, is expected to improve the individual evaluation and management of CRC patients at a high risk of occult liver metastasis. In addition, the precise mechanism whereby Gankyrin plays a regulatory role in liver metastasis of CRC requires further experimental study.

ETHICS STATEMENT

The studies involving human participants were reviewed and approved by Medical ethics committee of Jiangmen Central Hospital. The patients/participants provided their written informed consent to participate in this study. Written informed consent was obtained from the individual(s) for the publication of any potentially identifiable images or data included in this article.

AUTHOR CONTRIBUTIONS

CW and YH designed the study. CW, XL and YH wrote the manuscript. XL, XZ, CM, LR, MW, WL, SL, YL and LS contributed to collection of the data. YH, QT, XZ and JZ contributed to the critical revision of the manuscript. All authors contributed to the article and approved the submitted version.

ACKNOWLEDGMENTS

All authors would like to express their sincere thanks to the participants who provided colorectal tissue samples for this study and ensuring the successful completion of the study.

REFERENCES

1. Marx V. Tracking Metastasis and Tricking Cancer. *Nature* (2013) 494:133. doi: 10.1038/494131a
2. Chen W, Zheng R, Baade PD, Zhang S, Zeng H, Bray F, et al. Cancer Statistics in China, 2015. *CA Cancer J Clin* (2016) 66:115–32. doi: 10.3322/caac.21338
3. Otchy D, Hyman NH, Simmang C, Anthony T, Buie WD, Cataldo P, et al. Practice Parameters for Colon Cancer. *Dis Colon Rectum* (2004) 47:1269–84. doi: 10.1007/s10350-004-0598-8
4. Qin X, Wang X, Liu F, Morris LE, Wang X, Jiang B, et al. Gankyrin Activates Mtorc1 Signaling by Accelerating TSC2 Degradation in Colorectal Cancer. *Cancer Lett* (2016) 376:83–94. doi: 10.1016/j.canlet.2016.03.013
5. Xu X, Lou Y, Tang J, Teng Y, Zhang Z, Yin Y, et al. The Long non-Coding RNA Linc-GALH Promotes Hepatocellular Carcinoma Metastasis *via* Epigenetically Regulating Gankyrin. *Cell Death Dis* (2019) 10:86. doi: 10.1038/s41419-019-1348-0
6. Jahangiri R, Mosaffa F, EmamiRazavi A, Gharib M, Jamialahmadi K. Increased Expression of Gankyrin and Stemness Factor Oct-4 Are Associated With Unfavorable Clinical Outcomes and Poor Benefit of Tamoxifen in Breast Carcinoma Patients. *Pathol Oncol Res* (2020) 26:1921–34. doi: 10.1007/s12253-019-00766-2
7. Guo X, Piao H, Xue Y, Liu Y, Zhao H. LMX1B-Associated Gankyrin Expression Predicts Poor Prognosis in Glioma Patients. *J Int Med Res* (2020) 48:300060520954764. doi: 10.1177/0300060520954764
8. Camacho-Moll ME, Macdonald J, Looijenga LHJ, Rimmer MP, Donat R, Marwick JA, et al. The Oncogene Gankyrin is Expressed in Testicular Cancer and Contributes to Cisplatin Sensitivity in Embryonal Carcinoma Cells. *BMC Cancer* (2019) 19:1124. doi: 10.1186/s12885-019-6340-7
9. Wang Q, Wei J, Wang C, Zhang T, Huang D, Wei F, et al. Gambogic Acid Reverses Oxaliplatin Resistance in Colorectal Cancer by Increasing Intracellular Platinum Levels. *Oncol Lett* (2018) 16:2366–72. doi: 10.3892/ol.2018.8916
10. Chen J, Liu A, Wang Z, Wang B, Chai X, Lu W, et al. LINC00173.v1 Promotes Angiogenesis and Progression of Lung Squamous Cell Carcinoma by Sponging miR-511-5p to Regulate VEGFA Expression. *Mol Cancer* (2020) 19:98. doi: 10.1186/s12943-020-01217-2
11. Chen J, Liu A, Lin Z, Wang B, Chai X, Chen S, et al. Downregulation of the Circadian Rhythm Regulator HLF Promotes Multiple-Organ Distant Metastases in Non-Small Cell Lung Cancer Through PPAR/NF-KappaB Signaling. *Cancer Lett* (2020) 482:56–71. doi: 10.1016/j.canlet.2020.04.007
12. Viola P, Maurya M, Croud J, Gazdoza J, Suleman N, Lim E, et al. A Validation Study for the Use of ROS1 Immunohistochemical Staining in Screening for ROS1 Translocations in Lung Cancer. *J Thorac Oncol* (2016) 11:1029–39. doi: 10.1016/j.jtho.2016.03.019
13. Al-Temaimi RA, Jacob S, Al-Ali W, Thomas DA, Al-Mulla F. Reduced FHIT Expression is Associated With Mismatch Repair Deficient and High CpG Island Methylator Phenotype Colorectal Cancer. *J Histochem Cytochem* (2013) 61:627–38. doi: 10.1369/0022155413497367
14. Sun Y, Tan Y, Lu Z, Li B, Sun C, Li T, et al. Arctigenin Inhibits Liver Cancer Tumorigenesis by Inhibiting Gankyrin Expression *via* C/Ebpα and Pparα. *Front Pharmacol* (2018) 9:268. doi: 10.3389/fphar.2018.00268
15. Zhang J, Yang Y, Zhang Z, He Y, Liu Z, Yu Y, et al. Gankyrin Plays an Essential Role in Estrogen-Driven and GPR30-Mediated Endometrial Carcinoma Cell Proliferation *via* the PTEN/PI3K/AKT Signaling Pathway. *Cancer Lett* (2013) 339:279–87. doi: 10.1016/j.canlet.2012.10.037
16. Zheng T, Hong X, Wang J, Pei T, Liang Y, Yin D, et al. Gankyrin Promotes Tumor Growth and Metastasis Through Activation of IL-6/STAT3 Signaling in Human Cholangiocarcinoma. *Hepatology* (2014) 59:935–46. doi: 10.1002/hep.26705
17. Wang C, Li Y, Chu C, Zhang X, Ma J, Huang H, et al. Gankyrin Is a Novel Biomarker for Disease Progression and Prognosis of Patients With Renal Cell Carcinoma. *EBioMedicine* (2019) 39:255–64. doi: 10.1016/j.ebiom.2018.12.011
18. Gao L, Xie H, Dong L, Zou J, Gao X, Ou L, et al. Gankyrin is Essential for Hypoxia Enhanced Metastatic Potential in Breast Cancer Cells. *Mol Med Rep* (2014) 9:1032–6. doi: 10.3892/mmr.2013.1860
19. Sakurai T, Komeda Y, Nagai T, Kamata K, Minaga K, Yamao K, et al. Gankyrin Contributes to Tumorigenesis and Chemoresistance in Sporadic Colorectal Cancer. *Digestion* (2019) 100:192–200. doi: 10.1159/000494969
20. Krzywda S, Brzozowski AM, Higashitsuji H, Fujita J, Welchman R, Dawson S, et al. The Crystal Structure of Gankyrin, an Oncoprotein Found in Complexes With Cyclin-Dependent Kinase 4, a 19S Proteasomal ATPase Regulator, and the Tumor Suppressors Rb and P53. *J Biol Chem* (2004) 279:1541–5. doi: 10.1074/jbc.M310265200
21. Mahajan A, Guo Y, Yuan C, Weghorst CM, Tsai MD, Li J. Dissection of Protein-Protein Interaction and CDK4 Inhibition in the Oncogenic Versus Tumor Suppressing Functions of Gankyrin and P16. *J Mol Biol* (2007) 373:990–1005. doi: 10.1016/j.jmb.2007.08.038
22. Qiu W, Wu J, Walsh EM, Zhang Y, Chen C, Fujita J, et al. Retinoblastoma Protein Modulates Gankyrin-MDM2 in Regulation of P53 Stability and Chemosensitivity in Cancer Cells. *Oncogene* (2008) 27:4034–43. doi: 10.1038/onc.2008.43
23. Jin B, He K, Wang H, Bai B, Zhou T, Li H, et al. Proteomics Analysis Reveals Insight Into the Mechanism of H-Ras-Mediated Transformation. *J Proteome Res* (2006) 5:2815–23. doi: 10.1021/pr060283f
24. Man J, Liang B, Gu Y, Zhou T, Li A, Li T, et al. Gankyrin Plays an Essential Role in Ras-Induced Tumorigenesis Through Regulation of the RhoA/ROCK Pathway in Mammalian Cells. *J Clin Invest* (2010) 120:2829–41. doi: 10.1172/JCI42542
25. Bai Z, Tai Y, Li W, Zhen C, Gu W, Jiang Z, et al. Gankyrin Activates IL-8 to Promote Hepatic Metastasis of Colorectal Cancer. *Cancer Res* (2013) 73:4548–58. doi: 10.1158/0008-5472.CAN-12-4586
26. Liu R, Li Y, Tian L, Shi H, Wang J, Liang Y, et al. Gankyrin Drives Metabolic Reprogramming to Promote Tumorigenesis, Metastasis and Drug Resistance Through Activating β-Catenin/C-Myc Signaling in Human Hepatocellular Carcinoma. *Cancer Lett* (2019) 443:34–46. doi: 10.1016/j.canlet.2018.11.030

6

An Essential NRP1-Mediated Role for Tagln2 in Gastric Cancer Angiogenesis

Hongwei Jin[1*†], *Wei Zheng*[2,3†], *Jingjing Hou*[2,3], *Huifang Peng*[4*] and *Huiqin Zhuo*[2,3*]

[1] Xiamen Key Laboratory of Biomarker Translational Medicine, Medical Laboratory of Xiamen Humanity Hospital Fujian Medical University, Xiamen, China, [2] Department of Gastrointestinal Surgery, The Affiliated Zhongshan Hospital, Xiamen University, Xiamen, China, [3] Department of Gastrointestinal Surgery, Xiamen Municipal Key Laboratory of Gastrointestinal Oncology, Xiamen, China, [4] Department of Endocrinology, The First Affiliated Hospital and College of Clinical Medicine of Henan University of Science and Technology, Luoyang, China

***Correspondence:**
Hongwei Jin
jhw@xmu.edu.cn
Huifang Peng
penghuifang_sky@163.com
Huiqin Zhuo
zhuohuiqin@xmu.edu.cn

†These authors have contributed equally to the work

Knowledge about the precise biological role and underlying mechanism of Tagln2 in tumor progression is relatively limited, especially in angiogenesis focused on tumor derived endothelial cells (ECs) has rarely been reported. Here, the function, molecular mechanism and potential clinical value of Tagln2 in gastric cancer (GC) angiogenesis were investigated. GC tissue microarrays were used to assess the expression of Tagln2 in ECs. The relationships between expression and clinicopathological features were analyzed to evaluate the clinical value of Tagln2. Gain- and loss-of-function approaches were performed in ECs to investigate the functions of Tagln2 in angiogenesis. A combination of angiogenesis antibody array, RNA-Seq analyses and a series of *in vitro* experiments were performed to reveal the proangiogenic mechanism mediated by NRP1. Immunohistochemistry performed on an independent tissue chip (n=75) revealed significant upregulation of Tagln2 in tumor-derived ECs which were specifically immunolabeled with CD34. Additionally, high Tagln2 levels correlated significantly with the presence of lymph node as well as distant metastases. Gain- and loss-of-function approaches highlighted the function of Tagln2 in promoting EC proliferation, motility, and capillary-like tube formation and in reducing apoptosis. Tagln2 upregulation led to significantly increased mRNA and protein levels of NRP1 and subsequently activated the NRP1/VEGFR2 and downstream MAPK signaling pathways. These data indicate the importance of Tagln2 in angiogenesis, as a potential therapeutic target, and as a candidate prognostic marker in GC.

Keywords: Tagln2, NRP1, gastric cancer, angiogenesis, tumor-derived endothelial cell

INTRODUCTION

Gastric cancer (GC) is one of the most common malignant tumors worldwide. Its morbidity and mortality rate ranked fifth and fourth, respectively, in 2020 (1). The incidence of GC is high in China, and the number of new cases (679,100) and deaths (498,000) in 2015 ranked second only to lung cancer (LC) among all types of tumors (2). In the last decade, several antiangiogenic drugs based on the VEGF-VEGFR2 signaling axis (the most highly recognized target for current antiangiogenic therapy), including bevacizumab (a monoclonal antibody against VEGF), ramucirumab (a monoclonal antibody against VEGFR2) and apatinib (a tyrosine kinase inhibitor targeting VEGFR2), have been introduced for GC treatment. However, the survival benefit leads only to short survival benefits, and the need to investigate molecular mechanisms and potential therapeutic targets for combating angiogenesis in GC.

Tagln2 is a 22-kDa actin stress fiber-associated protein that stabilizes actin filaments, with ~70% amino acid sequence homology to two of its isoforms, Tagln1 and Tagln3. The function of Tagln2 has not yet been clarified, but recent reports have demonstrated that certain tumors, including those of colorectal cancer (3), bladder cancer (4), uterine cervical squamous cell carcinoma (5), esophageal squamous cell carcinoma (6) and gliomas (7), exhibit Tagln2 overexpression. Tagln2 upregulation is associated with lymph node and distant metastasis, advanced stage, and poor survival in colorectal carcinoma (3). In addition, suppression of Tagln2 markedly decreased cell viability by inducing apoptosis in bladder cancer cell lines (4). Moreover, *TAGLN2* is the target of certain tumor-suppressive miRNAs, such as miR-1, miR-133a (4, 6), miR-145-5p (8) and miR-133b (9). These findings suggest the roles of Tagln2 in tumor progression or metastasis. Conversely, Tagln2 is frequently downregulated in breast and prostate cancers (10). In addition, a role has been suggested for Tagln2 in impeding metastasis in metastasized Barrett's adenocarcinoma (11). In hepatocellular carcinoma cells with PFTK1 suppression, unphosphorylated Tagln2 inhibits cell motility through its strong actin-binding ability, which possibly abolishes actin cytoskeleton dynamics (12), thereby suggesting a role as a tumor suppressor. These contradictory results reveal a complex role for Tagln2 in tumorigenesis.

Knowledge about the precise biological role and underlying mechanism of Tagln2 in tumor progression is relatively limited compared to knowledge about other Tagln isoforms. As described in previous reports, Tagln2 is essential for the formation of stable immunological synapses between cytotoxic T cells and cancer cells (13), and Tagln2-actin-lymphocyte function-associated antigen-1 (LFA-1) axis for the effects of adoptive T cell therapy (14). Tagln2 is significantly induced in hypoxic lung cancer cells, accompanied by an increase in epithelial-mesenchymal transition (EMT) and resistance to γ-radiation *via* activation of the IGF1Rβ/PI3K/AKT pathway (15). Our group found that Tagln2 expression was significantly higher in microvascular endothelial cells (ECs) from lung cancer tumor tissues than in their paired normal counterparts, which was associated with advanced clinical stage, increased tumor size, and histological neural invasion (16). These findings demonstrated the essential function of Tagln2 in tumor angiogenesis for the first time, but the precise molecular mechanism involved in this process has not yet been reported.

Here, GC tissue microarrays containing 75 tumor tissues and paired normal counterparts were used to assess the expression of Tagln2 in ECs, in which CD34 was used to specifically label ECs. The relationship between expression and clinicopathological features was analyzed to evaluate the clinical value of Tagln2. Gain- and loss-of-function experiments of Tagln2 in angiogenesis were performed in ECs, with a focus on proliferation, motility, apoptosis, and capillary-like tube formation. A combination of angiogenesis antibody array, RNA-Seq analyses and a series of cell-based functional experiments were performed to reveal the critical role of Neuropilin-1 (NRP1, the coreceptor with VEGFR2 for the $VEGF_{165}$ isoform of VEGF-A) and downstream MAPK signaling pathways in the angiogenic activity of Tagln2.

MATERIALS AND METHODS

Cells and Arrays

EC lines (Ealy926 and ED-25) were purchased from the Institute of Cell Biology (Shanghai, China) and cultured in DMEM-F12 medium supplemented with 10% fetal bovine serum (FBS, HyClone, Logan, UT). Primary human umbilical vein endothelial cells (HUVECs) were prepared by our laboratory and cultured in Medium 131 supplemented with 10% microvascular growth supplement, 50 U/ml penicillin, and 50 µg/ml streptomycin (Invitrogen, CA, USA). Cells were maintained in a humidified chamber at 37°C in 5% CO_2.

A RayBiotech Human Angiogenesis Antibody Array 1000 and an Adhesion Molecule Array Q1 (Cat#QAH-ANG-2 and QAH-CAM-1) were purchased from RayBiotech Inc. (Norcross, GA, USA). Tissue microarrays of GC and paired normal counterpart tissues were obtained from Shanghai Outdo Biotech Company (Shanghai, China; Cat# HstmA150CS02).

In Vitro Assays of the Angiogenic Function of Tagln2

Full-length cDNA encoding human *TAGLN2* was amplified by PCR and was cloned into the pLVX-IRES-NEO vector and verified by DNA sequencing (Invitrogen). Small interfering RNA (siRNA) targeting *TAGLN2* was synthesized by Sigma. The siRNA sequences that resulted inefficient *TAGLN2* knockdown were as follows: si*TAGLN2*#1: 5′-CCAACUGG UUCCCUAAGAA-3′, si*TAGLN2*#2: 5′-GGCAUUAACACC ACUGACA-3′, and si*TAGLN2*#3: 5′-CCAACUGGCCUCU UCCUUU-3′. Plasmids (pLVX-*TAGLN2* or control vector) or siRNAs (siRNA targeting *TAGLN2* or a nontargeting siCtrl) were transfected for 36 h into EC cells *via* Lipofectamine 2000 or Lipofectamine™ RNAi MAX (Thermo, USA), respectively. Stably transfected clones were infected with lentiviral expression vector and established by G418 selection. The overexpression or knockdown efficiency was evaluated by western blotting. si*TAGLN2*#3 was used for the *in vitro* functional assays.

Cell proliferation was quantified using a CCK8 cell proliferation assay kit according to the manufacturer's instructions. Cells were harvested and prepared for apoptosis analysis using Annexin V-FITC and propidium iodide (PI) in accordance with the instructions of the cellular apoptosis detection kit (BD) and evaluated by FACS. For Transwell migration, ECs (1× 10^6 cells/ml in serum-free DMEM-F12) were added to the upper chambers, and DMEM-F12 supplemented with 10% fetal bovine serum (FBS) was added to the lower chambers. After 19 h, cells on the underside of the lower membrane were fixed, stained with crystal violet, and photographed.

To assess the tube-forming activity of ECs, 200 µl of Matrigel (BD Biosciences) was added to the wells and allowed to polymerize for at least 2 h at 37°C. ECs (2×10^4) were resuspended in serum-free medium and added to the Matrigel, allowed to form polygonal structures for 6 h at 37°C, and imaged by light microscopy. Vascular branch crossing was counted in five nonoverlapping microscopic fields under 40× magnification for each condition. All experiments were performed in triplicate.

RNA-Seq Analysis

Total RNA was extracted from HUVECs infected with lentiviral expression vector directing the expression of *TAGLN2* or with mock vectors (three replicates per group). mRNA libraries were sequenced on an Illumina sequencing platform, and bioinformatic analysis was performed by Genedenovo Biotechnology Co., Ltd. (Guangzhou, China). Differentially expressed genes (DEGs) were identified with two criteria: a false discovery rate (FDR) of < 0.05 and a $|\log_2\text{fold change}|$ of > 1. To gain insight into the functional distribution of the DEGs, various bioinformatic analysis approaches, including heatmap analysis, Gene Ontology (GO) analysis, and Kyoto Encyclopedia of Genes and Genomes (KEGG) pathway enrichment analysis were used. A protein-protein interaction (PPI) network was constructed based on the STRING website (https://string-db.org/).

Array Assays

HUVECs infected with lentiviral expression vector directing the expression of TAGLN2 or with mock vectors were harvested and analyzed for protein expression *via* the Human Antibody Array 1000 and Adhesion Molecule Array Q1, according to the manufacturer's instructions. Blots were scanned with an InnoScan 300 Microarray Scanner and analyzed with ImageJ software (RayBiotech, USA). Proteins with blots densities exhibiting a fold increase of greater than 1.5 or a fold decrease of greater than 0.67 were defined as differentially expressed proteins.

Identification of the Mechanism Mediating the Proangiogenic Function of Tagln2

To identify the important roles of the NRP1 and MAPK signaling pathways in the proangiogenic function of Tagln2, the expression levels of NRP1, two major MAPK signaling pathway molecules (extracellular signal-regulated kinase (ERK) and c-Jun N-terminal kinase (JNK)), and some differentially expressed proteins or markers involved in angiogenesis, migration and apoptosis were measured. The expression levels of *NRP1* and *TAGLN2* were modulated with siRNA or plasmid vector in Ealy926 cells stably expressing TAGLN2 and control cells, as appropriate. Then, the corresponding functional assays, including cell migration and tube formation assays, were conducted. EC samples (Ealy926 cell) with *TAGLN2* or *NRP1* expression modulation were harvested and prepared for western blot analysis. Blots were incubated with primary antibodies against Tagln2, VEGFR2, VWF, E-Cadherin, NrCAM, P-selectin, Caspase 3/cleaved Caspase 3, PARP1/cleaved PARP1 (ProteinTech, Cat#15508-1-AP, 67407-1-AP, 11778-1-AP, 60335-1-AP, 21608-1-AP, 60322-1-AP, 19677-1-AP and 13371-1-AP), NRP1, Phospho-ERK1/2, Total ERK1/2 (Abcam, Cat#ab25998, ab50011 and ab54230), Phospho-JNK, and Phospho-C-JUN (Cell Signaling Technology, Cat#4668 and 3270), respectively. Targeted proteins were detected with enhanced chemiluminescence (ECL, Millipore, USA).

Tissue Microarray Analysis

GC tissue microarrays containing a total of 75 tumor tissues and their paired normal counterparts was used to assess the expression of Tagln2 in ECs. Immunohistochemical (IHC) staining was performed using EnVision + System-HRP kits. A transgelin-2-specific polyclonal antibody was used at a 1:7500 dilution, and antibody against CD34 (Ready-to-use, DAKO, Denmark, Cat#IS632) was used to specifically label ECs. Analysis/scoring of IHC data was performed by two certified pathologists from our hospital, and the scores were averaged. In order to evaluate microvessel density (MVD), all stained sections were screened at 40×, and vessels were counted in three spots for CD34. Any brown-stained cells or in small clusters and separate from other connective tissue elements were counted as a single microvessel, even in the absence of vessel lumen. Large vessels containing muscular walls were excluded. MVD was expressed as the mean number of counted microvessels per high power field (HPF). The expression of Tagln2 in ECs identified by CD34-positive staining was scored at 40× magnification as follows: one hundred ECs were counted per slice, and the percentage of positive cells (PP) was calculated. The intensity of staining (IS) was scored as 0: negative, 1: weak, 2: moderate and 3: strong. The results were scored by multiplying the PP by the IS (immunoreactive score = PP × IS). The relationships between the expression level and clinicopathological features were analyzed to evaluate the potential clinical value of Tagln2.

Statistical Analysis

Statistical analysis was performed using SPSS Viewer 18.0 (SPSS, IL, USA) and GraphPad (version 5.0). Qualitative variables were analyzed by using the Kruskal-Wallis H test, the t-test and the Mann-Whitney U test. Two-tailed *P*-values of ≤0.05 were considered statistically significant. Clinical data were analyzed with Pearson correlation tests and one-way ANOVA.

RESULTS

Tagln2 Protein Expression Was Aberrantly Increased in GC-Derived ECs

GC tissue microarrays containing 75 tumor tissues and paired normal counterparts from patients with available clinical data was used for IHC analysis of CD34 and Tagln2 (**Table 1**). IHC

TABLE 1 | Clinical data related to 75 gastric cancer specimens on the tissue microarray chip.

NO.	Gender	Age (years)	Histological grade	Size	T Stage	N Stage	M Stage	Stage
1	M	67	III	4.0×3.0×1.0cm	T1b	N0	M0	1A
2	M	63	II-III	2.5×2.0×3.0cm	T1b	N0	M0	1A
3	M	43	II	4.0×3.0×0.5cm	T1b	N0	M0	1A
4	M	69	II-III	5.0×4.5×1.5cm	T2	N0	M0	1B
5	M	57	I-II	3.0×3.0×1.0cm	T2	N0	M0	1B
6	F	50	II-III	5.0×5.0×1.0cm	T2	N0	M0	1B
7	M	74	II	2.0×1.2×1.0cm	T1b	N1	M0	1B
8	M	53	II-III	7.0×6.0×2.0cm	T3	N0	M0	2A
9	M	53	II	6.0×4.0×1.5cm	T3	N0	M0	2A
10	M	69	II	5.5×5.0×1.1cm	T3	N0	M0	2A
11	F	63	III	6.0×5.0×2.0cm	T3	N0	M0	2A
12	M	67	II	6.0×6.0×2.0cm	T3	N0	M0	2A
13	M	77	II	6.0×5.0×1.0cm	T3	N0	M0	2A
14	M	76	II-III	5.0×4.0cm	T3	N0	M0	2A
15	M	77	II	6.0×4.0×2.0cm	T3	N0	M0	2A
16	M	47	I-II	3.0×2.5×1.0cm	T3	N0	M0	2A
17	M	69	II	8.0×6.0×1.0cm	T3	N0	M0	2A
18	M	75	II	3.0×4.0×1.6cm	T2	N1	M0	2A
19	–	–	II	5.0×4.0×0.6cm	T2	N1	M0	2A
20	F	47	II-III	3.0×3.0×1.0cm	T2	N1	M0	2A
21	M	68	II	3.0×3.0×0.8cm	T3	N0	M0	2A
22	M	62	III	3.0×3.0×1.0cm	T3	N0	M0	2A
23	F	72	III	5.0×3.5×1.5cm	T3	N0	M0	2A
24	F	63	III	8.0×6.5×2.0cm	T4a	N0	M0	2B
25	F	73	III	4.0×3.0×1.0cm	T4a	N0	M0	2B
26	M	51	III	2.5×3.0×1.5cm	T4a	N0	M0	2B
27	F	78	II	2.0×2.0×1.0cm	T4a	N0	M0	2B
28	M	61	II-III	4.0×4.0×2.0cm	T4a	N0	M0	2B
29	M	75	III	4.0×3.0×0.6cm	T3	N1	M0	2B
30	M	55	II	4.0×2.0×1.0cm	T3	N1	M0	2B
31	M	60	II	3.6×3.5cm	T3	N1	M0	2B
32	M	61	II	6.0×5.0×0.5cm	T3	N1	M0	2B
33	M	55	II-III	2.0×2.0×0.8cm	T3	N1	M0	2B
34	M	78	III	5.0×4.0×2.0cm	T3	N1	M0	2B
35	F	50	II	2.0×1.0×0.5cm	T2	N2	M0	2B
36	M	65	III	2.5×1.5×1.0cm	T3	N1	M0	2B
37	M	80	II-III	4.2×3.5×1.5cm	T3	N1	M0	2B
38	M	68	III	5.0×4.0×1.5cm	T3	N1	M0	2B
39	M	60	II-III	5.0×4.0×1.5cm	T3	N2	M0	3A
40	F	64	II-III	4.0×2.0×1.5cm	T3	N2	M0	3A
41	M	50	II-III	4.0×4.0×2.5cm	T3	N2	M0	3A
42	F	47	III	8.0×7.0×2.0cm	T3	N2	M0	3A
43	M	55	III	5.0×5.0×1.5cm	T3	N2	M0	3A
44	M	55	II-III	4.0×3.5×2.5cm	T3	N2	M0	3A
45	M	57	II-III	13.0×6.0cm	T2	N3a	M0	3A
46	M	46	III	4.0×3.0×1.0cm	T2	N3b	M0	3A
47	M	66	III	12.0×7.0×1.5cm	T3	N2	M0	3A
48	M	55	II	5.5×4.0×2.0cm	T4a	N1	M0	3A
49	M	76	II	11.0×9.0×1.5cm	T3	N2	M0	3A
50	M	72	III	6.0×4.0×1.0cm	T3	N2	M0	3A
51	F	59	II-III	7.0×6.0×1.5cm	T4b	N0	M0	3B
52	F	64	II-III	5.0×4.0×1.3cm	T4b	N1	M0	3B
53	F	69	II-III	3.5×2.5×1.3cm	T4a	N2	M0	3B
54	M	68	II	2.0×2.0×1.5cm	T3	N3a	M0	3B
55	M	50	II-III	4.0×3.0×1.0cm	T3	N3a	M0	3B
56	M	56	III	6.0×3.5×1.5cm	T3	N3a	M0	3B
57	M	69	II-III	7.0×5.5×2.0cm	T3	N3a	M0	3B
58	M	80	II-III	8.0×7.0×4.0cm	T3	N3b	M0	3B
59	M	67	II	3.0×3.0×1.0cm	T3	N3a	M0	3B
60	M	56	III	4.0×3.0×1.0cm	T3	N3a	M0	3B
61	F	67	III	4.5×2.0×1.5cm	T3	N3a	M0	3B
62	M	72	III	8.0×6.0×1.0cm	T4a	N3a	M0	3C
63	M	65	III	4.5×3.0×1.0cm	T4b	N3b	M0	3C

(Continued)

TABLE 1 | Continued

NO.	Gender	Age (years)	Histological grade	Size	T Stage	N Stage	M Stage	Stage
64	M	51	III	8.0×7.0×1.0cm	T4b	N3b	M0	3C
65	F	65	II-III	4.0×4.0×1.5cm	T4b	N3a	M0	3C
66	M	67	II-III	6.0×4.0×2.0cm	T4a	N3a	M0	3C
67	M	30	II-III	5.0×2.5×1.0cm	T4a	N3a	M0	3C
68	M	69	II-III	5.0×4.5×2.0cm	T3	N2	M1	4
69	F	75	III	5.5×4.5×3.5cm	T3	N3a	M1	4
70	M	61	II	7.0×5.0×1.5cm	–	N2	M1	4
71	M	50	II-III	10.0×8.0×2.8cm	T3	N3a	M1	4
72	M	70	III	4.0×4.0×2.0cm	T4b	N3a	M1	4
73	M	58	II	5.5×4.0×1.0cm	T4a	N3a	M1	4
74	M	52	III	5.0×4.0×1.0cm	T3	N3a	M1	4
75	M	54	II-III	4.8×4.3×3.5cm	T4b	N2	M1	4

Gender: female (F), male (M); histological grade: high differentiation (I), moderate differentiation (II), low differentiation (III).

images from three patients with weak, moderate and strong Tagln2 expression in ECs from gastric cancer were shown (**Figure 1A**). The level of $CD34^+$ MVD was 26.88 ± 1.30 and 22.56 ± 0.65 in tumors and paired adjacent normal tissues, respectively (P = 0.004). Significant Tagln2 staining was observed in ECs from tumors (score: 2.00 ± 0.92) compared with that from normal tissues (score: 0.66 ± 0.07; P< 0.0001, **Figure 1B**). High Tagln2 expression (score >2) was more frequently observed in ECs from tumor tissues (68%) than in ECs from normal tissues (6%). Statistical analysis of clinical data for patients with GC revealed that sex, age, histological grade, tumor size, T stage and overall cancer stage (Stage I-IV) were not significantly correlated with the Tagln2 expression in ECs. However, the expression of Tagln2 in ECs was significantly correlated with the presence of lymph node as well as distant metastases of patients (**Figure 1C**). Tagln2 expression was positively correlated with the N stage (scores for N stage N0, N1, N2 and N3: 1.66 ± 0.17, 1.93 ± 0.22, 2.20 ± 0.13, and 2.23 ± 0.14, respectively) and M stage (scores for M0 and M1: 1.93 ± 0.10 and 2.63 ± 0.16, respectively). On the other hand, in case of the $CD34^+$ MVD, no association with lymph node status or distant metastases was observed. Results demonstrated the essential function of Tagln2 in GC tumor angiogenesis, and the proangiogenic activity and mechanism involved in the process were necessary to be studied.

Proangiogenic activity of Tagln2

The overexpression and knockdown efficiencies of Tagln2 in the Ealy926 and ED-25 cell lines were confirmed by western blotting (**Figure 2A**). The results of survival assays revealed that the influence of Tagln2 to the proliferation of ECs was not very significant, unless the observation time was up to 48 h. The proliferation was significantly decreased at 48 h in both cell lines after Tagln2 knockdown, but was significantly increased at 96 h in the Ealy926 cell line, or at 72 h in the ED-25 cell line after Tagln2 overexpression, respectively. Silencing endogenous Tagln2 increased the percentage of apoptotic cells ($FITC^+PI^-$ and $FITC^+PI^+$), while overexpression had the opposite effect (**Figure 2B**) at 48 h. Cell migration was significantly increased upon Tagln2 overexpression (by approximately two folds), whereas the opposite result was observed in knockdown cells. In the *in vitro* tube formation assay, with Tagln2 upregulation, the intercellular space became narrower, and many more capillary-like structures were formed; however, silencing endogenous Tagln2 resulted in abrogation of the capillary-like structures and loosening of ECs (**Figures 2C, D**).

Tagln2-Associated Molecular Mechanism

To obtain a comprehensive picture of the Tagln2-associated molecular mechanism, RNA-Seq analysis was performed for transcriptomic profiling. An average of 7.28 Gb of clean data were collected from each sample. The overall Q30 percentage was greater than 90.49%, and more than 92.76% of the reads were mapped to reference genes in all groups. The gene expression levels are presented as fragments per kilobase of transcript per million mapped reads (FPKM) values, and a correlation coefficient of greater than 0.99 was observed between samples from the same group. Overall, compared to the control, 86 DEGs (40 downregulated and 46 upregulated genes, **Figure 3A** and **Table 2**) were identified in *TAGLN2* overexpression group, in which 39 DEGs were upregulated by more than 8-fold. The heatmap of RNA-Seq data shows that the expression patterns were very similar across the three samples in each group (**Figure 3B**). DEGs were further analyzed by the GO and KEGG databases for functional and pathway annotations. The GO analysis results indicated that *TAGLN2*-associated genes were most enriched in the terms methyltransferase activity, protein binding, ATPase activity, ion binding, and cytoskeletal protein binding. The top 15 KEGG pathways most significantly enriched in DEGs are displayed in **Figure 3C**; the greatest proportions of DEGs were enriched in the following pathways: MAPK signaling pathway, Lysine degradation, Synaptic vesicle cycle, and GABAergic synapse.

Tagln2-Derived Expression of Angiogenesis Factors and Adhesion Molecular in ECs

To detect the Tagln2-deraived changes in two main functions of ECs, namely growth factors expression and cell adhesion, angiogenesis antibody array (**Figure 4A**) and adhesion molecule array (**Figure 4B**) analyses were performed in primary HUVECs. Totally 60 angiogenesis and 17 adhesion molecular were detected,

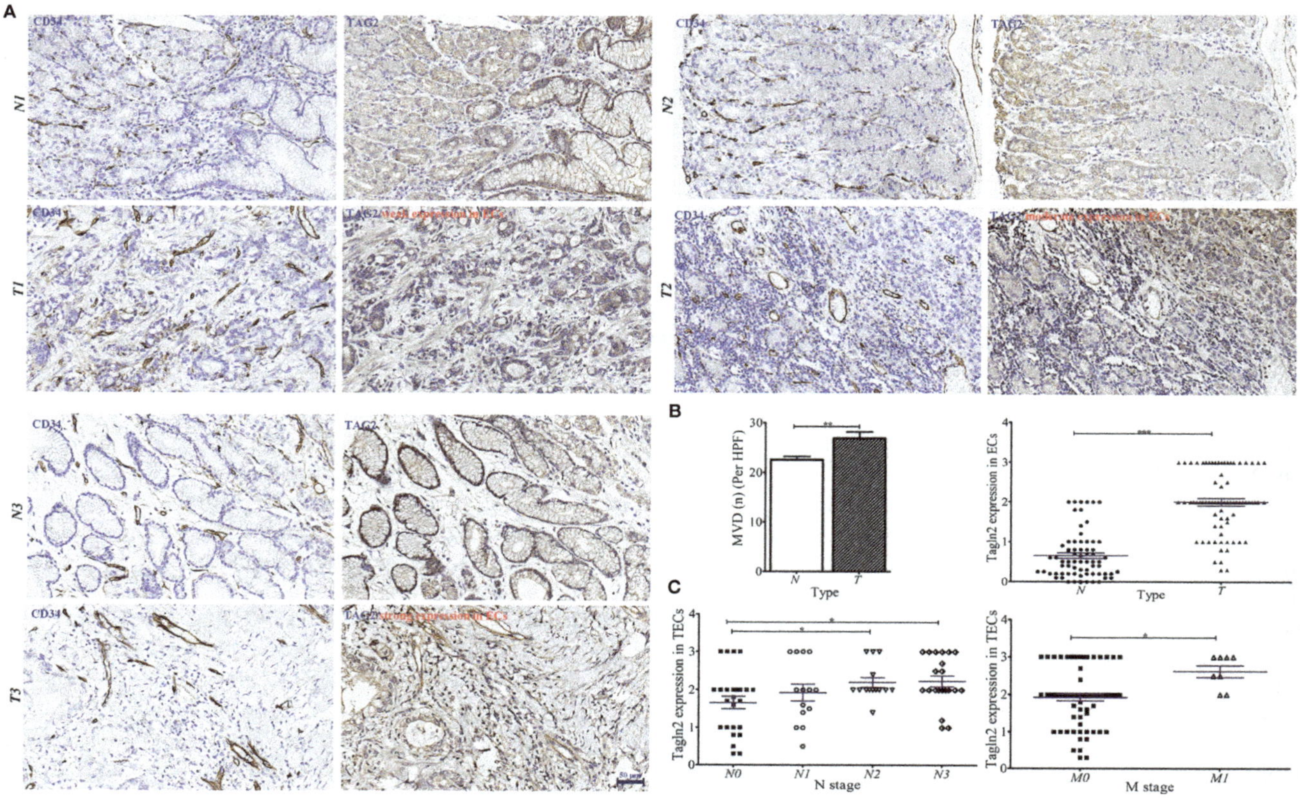

FIGURE 1 | Aberrantly increased Tagln2 protein expression in tumor-derived endothelial cells (ECs) was assessed by immunohistochemical (IHC) analysis of a gastric cancer (GC) tissue microarray (TMA) chip containing 75 tumor tissues and their paired normal counterparts. **(A)** IHC images from three patients with weak, moderate and strong Tagln2 expression in ECs from GC were shown, in which CD34 was used to specifically label ECs. **(B)** The microvessel density (MVD) and IHC scores of Tagln2 expression in ECs from gastric tumor tissues (t) and paired normal counterparts (N). **(C)** The significantly positive relationship between the expression of Tagln2 in tumor-derived ECs from GC tissues and the presence of lymph node (N stage) as well as distant metastases (M stage) of patients. For the calculation of MVD, all stained sections were screened at 40×, and vessels were counted in three spots. MVD was expressed as the mean number of counted microvessels per high power field (HPF). The expression of Tagln2 in ECs identified by CD34-positive staining was scored at 40× magnification as follows: one hundred ECs were counted per slice, and the percentage of positive cells (PP) was calculated. The intensity of staining (IS) was scored as 0: negative, 1: weak, 2: moderate and 3: strong. The results were scored by multiplying the PP by the IS (immunoreactive score = PP × IS). **P* < 0.05, ***P* < 0.01, ****P* < 0.001.

and the significantly expressed molecular were shown in **Figures 4A, B**, respectively. Five proteins involved in leukocyte recruitment (uPAR, RANTES, ENA-78, ANG-2 and LIF), were downregulated after Tagln2 overexpression. The levels of angiogenic cytokines and chemokines (TNFα, IL-8, IL-1b, IL-6, IL-1a, IL-12p40, IL-12p70, TGFα, IGF-1, PDGF-BB, EGF, HGF, G-CSF and GRO), and EC markers (PECAM1 (CD31), VEGFR2 and Tie-2) were upregulated by Tagln2 overexpression. Adhesion molecule including CEACAM-1, NrCAM (implicated in pro-angiogenic signaling, and enhance of vasculature permeability), ALCAM (acted in invasion and metastasis of several primary tumors), and ICAM-3 (identified on vessels in malignant tumors, correlated with the level of vascular differentiation) (17–19) were upregulated. However, E-cadherin (essential for morphogenetic movements), Leukocyte migration related P-selectin and vascular cell adhesion protein 1 (VCAM-1) were downregulated by Tagln2 overexpression (**Figure 4B**).

The Most Critical Molecule and Signaling Pathway Identification

To identify the most critical molecule and signaling pathway related to the angiogenic function of Tagln2, the relationship between 46 upregulated DEGs (identified by RNA-Seq) and 26 differentially expressed angiogenesis molecules, was analyzed and deeply mined using the STRING website. A protein-protein interaction network was constructed (**Figure 4C**). The corresponding top10 enriched biological processes and KEGG pathways were also determined and are shown in **Figure 4D**. The analyzed proteins were enriched in the terms positive regulation of cell migration, signaling receptor activity, proliferation, phosphorylation, MAPK cascade, PI3K signaling, vasculature development, angiogenesis and negative regulation of cell death and were enriched mainly in the MAPK, IL-17, TNF, PI3K-Akt, Ras, Rap1, Jak-STAT and HIF-1 signaling pathways. The MAPK signaling pathway, the most important enriched

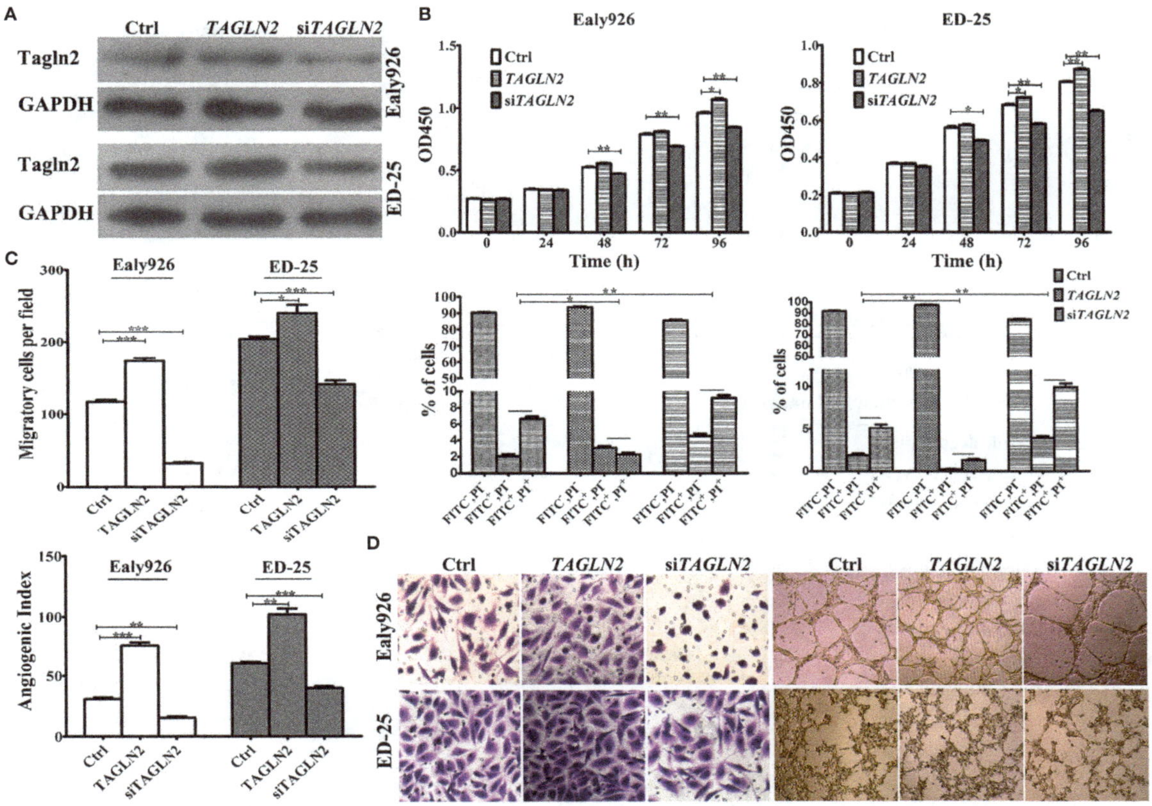

FIGURE 2 | *In vitro* assays of Tagln2 functions in the Ealy926 and ED-25 cell lines with Tagln2 overexpression or knockdown. **(A)** Efficient Tagln2 overexpression or knockdown was confirmed by western blotting. **(B)** Survival and apoptosis assays with Ealy926 and ED-25 cells after Tagln2 overexpression or knockdown. **(C, D)** Migration and *in vitro* tube-forming activity of Ealy926 and ED-25 cells after Tagln2 overexpression or knockdown. Cell numbers were counted in five randomly selected fields under a microscope. *$P < 0.05$, **$P < 0.01$, ***$P < 0.001$.

pathway identified through RNA-Seq and network analysis, has been demonstrated to play crucial roles in tumor angiogenesis in previous studies (20, 21). Thirteen of the upregulated DEGs, including *HIVEP2, CASP10, PTPRK, MEF2C, NRP1, NUMA1, NSF, PTPRM, NCOR2, SEMA4D, NUP88, LMNA* and *RPL23A* were involved in this network. Moreover, NRP1, the node with the highest degree in the network, was involved in 9 of the top 10 biological processes and had the closest relation among the proteins encoded by the above mentioned 13 genes with proteins from the angiogenesis antibody array.

In comparison the Tagln2 associated transcriptomic profiling with that of NRP1 in our previous study (22), 20 common DEGs (23%) were obtained with the similar change trends, including 11 upregulated genes (*HIVEP2, SLC38A2, CASP10, ATP2C1, NSD2, PTPRK, ZNF462, SEMA4D, ELP5, NCOA4* and *DNPEP*), and 10 downregulated genes (*SFXN3, NAGK, GPSM1, TNIP1, ATP6V0E2, ZNF839, NBPF14, PJA1, TUBGCP2* and *PLEKHM1*). Moreover, four genes (*HIVEP2, CASP10, PTPRK* and *SEMA4D*) were implicated in the mentioned network. Overall, these data suggested that NRP1 may be a critical molecule and MAPK signaling pathway is likely to be the most important enriched pathway mediating the angiogenic activity of Tagln2.

NRP1 Mediated the Angiogenic Function of Tagln2

To examine whether NRP1 mediated the angiogenic function of TAGLN2, a control Ealy926 cell line (pLVX-ctrl) and an Ealy926 cell line stably expressing TAGLN2 (pLVX-*TAGLN2*) were subjected to a series of treatments and prepared for migration and capillary-like tube formation assays (**Figure 5A**). Knockdown of endogenous NRP1 or Tagln2 greatly decreased the number of migratory cells, and the decrease was more significant with the Tagln2 knockdown treatment. Moreover, the decrease was partially or mostly ablated by exogenous replenishment of NRP1or Tagln2 in both pLVX-ctrl and pLVX-*TAGLN2* cells. As expected, similar results were observed in the *in vitro* tube formation assay.

After modulation of *TAGLN2* and *NRP1* expression in ECs, levels of proteins involved in angiogenesis, migration and apoptosis were measured. As shown in **Figure 5B**, forced expression of Tagln2 in Ealy926 cell resulted in significant increase of NRP1, as well as VEGFR2, VWF (markers of endothelial cells) and NrCAM (mediating capillary outgrowth) protein levels by western blotting. However, corresponding levels of E-cadherin and P-selectin (related to ECs adhesion and

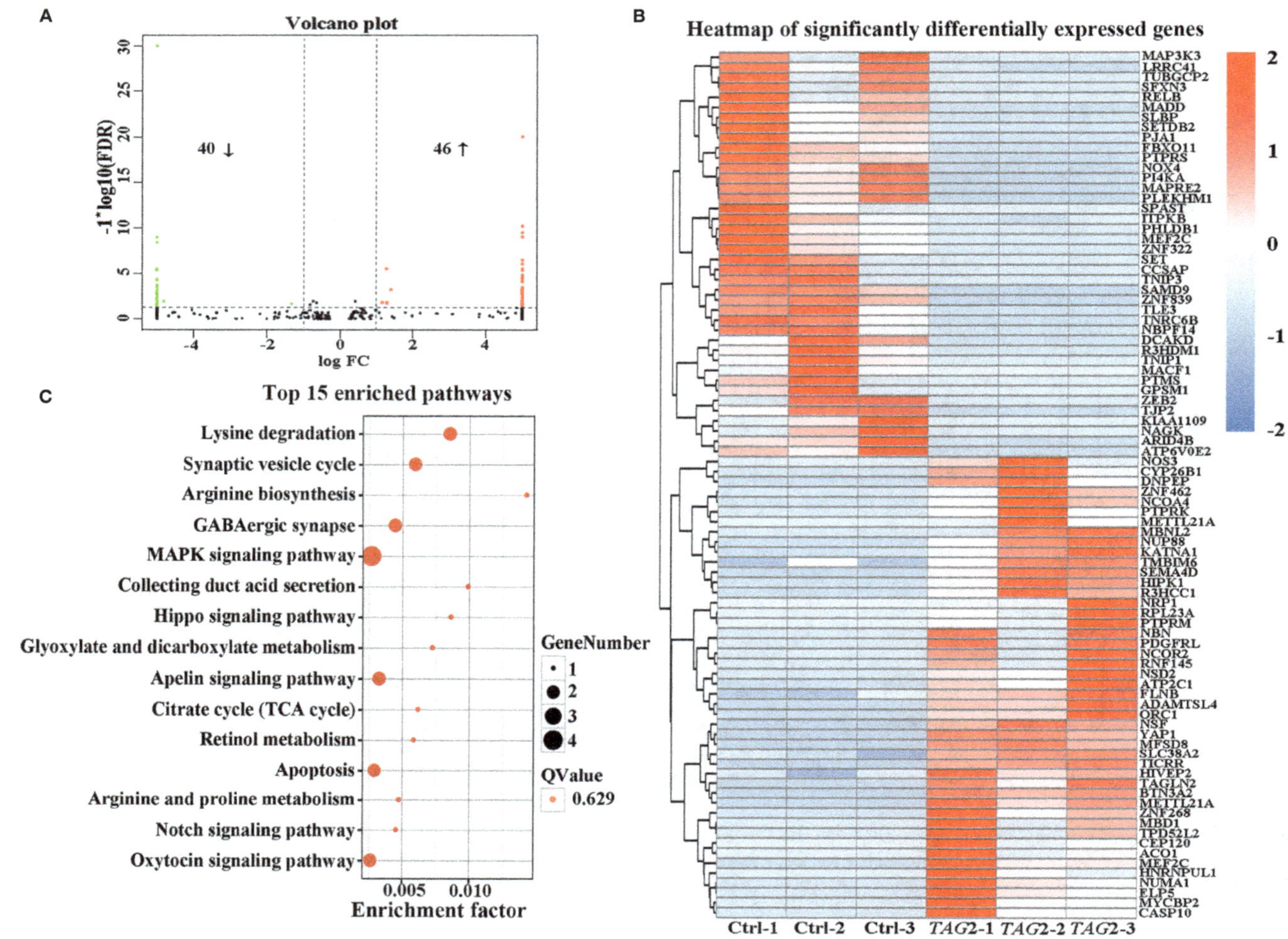

FIGURE 3 | Identification the potential mechanism involved in the proangiogenic activity of Tagln2 by RNA-Seq analyses. Primary HUVECs infected with lentiviral expression vector directing the expression of TAGLN2 or with mock vectors were prepared. mRNA libraries were sequenced on an Illumina sequencing platform, and bioinformatic analysis was performed by Genedenovo Biotechnology Co., Ltd. (Guangzhou, China). DEGs were identified with two criteria: a false discovery rate (FDR) of < 0.05 and a $|log_2fold\ change|$ of > 1. A volcano plot **(A)**, heatmap **(B)** and top15 KEGG pathways enriched in the significant DEGs identified by RNA-Seq **(C)** were shown.

migration), as well as cleaved Caspase 3 and cleaved PARP1 (markers of apoptosis) were decrease. As expected, inhibition of endogenous Tagln2 expression resulted in significant decrease of NRP1, VEGFR2, VWF and NrCAM, but protein levels of E-cadherin, P-selectin, cleaved Caspase 3 and cleaved PARP1 were all upregulated. These were consistent with the pro-angiogenic, pro-migration and anti-apoptotic functions of Tagln2 in ECs mentioned above. Inhibition or overexpression of NRP1 came with the consistent results, except that modulation of NRP1 expression had no impact on the protein levels of Tagln2 and P-selectin. Moreover, in NRP1 or Tagln2 silencing group, the expression of VEGFR2, VWF, and NrCAM was recovered with exogenous replenishment of Tagln2 or NRP1, and the expression of E-cadherin, cleaved Caspase and cleaved PARP1 was downregulated again, respectively. In addition, the phosphorylation levels of downstream targets, including ERK1/2, JNK, and C-Jun, were significantly increased after Tagln2 overexpression in ED-25 and Ealy926 cells, while the inverse results were found in si-*TAGLN2* cells (**Figure 5C**). Taken together, these results revealed that the molecular mechanism underlying the angiogenic activity of Tagln2—namely, Tagln2 upregulation—led to a significant increase in NRP1, which mediated the NRP1/VEGFR2 pathway and the downstream MAPK/ERK and MAPK/JNK signaling pathways.

DISCUSSION

The function of Tagln2 in tumor progression has not yet been clarified; importantly, the precise biological role and underlying mechanism of this molecule in tumor angiogenesis has rarely been reported. In our previous report, we found that Tagln2 was

TABLE 2 | DEGs related to *TAGLN2* overexpression in HUVECs identified using RNA-Seq analysis.

NO.	Symbol	Description	$log_2^{(FC)}$
1	PTMS	Parathymosin	-12.46
2	FBXO11	F-box protein 11	-12.24
3	SET	SET nuclear proto-oncogene	-12.00
4	RELB	RELB proto-oncogene, NF-kB subunit	-11.82
5	TJP2	Tight junction protein 2	-11.76
6	SFXN3	Sideroflexin 3	-11.68
7	SLBP	Stem-loop binding protein	-10.92
8	NAGK	N-acetylglucosamine kinase	-10.81
9	GPSM1	G protein signaling modulator 1	-10.66
10	TNIP1	TNFAIP3 interacting protein 1	-10.59
11	TNIP3	TNFAIP3 interacting protein 3	-10.49
12	MAP3K3	Mitogen-activated protein kinase kinasekinase 3	-10.04
13	ATP6V0E2	ATPase H+ transporting V0 subunit e2	-10.04
14	CCSAP	Centriole, cilia and spindle associated protein	-9.91
15	NOX4	NADPH oxidase 4	-9.81
16	SPAST	Spastin	-9.53
17	ZNF839	Zinc finger protein 839	-9.51
18	SAMD9	Sterile alpha motif domain containing 9	-9.39
19	NBPF14	Neuroblastoma breakpoint family member 14	-9.34
20	DCAKD	Dephospho-CoA kinase domain containing	-9.23
21	SEPT9	Septin 9	-9.22
22	PJA1	Praja ring finger ubiquitin ligase 1	-9.05
23	TUBGCP2	Tubulin gamma complex associated protein 2	-9.04
24	ZEB2	Zinc finger E-box binding homeobox 2	-8.76
25	R3HDM1	R3H domain containing 1	-8.63
26	MAPRE2	Microtubule associated protein RP/EB family member 2	-8.57
27	PTPRS	Protein tyrosine phosphatase, receptor type S	-8.44
28	SETDB2	SET domain bifurcated 2	-8.38
29	ZNF322	Zinc finger protein 322	-8.26
30	TLE3	Transducin like' enhancer of split 3	-8.23
31	PHLDB1	Pleckstrin homology like domain family B member 1	-8.20
32	MADD	MAP kinase activating death domain	-8.15
33	KIAA1109	Fragile Site-Associated Protein	-7.59
34	PLEKHM1	Pleckstrin homology domain-containing family M member 1	-7.59
35	TNRC6B	Trinucleotide repeat containing 6B	-7.06
36	MACF1	Microtubule-actin crosslinking factor 1	-6.87
37	PI4KA	PREDICTED: phosphatidylinositol 4-kinase alpha isoform X3	-6.57
38	ARID4B	AT-rich interaction domain 4B	-5.02
39	LRRC41	Leucine-rich repeat-containing protein 41	-4.80
40	ITPKB	Inositol-trisphosphate 3-kinase B	-1.31
41	TMBIM6	Transmembrane BAX inhibitor motif containing 6	1.17
42	FLNB	Filamin B	1.28
43	HIVEP2	Human immunodeficiency virus type I enhancer binding protein 2	1.30
44	SLC38A2	Solute carrier family 38 member 2	1.42
45	KATNA1	Katanin catalytic subunit A1	5.66
46	TICRR	TOPBP1 interacting checkpoint and replication regulator	7.06
47	CASP10	Caspase 10	7.98
48	ADAMTSL4	ADAMTS like 4	8.18
49	CYP26B1	Cytochrome P450 family 26 subfamily B member 1	8.20
50	ATP2C1	ATPase secretory pathway Ca2+ transporting 1	8.42
51	TAGLN2	Transgelin 2	8.50
52	NSD2	Nuclear receptor binding SET domain protein 2	8.54
53	YAP1	Yes associated protein 1	8.57
54	PTPRK	Protein tyrosine phosphatase, receptor type K	8.74
55	MEF2C	Myocyte enhancer factor 2C	8.74
56	ZNF462	Zinc finger protein 462	8.87
57	NRP1	Neuropilin 1	8.98
58	ORC1	Origin recognition complex subunit 1	9.06
59	NUMA1	Nuclear mitotic apparatus protein 1	9.09
60	HIPK1	Homeodomain interacting protein kinase 1	9.18
61	MBNL2	Muscleblind like splicing regulator 2	9.28
62	NSF	N-ethylmaleimide sensitive factor, vesicle fusing ATPase	9.34
63	PTPRM	Protein tyrosine phosphatase, receptor type M	9.40

(Continued)

TABLE 2 | Continued

NO.	Symbol	Description	$log_2^{(FC)}$
64	BTN3A2	Butyrophilin subfamily 3 member A2	9.46
65	CEP120	Centrosomal protein 120	9.54
66	NCOR2	Nuclear receptor corepressor 2	9.60
67	NOS3	Nitric oxide synthase 3	9.61
68	ZNF268	Zinc finger protein 268	9.75
69	METTL21A	Methyltransferase like 21A	9.87
70	MBD1	Methyl-CpG binding domain protein 1	10.04
71	SEMA4D	Semaphorin 4D	10.07
72	ELP5	Elongator acetyltransferase complex subunit 5	10.10
73	RNF145	Ring finger protein 145	10.16
74	NUP88	Nucleoporin 88	10.20
75	NCOA4	Nuclear receptor coactivator 4	10.21
76	R3HCC1	R3H domain and coiled-coil containing 1	10.22
77	TPD52L2	Tumor protein D54	10.31
78	HNRNPUL1	Heterogeneous nuclear ribonucleoprotein U like 1	10.34
79	LMNA	Lamin A/C	10.43
80	MFSD8	Major facilitator superfamily domain-containing protein 8	10.43
81	MYCBP2	MYC binding protein 2, E3 ubiquitin protein ligase	10.52
82	NBN	Nibrin	10.80
83	ACO1	Aconitase 1	11.11
84	DNPEP	Aspartyl aminopeptidase	11.73
85	PDGFRL	Platelet derived growth factor receptor like	12.31
86	RPL23A	Ribosomal protein L23a	12.39

significantly overexpressed in ECs from lung cancer tumor tissues and that its high expression was associated with advanced clinical stage, increased tumor size, and histological neural invasion (16). These data indicated the important role of Tagln2 in tumor angiogenesis, so we further explored its function specifically in GC. Recently, antiangiogenic strategies have primarily focused on targeting tumor-derived ECs, which, within the tumor microenvironment, exhibit unique characteristics during tumor progression (16). The proangiogenic functions of Tagln2 were first studied in ECs. Tagln2 overexpression significantly promoted EC proliferation, motility and capillary-like tube formation, but these processes were obviously inhibited after Tagln2 downregulation. These processes are integral components of angiogenesis and prerequisites for malignant tumor growth. Tagln2 elevated the levels of angiogenic cytokines and chemokines in ECs, including TNFα, GRO, IL-8, HGF, IL-6, IL-1, PDGF-BB, and so on, which are characterized as important promoters of angiogenesis (23–26). The increased expression of the EC markers PECAM1, VEGFR2 and Tie-2 detected in the array, confirmed the Tagln2-derived angiogenesis. VEGFR2 activation is the most potent inducer of angiogenesis and is associated with enhanced EC migration and survival (27). The Tie-2 tyrosine kinase receptor, which has been shown to be the first validated tumor vascular response biomarker for VEGF inhibitor efficacy in metastatic colorectal cancer, is expressed mainly on vascular ECs and is essential for vascular maturation (28). Upregulation of the adhesion molecules CEACAM1, and ALCAM plays an important role in regulating EC network formation, migration and permeability, implicating the function of Tagln2 in the pro-angiogenesis and invasion/metastasis of tumors (17, 29). Downregulation of proteins involved in leukocyte recruitment (uPAR, RANTES, ENA-78, ANG-2 and LIF), and leukocyte trans endothelial migration (P-selectin and VCAM-1) (30), indicated the Tagln2 associated interaction decrease between leukocyte and ECs.

Furthermore, the results of integrated analysis of antibody array and RNA-Seq data suggested that NRP1 may be the critical molecule mediating the angiogenic activity of Tagln2. NRP1, a transmembrane protein, promotes both physiological and pathological angiogenesis in ECs (31). Studies in endothelial- and VEGF binding-specific NRP1 knock-in mice demonstrate that VEGF-NRP1 signaling pathways in ECs are essential for angiogenesis (32). NRP1 has been investigated mainly as a coreceptor with VEGFR2 for the $VEGF_{165}$ isoform of VEGF-A, and its overexpression enhances the affinity labeling of $VEGF_{165}$ (33). Then, the complex formed by NRP1 and phosphorylated VEGFR2 trigger activation of the downstream focal adhesion kinase PI3K/Akt and the MAPK pathway to promote EC proliferation and migration and angiogenic sprout formation (34). NRP1 also acts as a receptor for class III/IV semaphorins (35) and several other growth factors, such as HGF, FGF, TGF-β, and PDGFB (36, 37). NRP1 expression was upregulated in primary tumor tissue than normal tissue of stomach adenocarcinoma from TCGA data, which was related to tumor stage, and high expression of NRP1 was significantly related to a shorter overall survival (22). Recent studies have supported NRP1 as a potential tumor anti-angiogenesis therapeutic target, and NRP1-neutralizing antibodies or small-molecule antagonists have been shown to suppress tumor growth in an additive manner to VEGF neutralization (38). In the present study, the expression of NRP1 as well as that of multiple downstream signaling mediators, including phosphorylated ERK1/2, JNK and c-Jun, was significantly upregulated by Tagln2 overexpression. In addition, cells stably expressing TAGLN2 and subjected to a series of treatments, including

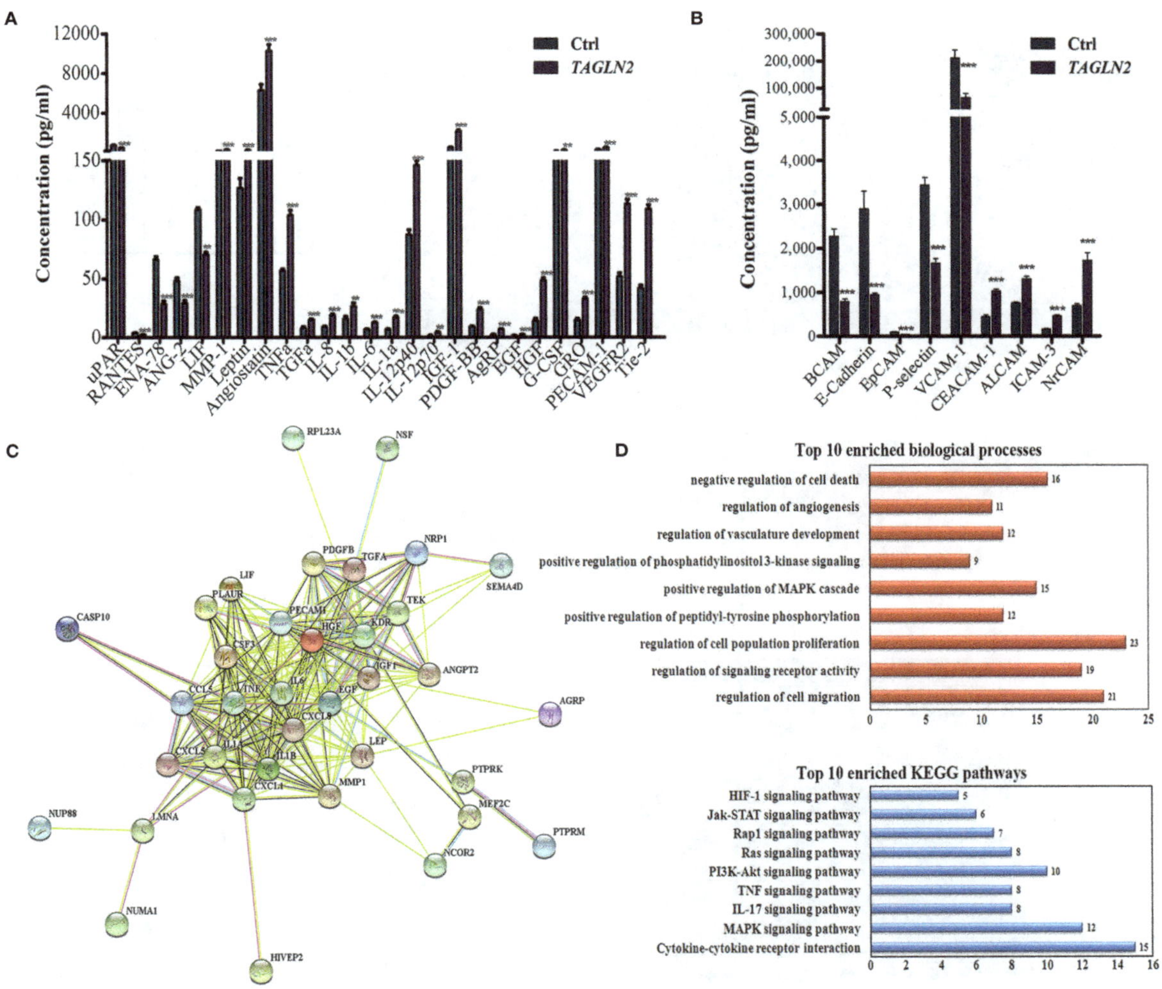

FIGURE 4 | The critical molecule and signaling pathway related to the angiogenic function of Tagln2. **(A, B)** Tagln2-derived expression of angiogenesis factors and adhesion molecular in ECs. Primary HUVECs infected with lentiviral expression vector directing the expression of TAGLN2 or with mock vectors were prepared. The RayBiotech Human Angiogenesis Antibody Array 1000 and Adhesion Molecule Array Q1 (Cat#QAH-ANG-2 and QAH-CAM-1) were purchased from RayBiotech Inc. (Norcross, GA, USA). Blots were scanned with an InnoScan 300 Microarray Scanner and analyzed using ImageJ software. Proteins with band densities exhibiting a fold increase of greater than 1.5 or a fold decrease of greater than 0.67 were defined as differentially expressed proteins. The relationship between 26 differentially expressed proteins from the angiogenesis antibody array and 47 upregulated DEGs identified by RNA-Seq were analyzed and deeply mined using the STRING website (https://string-db.org/). A protein-protein interaction network was constructed **(C)**, and the corresponding Top 10 enriched biological processes and KEGG pathways **(D)** were shown. $^{**}P < 0.01$, $^{***}P < 0.001$.

simultaneous knockdown of TAGLN2 and NRP1, TAGLN2 knockdown with exogenous replenishment of NRP1, or NRP1 knockdown with exogenous replenishment of TAGLN2 were prepared for migration, capillary-like tube formation and protein detection assays. The results of these assays further revealed the critical role of NRP1 in the angiogenic activity of Tagln2 and the activation of MAPK/ERK and MAPK/JNK signaling pathways. These findings indicate the potential therapeutic value of Tagln2 in combating angiogenesis in GC.

Tagln2 has been demonstrated to be upregulated and possess oncogenic functions in various solid cancers (3–7), but only one study mentioned the elevated expression of Tagln2 in GC as the target of microRNA-133a (39). High expression of Tagln2 in tumor-derived ECs from lung cancer was observed in our previous research and was associated with stage, tumor size, and histological neural invasion (16). Moreover, elevated expression of Tagln2 in tumor-derived ECs but not in the whole mixed tumor tissue was reported for the first time. In this study, Tagln2 expression was significantly upregulated in ECs from gastric tumor tissues compared with that from normal tissues, and significantly correlated with the presence of lymph node as well as distant metastases. Given the substantial resources invested in NRP1-targeted anti-angiogenesis therapies for cancer, our results will provide new insights into the regulate mechanisms of NRP1 related angiogenesis and ultimately may be integral for developing new treatment strategies.

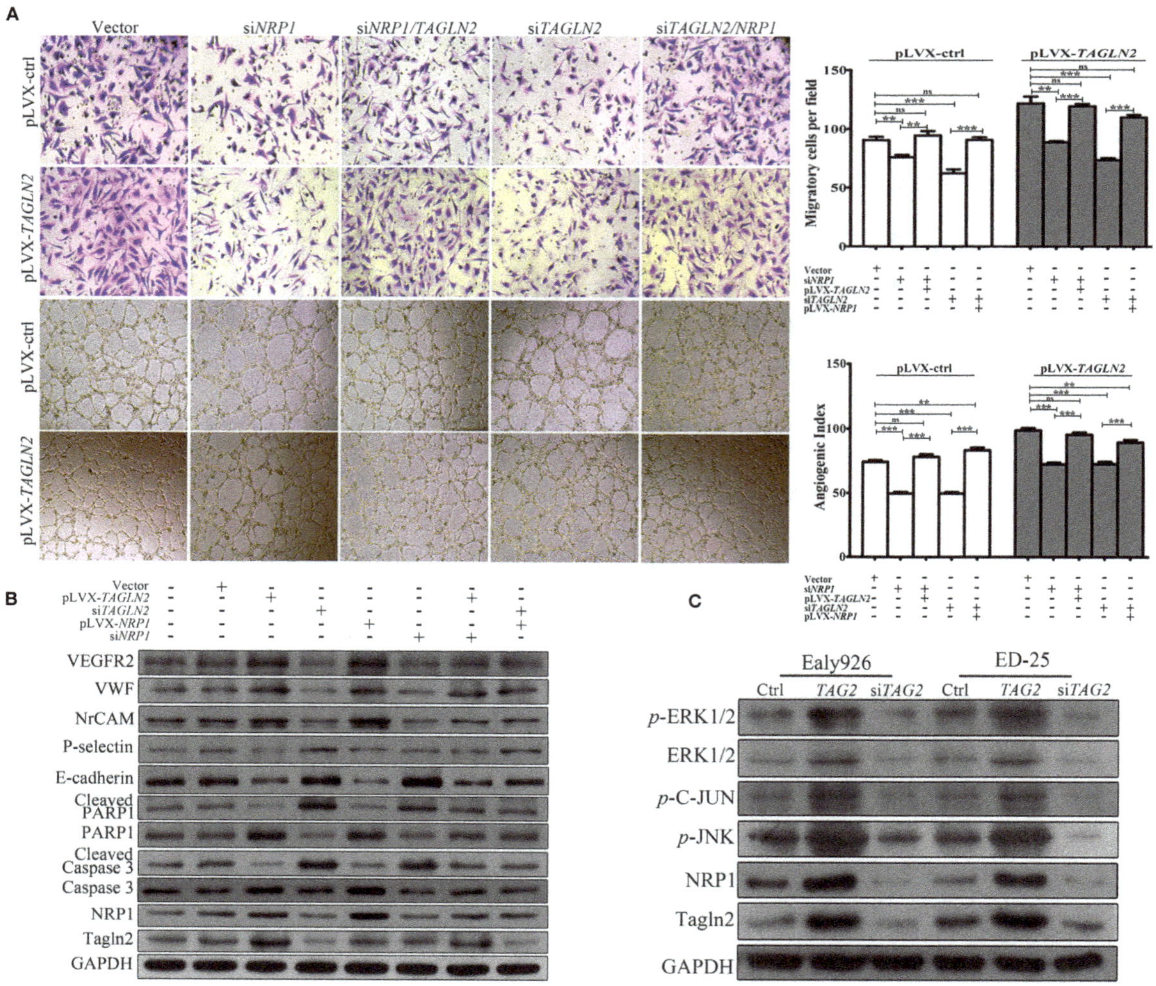

FIGURE 5 | NRP1 mediated the angiogenic function of Tagln2. **(A)** Migration and *in vitro* tube-forming activity of control Ealy926 cells (pLVX-ctrl) and Ealy926 cells with stable expression of TAGLN2 (pLVX-*TAGLN2*) subjected to a series of treatments, including knockdown of endogenous NRP1, knockdown of endogenous Tagln2, knockdown of endogenous NRP1 with exogenous replenishment of Tagln2 or knockdown of endogenous Tagln2 with exogenous replenishment of NRP1. **(B, C)** After modulation of *TAGLN2* and *NRP1* expression in ECs, levels of VEGFR2, VWF (markers of endothelial cells), NrCAM (mediating capillary outgrowth), E-cadherin, P-selectin (related to ECs adhesion and migration), Caspase 3/cleaved Caspase 3 and PARP1/cleaved PARP1 (markers of apoptosis), as well as downstream targets, including phosphorylated ERK1/2, JNK, and C-Jun, were measured by western blotting. GAPDH was used as the loading control. $^{**}P < 0.01$, $^{***}P < 0.001$. ns, not significant.

In conclusions, we demonstrated that Tagln2 expression was significantly upregulated in ECs from gastric tumor tissues compared with ECs from normal tissues and was significantly correlated with the presence of lymph node as well as distant metastases. The results of gain- and loss-of-function approaches emphasized the function of Tagln2 in promoting EC proliferation, motility, and capillary-like tube formation and in reducing apoptosis. Tagln2 upregulation led to significantly increased mRNA and protein levels of NRP1 and subsequently activated the NRP1/VEGFR2 and downstream MAPK signaling pathways to promote angiogenesis. Tagln2 may therefore be both a therapeutic target in combination with current antiangiogenic strategies targeting VEGF-mediated pathways and a candidate prognostic marker for GC.

AUTHOR CONTRIBUTIONS

HZ and HJ conceived and designed the research. HZ, JH, HJ, WZ, and HP developed the methodology. JH and HP analyzed/scored the IHC results. WZ and HP analyzed and interpreted the data (e.g., statistical analysis, biostatistics, and computational analysis). HZ and HJ wrote and reviewed the manuscript. JH and HP provided administrative, technical, or material support (i.e., reporting or organizing data and constructing databases). HZ and JH supervised this study. All authors contributed to the article and approved the submitted version.

REFERENCES

1. Sung H, Ferlay J, Siegel RL, Laversanne M, Soerjomataram I, Jemal A, et al. Global Cancer Statistics 2020: GLOBOCAN Estimates of Incidence and Mortality Worldwide for 36 Cancers in 185 Countries. *CA Cancer J Clin* (2021) 0:1–41. doi: 10.3322/caac.21660
2. Chen WQ, Zheng RS, Baade PD, Zhang SW, Zeng HM, Bray F, et al. Cancer Statistics in China 2015. *CA Cancer J Clin* (2016) 66(2):115–32. doi: 10.3322/caac.21338
3. Zhang Y, Ye Y, Shen D, Jiang K, Zhang H, Sun W, et al. Identification of Trasgelin-2 as Biomarker of Colorectal Cancer by Laser Capture Microdissection and Quantitative Proteome Analysis. *Cancer Sci* (2010) 101 (2):523–9. doi: 10.1111/j.1349-7006.2009.01424.x
4. Yoshino H, Chiyomaru T, Enokida H, Kawakami K, Tatarano S, Nishiyama K, et al. The Tumor-Suppressive Function of miR-1 and miR-133a Targeting TAGLN2 in Bladder Cancer. *Br J Cancer* (2011) 104(5):808–18. doi: 10.1038/bjc.2011.23
5. Fukushima C, Murakami A, Yoshitomi K, Sueoka K, Nawata S, Nakamura K, et al. Comparative Proteomic Profiling in Squamous Cell Carcinoma of the Uterine Cervix. *Proteomics Clin Appl* (2011) 5(3-4):133–40. doi: 10.1002/prca.201000077
6. Du YY, Zhao LM, Chen L, Sang MX, Li J, Ma M, et al. The Tumor-Suppressive Function of miR-1 by Targeting LASP1 and TAGLN2 in Esophageal Squamous Cell Carcinoma. *J Gastroenterol Hepatol* (2016) 31 (2):384–93. doi: 10.1111/jgh.13180
7. Han MZ, Xu R, Xu YY, Zhang X, Ni SL, Huang B, et al. TAGLN2 is a Candidate Prognostic Biomarker Promoting Tumorigenesis in Human Gliomas. *J Exp Clin Cancer Res* (2017) 36(1):155. doi: 10.1186/s13046-017-0619-9
8. Zhang H, Jiang M, Liu Q, Han Z, Zhao Y, Ji S. miR-145-5p Inhibits the Proliferation and Migration of Bladder Cancer Cells by Targeting TAGLN2. *Oncol Lett* (2018) 16(5):6355–60. doi: 10.3892/ol.2018.9436
9. Zhao F, Zhou LH, Ge YZ, Ping WW, Wu X, Xu ZL, et al. MicroRNA-133b Suppresses Bladder Cancer Malignancy by Targeting TAGLN2-Mediated Cell Cycle. *J Cell Physiol* (2019) 234(4):4910–23. doi: 10.1002/jcp.27288
10. Xu SG, Yan PJ, Shao ZM. Differential Proteomic Analysis of a Highly Metastatic Variant of Human Breast Cancer Cell Using Two-Dimensional Differential Gel Electrophoresis. *J Cancer Res Clin Oncol* (2010) 136:1545–56. doi: 10.1007/s00432-010-0812-0
11. Elsner M, Rauser S, Maier S, Schone C, Balluff B, Meding S, et al. MALDI Imaging Mass Spectrometry Reveals COX7A2, TAGLN2 and S100-A10 as Novel Prognostic Marker in Barret's Adenocarcinoma. *J Proteomics* (2012) 75 (15):4693–704. doi: 10.1016/j.jprot.2012.02.012
12. Leung WKC, Ching AKK, Chan AWH, Poon TCW, Mian H, Wong AST, et al. A Novel Interplay Between Oncogenic PFTK1 Protein Kinase and Tumor Suppressor TAGLN2 in the Control of Liver Cancer Cell Motility. *Oncogene* (2011) 30(44):4464–75. doi: 10.1038/onc.2011.161
13. Na BR, Jun CD. TAGLN2-Mediated Actin Stabilization at the Immunological Synapse: Implication for Cytotoxic T Cell Control of Target Cells. *BMB Rep* (2015) 48(7):369–70. doi: 10.5483/bmbrep.2015.48.7.132
14. Jeon BN, Kim HR, Chung YS, Na BR, Park H, Hong C, et al. Actin Stabilizer TAGLN2 Potentiates Adoptive T Cell Therapy by Boosting the Inside-Out Costimulation Via Lymphocyte Function-Associated Antigen-1. *Oncoimmunology* (2018) 7(12):e1500674. doi: 10.1080/2162402X.2018.1500674
15. Kim IG, Lee JH, Kim SY, Hwang HM, Kim TR, Cho EW. Hypoxia-Inducible Transgelin 2 Selects Epithelial-to-Mesenchymal Transition and γ-Radiation-Resistant Subtypes by Focal Adhesion Kinase-Associated Insulin-Like Growth Factor 1 Receptor Activation in Non-Small-Cell Lung Cancer Cells. *Cancer Sci* (2018) 109(11):3519–31. doi: 10.1111/cas.13791
16. Jin H, Cheng X, Pei Y, Fu J, Lyu Z, Peng H, et al. Identification and Verification of Transgelin-2 as a Potential Biomarker of Tumor-Derived Lung-Cancer Endothelial Cells by Comparative Proteomics. *J Proteomics* (2016) 136:77–88. doi: 10.1016/j.jprot.2015.12.012
17. Nouvion AL, Oubaha M, Leblanc S, Davis EC, Jastrow H, Kammerer R, et al. CEACAM1: A Key Regulator of Vascular Permeability. *J Cell Sci* (2010) 123 (Pt 24):4221–30. doi: 10.1242/jcs.073635
18. Münsterberg J, Loreth D, Brylka L, Werner S, Karbanová J, Gandrass M, et al. ALCAM Contributes to Brain Metastasis Formation in Non-Small-Cell Lung Cancer Through Interaction With the Vascular Endothelium. *Neuro Oncol* (2020) 22(7):955–66. doi: 10.1093/neuonc/noaa028
19. Appleby SL, Cockshell MP, Pippal JB, Thompson EJ, Barrett JM, Tooley K, et al. Characterization of a Distinct Population of Circulating Human Non-Adherent Endothelial Forming Cells and Their Recruitment Via Intercellular Adhesion Molecule-3. *PloS One* (2012) 7(11):e46996. doi: 10.1371/journal.pone.0046996
20. Tang X, Zhang Q, Shi S, Yen Y, Li X, Zhang Y, et al. Bisphosphonates Suppress Insulin-Like Growth Factor 1-Induced Angiogenesis Via the HIF-1alpha/VEGF Signaling Pathways in Human Breast Cancer Cells. *Int J Cancer* (2010) 126:90–103. doi: 10.1002/ijc.24710
21. Zhuo H, Zhao Y, Cheng X, Xu M, Wang L, Lin L, et al. Tumor Endothelial Cell-Derived Cadherin-2 Promotes Angiogenesis and Has Prognostic Significance for Lung Adenocarcinoma. *Mol Cancer* (2019) 18(1):34. doi: 10.1186/s12943-019-0987-1
22. Lyu Z, Jin HW, Yan ZJ, Hu KY, Jiang HW, Peng HF, et al. Effects of NRP1 on Angiogenesis and Vascular Maturity in Endothelial Cells Are Dependent on the Expression of SEMA4D. *Int Mol Med* (2020) 46(4):1321–34. doi: 10.3892/ijmm.2020.4692
23. Pappa CA, Tsirakis G, Kanellou P, Kaparou M, Stratinaki M, Xekalou A, et al. Monitoring Serum Levels ELR$^+$CXC Chemokines and the Relationship Between Microvessel Density and Angiogenic Growth Factors in Multiple Myeloma. *Cytokine* (2011) 56(3):616–20. doi: 10.1016/j.cyto.2011.08.034
24. Huang Q, Duan L, Qian X, Fan J, Lv Z, Zhang X, et al. Il-17 Promotes Angiogenic Factors IL-6, Il-8, and Vegf Production Via Stat1 in Lung Adenocarcinoma. *Sci Rep* (2016) 6:36551. doi: 10.1038/srep36551
25. Mantovani A, Barajon I, Garlanda C. IL-1 and IL-1 Regulatory Pathways in Cancer Progression and Theapy. *Immunol Rev* (2018) 281(1):57–61. doi: 10.1111/imr.12614
26. Xue Y, Lim S, Yang Y, Wang Z, Jensen LD, Hedlund EM, et al. Pdgf-BB Modulates Hematopoiesis and Tumor Angiogenesis by Inducing Erythropoietin Production in Stromal Cells. *Nat Med* (2011) 18(1):100–10. doi: 10.1038/nm.2575
27. Njah K, Chakraborty S, Qiu B, Arumugam S, Raju A, Pobbati AV, et al. A Role of Agrin in Maintaining the Stability of Vascular Endothelial Growth Factor Receptor-2 During Tumor Angiogenesis. *Cell Rep* (2019) 28(4):949–65. doi: 10.1016/j.celrep.2019.06.036
28. Jayson GC, Zhou C, Backen A, horsley L, Marti-Marti K, Shaw D, et al. Plasma Tie2 Is a Tumor Vascular Response Biomarker for VEGF Inhibitors in Metastatic Colorectal Cancer. *Nat Commun* (2018) 9(1):4672. doi: 10.1038/s41467-018-07174-1
29. Poissonnier L, Villain G, Soncin F, Mattot V. miR126-5p Repression of ALCAM and SetD5 in Endothelial Cells Regulates Leucocyte Adhesion and Transmigration. *Cardiovasc Res* (2014) 102(3):436–47. doi: 10.1093/cvr/cvu040
30. Goswami D, Vestweber D. How Leukocytes Trigger Opening and Sealing of Gaps in the Endothelial Barrier. *F1000Res* (2016) 2016:5. doi: 10.12688/f1000research.9185.1
31. Fantin A, Lampropoulou A, Gestri G, Raimondi C, Senatore V, Zachary I, et al. NRP1 Regulates CDC42 Activation to Promote Filopodia Formation in Endothelial Tip Cells. *Cell Rep* (2015) 11(10):1577–90. doi: 10.1016/j.celrep.2015.05.018
32. Gu C, Rodriguez ER, Reimert DV, Shu T, Fritzsch B, Richards LJ, et al. Neuropilin-1 Conveys Semaphorinand VEGF Signaling During Neural and Cardiovascular Development. *Dev Cell* (2003) 5(1):45–57. doi: 10.1016/s1534-5807(03)00169-2
33. Fantin A, Vieira JM, Plein A, Denti L, Fruttiger M, Pollard JW, et al. NRP1 Acts Cell Autonomously in Endothelium to Promote Tip Cell Function During Sprouting Angiogenesis. *Blood* (2013) 121(12):2352–62. doi: 10.1182/blood-2012-05-424713
34. Nienhuser H, Schmidt T. Angiogenesis and Anti-Angiogenic Therapy in Gastric Cancer. Int. *J Mol Sci* (2018) 19(1):43. doi: 10.3390/ijms19010043
35. Janssen BJ, Mailinauskas T, Weir GA, Cader MZ, Siebold C, Jones EY. Neuropilins Lock Secreted Semaphorins Onto Plexins in a Ternary Signaling Complex. *Nat Struct Mol Biol* (2012) 19(12):1293–9. doi: 10.1038/nsmb.2416
36. Dhar K, Dhar G, Majumder M, Haque I, Mehta S, Van Veldhuizen PJ, et al. Tumor Cell-Derived PDGF-B Potentiates Mouse Mesenchymal Stem Cells-Pericytes Transition and Recruitment Through an Interaction With NRP-1. *Mol Cancer* (2010) 9:209. doi: 10.1186/1476-4598-9-209
37. Glinka Y, Stoilova S, Mohammed N, Prud'homme GJ. Neuropilin-1 Exerts Co-Receptor Function for TGF-Beta-1 on the Membrane of Cancer Cells and

Enhances Responses to Both Latent and Active TGF-Beta. *Carcinogenesis* (2011) 32(4):613–21. doi: 10.1093/carcin/bgq281

38. Powell J, Mota F, Steadman D, Soudy C, Miyauchi JT, Crosby S, et al. Small Molecule Neuropilin-1 Antagonists Combine Antiangiogenic and Antitumor Activity With Immune Modulation Through Reduction of Transforming Growth Factor Beta (Tgfβ) Production in Regulatory T-Cells. *J Med Chem* (2018) 61(9):4135–54. doi: 10.1021/acs.jmedchem.8b00210
39. Xu XC, Zhang YH, Zhang WB, Li T, Gao H, Wang YH. MicroRNA-133 a Functions as Tumor Suppressor in Gastric Cancer. *J Biol Regul Homeost Agents* (2014) 28(4):615–24. doi: 10.1007/s13277-015-3749-8

7

Positive Crosstalk Between Hedgehog and NF-κB Pathways Is Dependent on KRAS Mutation in Pancreatic Ductal Adenocarcinoma

Yuqiong Wang[1†], Dan Wang[2†], Yanmiao Dai[3†], Xiangyu Kong[4], Xian Zhu[4], Yunxia Fan[2], Yaodong Wang[3], Hongyu Wu[4], Jing Jin[4], Wenzhu Yao[5], Jun Gao[2], Kaixuan Wang[4*] and Hongwei Xu[3*]*

[1] Department of Gastroenterology, the Hospital of 92608 People's Liberation Army of China (PLA) Troops, Shanghai, China, [2] Institute of Oncology, Second Affiliated Hospital, Xi'an Medical University, Xi'an, China, [3] Department of Gastroenterology, Kunshan Affiliated Hospital of Nanjing University of Chinese Medicine, Suzhou, China, [4] Department of Gastroenterology, Changhai Hospital, Second Military Medical University, Shanghai, China, [5] Bureau of headmaster, Xi'an Medical University, Xi'an, China

***Correspondence:**
Jun Gao
13816012151@163.com
Kaixuan Wang
wangkaixuan224007@163.com
Hongwei Xu
niannian5727@126.com

†These authors share first authorship

It has been shown that aberrant activation of the Hedgehog (Hh) and nuclear factor-kappa B (NF-κB) signaling pathways plays an important role in the pancreatic carcinogenesis, and KRAS mutation is a hallmark of pancreatic ductal adenocarcinoma (PDAC). Until now, the role of KRAS mutation in the context of crosstalk between Hh and NF-κB signaling pathways in PDAC has not been investigated. This study was to determine whether the crosstalk between the Hh and NF-κB pathways is dependent on KRAS mutation in PDAC. The correlation between Gli1, Shh, NF-κB p65 expression and KRAS mutation in PDAC tissues was firstly examined by immunohistochemistry. Next, Western blotting, qPCR, and immunofluorescence were conducted to examine the biological effects of interleukin-1β (IL-1β) and tumor necrosis factor-alpha (TNF-α) as NF-κB signaling agonists, Shh as an Hh ligand alone or in combination with KRAS small interfering RNA (si-KRAS) in KRAS-mutant PDAC cells (MT-KRAS; SW1990 and Panc-1), wild-type KRAS PDAC cells (WT-KRAS; BxPC-3) and mutant KRAS knock-in BxPC-3 cells *in vitro* as well as tumor growth *in vivo*. KRAS mutation-dependent crosstalk between Hh and NF-κB in PDAC cells was further assessed by Ras activity and luciferase reporter assays. The aberrant Hh and NF-κB pathway activation was found in PDAC tissues with KRAS mutation. The same findings were confirmed in MT-KRAS PDAC cells and MT-KRAS knock-in BxPC-3 cells, whereas this activation was not observed in WT-KRAS PDAC cells. However, the activation was significantly down-regulated by KRAS silencing in MT-KRAS PDAC cells. Furthermore, MT-KRAS cancer cell proliferation and survival *in vitro* and tumor growth after inoculation with MT-KRAS cells *in vivo* were promoted by NF-κB and Hh signaling activation. The pivotal factor for co-activation of NF-κB and Hh signaling is MT-KRAS protein upregulation, showing that positive crosstalk between Hh and NF-κB pathways is dependent upon KRAS mutation in PDAC.

Keywords: KRAS mutation, hedgehog pathway, NF-κB pathway, crosstalk mechanism, pancreatic ductal adenocarcinoma

INTRODUCTION

Pancreatic ductal adenocarcinoma (PDAC) is one of the most lethal malignancies, with an overall 5-year relative survival rate below 9% (1). Its development and progression are multistep processes involving numerous aberrant genes and signaling pathways (2). Based on global genomic analyses, 12 core signaling pathways and processes have been identified as having clear involvement in PDAC carcinogenesis, suggesting that deregulation of these core pathways are involved in the tumorigenesis of pancreatic cancer (3–5). Among these pathways, the Hedgehog (Hh), nuclear factor-kappa B (NF-κB), and KRAS signaling pathways have been the most studied and their aberrant activation has been shown to play an important role in the pancreatic carcinogenesis (6, 7).

Hh signaling was first discovered in the Drosophila fruit fly by Nusslein-Volhard and Wieschaus, and has since been linked to many aspects of tumor development and disease (8). Specifically, the Hh signaling pathway plays a critical role in pancreatic embryological development, but is inhibited in the mature pancreas. In addition, the Hh signaling pathway is aberrantly activated in the tumor microenvironment of pancreatic cancer to promote the growth of tumor stroma (9). Recent studies, including ours, have suggested that the activation of the Hh pathway has malignant characteristics of the canonical Hh pathway in the tumor stroma and non-canonical Hh-pathway in tumor cells (10–14). Sonic hedgehog (Shh) is the key molecule in the Hh signaling pathway, exerting its role by binding to the target cell member receptor. Shh can induce the activation of the Gli family of transcription factors including Gli1, by the classical pathway as well as the nonclassical pathway (15).

KRAS mutation is a hallmark of PDAC and is detected in 75–95% of these malignancies (16, 17). The role of aberrant KRAS signaling caused by mutation in pancreatic cancer has been clearly demonstrated in genetically engineered mouse models, with the oncogene KRAS G12D mutation conditionally activated in the embryonic pancreas (7). However, in pancreatic epithelial cells, the KRAS G12D activation can induce the development of pancreatic intraepithelial neoplasia (PanIN) precursor lesions, which eventually progress to invasive PDAC after a long period of latency (18–20). If the expression of oncogenic KRAS transgenes is silenced during pancreas development and only activated in adult animals, neither PanIN development nor tumor will develop (21). In addition, KRAS mutations arise presumably in the adult pancreas (2). In that case, KRAS mutation may facilitate or amplify the aberrant activation of other genes or pathways and their interactions, leading to PDAC progression (16, 22, 23).

Stromal hyperplasia is the distinct pathological feature of PDAC, which results in a pronounced pro-inflammatory microenvironment which is driven by the secretion of multiple tumor-derived pro-inflammatory cytokines for cancer cells (18, 24). Indeed, pivotal pro-inflammatory cytokines, including tumor necrosis factor-α (TNF-α) and interleukin-1β (IL-1β), may be secreted by tumor-associated macrophages to further promote tumor cell growth, migration, invasion, and the epithelial to mesenchymal transition, mainly *via* the NF-κB pathway (10, 24–26).

Our previous study indicated that pro-inflammatory cytokines, mainly TNF-α and IL-1β, played a key role in the activation of both canonical and non-canonical Hh pathways in an NF-κB activation-dependent manner in PDAC (10). Intrigued by and built upon these previous findings, we attempted to illuminate the specific mechanisms for the KRAS dependent mutual activation of NF-κB and Hh signaling in PDAC.

MATERIALS AND METHODS

Patients and Samples

Forty patients diagnosed with PDAC and confirmed by histopathology were selected for this study. The study included 14 females and 26 males with a median age at surgery of 58.30 years (range, 50–65 years). Tissue samples were obtained from 2012–2014 at the time of surgery at Changhai Hospital (Shanghai, China). Informed consents were obtained from all patients, and the study was approved by Changhai Hospital Ethics Review Committee. Tissue samples were formalin-fixed and paraffin-embedded, sliced in 3 μm sections, and stained with hematoxylin and eosin (H&E) for routine pathological examination.

Immunohistochemistry

For immunohistochemical (IHC) staining, tissue sections were deparaffinized in xylene, hydrated in a series of diluted ethanol, and subsequently immersed in 3% hydrogen peroxide for 10 min to inactivate endogenous peroxidases. After antigen retrieval, slides were incubated at 4°C overnight with primary antibodies, including rabbit anti-Gli1 polyclonal antibody (1:100, ab49314; Abcam), mouse anti-NF-κB p65 monoclonal antibody (1:50, SC-8008; Santa Cruz), or rabbit anti-Shh monoclonal antibody (1:200, ab53281; Abcam). The next day, slides were washed three times with phosphate-buffered saline (PBS) and incubated for 45 min at room temperature with the appropriate goat anti-rabbit secondary antibody (1:500, ab7090; Abcam) or goat anti-mouse secondary antibody (1:500, ab97040; Abcam). Then the slides were washed with PBS, immersed in liquid 3,3'-diaminobenzidine (DAB) for 5 min, and counterstained with hematoxylin. PBS instead of primary antibody was used for the negative controls. Nuclear expression of Gli1, NF-κB p65, and Shh expression were assessed independently by two pathologists. Staining intensity and distribution were quantified by semi-quantitative scoring. Staining intensity was defined as weak, moderate, or intense while staining distribution was defined as focal (≤10%), regional (11–50%), or diffuse (>50%).

Abbreviations: H&E, hematoxylin and eosin; Hh, Hedgehog; si-KRAS, Human KRAS small interfering RNA; IHC, immunohistochemical; IL-1β, interleukin-1-beta; ip, intraperitoneally; DAB, liquid 3,3'-diaminobenzidine; NF-κB, nuclear factor-kappa B; PDAC, pancreatic ductal adenocarcinoma; PBS, phosphate-buffered saline; PVDF, polyvinylidene difluoride membranes; TNF-α, tumor necrosis factor-alpha.

Cell Culture and Treatment

PDAC cell lines (SW1990, Panc-1, and BxPC-3) were purchased from the Type Culture Collection of the Chinese Academy of Sciences (Shanghai, China). Cells were cultured in Dulbecco's Modified Eagle Medium (DMEM; Gibco, USA) supplemented with 10% fetal bovine serum (FBS; Gibco, USA) and 100 U/mL penicillin-100 ng/mL streptomycin solution (Hyclone, USA). Recombinant human sonic hedgehog (rh-Shh; 1845-SH-100), recombinant human IL-1β (rh-IL-1β; 201-LB-025), and recombinant human TNF-α (rh-TNF-α; 210-TA-100) were purchased from R&D Systems (USA). Human KRAS small interfering RNA (si-KRAS) was purchased from Dharmacon Company. In brief, 2×106 cells were seeded in 10 cm dishes (Corning, USA). When a 50% cell density was reached, cells were starved with 1% FBS-DMEM and then treated with 100 ng/mL Shh, 5 ng/mL IL-1β, 10 ng/mL TNF-α (in 1% FBS-DMEM), and si-KRAS alone or in combination for 48 h, while the medium was freshly replaced every 6 h.

Detection of KRAS Mutations in Codons 12 and 13

For further testing of KRAS mutations, Genomic DNA was extracted from tissue samples using the DNeasy Blood & Tissue Kit (Qiagen, Germany). DNA quantification was done with the Qubit 2.0 Fluorimeter with dsDNA High Sensitivity Assay Kit (Thermo, Germany). Sequencing of KRAS codons 12/13 was performed by Shanghai Life Technologies Biotechnology Co., Ltd in China.

RNA Extraction and Quantitative PCR

For analysis of mRNA expression, total RNA was extracted from PDAC cells using trizol reagent and purified through digestion with DNase I for 15 min. RNA was recovered using the RNeasy Kit (Qiagen, Germany). Reverse transcription of 1 μg purified RNA was conducted in a 20 μL reverse transcription system for 15 min at 37°C according to the manufacturer's protocol. Gli1, NF-κB, Shh, KRAS, and GAPDH Taqman primers were purchased from Invitrogen (Shanghai Life Technologies Biotechnology Co., Ltd.). For quantitative PCR (qPCR), 20 μL mixture reactions including gene-specific taqman primers were run the Roche LightCycler® 480 instrument (Roche, Switzerland). The amount of each target gene in a given sample was normalized to the level of GAPDH in that sample. All experiments were run in triplicate.

Extraction of Nuclear and Cytoplasmic Proteins and Western Blotting

For protein analysis, adherent cells were collected with 0.25% trypsin (Gibco; USA) and centrifuged at 1,000 rpm for 5 min. Next, cells were washed twice with PBS and nuclear and cytoplasmic proteins were extracted with the NE-PER Nuclear and Cytoplasmic Extraction Reagents Kit (Thermo, USA). Protein concentration was then determined using the bicinchoninic acid (BCA) protein assay kit (Thermo, USA) according to the manufacturer's instructions. Both nuclear and cytoplasmic proteins were separated on sodium dodecyl sulfate-polyacrylamide gel electrophoresis (SDS-PAGE), transferred to 0.45 μm polyvinylidene difluoride membranes (PVDF, Bio-Rad; USA), and blocked with 1% bovine serum albumin for 1 h. Then, membranes were incubated overnight at 4°C with rabbit anti-Shh monoclonal antibody (1:2000, ab53281; Abcam), rabbit anti-Gli1 polyclonal antibody (1:1000, ab49314; Abcam), mouse anti-NF-κB p65 monoclonal antibody (1:500, SC-8008; Santa Cruz), rabbit anti-KRAS polyclonal antibody (1:1000, ab180772; Abcam), rabbit anti-GAPDH polyclonal antibody (1:2000, ab9485; Abcam), rabbit anti-phosphorylated ERK1/2 (p-ERK1/2) (1:2000, #4376; CST) and anti-total ERK1/2 (t-ERK1/2) monoclonal antibodies (1:2000, #4695; CST), rabbit anti-phosphorylated AKT1 (p-AKT1) (1:1000, #9018; CST) and anti-total-AKT1 (t-AKT1) monoclonal antibodies (1:1000, #2938; CST) and rabbit anti-histone H3 polyclonal antibody (1:3000, ab1791; Abcam), followed by secondary antibody with a dilution of 1:2000 (goat anti-rabbit antibody, ab7090, Abcam; goat anti-mouse antibody, ab97040, Abcam). The amount of each target gene was normalized to GAPDH or histone H3 in each sample. The blots were visualized using an enhanced chemiluminescence reagent (Thermo, USA).

Immunofluorescence Analysis

For immunofluorescence analysis, SW1990, Panc-1 and BxPC-3 cells were seeded in 24-well plates containing a sterile glass slide. Cells were treated with different stimuli: 100 ng/mL Shh, 5 ng/mL IL-1β, 10 ng/mL TNF-α (in 1% FBS-DMEM) and si-KRAS alone or in combination for 48 h, and then washed three times with ice-cold PBS, fixed in 4% paraformaldehyde for 20 min at room temperature, and finally treated with 0.1% triton for 30 min. After blocking in 1% bovine serum albumin for 1 h at room temperature, the slides were incubated at 4°C overnight with the indicated primary antibody, including rabbit anti-Gli1 (1:100, ab49314; Abcam), rabbit anti-NF-κB p65 subunit (1:50, SC-8008; Santa Cruz) and rabbit anti-Shh (1:200, ab53281; Abcam). Subsequently, fluorescein Dylight 488 or Dylight 594 conjugated donkey anti-rabbit secondary antibody (Jackson Laboratories, USA) at a dilution of 1: 200 was added into cells for 1 h at room temperature. Finally, slides were washed and examined under a fluorescence microscope (Olympus, Japan).

Ras Activity Assay

Ras activity was measured using Ras Activation Assay Kit (Millipore, USA) according to the manufacturer's protocol. Briefly, cells were homogenized in 1× lysis buffer on ice, then sonicated and centrifuged at 12,000 rpm at 4°C for 10 min. Protein concentration was determined by the BCA Protein Assay Kit. Then 1/10 of the lysate was set aside to allow quantification of total Ras and protein concentration. GAPDH was used as an internal control. Equal amounts of lysate were incubated for 1 h at 4°C with agarose beads coated with the Raf-Ras binding domain provided in the kit. Beads were washed three times with ice-cold lysis buffer, and then boiled for 5 min with loading buffer.

Luciferase Assay

For the luciferase assay, cells in 6-well plates were co-transfected with 10 ng pRL-TK (Promega, USA) and 500 ng pGL3-8×Gli1 binding site (BS) luciferase reporter plasmids (wild-type, WT or mutant-type, MT) by FuGENE HD Transfection (Promega,

USA). After 8 h, the medium was changed to 1% FBS-DMEM (control), 100 ng/mL Shh, 5 ng/mL IL-1β, or 10 ng/mL TNF-α in 1% FBS-DMEM for treatment. Luciferase assays were performed 48 h later according to the protocol of the Dual Luciferase Assay Kit (Promega, USA). The luciferase activities were normalized to the Renilla luciferase activity. MT pGL3-8×Gli1 BS luciferase report plasmids were used as control. pGL3-8×Gli1 BS luciferase reporter plasmids (WT or MT) were kindly gifted by Doctor Lei Li from the Shanghai Changhai Hospital.

Cell Counting Kit-8 Assay

Cell viability was determined using the Cell Counting Kit-8 Assay Kit (Dojindo, Japan). Briefly, cells were seeded into 96-well plates at a density of 2×104 cells per well overnight and treated with 1% FBS-DMEM, 100 ng/mL Shh, 5 ng/mL IL-1β, 10 ng/mL TNF-α or si-KRAS (0.15 ng) transfected alone or in combination. At 0, 24, 36, and 48 h post-stimulation, cells were treated with 2-(2-methoxy-4-nitrophenyl)-3-(4-nitrophenyl)-5-(2,4-disulfophenyl)-2H-tetrazolium mono-sodium salt (WST-8) in the dark according to the protocol. Absorbance values were measured at 450 nm by an enzyme-linked immunosorbent assay. All experiments were performed in triplicate.

Apoptosis Assay

Apoptosis was detected and quantified using the Annexin V/FITC staining kit (eBioscience, USA). At 48 h after stimulation, cells were collected and washed twice with PBS. Then cells were centrifuged, resuspended in 100 μL binding buffer, and stained with Annexin V (5 μL) for 15 min at room temperature in the dark. Next, samples were stained with propidium iodide (10 μL) for 5 min in the dark before flow cytometry (Miltenyi Biotec, Germany). The results were analyzed by FlowJo software (Tree Star Inc., USA).

MT-KRAS Plasmid Transfection

MT-KRAS plasmid (KRAS (G12D) mutation) was purchased from Addgene (Watertown, USA). Cells in 6-well plates were transfected with MT-KRAS plasmid using FuGENE HD Transfection Reagent (Promega, USA). Specifically, cells in each well were transfected with 2 μg plasmid, and vehicle was used as control. After 8 h, cells were treated with 1% FBS-DMEM, 100 ng/mL Shh, 5 ng/mL IL-1β, or 10 ng/mL TNF-α in 1% FBS-DMEM. After 48 h, cells were collected for further analysis.

Mouse Xenograft Models

All animal procedures were approved by the Institutional Animal Care and Use Committee of Shanghai Changhai Hospital and conducted in accordance with NIH guidelines for the care and use of laboratory animals. Four-week-old male athymic nude mice were purchased from the Shanghai Laboratory Animal Center in China and raised under specific pathogen-free conditions. SW1990, Panc-1, and BxPc-3 cells (4×106) were respectively resuspended in 100 μL PBS, and then injected subcutaneously into the right flank of mice. After mice developed tumors (for SW1990 and BxPC-3 after 1 week, and for Panc-1 after around 4 weeks), they were randomly assigned into control group (n = 5), Shh group (n = 5), IL-1β group (n = 5), or TNF-α group (n = 5). The administered treatments were as follows: the control group received 200 μL PBS intraperitoneally (ip) daily (QOD); the Shh group received 300 ng Shh (200 μL ip QOD); the IL-1β group received 10 ng IL-1β (200 μL ip QOD); and the TNF-α group received 500 ng TNF-α (200 μL ip QOD) (27–29). After 2 weeks, mice were sacrificed and tumor volumes (V) were calculated (V = [L × W2] × 0.5, [L - length, W - width]) (30). Next, tumor tissues were fixed in formalin for IHC staining, and staining intensity was scored as follows: 0, no staining; 1, mild staining, weak yellow; 2, moderate staining, dark yellow; 3, strong staining, brown; 4, very strong staining, dark brown. The percentage of stained cells was also determined. Finally, the immunoscore was obtained by calculating the product of the proportion of positive cells at each intensity and the corresponding intensity value (31, 32).

Statistical Analysis

All calculations were performed using the Statistical Package for the Social Sciences (version 18.0; USA). The Student's t-test was used to compare the groups and determine the statistical significance. Pearson's correlation was used to calculate the correlation coefficient. All data are expressed as the mean ± standard deviation. $P < 0.05$ was considered statistically significant.

RESULTS

Positive Correlation of Hh and NF-κB Pathway Activation on the Presence of KRAS Mutations in PDAC Tissues

In 40 PDAC tissue samples, KRAS codons 12 and 13 were sequenced and the IHC expression of Shh, Gli1, and NF-κB p65 was examined. KRAS mutation (MT-KRAS) in 32 PDAC tissue samples was detected and no mutation (WT-KRAS) in 8 PDAC tissue samples was detected by sequencing technology. Meanwhile, a significant positive correlation in Gli1, Shh, and NF-κB p65 expression in MT-KRAS tissues was observed, whereas there was no correlation in WT-KRAS tissues by IHC staining (**Figure 1**). These results suggest that there is a KRAS mutation-dependent positive correlation in aberrant activation of Hh and NF-κB pathways in PDAC.

Crosstalk Between Hh and NF-κB Pathways Relies on KRAS Mutation as a Type of Switch in PDAC Cells

To further determine whether crosstalk between Hh and NF-κB pathways is indeed dependent on the presence or absence of KRAS mutation, three different PDAC cell lines (SW1990, Panc-1, and BxPC-3) were chosen based on their specific traits. SW1990 and Panc-1 cell lines have the G12D KRAS mutation whereas the BxPC-3 cell line is negative for KRAS mutation (**Figure S1**). In addition, Shh, Gli1, and NF-κB p65 mRNA and protein expression were detected in all cell lines (**Figure S2**). In this study, cells were treated with IL-1β, TNF-α and Shh and

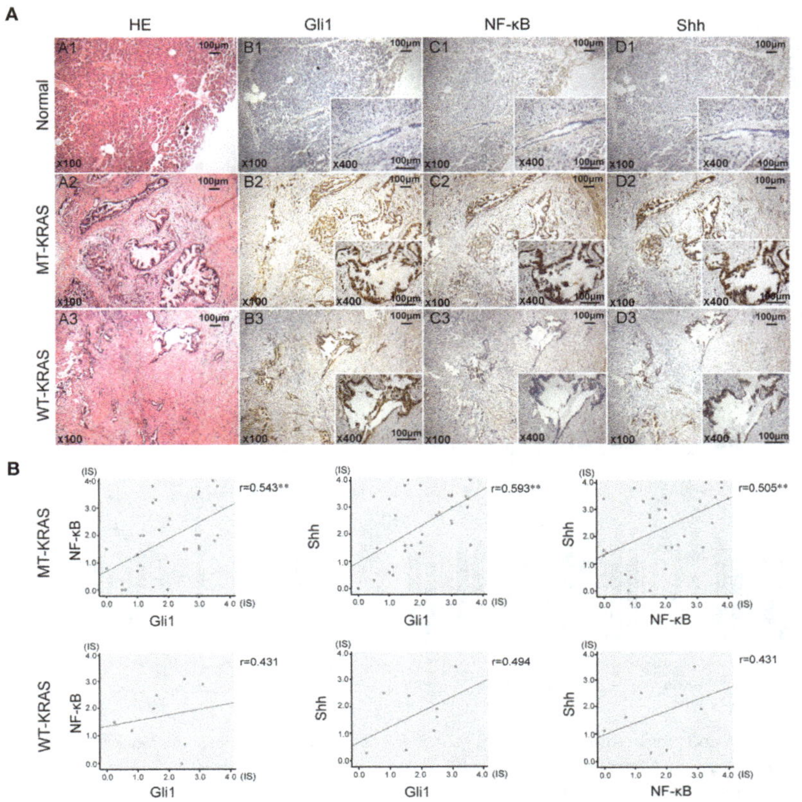

FIGURE 1 | Gli1, NF-κB p65 and Shh protein expression in PDAC tissues with or without KRAS mutation. **(A)** Typical serial PDAC tissue section. HE staining and IHC staining for Gli1, NF-κB p65 and Shh proteins in the normal tissue (A1, B1, C1 and D1), MT-KRAS PDAC tissues (A2, B2, C2 and D2) and WT-KRAS PDAC tissues (A3, B3, C3 and D3). **(B)** Correlation of Gli1, NF-κB p65 and Shh protein expressions in the MT-KRAS and WT-KRAS PDAC tissues. $^{**}p < 0.01$, n=40.

different responses were observed based on the presence or absence of KRAS mutation. Treatment with IL-1β and TNF-α, NF-κB signaling agonists, significantly upregulated NF-κB p65, Shh, and Gli1 mRNA [**Figures 2A(a, b)**], nuclear Gli1 and NF-κB protein, and Shh protein [**Figures 2B (a, b)**] expression in SW1990 and Panc-1 cells. After we demonstrated that si-KRAS transfections are effective in downregulating KRAS expression in the chosen cell lines (**Figure S4**), the combined treatment of si-KRAS with either IL-1β and TNF-α significantly downregulated the stimulatory effects caused by either stimulus alone [**Figures 2A(a, b)** and **2B (a, b)**]. However, no significant changes in the mRNA and protein expression of Gli1, NF-κB, and Shh were observed in BxPC-3 cells treated with IL-1β, TNF-α, or the combination of si-KRAS with either of these two cytokines [**Figures 2A(c)** and **2B(c)**]. The above original Western blots images were shown in **Figure S3**. Next, Shh as an Hh signaling ligand not only significantly upregulated the mRNA and protein expression of Shh and nuclear Gli1 but also NF-κB p65 mRNA and nuclear protein expression in SW1990 and Panc-1 cells, whereas the combined treatment with si-KRAS significantly abrogated the observed stimulatory effects [**Figures 3A(a, b), 3B(a, b)**]. However, no significant changes in Gli1, NF-κB, and Shh mRNA and protein expression were observed in BxPC-3 cells treated with Shh alone or in combination with si-KRAS [**Figures 3A(c), 3B(c)**]. The above original Western blots images were shown in **Figure S5** Similar effects on NF-κB p65 expression were observed with combined treatment of Shh and si-KRAS as detected by immunofluorescence staining in MT-KRAS cell lines SW1990 and Panc-1 and WT-KRAS cell line BxPC-3 (**Figure S6**). In addition, the pGL3-8×Gli1 BS luciferase reporter assay showed that the observed Gli1 gene promoter enhancement after this combined treatment was due to upregulated Gli1 gene expression in MT-KRAS cell lines SW1990 and Panc-1 whereas no significant changes were observed in BxPC-3 (**Figure 4**). To determine whether introduction of KRAS mutation in WT-KRAS PDAC cells could result in positive crosstalk between Hh and NF-κB signaling pathways in a similar manner as seen in MT-KRAS cells, an expression plasmid with KRAS (G12D) mutation (MT-KRAS) was constructed and its potency was validated in BxPC-3 cells (**Figure S7**). Subsequently, transfected cells were treated with IL-1β, TNF-α, or Shh. The results showed that IL-1β and TNF-α could upregulate Gli1 and Shh mRNA expression, and Shh stimulation enhanced NF-κB p65 mRNA expression in BxPC-3 transfected cells (**Figure S8**). But no significant protein expression changes were observed (Data not shown). These

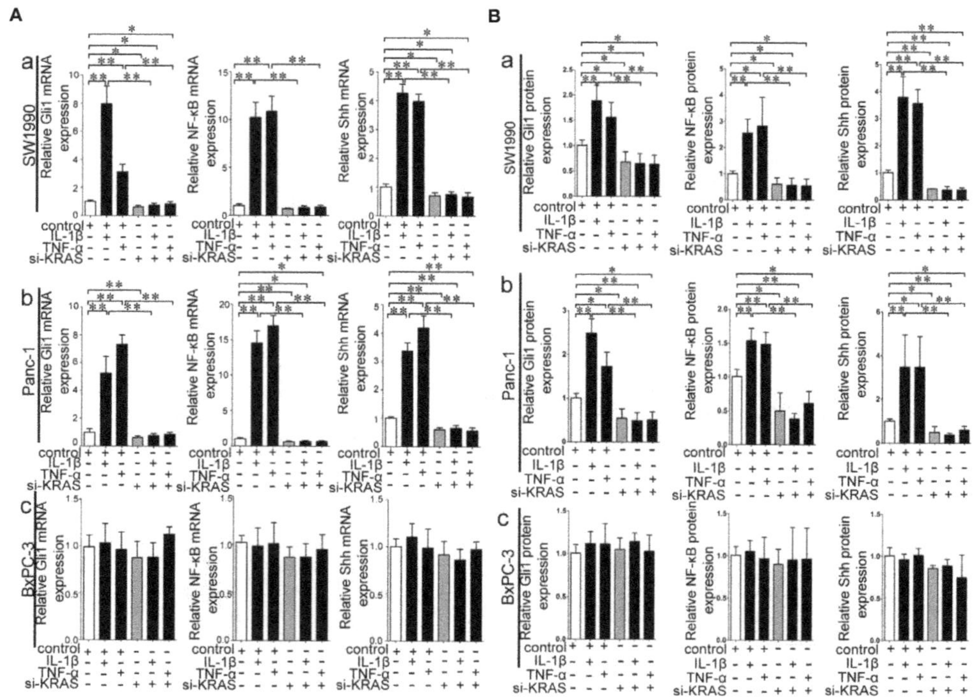

FIGURE 2 | Stimulatory effects on mRNA and protein expression of Gli1, NF-κB and Shh on PDAC cell lines treated with IL-1β and TNF-α alone or in combination with si-KRAS. **(A)** represented mRNA expression in three PDAC cell lines; **(B)** represented gray analysis of relative protein expression; [a. SW1990, b Panc-1, c BxPC-3]. All data were obtained from three independent experiments. *p < 0.05; **p < 0.01.

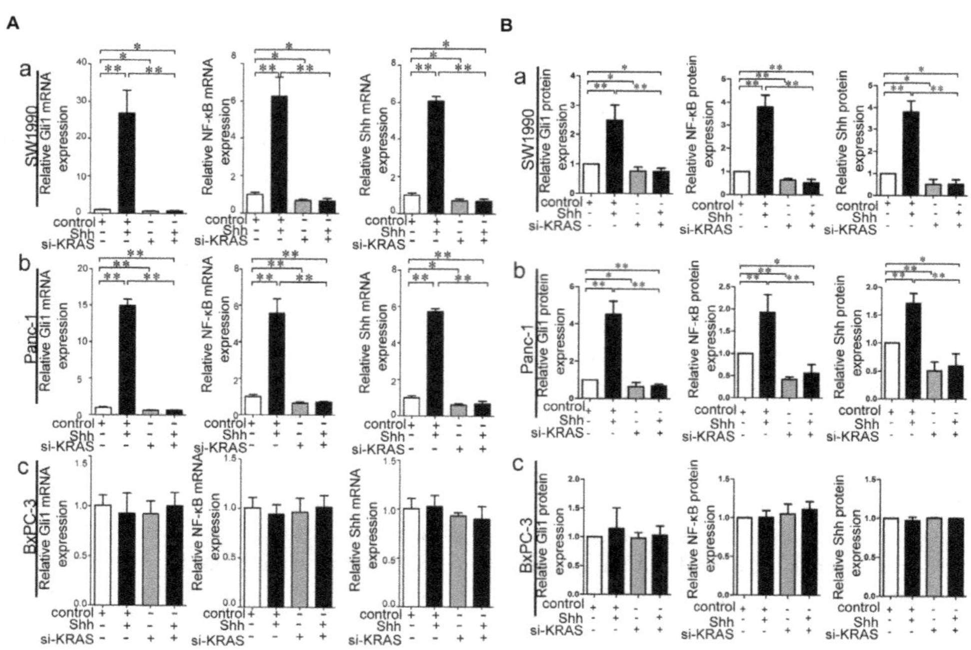

FIGURE 3 | Stimulatory effects on mRNA and protein expression of Gli1, NF-κB and Shh on PDAC cell lines treated with Shh as Hh activating ligand treatment alone or in combination with si-KRAS transfection. **(A)** mRNA expression of Gli1, NF-κB and Shh in three PDAC cell lines; **(B)** Gray analysis of relative protein expression [a. SW1990, b. Panc-1, c. BxPC-3]. All data were obtained in three independent experiments. *p < 0.05; **p < 0.01.

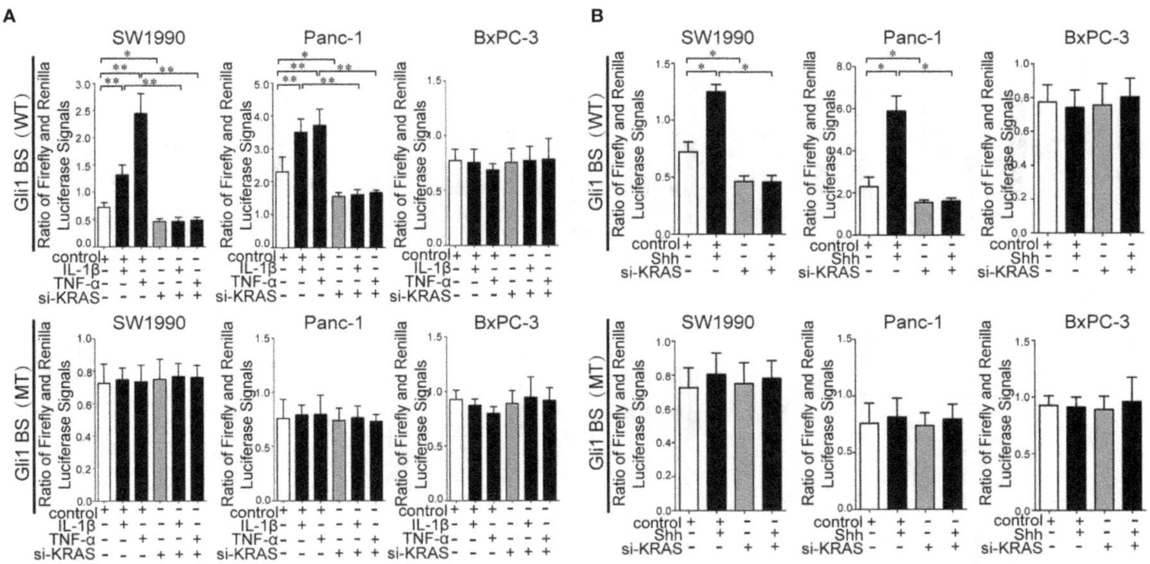

FIGURE 4 | Results of the pGL3-8×Gli1 BS luciferase reporter assay in the MT-KRAS cells (SW1990 and Panc-1) and WT-KRAS cells (BxPC-3) after treatment with: IL-1β, TNF-α alone or in combination with si-KRAS transfection **(A)**. Shh alone or in combination with si-KRAS transfection **(B)**. All data were obtained in three independent experiments. *$p < 0.05$; **$p < 0.01$.

results suggest that the KRAS mutation knock-in can confer the WT-KRAS cell line BxPC-3 with similar traits as those of MT-KRAS cell lines SW1990 and Panc-1. These data indicate the positive crosstalk between Hh and NF-κB signaling pathways in PDAC cells, which is dependent upon the gain-of-function KRAS mutation.

KRAS Protein Activity Is Essential for the Positive Interaction Between Hh and NF-κB Signaling Pathways

KRAS protein acts like a binary molecular switch, and can regulate cell activities only when bound to guanosine triphosphate (GTP). Mutations in KRAS protein render it insensitive to the function of GTP and lead to its constitutive activation (33). Therefore, the alteration of KRAS downstream signaling, such as p-/t-ERK1/2 and p/t-AKT1, and the Ras enzymatic activity were detected in MT-KRAS cells (SW1990 and Panc-1) and WT-KRAS cells (BxPC-3) treated with IL-1β, TNF-α, or Shh alone or in combination with si-KRAS. The expression of p-/t-ERK1/2 and p-/t-AKT1 was increased in SW1990 and Panc-1 cells after either IL-1β, TNF-α, or Shh stimulation, whereas the stimulating effects were significantly decreased by si-KRAS transfection in the combination treatments [(**Figures 5A (a, b), 5B (a, b)**]. However, the effects of IL-1β, TNF-α, and Shh stimulation on KRAS downstream effector molecules were not clearly observed in BxPC-3 cells treated either with IL-1β, TNF-α, Shh alone or in combination with si-KRAS [(**Figures 5A (c), 5B (c)**]. In addition, the stimulatory effects of IL-1β, TNF-α, Shh, and si-KRAS as combination treatments on Ras enzymatic activity were similar to alterations in KRAS downstream effector molecules under the same stimulus (**Figures 5C, D**). Original Western blots images were shown in **Figure S9**. Taken together, these data indicate that KRAS protein activity caused by KRAS mutation is an essential factor for the positive interaction between Hh and NF-κB signaling pathways in PDAC cells.

KRAS Mutation Supports the Malignant Features of PDAC Cells Promoted by IL-1β, TNF-α, or Shh Treatment

Next, we examined the effects of IL-1β, TNF-α, and Shh treatment alone or in combination with si-KRAS on the cellular processes of the three PDAC cell lines. As shown in **Figure 6**, in SW1990 and Panc-1 cells, malignant features such as cell proliferation and survival as indicated by apoptosis were significantly promoted by IL-1β, TNF-α, and Shh treatment compared with the controls. By contrast, malignant features were significantly less induced when cells were treated with those agents in combination with si-KRAS. Furthermore, although si-KRAS transfection in combination with those agents inhibited the features of malignant cells, treatment of SW1990 cells with Shh and Panc-1 cells with TNF-α still had a little effect on promoting malignant features such as proliferation and survival. However, all malignant features were unaltered in BxPC-3 cells treated with either IL-1β, TNF-α, Shh alone or in combination with si-KRAS, except for apoptosis in TNF-α treated Panc-1 cells, which may be caused by TNF-α specialty. These results suggest that the malignant features of PDAC cells are correlated with KRAS mutation, which acts through positive interaction between Hh and NF-κB signaling pathways.

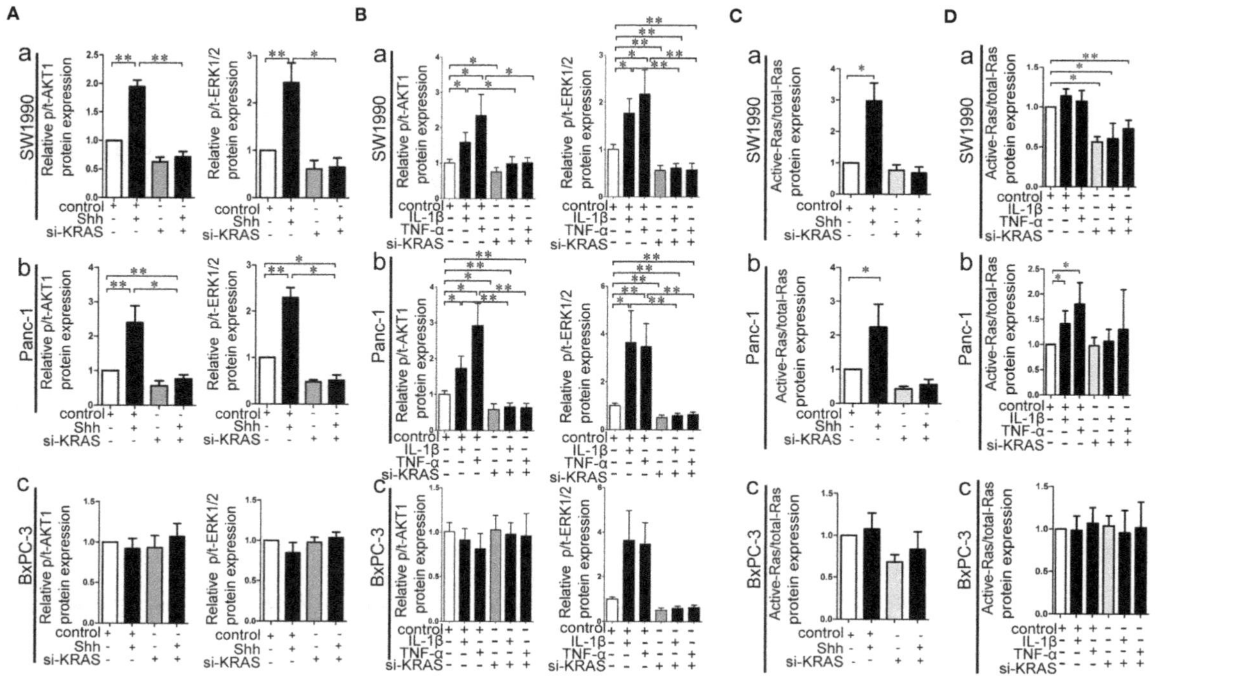

FIGURE 5 | The effect of IL-1β, TNF-α, Shh treatment in combination with si-KRAS on KRAS down-stream molecules (p-/t-ERK1/2 and p-/t-AKT1) and Ras enzymatic activity in the MT-KRAS cell lines (SW1990 and Panc-1) and WT-KRAS cell line (BxPC-3). The protein expression of p-/t-ERK1/2 and p-/t-AKT1 at Shh treatment in combination with si-KRAS treatment **(A)**; The effect of combined IL-1β or TNF-α with si-KRAS transfection on p-/t-ERK1/2 and p-/t-AKT1 **(B)**; Ras enzymatic activity at Shh treatment in combination with si-KRAS treatment **(C)**; The effect of combined IL-1β or TNF-α with si-KRAS transfection on Ras enzymatic activity **(D)** [a. SW1990, b. Panc-1, c. BxPC-3]. All data were obtained in three independent experiments. *p < 0.05; **p < 0.01.

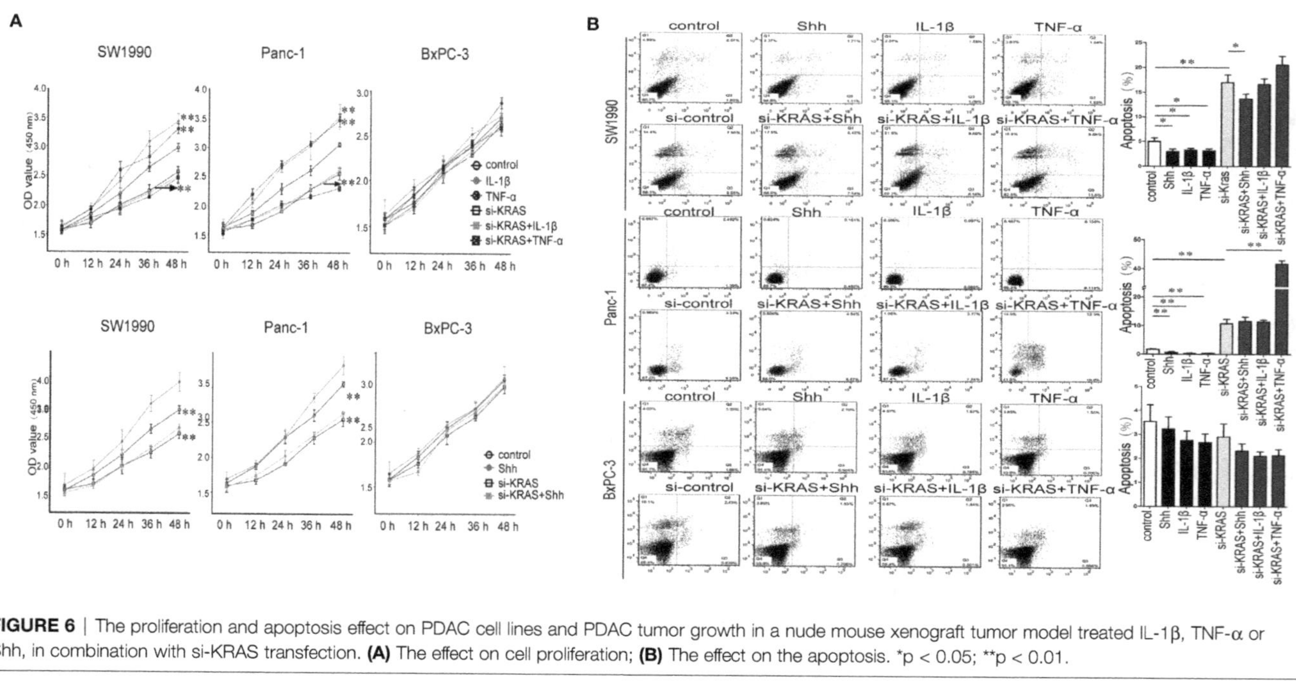

FIGURE 6 | The proliferation and apoptosis effect on PDAC cell lines and PDAC tumor growth in a nude mouse xenograft tumor model treated IL-1β, TNF-α or Shh, in combination with si-KRAS transfection. **(A)** The effect on cell proliferation; **(B)** The effect on the apoptosis. *p < 0.05; **p < 0.01.

KRAS Mutation Induces PDAC Tumor Growth Promoted by IL-1β, TNF-α, and Shh Stimulation in a Xenograft Tumor Model

The nude mouse xenograft tumor model was used to further validate the KRAS mutation-dependent PDAC tumor growth promoted by IL-1β, TNF-α, and Shh stimulation. After mice were inoculated with specific PDAC cells and developed tumors, they were treated with PBS Shh, IL-1β, or TNF-α, and the tumor size was measured every week. After IL-1β, TNF-α, and Shh treatment, tumor growth from the MT-KRAS cell lines SW1990 and Panc-1 was significantly induced compared to the control animals, whereas tumor growth from BxPC-3 cells was not stimulated (**Figure 7**). Similarly, nuclear protein expression of Gli1 and NF-κB p65 was significantly enhanced in tumor tissues from SW1990 cells treated with IL-1β, TNF-α and Shh, whereas no significant expression was observed in the tissues from BxPC-3 cells (**Figure S10**). These results confirm that the dependence of PDAC tumor growth on KRAS mutation is promoted by positive crosstalk between Hh and NF-κB signaling pathways.

DISCUSSION

KRAS gene mutations are quite common in PDAC and appear early in pancreatic carcinogenesis (16). In our study, KRAS mutation was present in 80% (32 of 40) of PDACs. However, KRAS mutation alone in the mature pancreas is not enough to induce PDAC formation (21). In addition, a recent study showed that Hh signaling is required for KRAS-induced pancreatic tumorigenesis (34). Moreover, NF-κB expression is positively associated with Shh expression in PDAC, and NF-κB activation induces the upregulation of Hh signaling (6). In this study we stratified tumor samples according to the KRAS mutation status, and found that Hh signaling and NF-κB were positively correlated only in tumors with KRAS mutation. Thus, our findings support the importance of KRAS mutation in PDAC development, and demonstrate it in another yet not presented context of signaling crosstalk between the Hh and NF-κB pathways.

Based on the results in PDAC tissues, we assumed that KRAS mutation may provide a facilitating environmental milieu for the

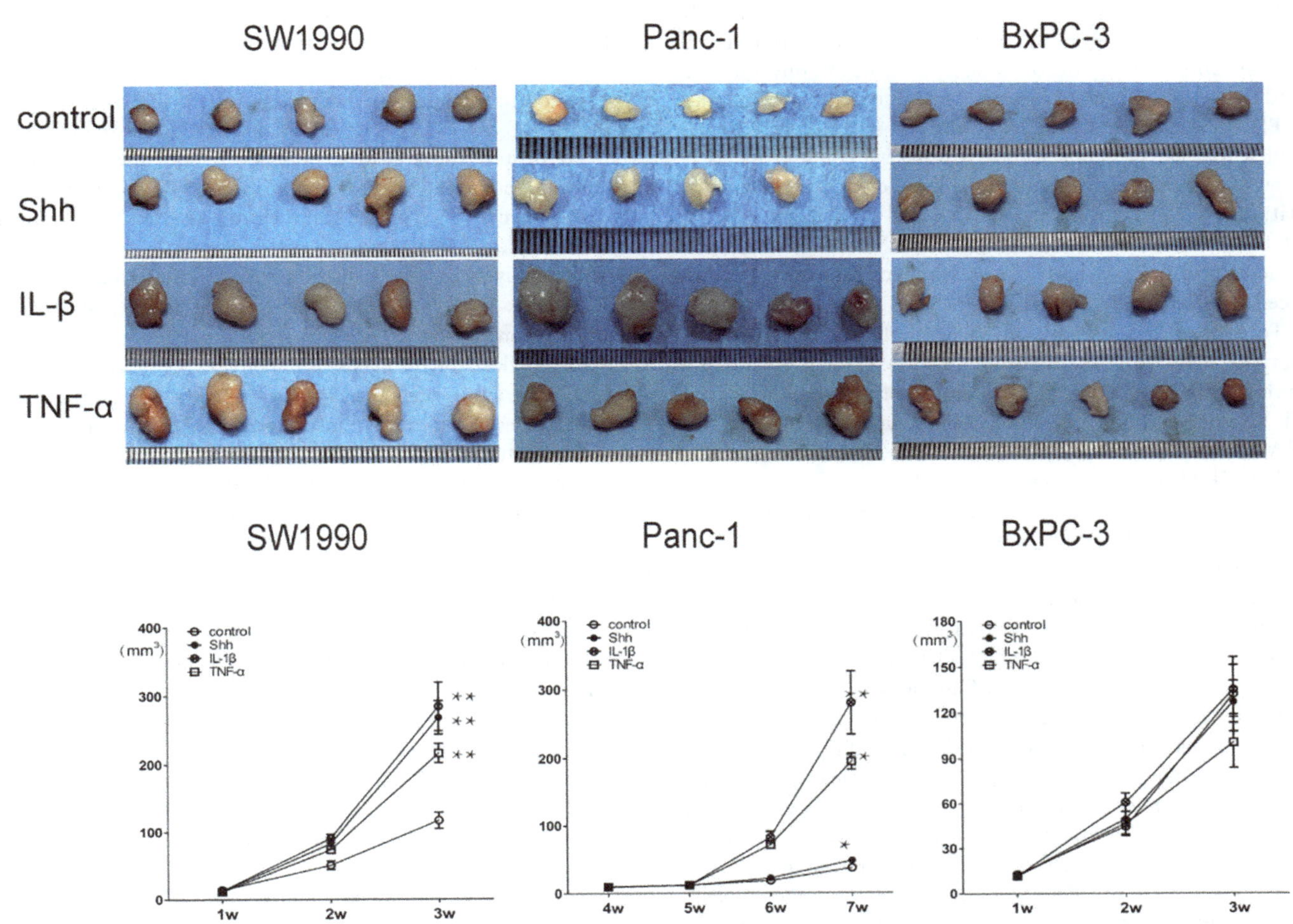

FIGURE 7 | Tumor growth was significantly promoted by IL-1β, TNF-α, and Shh in mice inoculate d with MT-KRAS cells compared with those inoculated with WT-KRAS cells; $^*p < 0.05$; $^{**}p < 0.01$.

aberrant activation and interaction of signaling pathways in the stromal cells as well. Desmoplasia or dense fibrotic stroma is atypical feature of PDAC tissues, and stromal activation is usually found around precancerous lesions (35). Indeed, stromal tissue is not a mere bystander in tumor progression since it has been established that tumor–stroma interactions affect tumorigenesis, angiogenesis, therapy resistance, and possibly the metastatic spread of tumor cells (35). Cells that constitute the tumor stroma provide many factors to initiate and/or support tumorigenesis, including the pro-inflammatory cytokines IL-1β and TNF-α.

Whether Hh pathway activation can up-regulate NF-κB expression has rarely been reported, and the influence of KRAS mutation in this context has not been explored. To verify our hypothesis, we first used rh-IL-1β and rh-TNF-α to stimulate PDAC cells, and tested Hh pathway expression in cell lines with different KRAS mutation status. Our data showed that only in cells with KRAS mutation, rh-IL-1β and rh-TNF-α could initiate Hh pathway activation. These findings suggest that KRAS mutation is a necessary condition for NF-κB/Hh pathway interaction, in keeping with our results obtained from patients' tumor samples.

Embryonic patterning and organ morphogenesis can be regulated by Hh signaling, which is also involved in the regeneration and repair of tissues in normal physiological conditions (11). Aberrant Hh pathway activation is a hallmark of PDAC. Hh pathway activation is mostly induced by Hh ligands that can generate tumor-stromal signaling crosstalk in an autocrine or paracrine manner (36). To further explore the relationship between the Hh pathway and NF-κB, we used rh-Shh to stimulate all three PDAC cell lines. Not surprisingly, NF-κB activation induced by Hh overexpression was only achieved in cell lines with KRAS mutation.

To confirm the necessity of KRAS mutation for Hh/NF-κB interplay in PDAC, we performed knocked down KRAS gene expression in all PDAC cell lines and constructed a knock-in of MT-KRAS plasmid in WT-KRAS cells. Our results showed that KRAS downregulation almost blocked the Hh/NF-κB interplay in MT-KRAS cells, whereas in WT-KRAS cells, MT-KRAS knock-in showed Hh/NF-κB interplay. Collectively, these data suggest that MT-KRAS expression is the key to Hh/NF-κB interplay in PDAC.

The MT-KRAS gene leads to constitutively active KRAS protein (33). Therefore, we decided to examine the expression of KRAS downstream genes and Ras enzymatic activity in PDAC cells treated with IL-1β, TNF-α, Shh alone or in combination with si-KRAS. As a result, KRAS activity was unaltered in WT-KRAS cells but not in MT-KRAS cells. In addition, we did not observe any change in protein expression of nuclear Gli1, nuclear NF-κB, and Shh when MT-KRAS plasmid was knocked into WT-KRAS cells. This might be due to the low level of MT-KRAS protein, which was not sufficient to enhance KRAS activity.

Interestingly, once KRAS was knocked down in Panc-1 cells, TNF-α reduced rather than promoted cell growth. This may be related to the effects of TNF-α, since TNF-α not only activates NF-κB to enhance cell proliferation, but also increases apoptosis. In this study, when KRAS was downregulated, TNF-α was more likely to increase apoptosis than promote cell growth.

Another interesting finding was that when Hh pathway was activated by rh-Shh, other than enhanced nuclear Gli1 and NF-κB expression, Shh itself was also upregulated. Shh is not a target gene of the Hh pathway, so increased Shh expression might be induced by NF-κB expression or some other non-classical Hh activation pathway. Thus, this finding may also be attributed to KRAS mutation in PDAC cells.

In our research, the correlation coefficients between Gli1 and NF-κB, Shh and NF-κB were only slightly over 0.5 in PDAC tissues, and this may be due to inter- and intra-tumor heterogeneity. Hh and NF-κB pathways are crucial in MT-KRAS PDACs, but there are also other pathways involved in PDAC progression. These findings need to be confirmed in a larger patient group.

In a nude mouse xenograft tumor model, tumor developed from SW1990 and Panc-1 cells stimulated with IL-1β, TNF-α, and Shh was significantly promoted compared to control animals, whereas no stimulating effect was observed on tumor development from BxPC-3 cells. This finding suggests that Hh and NF-κB pathways interact in MT-KRAS PDAC. In addition, tumors developed from BxPC-3 were smaller than those from MT-KRAS PDACs, which may suggest the importance of the KRAS gene in PDAC development. Similar alteration on SW1990 cells derived tumors' Gli1 and NF-kB nuclear protein expression in the nucleus were observed with IL-1β, TNF-α and Shh by IHC assay. However, BxPC-3 derived tumors' Gli1 and NF-kB protein were also expressed in the nucleus but no alteration was founded on the condition of IL-1β, TNF-α and Shh treatment. This suggests that the progress of BxPC-3 is much more complex than previous thought.

This study may have limitations. Firstly, we found that mut-KRAS knock-in led to significant increases in the Gli1, NF-kappaB, and Shh expression at the RNA level but not at protein level. With the existing data, the mechanisms underlying the differential effects on the RNA and protein levels remain unclear. Secondly, BxPC-3 cells displayed a constitutive intra-nuclear localization of NF-κB/p65, future study on the expression levels of phospho-p65 is needed to help in assessing the effect of mut-KRAS knock-in in WT-KRAS BxPC-3 cells. Thirdly, it was of note in this study that TNF-α treatment in combination with si-KRAS showed a significant increase of apoptosis compared with si-KRAS alone in Panc-1 cells, but not in SW1990 and BxPC-3 cells. At this point, we could not explain why the differential effects exist in various cells. It has also to be pointed out that the significant difference in the total number of cases with or without KRAS mutation may represent a bias in statistical interpretation. This is mainly because that KRAS mutation occurred in a majority of PDAC patients, accounting for as high as 80% (32/40) in this study. Further study with a larger sample size is underway in our center.

In conclusion, KRAS mutation is important for PDAC progression but its effects are not sufficient to initiate PDAC. In addition to the pathways analyzed in this study, KRAS mutations may facilitate activation and positive crosstalk between other pathways in PDAC tumorigenesis, which will need to be examined in future studies.

ETHICS STATEMENT

The studies involving human participants were reviewed and approved by Changhai Hospital Ethics Review Committee. The patients/participants provided their written informed consent to participate in this study.

AUTHOR CONTRIBUTIONS

JG, KW, and HX designed the experiments. YuW and DW wrote the manuscript. YuW, YD, XK, XZ, and JJ performed experiments and animal work. DW, YF, YaW, and HW assisted in acquisition, analysis and interpretation of data for the work. WY, YaW, HW, and JJ provided administrative support. JG, KW, HX, YD and DW provided financial support. YuW, DW, and YF revised the manuscript. All authors contributed to the article and approved the submitted version.

ACKNOWLEDGMENTS

The authors wish to thank all study participants for taking part in the study.

SUPPLEMENTARY MATERIAL

Supplementary Figure 1 | SW1990 and Panc-1 cell lines are positive for KRAS G12D mutation (MT-KRAS) while BxPC-3 cell line is negative for KRAS mutation (WT-KRAS).

Supplementary Figure 2 | Detection of Shh, Gli1 and NF-κB p65 mRNA and protein expression in Panc-1, SW1990 and BxPC-3 cells. **(A)** The mRNA expression analysis of Gli1, NF-κB and Shh. Western blot protein expression analysis was repeated three times (1, 2 and 3). **(C)** Gray analysis of relative protein expression for the Gli1, NF–κB and Shh. $^*p<0.05$; $^{**}p<0.01$.

Supplementary Figure 3 | Original protein Western blots image about stimulatory effects on protein expression of Gli1, NF-κB and Shh on PDAC cell lines treated with IL-1β and TNF-α alone or in combination with si-KRAS.

Supplementary Figure 4 | Two kinds of si-KRAS were used to knock down KRAS expression in all three cell lines, Negative control (NC) siRNA was used as control. The mRNA **(A)** and protein **(B, C)** expression were significantly decreased by both the si-KRAS1 and si-KRAS2. The si-KRAS1 silencing was stronger than effects obtained with si-KRAS2, and thus si-KRAS1 was selected for further experiments. $^*p<0.05$; $^{**}p<0.01$.

Supplementary Figure 5 | Original protein Western blots image about stimulatory effects on protein expression of Gli1, NF-κB and Shh on PDAC cell lines treated with Shh as Hh activating ligand treatment alone or in combination with si-KRAS transfection.

Supplementary Figure 6 | Effect of the treatment of PDAC cells with Shh as the Hh signaling ligand depending upon the presence or absence of KRAS mutation. Shh upregulated the NF-κB p65 nuclear expression in the SW1990 and Panc-1 cell lines, while these effects were significantly decreased when cells were treated with Shh in combination with si-KRAS. However, no change was observed after treatment of BxPC-3 cell line either with Shh alone or in combination with Shh si-KRAS.

Supplementary Figure 7 | Plasmid expressing KRAS (G12D) mutation (MT-KRAS plasmid) was constructed and transfected into BxPC-3 cell line. The mRNA **(A)** and protein expression **(B, C)** were tested by qPCR and Western blotting, respectively. As shown, MT-KRAS plasmid transfection significantly increased KRAS expression in BxPC-3. $^*p<0.05$; $^{**}p<0.01$.

Supplementary Figure 8 | The effect of WT-KRAS BxPC-3 PDAC cell line treatment with IL-1β, TNF-α, Shh, in combination with mut-KRAS transfections on Gli1, NF-κB and Shh mRNA expression. All data were obtained in three independent experiments. $^*p<0.05$; $^{**}p<0.01$.

Supplementary Figure 9 | Original protein Western blots image about effect of IL-1β, TNF-α, Shh treatment in combination with si-KRAS on KRAS down-stream molecules (p-/t-ERK1/2 and p-/t-AKT1) and Ras enzymatic activity in the MT-KRAS cell lines (SW1990 and Panc-1) and WT-KRAS cell line (BxPC-3). The protein expression of p-/t-ERK1/2 and p-/t-AKT1 at Shh treatment in combination with si-KRAS treatment **(A)**; The effect of combined IL-1β or TNF-α with si-KRAS transfection on p-/t-ERK1/2 and p-/t-AKT1 **(B)**; Ras enzymatic activity at Shh treatment in combination with si-KRAS treatment **(C)**; The effect of combined IL-1β or TNF-α with si-KRAS transfection on Ras enzymatic activity **(D)** [a. SW1990, b. Panc-1, c. BxPC-3]. All data were obtained in three independent experiments

Supplementary Figure 10 | The nuclear protein expression of Gli1 and NF-κB p65 in mice inoculated with MT-KRAS cells compared with those inoculated with WT-KRAS cells. All data were obtained in three independent experiments. $^*p<0.05$; $^{**}p<0.01$.

REFERENCES

1. Siegel RL, Miller KD, Jemal A. Cancer Statistics, 2020. *CA Cancer J Clin* (2020) 70(1):7–30. doi: 10.3322/caac.21590
2. Singhi AD, Maitra A. The Molecular Pathology of Precursor Lesions of Pancreatic Cancer. In: J Neoptolemos, R Urrutia, J Abbruzzese, M Büchler, editors. *Pancreatic Cancer*, vol. vol. 1 . New York, NY: Springer (2018). p. 147–76. doi: 10.1007/978-1-4939-7193-0_5
3. Jones S, Zhang X, Parsons DW, Lin JC, Leary RJ, Angenendt P, et al. Core Signaling Pathways in Human Pancreatic Cancers Revealed by Global Genomic Analyses. *Science* (2008) 321(5897):1801–6. doi: 10.1126/science.1164368
4. Iacobuzio-Donahue CA. Genetic Evolution of Pancreatic Cancer: Lessons Learnt From the Pancreatic Cancer Genome Sequencing Project. *Gut* (2012) 61(7):1085–94. doi: 10.1136/gut.2010.236026
5. He Y, Liu Y, Gong J, Liu C, Zhang H, Wu H. Identification of Key Pathways and Candidate Genes in Pancreatic Ductal Adenocarcinoma Using Bioinformatics Analysis. *Oncol Lett* (2019) 17(4):3751–64. doi: 10.3892/ol.2019.10041
6. Nakashima H, Nakamura M, Yamaguchi H, Yamanaka N, Akiyoshi T, Koga K, et al. Nuclear Factor-Kappab Contributes to Hedgehog Signaling Pathway Activation Through Sonic Hedgehog Induction in Pancreatic Cancer. *Cancer Res* (2006) 66(14):7041–9. doi: 10.1158/0008-5472.CAN-05-4588
7. Mueller S, Engleitner T, Maresch R, Zukowska M, Lange S, Kaltenbacher T, et al. Evolutionary Routes and KRAS Dosage Define Pancreatic Cancer Phenotypes. *Nature* (2018) 554(7690):62–8. doi: 10.1038/nature25459
8. Nusslein-Volhard C, Wieschaus E. Mutations Affecting Segment Number and Polarity in Drosophila. *Nature* (1980) 287(5785):795–801. doi: 10.1038/287795a0
9. Fattahi S, Pilehchian LM, Akhavan-Niaki H. Hedgehog Signaling Pathway: Epigenetic Regulation and Role in Disease and Cancer Development. *J Cell Physiol* (2018) 233(8):5726–35. doi: 10.1002/jcp.26506
10. Wang Y, Jin G, Li Q, Wang Z, Hu W, Li P, et al. Hedgehog Signaling non-Canonical Activated by Pro-Inflammatory Cytokines in Pancreatic Ductal Adenocarcinoma. *J Cancer* (2016) 7(14):2067–76. doi: 10.7150/jca.15786
11. Shevde LA, Samant RS. Nonclassical hedgehog-GLI Signaling and its Clinical Implications. *Int J Cancer* (2014) 135(1):1–6. doi: 10.1002/ijc.28424

12. Honselmann KC, Pross M, Jung CM, Wellner UF, Deichmann S, Keck T, et al. Regulation Mechanisms of the Hedgehog Pathway in Pancreatic Cancer: A Review. *Jop* (2015) 16(1):25–32. doi: 10.6092/1590-8577/2894
13. Girardi D, Barrichello A, Fernandes G, Pereira A. Targeting the Hedgehog Pathway in Cancer: Current Evidence and Future Perspectives. *Cells-Basel* (2019) 8(2):153–72. doi: 10.3390/cells8020153
14. Faria A, Akyala AI, Parikh K, Bruggemann LW, Spek CA, Cao W, et al. Smoothened-Dependent and -Independent Pathways in Mammalian Noncanonical Hedgehog Signaling. *J Biol Chem* (2019) 294(25):9787–98. doi: 10.1074/jbc.RA119.007956
15. Dong H, Liu H, Zhou W, Zhang F, Li C, Chen J, et al. GLI1 Activation by non-Classical Pathway Integrin alphavbeta3/ERK1/2 Maintains Stem Cell-Like Phenotype of Multicellular Aggregates in Gastric Cancer Peritoneal Metastasis. *Cell Death Dis* (2019) 10(8):574. doi: 10.1038/s41419-019-1776-x
16. Bournet B, Dufresne M, Selves J, Torrisani J, Cordelier P, Buscail L. Kras Oncogene and Pancreatic Cancer: Thirty Years After. *Med Sci (Paris)* (2013) 29(11):991–7. doi: 10.1051/medsci/20132911015
17. Ene-Obong A, Clear AJ, Watt J, Wang J, Fatah R, Riches JC, et al. Activated Pancreatic Stellate Cells Sequester CD8+ T Cells to Reduce Their Infiltration of the Juxtatumoral Compartment of Pancreatic Ductal Adenocarcinoma. *Gastroenterology* (2013) 145(5):1121–32. doi: 10.1053/j.gastro.2013.07.025
18. Baumgart S, Chen NM, Siveke JT, Konig A, Zhang JS, Singh SK, et al. Inflammation-Induced NFATc1-STAT3 Transcription Complex Promotes Pancreatic Cancer Initiation by Krasg12d. *Cancer Discovery* (2014) 4 (6):688–701. doi: 10.1158/2159-8290.CD-13-0593
19. Hermann PC, Sancho P, Canamero M, Martinelli P, Madriles F, Michl P, et al. Nicotine Promotes Initiation and Progression of KRAS-induced Pancreatic Cancer Via Gata6-dependent Dedifferentiation of Acinar Cells in Mice. *Gastroenterology* (2014) 147(5):1119–33. doi: 10.1053/j.gastro.2014.08.002
20. Nishikawa Y, Kodama Y, Shiokawa M, Matsumori T, Marui S, Kuriyama K, et al. Hes1 Plays an Essential Role in Kras-driven Pancreatic Tumorigenesis. *Oncogene* (2019) 38(22):4283–96. doi: 10.1038/s41388-019-0718-5
21. Guerra C, Schuhmacher AJ, Canamero M, Grippo PJ, Verdaguer L, Perez-Gallego L, et al. Chronic Pancreatitis is Essential for Induction of Pancreatic Ductal Adenocarcinoma by K-Ras Oncogenes in Adult Mice. *Cancer Cell* (2007) 11(3):291–302. doi: 10.1016/j.ccr.2007.01.012
22. Chuvin N, Vincent DF, Pommier RM, Alcaraz LB, Gout J, Caligaris C, et al. Acinar-to-Ductal Metaplasia Induced by Transforming Growth Factor Beta Facilitates KRAS(G12D)-Driven Pancreatic Tumorigenesis. *Cell Mol Gastroenterol Hepatol* (2017) 4(2):263–82. doi: 10.1016/j.jcmgh.2017.05.005
23. Dey P, Li J, Zhang J, Chaurasiya S, Strom A, Wang H, et al. Oncogenic KRAS-Driven Metabolic Reprogramming in Pancreatic Cancer Cells Utilizes Cytokines From the Tumor Microvironment. *Cancer Discovery* (2020) 10 (4):608–25. doi: 10.1158/2159-8290.CD-19-0297
24. Baumgart S, Ellenrieder V, Fernandez-Zapico ME. Oncogenic Transcription Factors: Cornerstones of Inflammation-Linked Pancreatic Carcinogenesis. *GUT* (2013) 62(2):310–6. doi: 10.1136/gutjnl-2011-301008
25. Chen Q, Wang J, Zhang Q, Zhang J, Lou Y, Yang J, et al. Tumour Cell-Derived Debris and IgG Synergistically Promote Metastasis of Pancreatic Cancer by Inducing Inflammation Via Tumour-Associated Macrophages. *Br J Cancer* (2019) 121(9):786–95. doi: 10.1038/s41416-019-0595-2
26. Zhuang L, Zhan X, Bi Y, Ji B. Induction of Pancreatic Inflammation Accelerates Pancreatic Tumorigenesis in Mice. *Methods Mol Biol* (2019) 1882:287–97. doi: 10.1007/978-1-4939-8879-2_25
27. Xia YP, He QW, Li YN, Chen SC, Huang M, Wang Y, et al. Recombinant Human Sonic Hedgehog Protein Regulates the Expression of ZO-1 and Occludin by Activating Angiopoietin-1 in Stroke Damage. *PloS One* (2013) 8(7):e68891. doi: 10.1371/journal.pone.0068891
28. Song J, Wu C, Zhang X, Sorokin LM. In Vivo Processing of CXCL5 (LIX) by Matrix Metalloproteinase (MMP)-2 and MMP-9 Promotes Early Neutrophil Recruitment in IL-1beta-induced Peritonitis. *J Immunol* (2013) 190(1):401–10. doi: 10.4049/jimmunol.1202286
29. Clauss M, Grell M, Fangmann C, Fiers W, Scheurich P, Risau W. Synergistic Induction of Endothelial Tissue Factor by Tumor Necrosis Factor and Vascular Endothelial Growth Factor: Functional Analysis of the Tumor Necrosis Factor Receptors. *FEBS Lett* (1996) 390(3):334–8. doi: 10.1016/0014-5793(96)00690-4
30. Jimeno A, Feldmann G, Suarez-Gauthier A, Rasheed Z, Solomon A, Zou GM, et al. A Direct Pancreatic Cancer Xenograft Model as a Platform for Cancer Stem Cell Therapeutic Development. *Mol Cancer Ther* (2009) 8(2):310–4. doi: 10.1158/1535-7163.MCT-08-0924
31. Xu L, Kwon YJ, Frolova N, Steg AD, Yuan K, Johnson MR, et al. Gli1 Promotes Cell Survival and is Predictive of a Poor Outcome in ERalpha-negative Breast Cancer. *Breast Cancer Res Treat* (2010) 123(1):59–71. doi: 10.1007/s10549-009-0617-5
32. Li J, Ramani K, Sun Z, Zee C, Grant EG, Yang H, et al. Forced Expression of Methionine Adenosyltransferase 1A in Human Hepatoma Cells Suppresses In Vivo Tumorigenicity in Mice. *Am J Pathol* (2010) 176(5):2456–66. doi: 10.2353/ajpath.2010.090810
33. Rosa R, Melisi D, Damiano V, Bianco R, Garofalo S, Gelardi T, et al. Toll-Like Receptor 9 Agonist IMO Cooperates With Cetuximab in K-ras Mutant Colorectal and Pancreatic Cancers. *Clin Cancer Res* (2011) 17(20):6531–41. doi: 10.1158/1078-0432.CCR-10-3376
34. Rajurkar M, De Jesus-Monge WE, Driscoll DR, Appleman VA, Huang H, Cotton JL, et al. The Activity of Gli Transcription Factors is Essential for Kras-induced Pancreatic Tumorigenesis. *Proc Natl Acad Sci U S A* (2012) 109(17): E1038–47. doi: 10.1073/pnas.1114168109
35. Erkan M, Hausmann S, Michalski CW, Fingerle AA, Dobritz M, Kleeff J, et al. The Role of Stroma in Pancreatic Cancer: Diagnostic and Therapeutic Implications. *Nat Rev Gastroenterol Hepatol* (2012) 9(8):454–67. doi: 10.1038/nrgastro.2012.115
36. Das S, Samant RS, Shevde LA. Nonclassical Activation of Hedgehog Signaling Enhances Multidrug Resistance and Makes Cancer Cells Refractory to Smoothened-targeting Hedgehog Inhibition. *J Biol Chem* (2013) 288 (17):11824–33. doi: 10.1074/jbc.M112.432302

8

Calcium Channel Protein ORAI1 Mediates TGF-β Induced Epithelial-to-Mesenchymal Transition in Colorectal Cancer Cells

Qingjie Kang[1]*, Xudong Peng*[1]*, Xiangshu Li*[1]*, Denghua Hu*[1]*, Guangxu Wen*[1]*, Zhengqiang Wei*[1] *and Baohong Yuan*[2*]

[1] *Department of Gastrointestinal Surgery, The First Affiliated Hospital of Chongqing Medical University, Chongqing, China,*
[2] *Department of Anesthesiology, The First Affiliated Hospital of Chongqing Medical University, Chongqing, China*

Correspondence:
Baohong Yuan
yinuocqmu@126.com

Accumulating evidence suggested that calcium release-activated calcium modulator 1 (ORAI1), a key calcium channel pore-forming protein-mediated store-operated Ca2+ entry (SOCE), is associated with human cancer. However, its role in colorectal cancer (CRC) progression has not been well studied. Epithelial-mesenchymal transition (EMT) is a multistep process that occurs during the progression of cancers and is necessary for metastasis of epithelial cancer. Transforming growth factor-β (TGF-β) is a pleiotropic cytokine that has been shown to induce EMT. In this study, we are aimed at exploring the effects of ORAI1 on TGF-β1-induced EMT process in CRC cells. Herein, we confirmed ORAI1 expression was higher in CRC tissues than in adjacent non-cancerous tissues by using immunohistochemical staining and Western blot analysis. Higher ORAI1 expression was associated with more advanced clinical stage, higher incidence of metastasis and shorter overall survival. We compared ORAI1 expression in SW480 and SW620 cells, two CRC cell lines with the same genetic background, but different metastatic potential. We found ORAI1 expression was significantly higher in SW620 cells which exhibited higher EMT characteristics. Furthermore, knockdown of ORAI1 suppressed the EMT of SW620 Cells. After induced the EMT process in SW480 cells with TGF-β1, we found treatment of TGF-β1 showed a significant increase in cell migration along with the loss of E-cadherin and an increase in N-cadherin and Vimentin protein levels. Also, TGF-β1 treatment increased ORAI1 expression and was closely associated with the increase of SOCE. Silencing ORAI1 significantly suppressed Ca2+ entry, reversed the changes of EMT-relevant marks expression induced by TGF-β1, and inhibited TGF-β1-mediated calpain activation and cell migration. Finally, we blocked SOCE with 2-APB (2-Aminoethyl diphenylborinate), a pharmacological inhibitor. Interestingly, 2-APB and sh-ORAI1 both exhibited similar inhibition effects to the SW480 cells. In conclusion, our results demonstrated that ORAI1 could mediate TGF-β-Induced EMT by promoting Ca2+ entry and calpain activity in Colorectal Cancer Cells.

Keywords: ORAI1, SOCE, TGF-β, EMT, colorectal cancer

INTRODUCTION

Colorectal cancer (CRC) is the third most commonly diagnosed cancer in the world. The incidence and mortality show wide geographical variations (1). It has become a predominant type of cancer and now accounts for approximately 10% of cancer-related mortality in western countries (2). And in Asian countries, the incidence of colorectal cancer has experienced an increase of two to four times during the past few decades (3). According to 2015 data from the National Cancer Center, China ranks third in the incidence and fifth in mortality of colorectal cancer (4). A growing number of studies support the notion that metastasis rather than the primary tumor is the principal cause of cancer-associated deaths (5). However, the exact molecular mechanism of tumor metastasis is still poorly understood.

Metastasis is a multi-step process beginning with the invasion of the cancer cells into surrounding tissue, intravasation of cells into the blood stream, extravasation to the secondary site, and finally, regrowth of the tumor cells as secondary metastases (6, 7). For metastasis to occur, a tumor cell shifts from a polarized epithelial state to an invasive mesenchymal phenotype through a process known as Epithelial-to-Mesenchymal Transition (EMT) (8). The EMT morphological changes transform the cell from a stationery form to a motile form, and several studies show that EMT and cell movement are regulated by Ca2+ influx (9, 10). Ca2+ is a multifunctional secondary messenger. Intracellular Ca2+ homeostasis is required for the development and maintenance of many physiological functions, such as movement, secretion, and gene transcription (11). Intracellular Ca2+ imbalance caused by carcinogenesis has been known to deregulate cell proliferation, migration and suppression of apoptosis (12). In non-excitable cells, the predominant Ca2+ influx pathway is store-operated Ca2+ entry (SOCE) (13). Although SOCE was first proposed in 1986 to describe the process that the depletion of intracellular Ca2+ stores causes the influx of extracellular Ca2+ (14), the identity of the channels key molecular components: ORAI1 and stromal interacting molecule 1 (STIM1) were discovered during the last decade (15). ORAI1 is a pore-forming protein located on the plasma membrane and exhibits four transmembrane domains (16), which is activated by the endoplasmic Ca2+ sensor STIM1 upon Ca2+ store depletion, promoting Ca2+ influx for Ca2+ store refilling and the activation of key Ca2+-dependent processes (17, 18).

Interestingly, recent studies have shown that ORAI1 is overexpressed in many types of cancer, such as lung cancer (19), hepatocarcinoma (20), and gastric cancer (21). Clinically, ORAI1 overexpression is strongly linked to poor clinical outcomes in gastric cancer patients (21). Furthermore, the high expression of ORAI1 enhanced cell proliferation and is associated with poor prognosis in colorectal cancer (22). *In vitro*, EMT-like changes of the cellular phenotype were noticed in ORAI1-knockdown gastric cancer cells, EMT mark gene E-cadherin mRNA expression was upregulated by silencing ORAI1 (21). Earlier studies found that ORAI1 is shown to be critical for breast tumor cell migration and metastasis (23). Moreover, ORAI1-mediated SOCE is reported to play an important role in the progression of various cancers (24). SOCE regulates cellular functions by promoting the entry of extracellular Ca2+ to the cytosol and activating Ca2+-dependent proteinases (25). Some studies have shown that blocking SOCE by using a specific blocker or by applying siRNA that target ORAI1 can inhibit the migration, invasion, and cell movement of cancer cells (9, 21, 26). These results suggested that there should be a direct relationship between ORAI1 and EMT, but the internal mechanisms are yet to be fully clarified.

Transforming growth factor-β (TGF-β), a pleiotropic cytokine, is found in a variety of tissues and is important for cell proliferation, differentiation, and apoptosis (27). In the tumor microenvironment, TGF-β is a strong inducer of the EMT. After treatment with TGF-β, the cell undergoes rapid and dynamic changes in gene regulation with morphological and migratory changes (28). TGF-β induces EMT and promotes cell migration and invasion through the downregulation of epithelial factors and upregulation of mesenchymal factors (29, 30). Calcium signaling serves as a bridge to link signals from the tumor microenvironment with specific cellular responses. For example, TGF-β induced EMT in MCF7 breast cancer cells has also been shown to be associated with increased Ca2+ influx into the cell (9). TGF-β-treatment caused an increase in Ca2+-induced calpain activity, which reduced E-cadherin protein levels, thereby increasing cell migration (29). However, the relationship between TGF-β-induced EMT and Ca2+ signaling remains unclear, and the functions of ORAI1-mediated SOCE in the TGF-β-induced EMT in colorectal cancer cells have not been investigated sufficiently.

In this study, we investigated the expression of ORAI1 in CRC tissues and found that ORAI1 overexpression is associated with progression and poor prognosis of CRC. Knockdown of ORAI1 suppressed the EMT of SW620 Cells. Moreover, we explored the role of ORAI1 and SOCE in the TGF-β1-induced EMT of SW480 cells. By knockdown the ORAI1 expression and the use of SOCE inhibitor, we found that ORAI1 and ORAI1-mediated SOCE plays an important role in TGF-β1-induced EMT in SW480 cells. Thus, ORAI1 and SOCE may be candidates for CRC therapy.

MATERIALS AND METHODS

Patients and Clinical Samples

The human colorectal cancer samples (n=80) and corresponding non-tumor tissues for immunohistochemistry were collected from each patient immediately after the surgical process at the First Affiliated Hospital of Chongqing Medical University from January to November 2014. None had received neoadjuvant therapy before surgery. All of the patients had complete clinical and follow-up data for five years. For Western blot expression studies, 40 pairs of fresh samples were frozen in liquid nitrogen immediately after surgical removal and maintained at -80°C until use.

Cell Culture

The SW480 and SW620 human CRC cell lines were respectively provided by the Cancer Laboratory and Central Laboratory of the First Affiliated Hospital of Chongqing Medical University.

These cell lines were routinely maintained in RPMI-1640 medium (HyClone, Logan, UT, USA) supplemented with 10% fetal bovine serum (HyClone, Logan, UT, USA) at 37°C in a humidified air atmosphere containing 5% CO_2. Before stimulation with TGF-β1 (PeproTech, Rocky Hill, NJ, USA), cells were cultured with medium supplemented with 1% fetal bovine serum for 12h, and then treated with TGF-β1(10ng/ml) for 12, 24 and 36h.

siRNA and Lentiviral Vectors Transduction

The RNA duplexes for siRNA-mediated ORAI1 silencing were synthesized by RiboBio (Guangzhou, China), and the sequences used were: 5'-CGTGCACAATCTCAACTCG-3'(siRNA1) and 5'-CCAGCATTGAGTGTGTACA-3'(siRNA2) as described previously (23, 31); control siRNA: 5'-TTCTCCGAACGTGTCACGT-3'. Transduction of the siRNAs (50nM) in CRC cells was performed using ribo FECT^{TM} CP Reagent (RiboBio, Guangzhou, China) according to the manufacturer's protocol. Plates were incubated for 48h until ready for assays. ORAI1-shRNA lentiviral vector, and scrambled-shRNA lentiviral vector were designed and generated by Neuron Biotech (Shanghai, China). Cells were seeded at 6-well plates. After incubating for 24 hours, lentiviruses were added to the cells at a MOI of 20. Culture media were changed after 24h. 72h after transfection, cells were photographed under a fluorescent microscope (NikonTE2000-U, Japan). After selection with puromycin (2 μg/ml, Beyotime, Shanghai, China) for 2 weeks, the transduced cells were used in further experiments.

Transwell Chamber Assay

Cell migration assays were determined using the transwell chamber (8μm pore size). 5×10^4 cells with 400μl serum-free medium were plated in the upper chamber, the culture medium (600μl) containing 10% FBS was placed in the lower chamber. After incubation for 24 h, the cells were removed from the upper chamber by a cotton swab. Then the invading cells were fixed with 4% formaldehyde and stained with 0.1% crystal violet and quantified with a light microscope. Five random fields were analyzed for each insert. Cell invasion was determined with Matrigel matrix (BD Biosciences, CA, USA) coated on the upper surface of the transwell chamber. Cells were treated as described above.

Measurement of Calcium Entry

The store-operated Ca2+ influx was determined using the Ca2+ sensitive fluorescent indicator Rhod-2AM (AAT Bioquest Inc, CA, USA) and an inverted laser scanning confocal microscope (LEICA, TCS SP2, Germany). In brief, cells were grown on laser confocal petri dish until 70% confluent and incubated with 5 μM Rhod-2AM in Ca2+-free Hanks' Balanced Salt Solution (HBSS) (Sangon Biotech, Shanghai, China) at 37°C for 35 min in the dark, washed twice with Ca2+-free HBSS and incubated at room temperature for 20 min. For fluorescence measurements, 5μM nifedipine (Sigma Chemical Co, MO, USA) was included in the Ca2+-free HBSS to block voltage-dependent Ca2+ channels (VDCC) (32). After 30s of baseline recording, Ca2+-free HBSS with 2μM Thapsigargin (Tg) (Sigma Chemical Co, MO, USA) was added to deplete intracellular Ca2+ store thus trigger the opening of SOCE channels and activation of SOCE. Continue scanning every 6s until cell fluorescence intensity basically returns to baseline. Then, 5mM $CaCl_2$ was added to induce the Ca2+ influx. Experiments were performed for 600s in the presence of 5mM Ca2+. Fluorescence imaging was carried out at the excitation and emission wavelengths of 557nm and 581nm, respectively. In fluorescence imaging analyses, Ca2+ changes were calculated as F/F0 after background subtraction, where F is the change in fluorescence signal intensity and F0 is the baseline.

Calpain Activation Assay

A calpain activity assay kit (Abcam, Cambridge, UK) was used to determine calpain activity in the cell according to the manufacturer's instructions. In brief, cells were lysed in the lysis buffer at 4°C. Cell lysates were then incubated with Ac-LLY-AFC, a calpain substrate and reaction buffer for 1 h at 37°C in the dark. Fluorescence emission was measured at 505 nm using a fluorescence spectrometer with an excitation light at 400 nm.

Immunohistochemistry (IHC)

Immunohistochemical staining was carried out on formalin-fixed paraffin-embedded blocks, and a series of sections (4-mm-thick) were prepared. Endogenous peroxidase activity was blocked by 3% hydrogen peroxide. After antigen retrieval, non-specific binding was blocked with normal goat serum. Then, the sections were incubated with rabbit anti-ORAI1 antibody (1:100, Abcam, Cambridge, UK) at 4°C overnight. Next day, the sections were incubated with secondary antibody for 45min. After the sections were counterstained, dehydrated, and mounted, the results were evaluated by two independent operators. The staining intensity was evaluated as follows: 0 (negative), 1 (weak), 2 (moderate), or 3 (strong). The staining extent was scored based on the area percentage of positive cells: 0(0-5%), 1 (6–25%), 2 (26–50%), 3 (51–75%), or 4 (>75%). The final score was the sum of staining extent and intensity. ORAI1 expression was classified as high expression (IHC score ≥4) and low expression (IHC score ≤ 3).

Immunofluorescence Staining

Cells were grown on glass coverslips placed inside 24-well plates until 60% confluent, and then fixed with 4% formaldehyde for 15 min at room temperature, After washing, Immunostaining Permeabilization Solution with Saponin (Beyotime Biotech, Shanghai, China) was added and incubated for approximately 5min, and then blocked with 4% BSA for 1 h. Anti-E-cadherin (1:200, Santa Cruz, CA, USA) or anti-Vimentin (1:200, Santa Cruz, CA, USA) primary antibody was incubated with blocked cells overnight at 4°C. After removing the primary antibodies and washing with PBS for three times, cells were incubated with Cy3-conjugated secondary antibody (1:300, Proteintech, Wuhan, China) for 1h at room temperature, followed by incubation with DAPI (Sangon Biotech, Shanghai, China) for 5min. After washing with PBS, coverslips were sealed with anti-quenching fluorescent mounting medium. Images were captured using a fluorescence microscope (Nikon TE2000-U, Japan).

Quantitative RT-PCR

Total RNA was isolated using the Trizol reagent (Invitrogen, CA, USA) and cDNA was generated using the PrimeScript™ RT reagent Kit (Takara, Dalian, China). Quantitative real-time PCR was performed with SYBR Premix Ex Taq (Takara, Dalian, China) using CFX96 Real Time PCR System (Bio-Rad, CA, USA). The RT primers were as follows: ORAI1: forward 5'-GCTGCTCTGCTGGGTCAAGTT-3'and reverse 5'- CGATAAAGATCAGGCCGAAGG-3', GAPDH: forward 5'-CTTTGGTATCGTGGAAGGACTC-3' and reverse 5'-GTAGAGGCAGGGATGATGTTCT -3'. The cycling program was: Pre–denaturation at 95°C for 30 seconds, followed by 40 cycles of 95°C for 5 seconds, 60°C for 30 seconds, and extension at 65°C for 1min. Relative expression level of ORAI1 was normalized to GAPDH and calculated using the$2^{-\Delta\Delta Ct}$ method.

Western Blot

The tissue samples and cells were lysed using RIPA Lysis Buffer (Beyotime Biotech, Shanghai, China) containing PMSF (Beyotime Biotech, Shanghai, China). The protein concentration was detected using the BCA kits. Equal amounts of protein were separated by 10%SDS-PAGE and transferred onto polyvinylidene difluoride membranes. After blocking with 5% nonfat milk in Tris-buffered saline-Tween (TBST) for 2h at room temperature, membranes were incubated with primary antibodies against ORAI1(1:500, Proteintech, Wuhan, China), E-cadherin (1:1000, Santa Cruz, CA, USA), N-cadherin (1:1000, Cell Signaling Technology, MA, USA)), Vimentin (1:1000, Santa Cruz, CA, USA), β-actin (1:2000, Proteintech, Wuhan, China) overnight at 4°C. After washing with TBST, membranes were incubated with HRP-labeled secondary antibodies for 2h at room temperature. Protein bands were detected using an enhanced chemiluminescence detection kit (ECL). Densitometric analysis was performed using Fusion software (Vilber Lourmat, France). β-actin was used as loading control.

Statistical Analysis

All experiments were repeated three times and all of the data were analyzed by SPSS19.0 software. Measurement data are expressed as mean ± standard deviation (SD). Comparison was made by the Student's *t* test between two groups and by the one-way ANOVA among multiple groups. The χ^2 test was used to analyze the correlation between ORAI1 expression and clinicopathologic parameters. The survival curves were generated by Kaplan-Meier method and analyzed by the log-rank test. $P<0.05$ was considered statistically significant.

RESULTS

ORAI1 Is Highly Expressed in Human CRC Tissues and Indicates Poor Clinical Outcomes

To investigate the expression of ORAI1 in human CRC tissues, we first examined ORAI1 expression in 80 CRC tissue samples and non-tumor tissues by immunohistochemical staining (IHC). As shown in **Figure 1A**, the results of IHC revealed that ORAI1 was mainly expressed in the membrane and cytoplasm. High expression (IHC score≥4) was assessed in 64 of 80 (80%) primary CRC samples compared with only in 24 of 80 (30%) paired non-tumor tissues, average staining scores of 4.85 and 2.23, respectively (**Table 1**, **Figure 1C**). Furthermore, ORAI1 expression was significantly higher in stage III and IV patients than that in stage I and II patients (5.30 vs. 3.92) (**Figure 1D**). We further detected ORAI1 expression in an additional 40 fresh CRC tissues and the corresponding non-tumor tissues by Western blot analysis. Consistent with IHC observations, ORAI1 was expressed at higher levels in CRC tumors compared with matched adjacent non-tumor tissues (**Figures 1B, E**).

Furthermore, we analyzed the association between ORAI1 expression and clinicopathological parameters in 80 CRC patients by IHC staining (**Table 2**). The results showed that the patients with high ORAI1 expression had a higher tendency to be with advanced clinical stage, high incidence of metastasis. But there were no statistical connections between ORAI1 overexpression and age, gender, and tumor size. Finally, we analyzed the association between ORAI1 expression and survival of CRC patients. By Kaplan-Meier survival analysis, we found that patients with higher ORAI1 expression were likely to be with significantly shorter overall survival (**Figure 1F**). Taken together, these results suggest that high expression of ORAI1 is associated with tumor progression and poor clinical outcomes.

Expression of ORAI1 Is Different in Primary (SW480) and Metastatic (SW620) Colon Cancer Cell Lines

Having identified the expression properties of ORAI1 in human CRC tissues, we further evaluated its expression level in two human CRC cell lines SW480 and SW620. Interestingly, Western blot analysis showed ORAI1 expression was significantly higher in SW620 cells than in SW480 cells (**Figure 2A**). The SW480 cell line was obtained from a primary CRC lesion, and the SW620 cell line was established from a lymph node (LN) metastasis in the same patient a year later, which exhibited higher metastasis potential (33). Therefore, the two cell lines have the same genetic background but different metastatic potential. Transwell assay also showed that SW620 cells migrate and invade more aggressively than SW480 cells (**Figure 2B**).

Importantly, a key feature of cancer metastasis is the initiation of EMT. Therefore, we detected expression of EMT-relevant markers in the two cell lines. As expected, expression of E-cadherin, an epithelial marker, was substantially lower in SW620 cells than in SW480 cells, but a significantly higher expression of Vimentin and N-cadherin, two mesenchymal markers, was observed in SW620 cells (**Figure 2A**). These changes in E-cadherin and Vimentin expression were confirmed by an immunofluorescent assay (**Figure 2C**). Combined with the distinct migratory ability, expression levels of EMT-related markers and ORAI1 between the two cell lines, these results suggest that ORAI1 might be involved in the EMT-derived migration in CRC cells.

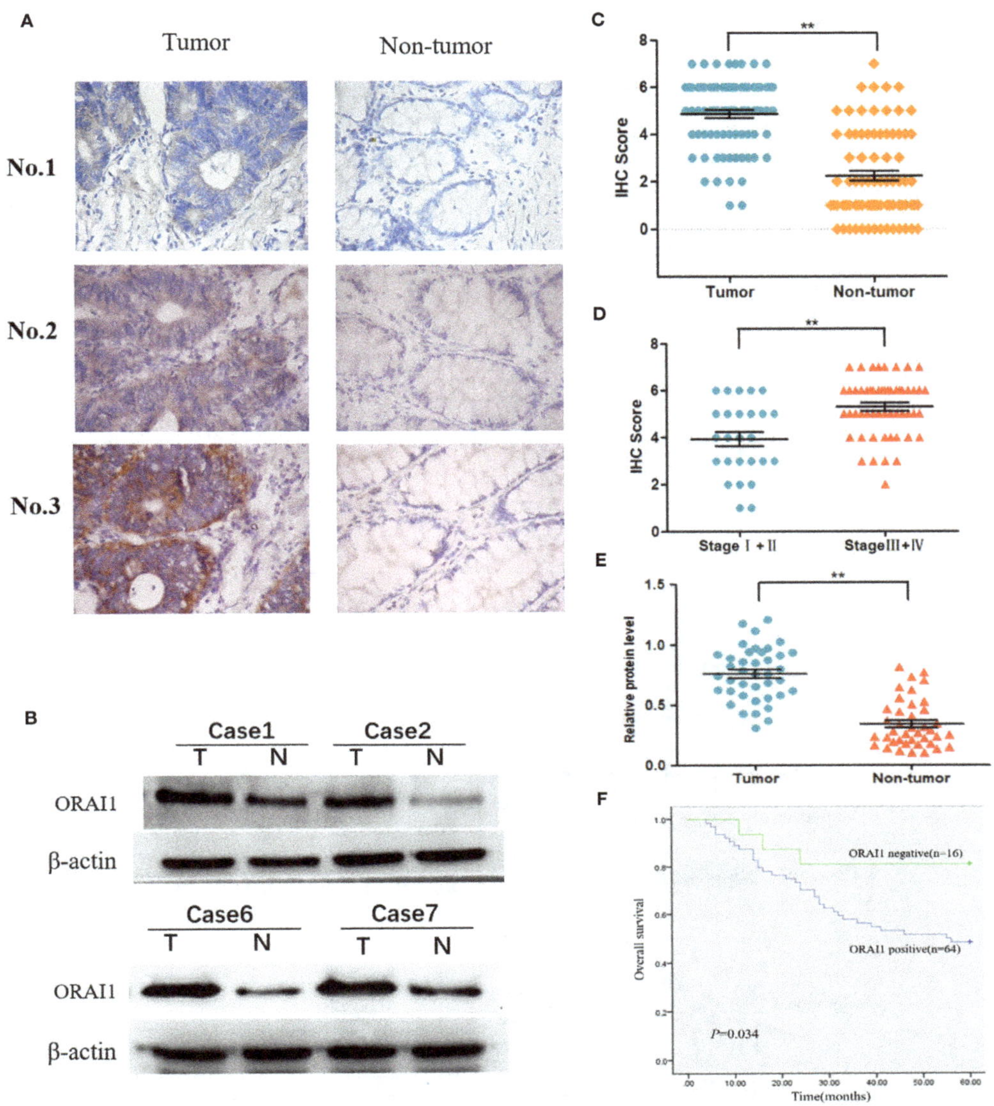

FIGURE 1 | Expression of ORAI1 is significantly upregulated in CRC tissues. **(A)** Representative immunohistochemistry staining of ORAI1 expression in 80 paired CRC tissues. magnification, ×400. **(B)** Western blot was applied to detect protein expression levels of ORAI1 in paired CRC tumor tissues (T) and non-tumor tissues (N). **(C)** Immunohistochemistry average staining scores of tumor tissues and matched non-tumor tissues. $^{**}P<0.01$. **(D)** IHC average staining scores of tumor tissues in stage I+II and stage III+IV patients. $^{**}P<0.01$. **(E)** The protein relative expression levels of ORAI1 in tumor tissues and non-tumor tissues of 40 patients by Western blot. $^{**}P<0.01$. **(F)** Kaplan–Meier's analysis of the correlation between ORAI1expression and overall survival (OS) of CRC patients.

Knockdown of ORAI1 Suppresses the EMT of SW620 Cells

As mentioned above, the SW620 cell line was obtained from a CRC lymph node (LN) metastasis, which exhibited higher EMT characteristics. To investigate the role of ORAI1 in the EMT of SW620 cells, SW620 cells were transduced with two ORAI1-specific siRNAs and a control siRNA, respectively, and we found that SW620-siRNA1 and SW620-siRNA2 cells exhibited 87% and 84% decrease in protein levels and 69% and 63% in mRNA levels (**Supplementary Figure S1A**). Transwell assays also showed that transduction with siRNA1 or siRNA2 in SW620 cells markedly decreased cell migration (**Supplementary Figure S1C**). Western blot analysis showed that both siRNA1 and siRNA2 transduction could suppress the EMT of SW620 cells (**Supplementary Figure S1D**). Given that siRNA1 has a slightly

TABLE 1 | Upregulation of ORAI1 in CRC tissues.

ORAI1 staining	Tumor	Adjacent non-tumor	χ^2	P
Positive	64	24	40.4	<0.01
Negative	16	56		

TABLE 2 | Correlation between ORAI1 and clinical parameters of CRC patients.

Variables	Case	ORAI1		χ^2	P
		-	+		
Age (years)					
≥60	32	6	26	0.052	0.819
<60	48	10	38		
Gender					
Male	55	10	45	0.364	0.546
Female	25	6	19		
Tumor size (cm)					
≥5	33	4	29	2.179	0.140
<5	47	12	35		
TNM stag					
I-II	26	11	15	11.980	0.001**
III-IV	54	5	49		
Lymph node metastasis (N_2)					
Yes	31	2	29	5.806	0.016*
No	49	14	35		

*P<0.05; **P<0.01.

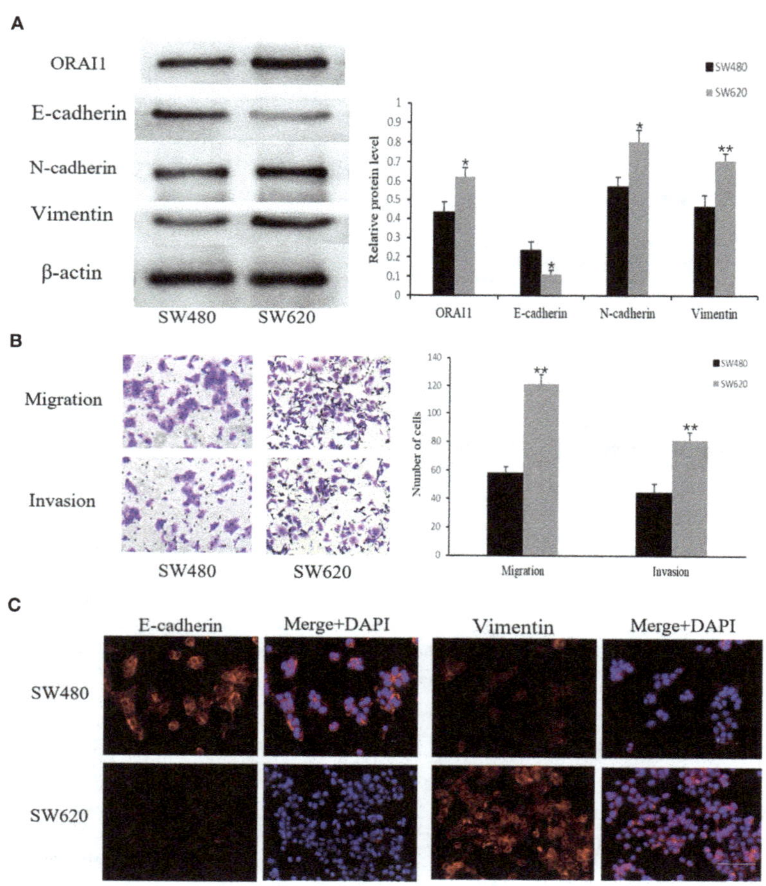

FIGURE 2 | SW480 and SW620 cells have different expression levels of ORAI1 and EMT-relevant markers. **(A)** Western blot analysis of ORAI1 and EMT-relevant markers expression in these two CRC cell lines. **(B)** The metastatic capability of these two cell lines was detected by transwell migration and invasion assays. magnification, ×200. **(C)** Immunofluorescence was performed to evaluate the expression of E-cadherin and Vimentin in these two CRC cell lines, Scale bar 75μm. All the experiments were repeated three times. *P<0.05; **P<0.01.

better knock-down effect, it was therefore selected as the target sequence for subsequent experiments. Accordingly, we used this sequence to construct the ORAI1-shRNA lentiviral vectors, and the expression of ORAI1 in the transfected cells was confirmed by QRT-PCR and Western blot. The results showed that cells transfected with ORAI1 shRNA exhibited 82% decrease in protein levels and 67% in mRNA levels (**Figure 3A**). By comparing the morphology of the cells under a light microscope, we observed that cells with ORAI1 shRNA showed highly organized cell-cell adhesion and cobblestone shape with epithelioid morphology appeared (**Figure 3B**). To further explore cell migration capacity after ORAI1 silencing, transwell assay was performed subsequently. The results showed the number of migrated cells was markedly decreased in ORAI1 silence cells compared to the negative control (**Figure 3B**).

Next, we assessed the effect of ORAI1 knockdown on the EMT-relevant molecules in these cell models. Western blot analysis showed that the expression of E-cadherin was significantly up-regulated, and the expression of N-cadherin and Vimentin was obviously down-regulated in SW620-shORAI1 cells, compared with control cells (**Figure 3C**). As ORAI1 is an essential component of SOCE channel, we further investigated SOCE initiation in these cells. When the medium was absent of Ca2+, addition of thapsigargin, an ER Ca2+-ATPase inhibitor, resulted in a rapid rise in intracellular Ca2+ level, consistent with depletion of ER Ca2+ stores. Subsequently, addition of Ca2+, which initiates Ca2+ influx, triggered another significant increase in the Ca2+ level (SOCE). As shown in **Figure 3D**, knockdown of ORAI1 decreased Ca2+ entry in SW620-shORAI1 cells compared with control cells. Following the inhibition of SOCE, decrease of the calpain activity was also observed in SW620-shORAI1 cells (**Figure 3E**). These results suggest that ORAI1 plays an important role in the acquisition of EMT in CRC cells. To further investigate the mechanism of ORAI1 in TGF-β induced EMT in CRC cells, we chose the SW480 cell line, which is characterized by a modest more mesenchymal characteristics, for the subsequent experiment.

TGF-β1 Induces EMT and Enhances ORAI1 Expression in SW480 Cells

Previous studies suggested that TGF-β1 is a powerful EMT stimulus (34), which is known to induce tumor cell invasion by activating EMT in metastatic cancer thereby enhancing invasiveness and metastasis (35). For this, we induced the EMT process in SW480 cells by treatment with 10ng/ml TGF-β1 for 0, 12, 24 or 36h. Time course responses to TGF-β1 were tested as well on the expression of E-cadherin, N-cadherin and Vimentin protein. Western blot analysis confirmed significant decreases in the levels of the E-cadherin protein and increases in the expression of Vimentin and N-cadherin protein in SW480 cells that had been treated with 10ng/ml TGF-β1 for 24 or 36 h (**Figure 4A**). These results suggest that TGF-β1 induces EMT most significantly after 24 h treatments in SW480 cells. Therefore, cells were incubated with 10ng/ml TGF-β1 for 24h in subsequent experiments.

By comparing the morphology of the cells under a light microscope, we observed that cells stimulated with TGF-β1 became an elongated morphology with losing polarity and cell–cell contacts (**Figure 4B**). Next, we further confirmed the effects of TGF-β1 on EMT in SW480 cells, using transwell assay and immunofluorescence. Transwell assay analysis showed that the number of cells migrated indeed had a significant increase in the migration of SW480 cells treated with TGF-β1 for 24h (**Figure 4B**). Based on the immunofluorescence staining for EMT-related molecules, E-cadherin expression was decreased and Vimentin expression was increased in TGF-β1-treated cells (**Figure 4C**). TGF-β has also been shown to regulate Ca2+ signaling (29), and thus we investigated whether store-operated Ca2+ entry (SOCE) initiation is altered upon treatment with TGF-β1. As shown in **Figure 4D**, SOCE activity was significantly increased in TGF-β1 treatment cells. Following the increased Ca2+ influx, overall calpain activity was measured, which showed a significant increase in SW480 cells after TGF–β1 treatment (**Figure 4E**). We then assessed whether TGF-β1 promotes Ca2+ influx accompanied by up-regulation of ORAI1 expression. Interestingly, Western blot analysis showed the expression of ORAI1 also increased with TGF-β1 treatment for 24 or 36h (**Figure 4A**). These results presented above suggest that TGF-β1-induced activation of ORAI1 and SOCE could be crucial for promoting EMT.

Knockdown of ORAI1 Attenuates the TGF-β1-Induced EMT in SW480 Cells

To verify whether ORAI1 is responsible for TGF-β1-induced EMT, SW480 cells were transduced with the two ORAI1-specific siRNAs. The knockdown efficiency was confirmed by QRT-PCR and Western blot, and we found that SW480-siRNA1 and SW480-siRNA2 cells showed 78% and 72% decrease in protein levels and 81% and 76% in mRNA levels (**Supplementary Figure S1B**). Transwell assays also showed that the number of migrated cells was significant reduction in SW480-siRNA1 or SW480-siRNA2 cells (**Supplementary Figure S1C**). Western blot analysis also showed that similar changes of EMT-relevant marks expression were found in these cells (**Supplementary Figure S1E**). These results indicated that siRNA1 also exhibited a slightly better knock-down effect in SW480 cells. Therefore, SW480 cells were infected with lentiviral vector expressing ORAI1 shRNA or a control shRNA lentivirus (NC), and we found that 61% decrease in protein levels and 79% in mRNA levels in SW480-shORAI1 cells, and without changes in SW480-NC cells (**Figure 5A**). These results suggest that we successfully silenced ORAI1 expression in SW480 cells with ORAI1-targeted shRNA. First, EMT-relevant markers were evaluated by Western blot. We found that ORAI1 knockdown induced a significant up-regulation of E-cadherin expression in parallel to a significant down-regulation of the N-cadherin and Vimentin expression, and ORAI1 downregulation could rescue E-cadherin inhibition after TGF–β1 treatment and alleviate the increase of N-cadherin and Vimentin expression induced by TGF-β1 (**Figure 5B**). To further establish that cell migration is also affected upon ORAI1 silencing, transwell assay was performed. The results showed the number of migrated cells was clearly decreased for ORAI1 silence cells, and knockdown of

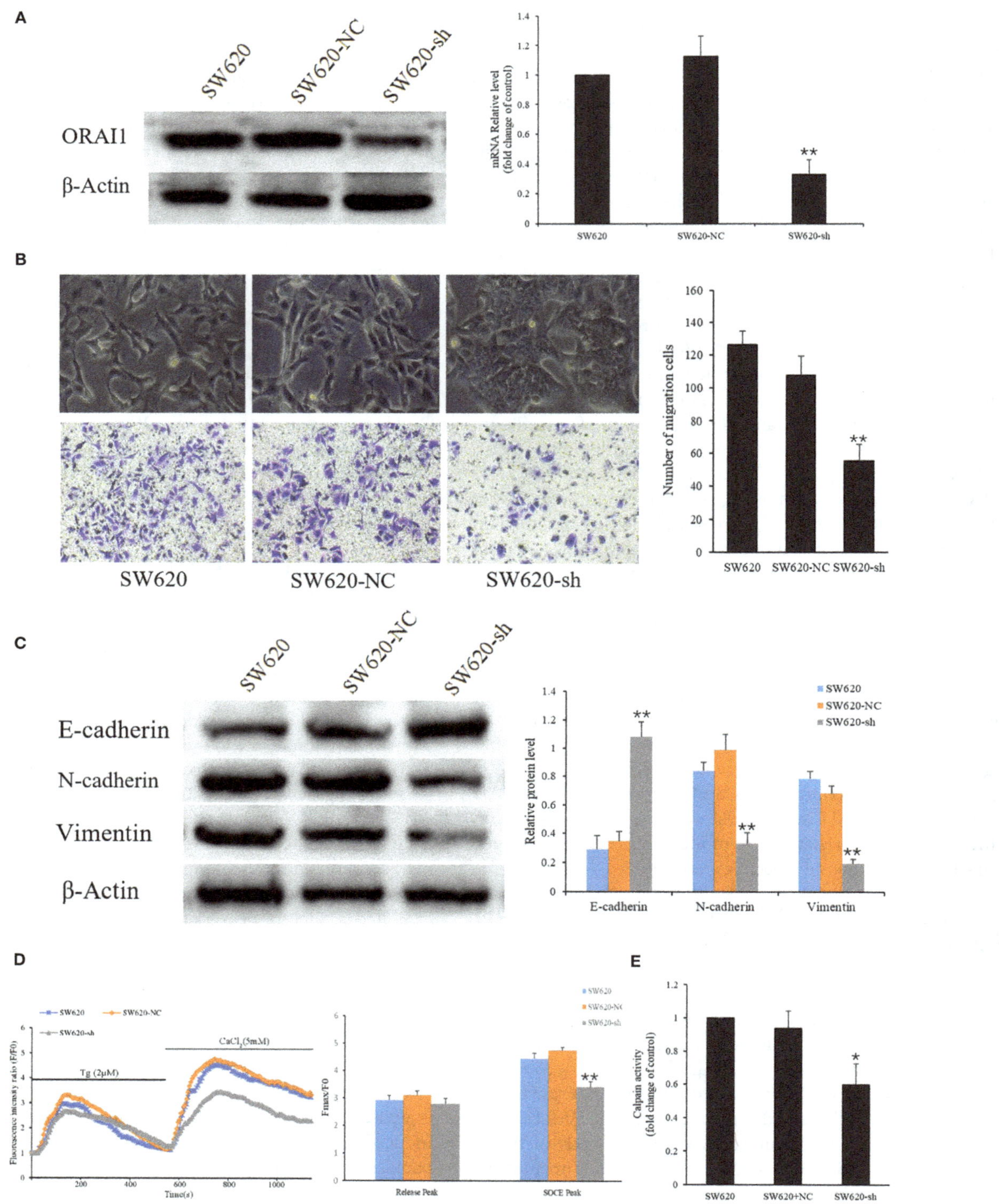

FIGURE 3 | ORAI1 knockdown suppresses the EMT of SW620 Cells. **(A)** SW620 cells were infected with lentivirus containing sh-ORAI1 or control sh-RNA lentivirus (NC) for 72 hours. Knockdown efficiency was confirmed by QRT-PCR (right panel) and Western blot (left panel). **(B)** Representative picture showed the morphological change of SW620 cells after infecting with lentivirus for 72 h. Cell migration was assessed by transwell assay. Magnification, ×200. **(C)** The protein levels of E-cadherin, N-cadherin and Vimentin were analyzed by Western blot. **(D)** Representative traces of intracellular Ca2+ signals were assessed by Rhod-2AM Ca2+ measurement. **(E)** Quantitative assessment of calpain activity in SW620 and the transfected cells. All the experiments were repeated three times. *P<0.05; **P<0.01.

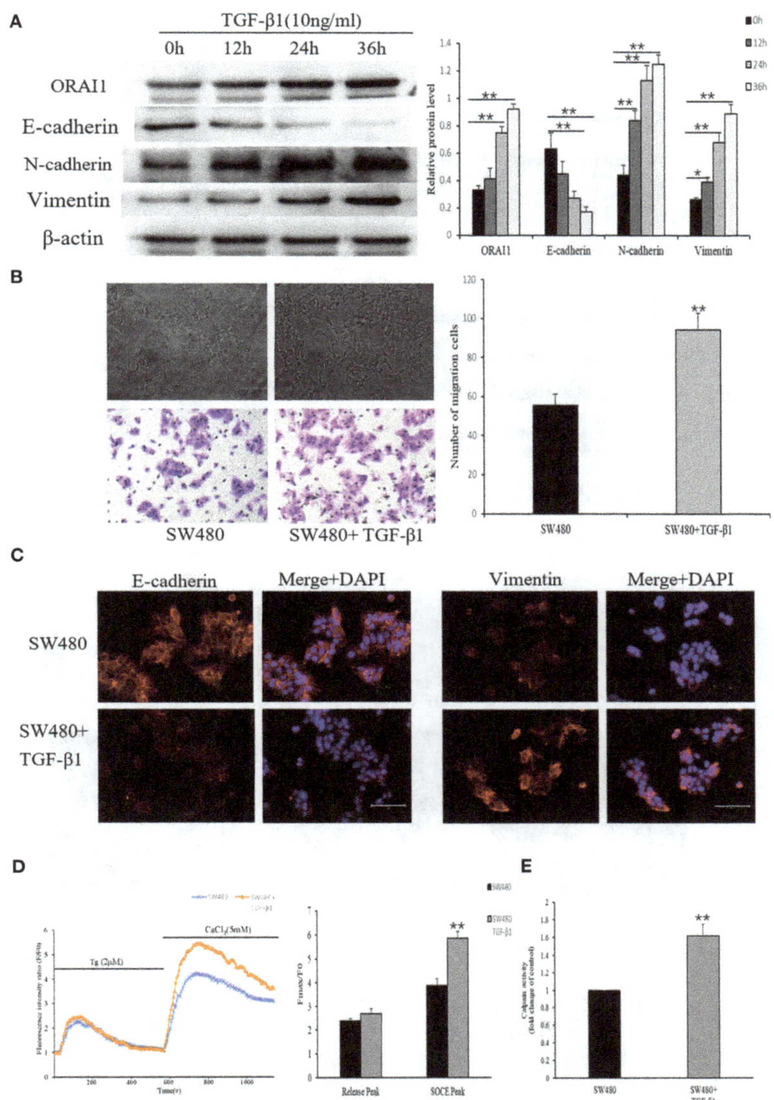

FIGURE 4 | TGF-β1 induces EMT and increases ORAI1-mediated Ca2+ entry in SW480 cells. **(A)** Western blot was performed to detect the expression of ORAI1 and EMT-relevant markers in SW480 cells treated with 10ng/ml TGF-β1 for 0,12,24 and 36h. **(B)** Representative picture showed the morphological change of SW480 cells after treatment with 10ng/ml TGF-β1 for 24 h. Cell migration was assessed by transwell assay. Magnification, ×200. **(C)** Immunofluorescence was performed to evaluate the expression of E-cadherin and Vimentin in SW480 cells after treatment with TGF-β1, Scale bar 75μm. **(D)** Representative traces of intracellular Ca2+ signals of SW480 cells with or without TGF-β1 treatment were assessed by Rhod-2AM Ca2+ measurement. **(E)** Quantitative assessment of calpain activity. All the experiments were repeated three times. **P*<0.05; ***P*<0.01.

ORAI1 significantly rescinded the increase in TGF-β1-induced migration (**Figure 5C**).

As ORAI1 can induce Ca2+ entry through SOCE mechanisms, we further detected SOCE initiation in SW480-shORAI1 cells and SW480-NC cells that were treated or not treated with TGF-β1 (**Figures 5D, E**). As shown in **Figure 5E**, TGF–β1 treatment also significantly increased Ca2+ entry in SW480-NC cells. Knockdown of ORAI1 not only decreased Ca2+ entry in SW480-shORAI1 cells, but also significantly attenuated TGF-β1-evoked Ca2+ entry compared with SW480-NC cells. Next we examined how a reduction in TGF-β1-induced activation of Ca2+ entry by shORAI1 affected Ca2+-dependent calpain activity. Decrease of the basal calpain activity levels was observed in SW480-shORAI1 cells, and silencing of ORAI1 abolished the increased calpain activity seen with TGF-β1 treatment (**Figure 5F**). These results strongly suggest ORAI1 downregulation was associated with a decrease of SOCE, and ORAI1 and ORAI1-mediated SOCE is involved in regulating TGF-β1-induced EMT.

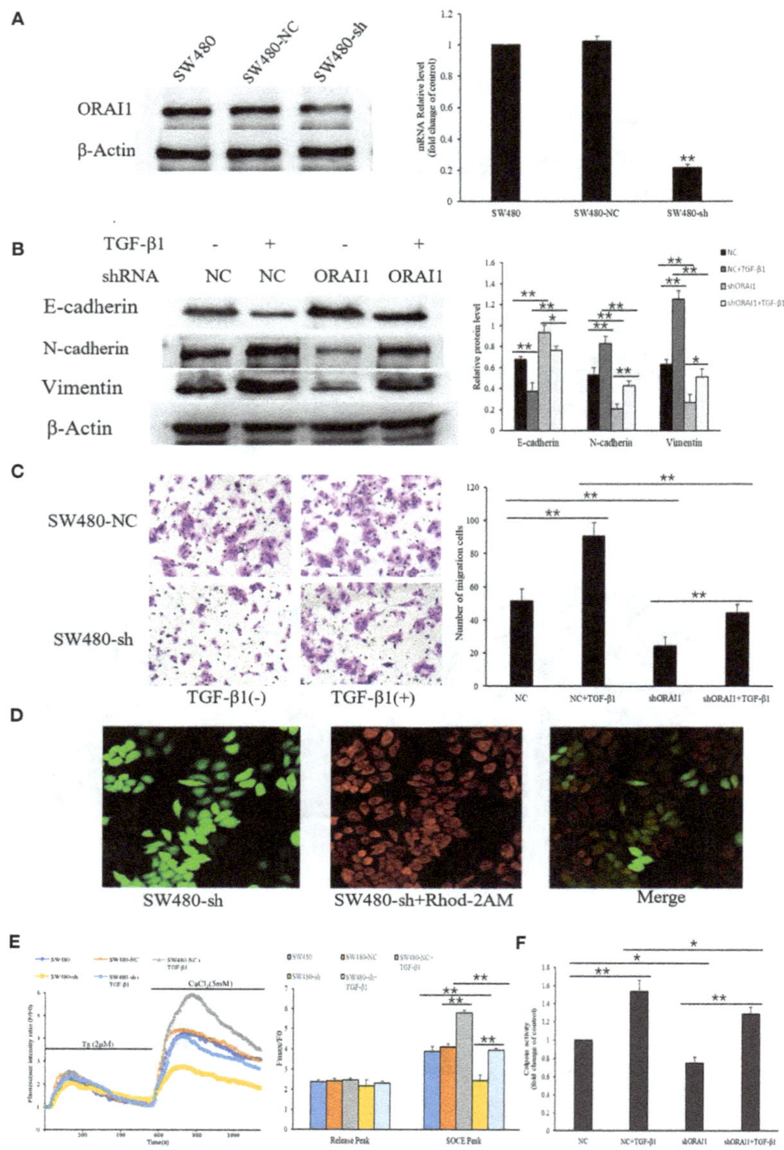

FIGURE 5 | ORAI1 silencing attenuates the TGF-β1-induced EMT in SW480 cells. **(A)** SW480 cells were infected with lentivirus containing shORAI1 or control shRNA lentivirus (NC) for 72 hours. Knockdown efficiency was confirmed by QRT-PCR (right panel) and Western blot (left panel). **(B)** SW480-shORAI1 cells and SW480-NC cells were stimulated with or without TGF-β1(10ng/ml) for 24h, and the protein levels of E-cadherin, N-cadherin and Vimentin were analyzed by Western blot. **(C)** Migration capacity of SW480-shORAI1 cells and SW480-NC cells was assessed by transwell assay. Magnification, ×200. **(D)** SW480 cells were treated with the Ca2+ sensitive fluorescent indicator Rhod-2AM, and fluorescence signals were detected by an inverted laser scanning confocal microscope, Scale bar 75μm. **(E)** Representative traces of intracellular Ca2+ signals were assessed by Rhod-2AM Ca2+ measurement. **(F)** Quantitative assessment of calpain activity in SW480-shORAI1 and SW480-NC cells with or without TGF-β1 treatment. All the experiments were repeated three times. $^{*}P<0.05$; $^{**}P<0.01$.

Blockade of SOCE Alleviates the TGF-β1-Induced EMT in SW480 Cells

The results mentioned above indicated that the effect of TGF-β1 on EMT may be related to increased SOCE-related Ca2+ influx. We therefore evaluated whether blocking store-mediated Ca2+ entry with 2-APB (2-Aminoethyl diphenylborinate), a pharmacologic inhibitor which has been previously shown to block calcium entry through ORAI channels (7), can alter the effects of TGF-β1. SW480 cells pretreated with or without TGF-β1were treated with 2-APB(100μM) for 30min. Ca2+ entry, transwell migration assay, and EMT-relevant markers were detected. As shown in **Figure 6A**, we found that cells treated with 2-APB showed a significant reduction in Ca2+ release (addition of thapsigargin) and Ca2+ entry (addition of Ca2+).

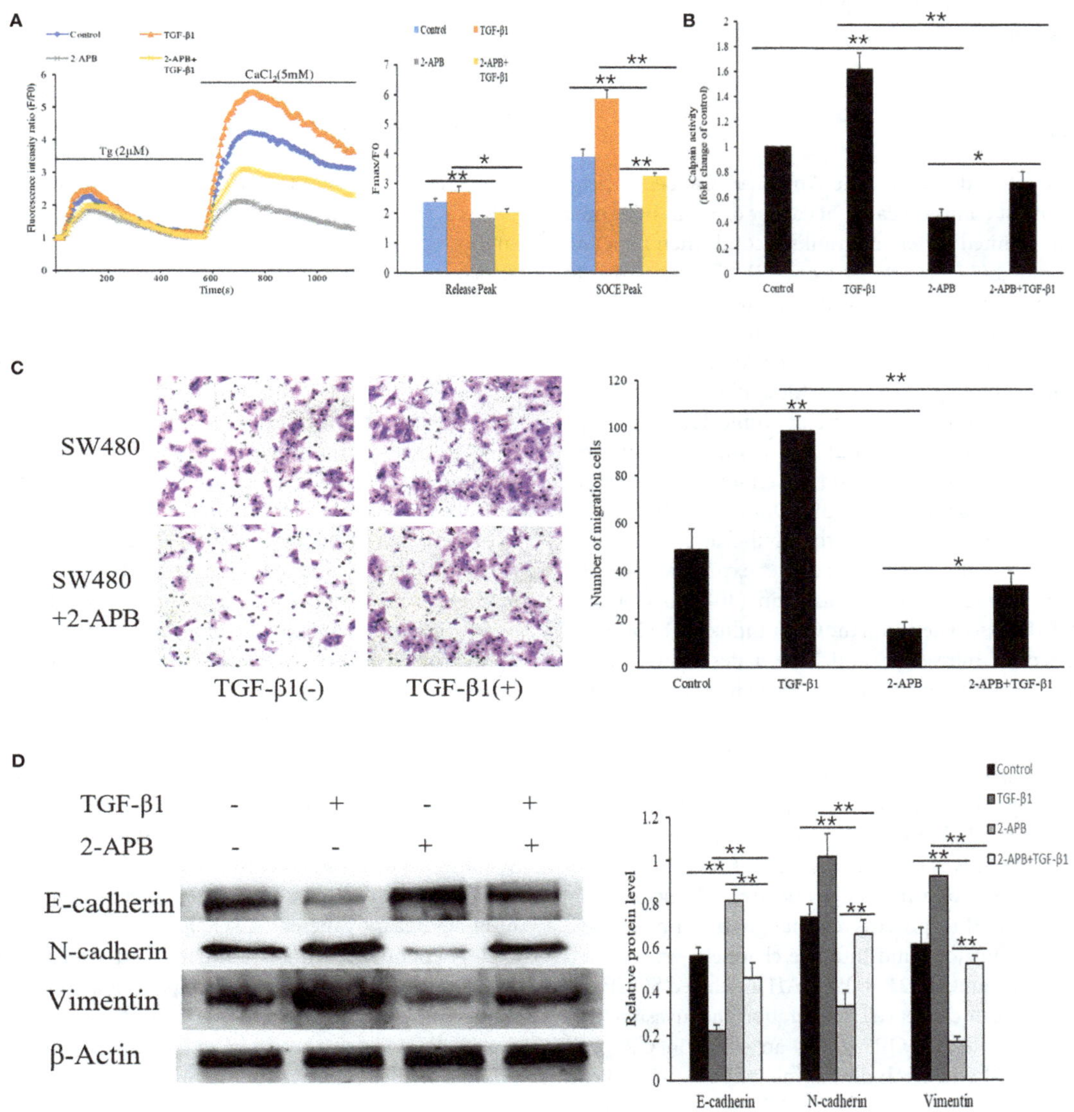

FIGURE 6 | Blockade of SOCE alleviates the TGF-β1-induced EMT in SW480 cells. **(A)** Representative traces of intracellular Ca2+ signals of SW480 cells with 2-APB and/or TGF-β1treatment were assessed by Rhod-2AM Ca2+ measurement. **(B)** Quantitative assessment of calpain activity in SW480 cells treated with 2-APB and/or TGF-β1. **(C)** SW480 cells were treated with 2-APB and/or TGF-β1, and cell migration was assessed by transwell assay. magnification, ×200. **(D)** Protein levels of E-cadherin, N-cadherin and Vimentin were analyzed by Western blot in SW480 pretreatment cells. All the experiments were repeated three times. **P*<0.05; ***P*<0.01.

Interestingly, a dramatic decrease in Ca2+ entry and Ca2+ release were also observed in the cells treated with TGF-β1 and 2-APB compared with TGF-β1 treatment cells. According to the calpain activity assays, treatment of 2-APB also repressed the TGF-β1-mediated Ca2+-dependent calpain activity (**Figure 6B**).

As blockade of SOCE has been previously shown to prevent cellular migration associated with EMT (36), to establish that cell migration is also affected upon Ca2+ influx in SW480 cells, transwell migration assay was performed which showed that treatment of 2-APB significantly inhibited cell migration in SW480 cells. Similarly, the increased migration seen with TGF-β1 treatment was attenuated by a blockage of Ca2+ entry with 2-APB (**Figure 6C**). Next, we further evaluated the effect of 2-APB treatment on EMT-relevant markers by Western blot. The results showed that 2-APB treatment of SW480 cells resulted in a pronounced increase in E-cadherin expression and a decrease in N-cadherin and Vimentin. Consistent with these results, TGF-β1-induced decrease in E-cadherin expression and increase in N-cadherin and Vimentin were also abolished by the addition of 2-APB (**Figure 6D**). Taken together, these results suggest that

SOCE-related Ca2+ influx also contributes to the EMT induced by TGF-β1 in SW480 cells. In addition, 2-APB and sh-ORAI1 both exhibited similar inhibition effects to the SW480 cells.

DISCUSSION

According to the latest data from the American Cancer Society, CRC is the third most common cause of cancer death in both men and women in the United States, and ranks second when men and women are combined (37). Mortality from CRC is mostly due to invasion and metastasis of neoplastic cells from the primary tumors to distant organ sites (29). Hence, understanding the mechanism regulating metastasis is critical to improving colon cancer survival. EMT is an important biological hallmark for epithelial cancer (38). Although EMT was first noticed during embryonic development, it is increasingly acknowledged that EMT makes a greater contribution to the tumor progression by enhancing migratory and invasive capabilities of cancer cells (39). During EMT processes, epithelial cells lose the expression of the epithelial characteristic marker, like E-cadherin and acquire the expression of the mesenchymal cell marker, such as Vimentin (40). This process has been shown to be associated with the Ca2+ influx (10). Ca2+ has versatility as a second messenger and it regulates many cellular functions by influencing various genes, proteins and signaling pathways (21). It regulates intracellular enzyme activity and protein-protein interactions through calmodulin or other calcium-binding proteins (26). Many types of cancer have been shown to have dysregulated expression of Ca2+ channels and other molecules involved in Ca2+ homeostasis (29). But the role of Ca2+ in EMT-associated metastasis is still not well understood. Ca2+ entry into tumor cells has been confirmed to be due to SOCE mediated by ORAI1 channels and this process in malignant tumors have fascinated many investigators, and thus the channels were already designated to “onco-channels” (21, 41). ORAI1-mediated SOCE has been confirmed to regulate cancer cell proliferation and invasion (24), and it has been reported that ORAI1 has an effect on CRC cell proliferation (22), but the research on the role of ORAI1-mediated SOCE in CRC is limited. Therefore, effects of ORAI1 on CRC should be warranted to investigate.

Emerging role of ORAI1 in human cancer has been reported. Upregulation of ORAI1 expression was observed in multiple human cancers, including non-small cell lung carcinoma (19), esophageal cancer (42) and gastric cancer (20). Consistent with these observations, we found that ORAI1 expression was markedly upregulated in CRC tissues compared with matched adjacent non-tumor tissues in this study. Moreover, we further examined the clinical relevance of ORAI1, and found that high expression of ORAI1 was closely associated with advanced clinical stage, high incidence of metastasis and shorter overall survival times. A previous study agreed with these conclusions demonstrating that ORAI1 overexpression was significantly correlated with poor prognosis in breast cancer (27). These results suggested that ORAI1 may be involved in CRC progression. In addition, since different cancer cell lines have distinct gene background, the genes that impact tumor progression may be differently expressed in these cells (43). Therefore, we further evaluated ORAI1 expression level in two human CRC cell lines SW480 and SW620, which have the same genetic background but different metastatic potential. In the present study, we provided evidence that ORAI1 expression differed in the two CRC cancer cell lines: SW620 cells, with more mesenchymal like characteristics and higher metastasis potential, express ORAI1 at higher levels than the SW480 cells with modest more epithelial characteristics. A recent study also demonstrated that STIM1 and ORAI3 are upregulated in metastatic CRC cells compared to primary CRC cells (44). Moreover, we also found that knockdown of ORAI1 suppressed the EMT of SW620 cells. These results suggest that ORAI1 might be involved in the EMT of CRC cells.

TGF-β1 is one of the most abundant growth factors stored and released by bone (45). Previous studies indicated that TGF-β1 can promote cancer cell invasion by regulating the induction of EMT (37). In our studies, when incubated with TGF-β1, SW480 cells underwent morphological changes from an “epithelial” polarized morphology to a mesenchymal fibroblastoid morphology and achieved increased migratory capabilities. This phenotypic transformation was accompanied by down-regulation of epithelial signature proteins including E–cadherin and increased expression of mesenchymal markers such as E–cadherin and Vimentin. However, the underlying mechanisms for TGF-β1 induced EMT of CRC cells are unclear. Previous studies demonstrated calcium signaling plays an important role in TGF-β signaling (46), and different mechanisms have been suggested to be involved in the regulation of Ca2+ homeostasis by TGF-β1 (38). Our studies show that TGF-β1 treatment enhanced the expression of ORAI1, an essential component of SOCE channel and promotes SOCE-related Ca2+ influx in SW480 cells. This result was similar with the result from a previous research that TGF-β1-induced EMT significantly increased SOCE in MCF7 breast cancer cells (9). Ca2+-dependent calpain contributes to many pathways that control cell migration, and M-calpain activity was shown to be significantly increased in CRC (47). In the present study, we show that TGF-β1 treatment amplified the calpain activity. These results provide further evidence for the importance of ORAI1, SOCE and calpain activity in TGF-β1-induced EMT of CRC cells.

To further verify the role of ORAI1 and ORAI1-mediated SOCE is critical for TGF-β1-induced EMT of CRC cells, we examined the effects of pharmacological inhibition for SOCE or gene silencing of ORAI1. 2-APB, a nonspecific pharmacological inhibitor, was previously shown to block SOCE through ORAI1 channels (48). Interestingly, blockade of SOCE markedly mitigated TGF-β1-induced migration and prevented reduced expression of E–cadherin protein after TGF–β1 treatment. Meanwhile, our results also showed that TGF-β1-induced increases in N-cadherin and Vimentin were decreased upon inhibition of Ca2+ influx by 2-APB, both of which are major cytoskeletal component of mesenchymal cells and necessary for motility seen in EMT. In addition, genetic studies using silencing method further established that ORAI1 is the major Ca2+ homeostasis channel in CRC cells. Our data confirmed that knockdown of ORAI1 led to decrease in Ca2+ influx, and significantly suppressed cell migration and changes of EMT-relevant marks expression induced by TGF-β1. This finding is consistent with the results of a previous study reporting that knockdown of ORAI1 in glioma can significantly reduce receptor-dependent Ca2+ influx and inhibit Pyke activity, thereby inhibiting glioma cell invasion and metastasis (49). Parallel phenomena were also observed for calpain activity. Importantly, a decrease in calpain activity was observed when Ca2+ influx was inhibited by 2-APB. Furthermore, knockdown of ORAI1 or inhibition of SOCE inhibited TGF-β1-induced increase in calpain activation. These results indicate that ORAI1 and ORAI1-mediated SOCE is involved in TGF-β1-induced EMT in SW480 cells.

CONCLUSION

In conclusion, our study indicated that ORAI1 expression was significantly upregulated in CRC, and ORAI1 overexpression was correlated with poor prognosis. we also had demonstrated that ORAI1 knockdown suppressed the EMT of SW620 Cells, and TGF-β1 treatment induced the EMT process in SW480 cells, increased ORAI1 expression, SOCE-mediated Ca2+ entry and calpain activity. Meanwhile, the effect of TGF-β1 treatment was obviously abolished by inhibiting Ca2+ influx with 2-APB and ORAI1 knockdown. Therefore, it can be inferred that TGF-β1induces EMT of SW480 cells by enhancing ORAI1 expression, promoting ORAI1-mediated Ca2+ entry and calpain activity. This is a possible mechanism for the TGF-β1-induced EMT in SW480 cells. Hence, ORAI1-mediated Ca2+ signaling may serve as a potential therapeutic target for CRC.

ETHICS STATEMENT

The studies involving human participants were reviewed and approved by Medical Ethics Review Committee of the First Affiliated Hospital of Chongqing Medical University. The patients/participants provided their written informed consent to participate in this study.

AUTHOR CONTRIBUTIONS

QK, BY, and ZW designed the study. QK and BY performed the main experiments. DH and GW collected patient specimens. XP and XL analyzed the data. QK wrote the manuscript. All authors contributed to the article and approved the submitted version.

ACKNOWLEDGMENTS

We would like to thank Professor Zheng Xiang and Hua Tang for their revision of this article.

REFERENCES

1. Navarro M, Nicolas A, Ferrandez A, Lanas A. Colorectal Cancer Population Screening Programs Worldwide in 2016: An Update. *World J Gastroenterol* (2017) 23:3632–42. doi: 10.3748/wjg.v23.i20.3632
2. Kuipers EJ, Grady WM, Lieberman D, Seufferlein T, Sung JJ, Boelens PG, et al. Colorectal Cancer. *Nat Rev Dis Primers* (2015) 1:15065. doi: 10.1038/nrdp.2015.65
3. Sung JJ, Lau JY, Goh KL, Leung WK. Asia Pacific Working Group on Colorectal Cancer. Increasing Incidence of Colorectal Cancer in Asia: Implications for Screening. *Lancet Oncol* (2005) 6:871–6. doi: 10.1016/S1470-2045(05)70422-8
4. Chen W, Zheng R, Baade PD, Zhang S, Zeng H, Bray F, et al. Cancer Statistics in China, 2015. *CA Cancer J Clin* (2016) 66:115–32. doi: 10.3322/caac.21338
5. Chaffer CL, Weinberg RA. A Perspective on Cancer Cell Metastasis. *Science* (2011) 331:1559–64. doi: 10.1126/science.1203543
6. Nieto MA. The Ins and Outs of the Epithelial to Mesenchymal Transition in Health and Disease. *Annu Rev Cell Dev Biol* (2011) 27:347–76. doi: 10.1146/annurev-cellbio-092910-154036
7. Bhattacharya A, Kumar J, Hermanson K, Sun Y, Qureshi H, Perley D, et al. The Calcium Channel Proteins ORAI3 and STIM1 Mediate TGF-β Induced Snail Expression. *Oncotarget* (2018) 9:29468–83. doi: 10.18632/oncotarget.25672
8. Kim JH, Lkhagvadorj S, Lee MR, Hwang KH, Chung HC, Jung JH, et al. Orai1 and STIM1 are Critical for Cell Migration and Proliferation of Clear Cell Renal Cell Carcinoma. *Biochem Biophys Res Commun* (2014) 448:76–82. doi: 10.1016/j.bbrc.2014.04.064
9. Hu J, Qin K, Zhang Y, Gong J, Li N, Lv D, et al. Downregulation of Transcription Factor Oct4 Induces an Epithelial-to-Mesenchymal Transition Via Enhancement of Ca2+ Influx in Breast Cancer Cells. *Biochem Biophys Res Commun* (2011) 411:786–91. doi: 10.1016/j.bbrc.2011.07.025
10. Beck A, Fleig A, Penner R, Peinelt C. Regulation of Endogenous and Heterologous Ca2+ Release-Activated Ca2+ Currents by Ph. *Cell Calcium* (2014) 56:235–43. doi: 10.1016/j.ceca.2014.07.011
11. Berridge MJ, Bootman MD, Roderick HL. Calcium Signalling: Dynamics, Homeostasis and Remodelling. *Nat Rev Mol Cell Biol* (2003) 4:517–29. doi: 10.1038/nrm1155
12. Villalobos C, Sobradillo D, Hernández-Morales M, Núñez L. Calcium Remodeling in Colorectal Cancer. *Biochim Biophys Acta Mol Cell Res* (2017) 1864:843–9. doi: 10.1016/j.bbamcr.2017.01.005
13. Chen YF, Hsu KF, Shen MR. The Store-Operated Ca(2+) Entry-Mediated Signaling is Important for Cancer Spread. *Biochim Biophys Acta* (2016) 1863:1427–35. doi: 10.1016/j.bbamcr.2015.11.030
14. Putney JW Jr. A Model for Receptor-Regulated Calcium Entry. *Cell Calcium* (1986) 7:1–12. doi: 10.1016/0143-4160(86)90026-6
15. Roberts-Thomson SJ, Peters AA, Grice DM, Monteith GR. ORAI-Mediated Calcium Entry: Mechanism and Roles, Diseases and Pharmacology. *Pharmacol Ther* (2010) 127:121–30. doi: 10.1016/j.pharmthera.2010.04.016
16. Derler I, Madl J, Schütz G, Romanin C. Structure, Regulation and Biophysics of I(CRAC), Stim/Orai1. *Adv Exp Med Biol* (2012) 740:383–410. doi: 10.1007/978-94-007-2888-2_16
17. Chalmers SB, Monteith GR. ORAI Channels and Cancer. *Cell Calcium* (2018) 74:160–7. doi: 10.1016/j.ceca.2018.07.011
18. Cantonero C, Sanchez-Collado J, Gonzalez-Nuñez MA, Salido GM, Lopez JJ, Jardin I, et al. Store-Independent Orai1-mediated Ca2+ Entry and Cancer. *Cell Calcium* (2019) 80:1–7. doi: 10.1016/j.ceca.2019.02.012
19. Zhan ZY, Zhong LX, Feng M, Wang JF, Liu DB, Xiong JP. Over-Expression of Orai1 Mediates Cell Proliferation and Associates With Poor Prognosis in Human non-Small Cell Lung Carcinoma. *Int J Clin Exp Pathol* (2015) 8:5080–8.

20. Yang N, Tang Y, Wang F, Zhang H, Xu D, Shen Y, et al. Blockade of Store-Operated Ca(2+) Entry Inhibits Hepatocarcinoma Cell Migration and Invasion by Regulating Focal Adhesion Turnover. *Cancer Lett* (2013) 330:163–9. doi: 10.1016/j.canlet.2012.11.040
21. Xia J, Wang H, Huang H, Sun L, Dong S, Huang N, et al. Elevated Orai1 and STIM1 Expressions Upregulate MACC1 Expression to Promote Tumor Cell Proliferation, Metabolism, Migration, and Invasion in Human Gastric Cancer. *Cancer Lett* (2016) 381:31–40. doi: 10.1016/j.canlet.2016.07.014
22. Gui L, Wang Z, Han J, Ma H, Li Z. High Expression of Orai1 Enhances Cell Proliferation and is Associated With Poor Prognosis in Human Colorectal Cancer. *Clin Lab* (2016) 62:1689–98. doi: 10.7754/Clin.Lab.2016.160131
23. Yang S, Zhang JJ, Huang XY. Orai1 and STIM1 are Critical for Breast Tumor Cell Migration and Metastasis. *Cancer Cell* (2009) 15:124–34. doi: 10.1016/j.ccr.2008.12.019
24. Liu X, Wan X, Kan H, Wang Y, Yu F, Feng L, et al. Hypoxia-Induced Upregulation of Orai1 Drives Colon Cancer Invasiveness and Angiogenesis. *Eur J Pharmacol* (2018) 832:1–10. doi: 10.1016/j.ejphar.2018.05.008
25. Deng W, Wang J, Zhang J, Cai J, Bai Z, Zhang Z. Orai1, a Direct Target of Microrna-519, Promotes Progression of Colorectal Cancer Via Akt/GSK3β Signaling Pathway. *Dig Dis Sci* (2016) 61:1553–60. doi: 10.1007/s10620-015-4029-6
26. Guo Y, Zhu J, Wang X, Li R, Jiang K, Chen S, et al. Orai1 Promotes Osteosarcoma Metastasis by Activating the Ras-Rac1-WAVE2 Signaling Pathway. *Med Sci Monit* (2019) 25:9227–36. doi: 10.12659/MSM.919594
27. Imamura T, Hikita A, Inoue Y. The Roles of TGF-β Signaling in Carcinogenesis and Breast Cancer Metastasis. *Breast Cancer* (2012) 19:118–24. doi: 10.1007/s12282-011-0321-2
28. Hao Y, Baker D, Ten Dijke P. Tgf-β-Mediated Epithelial-Mesenchymal Transition and Cancer Metastasis. *Int J Mol Sci* (2019) 20:2767. doi: 10.3390/ijms20112767
29. Schaar A, Sukumaran P, Sun Y, Dhasarathy A, Singh BB. Trpc1-STIM1 Activation Modulates Transforming Growth Factor β-Induced Epithelial-to-Mesenchymal Transition. *Oncotarget* (2016) 7:80554–67. doi: 10.18632/oncotarget.12895
30. Ge P, Wei L, Zhang M, Hu B, Wang K, Li Y, et al. TRPC1/3/6 Inhibition Attenuates the TGF-β1-Induced Epithelial-Mesenchymal Transition in Gastric Cancer Via the Ras/Raf1/ERK Signaling Pathway. *Cell Biol Int* (2018) 42:975–84. doi: 10.1002/cbin.10963
31. Wang Y, Li ZC, Zhang P, Poon E, Kong CW, Boheler KR, et al. Nitric Oxide-cGMP-PKG Pathway Acts on Orai1 to Inhibit the Hypertrophy of Human Embryonic Stem Cell-Derived Cardiomyocytes. *Stem Cells* (2015) 33:2973–84. doi: 10.1002/stem.2118
32. Gao YD, Zheng JW, Li P, Cheng M, Yang J. Store-Operated Ca2+ Entry is Involved in Transforming Growth Factor-β1 Facilitated Proliferation of Rat Airway Smooth Muscle Cells. *J Asthma* (2013) 50:439–48. doi: 10.3109/02770903.2013.778275
33. Zhang Z, Liu X, Feng B, Liu N, Wu Q, Han Y, et al. STIM1, a Direct Target of microRNA-185, Promotes Tumor Metastasis and is Associated With Poor Prognosis in Colorectal Cancer. *Oncogene* (2015) 34:4808–20. doi: 10.1038/onc.2014.404
34. Johansson J, Tabor V, Wikell A, Jalkanen S, Fuxe J. Tgf-β1-Induced Epithelial-Mesenchymal Transition Promotes Monocyte/Macrophage Properties in Breast Cancer Cells. *Front Oncol* (2015) 5:3. doi: 10.3389/fonc.2015.00003
35. Sun Y, Schaar A, Sukumaran P, Dhasarathy A, Singh BB. Tgf-β-Induced Epithelial-to-Mesenchymal Transition in Prostate Cancer Cells is Mediated Via TRPM7 Expression. *Mol Carcinog* (2018) 57:752–61. doi: 10.1002/mc.22797
36. Davis FM, Azimi I, Faville RA, Peters AA, Jalink K, Putney JW Jr, et al. Induction of Epithelial-Mesenchymal Transition (EMT) in Breast Cancer Cells is Calcium Signal Dependent. *Oncogene* (2014) 33:2307–16. doi: 10.1038/onc.2013.187
37. Siegel RL, Miller KD, Jemal A. Cancer Statistics, 2020. *CA Cancer J Clin* (2020) 70:7–30. doi: 10.3322/caac.21590
38. Zhang S, Miao Y, Zheng X, Gong Y, Zhang J, Zou F, et al. STIM1 and STIM2 Differently Regulate Endogenous Ca2+ Entry and Promote TGF-β-Induced EMT in Breast Cancer Cells. *Biochem Biophys Res Commun* (2017) 488:74–80. doi: 10.1016/j.bbrc.2017.05.009
39. Wu Y, Xu X, Ma L, Yi Q, Sun W, Tang L. Calreticulin Regulates TGF-β1-Induced Epithelial Mesenchymal Transition Through Modulating Smad Signaling and Calcium Signaling. *Int J Biochem Cell Biol* (2017) 90:103–13. doi: 10.1016/j.biocel.2017.07.023
40. Chei S, Oh HJ, Song JH, Seo YJ, Lee K, Lee BY. Magnolol Suppresses Tgf-β-Induced Epithelial-to-Mesenchymal Transition in Human Colorectal Cancer Cells. *Front Oncol* (2019) 9:752. doi: 10.3389/fonc.2019.00752
41. Ibrahim S, Dakik H, Vandier C, Chautard R, Paintaud G, Mazurier F, et al. Expression Profiling of Calcium Channels and Calcium-Activated Potassium Channels in Colorectal Cancer. *Cancers (Basel)* (2019) 11:561. doi: 10.3390/cancers11040561
42. Zhu H, Zhang H, Jin F, Fang M, Huang M, Yang CS, et al. Elevated Orai1 Expression Mediates Tumor-Promoting Intracellular Ca2+ Oscillations in Human Esophageal Squamous Cell Carcinoma. *Oncotarget* (2014) 5:3455–71. doi: 10.18632/oncotarget.1903
43. Xu Y, Zhang S, Niu H, Ye Y, Hu F, Chen S, et al. STIM1 Accelerates Cell Senescence in a Remodeled Microenvironment But Enhances the Epithelial-to-Mesenchymal Transition in Prostate Cancer. *Sci Rep* (2015) 5:11754. doi: 10.1038/srep11754
44. Zuccolo E, Laforenza U, Ferulli F, Pellavio G, Scarpellino G, Tanzi M, et al. Stim and Orai Mediate Constitutive Ca2+ Entry and Control Endoplasmic Reticulum Ca2+ Refilling in Primary Cultures of Colorectal Carcinoma Cells. *Oncotarget* (2018) 9:31098–119. doi: 10.18632/oncotarget.25785
45. Chen Y, Zhang K, Li Y, He Q. Estrogen-Related Receptor α Participates Transforming Growth Factor-β (Tgf-β) Induced Epithelial-Mesenchymal Transition of Osteosarcoma Cells. *Cell Adh Migr* (2017) 11:338–46. doi: 10.1080/19336918.2016.1221567
46. Cheng H, Wang S, Feng R. STIM1 Plays an Important Role in TGF-β-Induced Suppression of Breast Cancer Cell Proliferation. *Oncotarget* (2016) 7:16866–78. doi: 10.18632/oncotarget.7619
47. Guéguinou M, Harnois T, Crottes D, Uguen A, Deliot N, Gambade A, et al. SK3/TRPC1/Orai1 Complex Regulates SOCE-dependent Colon Cancer Cell Migration: A Novel Opportunity to Modulate anti-EGFR mAb Action by the Alkyl-Lipid Ohmline. *Oncotarget* (2016) 7:36168–84. doi: 10.18632/oncotarget.8786
48. DeHaven WI, Smyth JT, Boyles RR, Bird GS, Putney JW Jr. Complex Actions of 2-Aminoethyldiphenyl Borate on Store-Operated Calcium Entry. *J Biol Chem* (2008) 283:19265–73. doi: 10.1074/jbc.M801535200
49. Zhu M, Chen L, Zhao P, Zhou H, Zhang C, Yu S, et al. Store-Operated Ca(2+) Entry Regulates Glioma Cell Migration and Invasion Via Modulation of Pyk2 Phosphorylation. *J Exp Clin Cancer Res* (2014) 33:98. doi: 10.1186/s13046-014-0098-1

9

RAB10-ALK: A Novel *ALK* Fusion in a Patient with Gastric Cancer

Zhengqi Wen[1†], Dun Xiong[2†], Shurong Zhang[3†], Jiankun Liu[3], Bitao Li[4], Raomei Li[3] and Hushan Zhang[5]*

[1] Department of Oncology, The First Affiliated Hospital of Kunming Medical University, Kunming, China, [2] Department of Oncology, The People's Hospital of Puer City, Puer, China, [3] Department of Gastroenterology, The 920th Hospital of the Joint Logistics Support Force, PLA, Kunming, China, [4] Department of Prevention and Health Care, The First Affiliated Hospital of Kunming Medical University, Kunming, China, [5] The Medical Department, 3D Medicines Inc., Shanghai, China

***Correspondence:**
Hushan Zhang
15111010041@fudan.edu.cn

[†]These authors have contributed equally to this work

Gastric cancer is one of the most common cancers, while the current treatment options for gastric cancer are relatively scarce due to insufficient understanding of molecular characteristics and subtypes of gastric cancer. Different gene rearrangements of anaplastic lymphocyte kinase (*ALK*) have been reported in several types of cancer, especially in NSCLC. The first-generation *ALK* tyrosine kinase inhibitor (TKI) crizotinib, second-generation (ceritinib, alectinib, and brigatinib) and third-generation (lorlatinib) *ALK*-TKIs have been widely used for NSCLC patients with *ALK* rearrangement. However, little was reported about *ALK* mutation in gastric cancer (GC). Here we identified a novel form of *ALK* fusion, a case of GC with *RAB10-ALK* fusion, and this is the first report of *ALK* fusion in gastric cancer.

Keywords: anaplastic lymphocyte kinase fusion, anaplastic lymphocyte kinase-tyrosine kinase inhibitor, gastric cancer, next generation sequencing, cancer

INTRODUCTION

In recent years, *ALK* tyrosine kinase inhibitor (TKI) therapy has received great attention in solid tumors such as non-small cell lung cancer. However, few was reported about gene rearrangement of *ALK* in GC. Here we firstly present a case of GC with *RAB10-ALK* fusion, which is the first report of *ALK* fusion in GC.

CASE PRESENTATION

A 66-year-old male patient who is a minority (Lisu nationality) in Yunnan, China, was admitted to the hospital due to abdominal pain. The patient has no history of smoking and drinks alcohol occasionally. He has a history of hemorrhoids for many years without special treatment, has no history of infectious diseases such as hepatitis, tuberculosis, malaria, has no history of hypertension,

---

Abbreviations: *ALK*, anaplastic lymphocyte kinase; CAP, College of American Pathologists; CLIA, Clinical Laboratory Improvement Amendment; FISH, fluorescence *in situ* hybridization; GC, gastric cancer; IHC, immunocytochemistry; NGS, next-generation sequencing; NSCLC, non-small cell lung cancer; TKI, tyrosine kinase inhibitor.

and has no history of surgery. Both his parents are dead; the cause of death is unknown. He has no family history of infectious diseases and genetic diseases. The patient has symptoms of dry mouth, bitter mouth, no nausea, no acid reflux, no melena, mucus pus and blood in the stool, no fever. The mental state is fair, the physical strength is decreased, the appetite is poor, and the sleep is poor. There was no swelling and tenderness of superficial lymph nodes throughout the body.

Examination after admission showed a significant increase in serum biomarkers, including carcinoembryonic antigen, carbohydrate antigen, carbohydrate antigen CA199, carbohydrate antigen CA125, Cytokeratin-19-fragment CYFRA21-1. Gastroscopy revealed unevenness, ulcers, congestion, and edema at the lesser curvature and antrum of stomach (**Figure 1A**). Magnetic resonance examination displayed a large amount of fluid in the abdominal cavity and multiple lymph nodes adjacent to the abdominal aorta and enlarged (**Figure 1B**). Pathological examination revealed poorly differentiated adenocarcinoma of the stomach (signet ring cell carcinoma) (**Figure 1C**). In addition, the needle biopsy specimen was subjected to next generation sequencing (NGS) analysis in a laboratory accredited by the College of American Pathologists (CAP) and Clinical Laboratory Improvement Amendment (CLIA) (3D Medicines Inc., Shanghai, China), covering whole exon regions of 733 cancer related genes; as a result, fusion of *RAB10-ALK* with frequency of 15.23% and *ALK* amplification with frequency of 16% were detected in the stomach tissue of the patient (**Figures 2A, B**). In addition, several other genetic variants were also found, including KDM6A, TP53 mutation, and increased copy number of gene FGF19, BTK, IRS2, FGF3, EMSY (C11orf30), FGF4. Furthermore, immunocytochemistry (IHC) and fluorescence *in situ* hybridization (FISH) were also performed to verify the above mutation (**Figures 3A–E**). Immunohistochemical staining (Ventana Medical Systems, Tucson, AZ) showed an increased signal of *ALK* expression (**Figure 3C**), and *ALK* amplification was also verified by FISH (**Figure 3E**). However, the results of FISH excluded the common *ALK* fusion form EML4-*ALK* fusion (**Figures 3D, E**).

DISCUSSION

ALK is one of the membrane-bound receptor tyrosine kinases, which consist of an extra-cellular ligand binding domain, a single transmembrane domain, and a cytoplasmic tyrosine kinase domain.

In *ALK* fusions such as EML4-*ALK*, the amino-terminal fusion partner is fused to the intracellular tyrosine kinase domain of *ALK*, resulting in activation of downstream signaling. *ALK* signals activate numerous downstream pathways, including PI3K–Akt activation, MEKK2/3/MEK5/ERK5 pathway, RAS-MAPK, CRKL-C3G-RAP1, JAK-STAT and JUN pathway (1). In fact, almost all the *ALK* fusion proteins usually retain the cytoplasmic tyrosine kinase domain of *ALK* at the C-terminus, while the N-terminus is composed of a different protein. Several clinical trials have now confirmed that patients with *ALK* positive NSCLC can benefit from treatment with *ALK*-TKIs such as crizotinib, ceritinib, alectinib, brigatinib, and lorlatinib (2). Recent retrospective clinical researches in *ALK* positive NSCLC suggest different clinical outcomes based on the specific *ALK* fusion protein. That is, different *ALK* fusion form can mediate different downstream signaling and may exhibit different sensitivity to *ALK* tyrosine kinase inhibitors (TKIs) (2). The NGS method has expanded the different fusion partners identified in *ALK* positive NSCLC to 90, including Potential Fusion Partners RAB10 (3). However, except for EML4-*ALK*, which is the most prevalent *ALK* gene rearrangement in the *ALK*-positive NSCLC

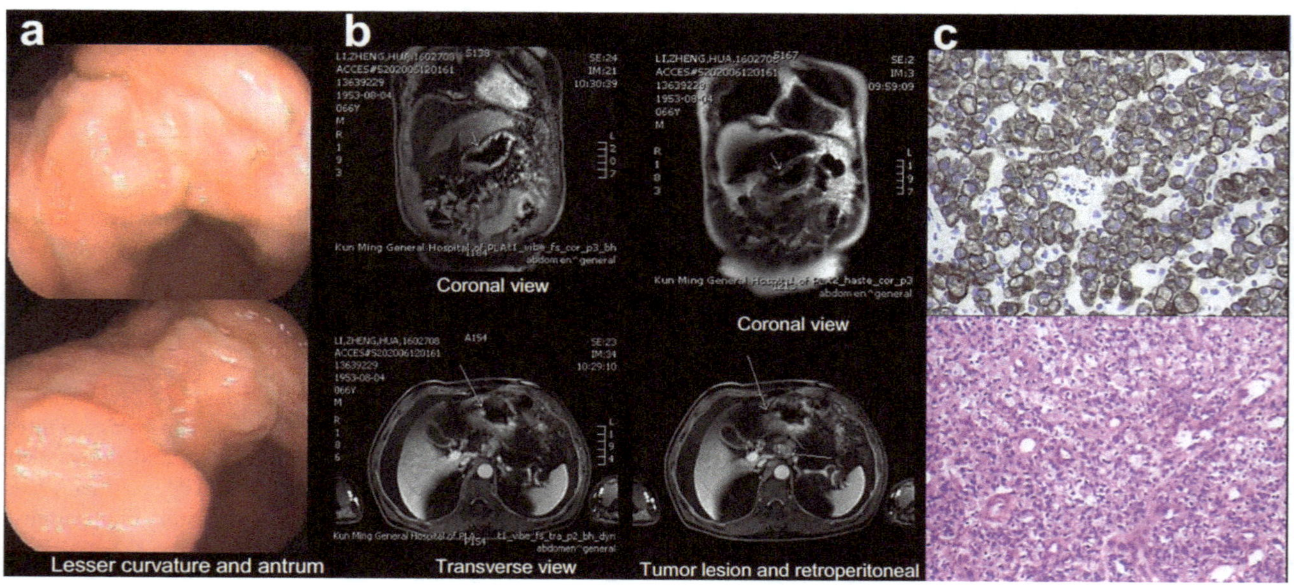

FIGURE 1 | Gastroscopy **(A)**, Magnetic Resonance Imaging (MRI) **(B)** displayed the tumor lesion, pathological diagnosis **(C)**, Immunohistochemical (IHC) staining for cytokeratin (CK) 6 and hematoxylin–eosin staining (HE).

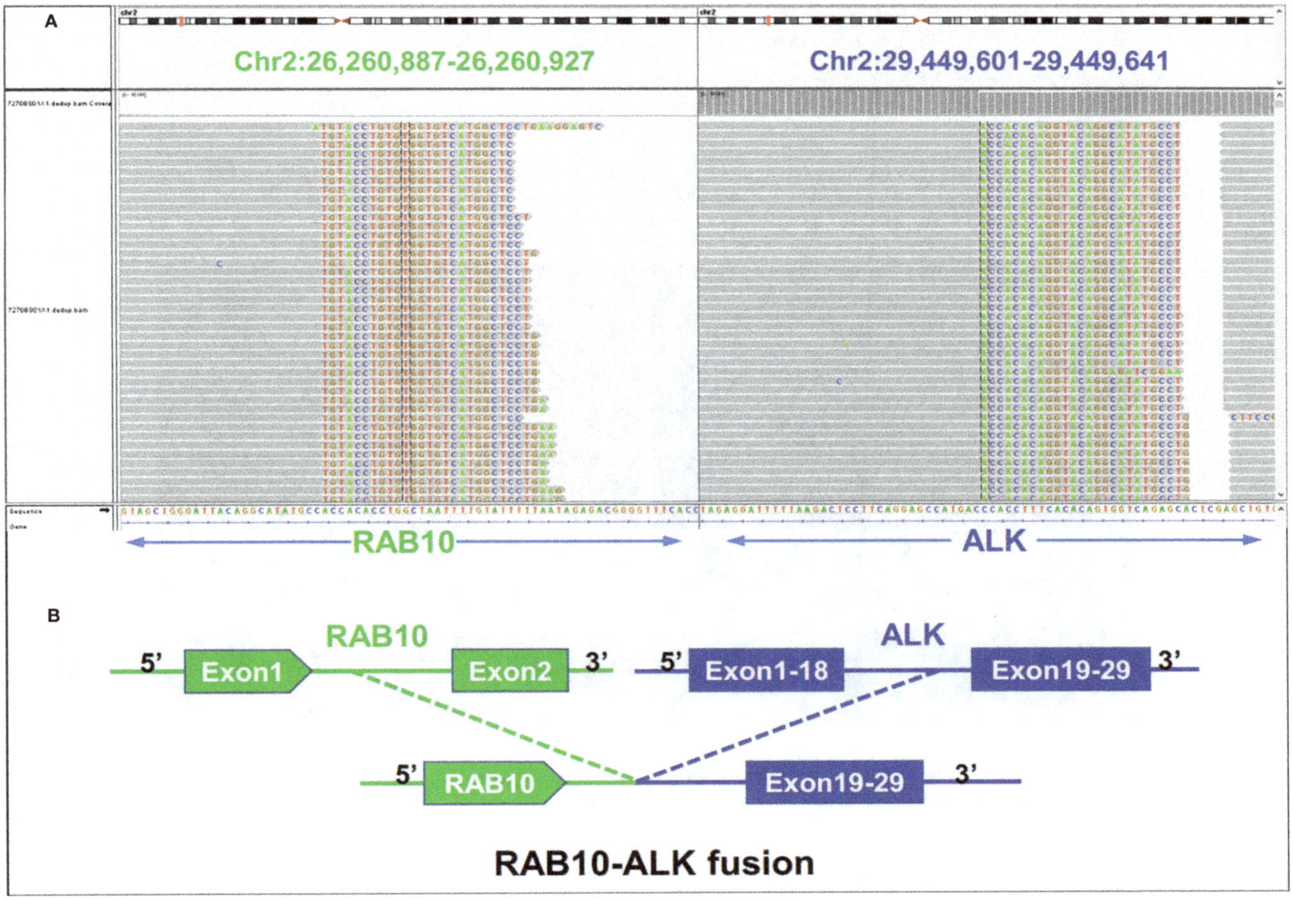

FIGURE 2 | Next-generation sequencing findings for the tumor tissue samples of the patient with gastric cancer. **(A)** *RAB10-ALK* fusion was validated manually using the Integrated Genomics Viewer (IGV); **(B)** a novel intergenic region between RAB10 and *ALK* exon 20 fusion variant was identified.

patients, there are few in-depth studies on most of other *ALK* fusions. The currently known evidence about *ALK* fusion proteins mainly originates from some of clinical cohorts of patients with *ALK*-positive NSCLC. Here, we firstly report the *RAB10-ALK* fusion and *ALK* amplification that are identified in patients with gastric cancer. This is the first report of an *ALK* fusion case in gastric cancer, and this is a novel type of *ALK* fusion. Regrettably, the patient refused to use the drug *ALK*-TKI of cross-indications, such as crizotinib, ceritinib *etc.*

Different *ALK* inhibitors have been used to the majority of *ALK*-positive patients, and all have shown a certain effect in controlling disease progression, especially in NSCLC (4). Well use of different *ALK*-TKIs will benefit the patient more. As reported, according to the different *ALK* mutation sites detected by NGS, a female patient with metastatic *ALK* rearrangement NSCLC received treatment of different *ALK*-TKIs, and finally the patient survived more than 48 months (5). However, rare cases of *ALK* mutations have been observed among GC patients, and there is no applications of *ALK*-TKIs in the GC treatment at present. For the efficacy of *ALK*-TKIs in NSCLC, crizotinib was also recommended to the patient reported in this case, but he refused because of his own reasons.

GC is one of the most common cancers worldwide. Although the incidence of GC has been steadily declining in the past few decades, due to the current lack of understanding of GC molecular characteristics and subtypes, the current treatment options for gastric cancer patients are relatively monotonous. Previous studies on the gene fusion mutations in gastric or signet ring adenocarcinoma are few, which may be related to the usual use of methods other than NGS in the past. For example, in 42 cases of signet ring cell carcinoma of the gastrointestinal tract, two different *ALK* antibody based IHC did not detect the "possibly positive" cases with *ALK* translocation detected by FISH (6). With the application of NGS technology and other genomic technologies, GC is currently being studied and typed in more detail at the molecular level. Gene fusions were also found in gastric cancer through NGS technology. Some researchers conducted whole-genome sequencing on 32 pairs of gastric signet ring cell carcinoma samples and found frequent CLDN18-ARHGAP26/6 fusion protein (25%), which was associated with a poor prognosis (7). Accordingly, based on the wider application of NGS detection technology, GC can be diagnosed and treated more accurately in the future. *ALK* rearrangements have been reported in several types of cancer,

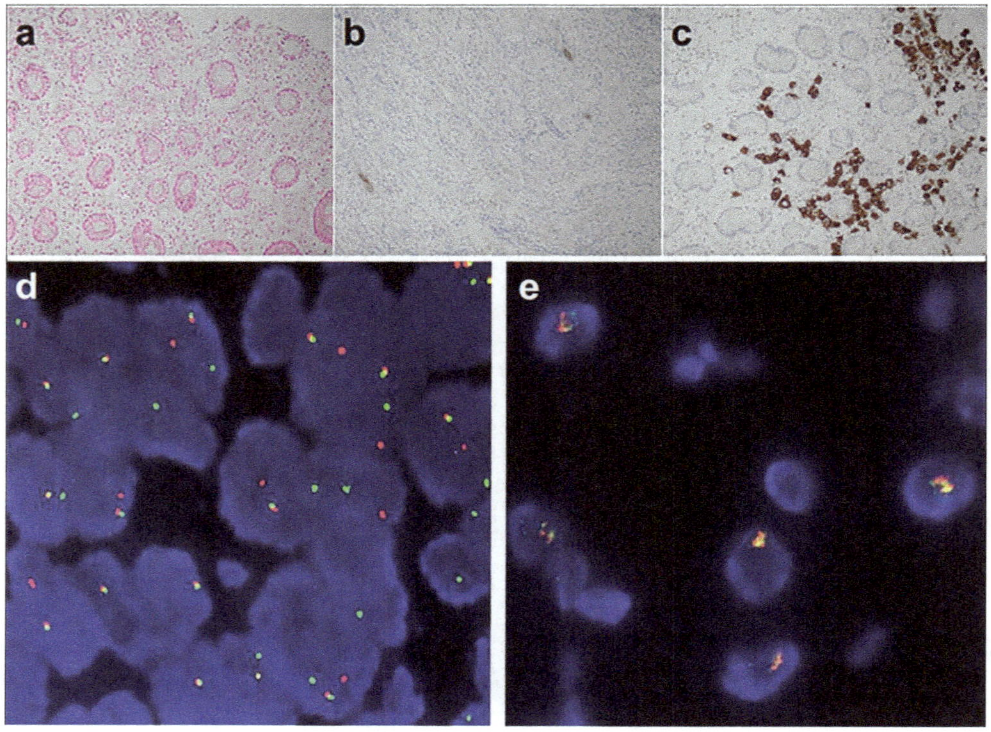

FIGURE 3 | *ALK* detected by Ventana-D5F3 IHC assay and FISH. **(A)** HE staining (200×); **(B)** *ALK* negative control 200×; **(C)** *ALK* IHC staining of the patient (200×), **(D)** EML4-*ALK* fusion positive control; **(E)** *ALK* detection of the patients, amplification of ALK was displayed (16%).

such as NSCLC, breast cancer, renal cell carcinoma (RCC), diffuse large B-cell lymphoma (DLBCL), serous ovarian carcinoma (SOC), inflammatory myofibroblastic tumor (IMT), renal medulla carcinoma (RMC), colon cancer, and to a lesser extent, esophageal squamous cell carcinoma (ESCC) (8); however, data on *ALK* rearrangement in GC is rare now.

About 90 different *ALK* fusion partners have been already identified, such as EML4, TPM-3/-4, TFG, CLTC, PRKAR1A, LMNA, KIF5B, RANBP2, FN1 (3). Although these partner genes have been described for *ALK*, little data is currently addressed on how different fusion partners affect the efficacy of *ALK*-TKIs. Therefore, the therapy of *ALK* positive cancers is currently determined regardless of which fusion partner is present. However, with the development of NGS technology and the advancement of precision medicine, more fusion partners will be identified and clinical evidence will be accumulated; based on these, different clinical strategies will be applied to patients with different *ALK* fusions. RAB10 is a novel *ALK* fusion partner that has been associated with cancer. RAB10 is a key regulator of endocytic recycling, belongs to the RAS oncogene superfamily, and it is reported to be an oncogene in HCC and is associated with poor prognosis (9). *ALK* fusion usually leads to abnormal activation of the *ALK* kinase domain and induces the activation of downstream signal transduction, leading to the growth of tumor cells. Since *RAB10-ALK* is a novel fusion mode, whether the domains reserved in RAB10 may contribute to the activation of *RAB10-ALK* remains unknown. Therefore, it is necessary to further research and verify the function of *RAB10-ALK* and the response to TKI.

CONCLUSION

This case provides a new reference for understanding *ALK* fusion mutations, discovers new molecular characteristics of GC patients, and provides the possibility for the future application of *ALK*-TKIs in GC patients. NGS can be performed as a routine test to explore more opportunities for treating GC patients.

ETHICS STATEMENT

The studies involving human participants were reviewed and approved by the Ethics Committee of the First Affiliated Hospital of Kunming Medical University. The patients/participants provided their written informed consent to participate in this study. Written informed consent was obtained from the individual(s) for the publication of any potentially identifiable images or data included in this article.

AUTHOR CONTRIBUTIONS

HZ and ZW put forward the content of the paper. HZ wrote the manuscript. DX, BL, JL, RL and SZ reviewed literature and clinical data. All authors contributed to the article and approved the submitted version.

ACKNOWLEDGMENTS

The authors thank the patient and his family for consenting to report this case information.

REFERENCES

1. Hallberg B, Palmer RH. The role of the ALK receptor in cancer biology. *Ann Oncol* (2016) 27 Suppl 3:iii4–iii15. doi: 10.1093/annonc/mdw301
2. Childress MA, Himmelberg SM, Chen H, Deng W, Lovly CM. ALK Fusion Partners Impact Response to ALK Inhibition: Differential Effects on Sensitivity, Cellular Phenotypes, and Biochemical Properties. *Mol Cancer Res* (2018) 16 (11):1724–36. doi: 10.1158/1541-7786.MCR-18-0171
3. Ou S-HII, Zhu VW, Nagasaka M. Catalog of 5' Fusion Partners in ALK-positive NSCLC Circa 2020. *Jto Clin Res Rep* (2020) 1(1):1–10. doi: 10.1016/j.jtocrr.2020.100015
4. Thai AA, Solomon BJ. Treatment of ALK-positive nonsmall cell lung cancer: recent advances. *Curr Opin Oncol* (2018) 30(2):84–91. doi: 10.1097/CCO.0000000000000431
5. Shaw AT, Friboulet L, Leshchiner I, Gainor JF, Bergqvist S, Brooun A, et al. Resensitization to Crizotinib by the Lorlatinib ALK Resistance Mutation L1198F. *N Engl J Med* (2016) 374(1):54–61. doi: 10.1056/NEJMoa1508887
6. Alese OB, El-Rayes BF, Sica G, Zhang G, Alexis D, La Rosa FG, et al. Anaplastic lymphoma kinase (ALK) gene alteration in signet ring cell carcinoma of the gastrointestinal tract. *Ther Adv Med Oncol* (2015) 7(2):56–62. doi: 10.1177/1758834014567117
7. Shu Y, Zhang W, Hou Q, Zhao L, Zhang S, Zhou J, et al. Prognostic significance of frequent CLDN18-ARHGAP26/6 fusion in gastric signet-ring cell cancer. *Nat Commun* (2018) 9(1):2447. doi: 10.1038/s41467-018-04907-0
8. Ducray SP, Natarajan K, Garland GD, Turner SD, Egger G. The Transcriptional Roles of ALK Fusion Proteins in Tumorigenesis. *Cancers (Basel)* (2019) 11 (8):1074. doi: 10.3390/cancers11081074
9. Wang W, Jia WD, Hu B, Pan YY. RAB10 overexpression promotes tumor growth and indicates poor prognosis of hepatocellular carcinoma. *Oncotarget* (2017) 8(16):26434–47. doi: 10.18632/oncotarget.15507

10

Analysis of the PD-1 Ligands Among Gastrointestinal Cancer Patients: Focus on Cancer Immunity

Lin Dai [1,2,3†], *Zilin Huang* [4†] *and Wang Li* [4*]

[1] *Cancer Prevention Center, Sun Yat-sen University Cancer Center, Guangzhou, China,* [2] *State Key Laboratory of Oncology in South China, Guangzhou, China,* [3] *Collaborative Innovation Center for Cancer Medicine, Guangzhou, China,* [4] *Department of Medical Imaging and Interventional Radiology, Sun Yat-sen University Cancer Center, Guangzhou, China*

Correspondence:
Wang Li
liwang@sysucc.org.cn

† *These authors have contributed equally to this work*

Many types of gastrointestinal cancer have shown promising outcomes after checkpoint blockade immunotherapy; however, it remains largely unclear about the expression profiles of programmed death 1 (PD-1) ligands (CD274 and PDCD1LG2) in the context of human pan-cancer. This work comprehensively analyzed the expression pattern of the PD-1 ligands and the clinical significance in the prognosis prediction among the seven types of gastrointestinal malignancies collected from The Cancer Genome Atlas (TCGA) and the Cancer Cell Line Encyclopedia (CCLE) database. Furthermore, the correlation of CD274/PDCD1LG2 with cancer immunity was also explored. The patients with liver hepatocellular carcinoma (LIHC) receiving cytokine-induced killer (CIK) cell immunotherapy at our cancer center were enrolled. CD274 and PDCD1LG2 displayed inconsistent gene expression levels among the diverse cancer cell lines. Typically, the abnormal expression level of CD274 and PDCD1LG2 was detected in both esophageal carcinoma (ESCA) and stomach adenocarcinoma (STAD), where PDCD1LG2 was related to the overall survival (OS) of the patients in ESCA (p = 0.015) and STAD (p = 0.025). High-serum CD274 and PDCD1LG2 levels predicted a worse survival in the patients with LIHC receiving CIK therapy. More importantly, the expression level of CD274 and PDCD1LG2 was significantly correlated with the degree of Estimation of STromal and Immune cells in MAlignant Tumor tissues using the Expression data (ESTIMATE). In addition, we found that CD274 and PDCD1LG2 were correlated with gene markers in tumor-infiltrating immune cells. Furthermore, the expression of CD274 and PDCD1LG2 was correlated with tumor mutation burden (TMB), microsatellite instability (MSI), mismatch repair (MMR), and DNA methyltransferase (DNMT) of different types of cancers. The present work comprehensively analyzed a RNA sequencing of the PD-1 ligands across the seven distinct types of gastrointestinal cancers, which provided clues for further studies in cancer immunity and development.

Keywords: gastrointestinal cancer, CD274, PDCD1LG2, prognosis, cancer immunity

INTRODUCTION

Gastrointestinal malignant tumor is a leading cause of death (1). The development of immunotherapy using immune checkpoint inhibitors has achieved breakthroughs in treating cancers. Programmed death 1 (PD-1) and its ligands, programmed death ligand 1 (PD-L1, or CD274) and PD-L2 (PDCD1LG2), are known as an immune checkpoint axis available to the cancer cells escaping from the immune destruction of T cells (2). In other words, PD-1 binds two ligands CD274 and PDCD1LG2 to inhibit the T-cell activation and invalidate immune surveillance. The results from experimental investigations and clinical studies showed that PD-1/PD-L1 blockers were demonstrated to be effective in gastrointestinal cancers (3, 4). However, a specific gene expression of CD274/PDCD1LG2 in gastrointestinal cancers at a pan-cancer level remains largely unknown.

A pan-cancer analysis is initially utilized in the field of cancer research to shed more light on the common features and heterogeneities of various human malignancies (5). A pan-cancer analysis, which is also referred to as an analysis of molecular abnormalities among several cancer types, is able to identify the common features and heterogeneities of some vital dysregulated biological processes in diverse cancer cell lineages. The project of a pan-cancer analysis, including Cancer Cell Line Encyclopedia (CCLE) and The Cancer Genome Atlas (TCGA), has been established based on the different human cancer cell lines and tissues at epigenomic, genomic, proteomic, and transcriptomic levels (6–8). Recently, a pan-cancer analysis is adopted to identify certain functional and pathway genes, which allows to specifically, comprehensively, and thoroughly understand human cancers. Considering as an example, the tumor hypoxia-associated multi-omic molecular characteristics were investigated, and some molecular alterations were suggested to be correlated with the sensitivity or resistance to antitumor agents. It contributed to a comprehensive understanding of tumor hypoxia at the molecular level and has certain implications for cancer treatment in clinical practice (9). The updated data regarding the frequency, etiology, and outcomes of the forkhead box protein M1 (FOXM1) upregulation in human cancers were defined among 33 cancer types derived from TCGA databases (10). Notably, the information obtained from these 33 TCGA-derived cancers had systemically revealed the long non-coding RNA- (lncRNA-) mediated dysregulation in cancers, which also provides the precious approach and resources to investigate the lncRNAs functions in cancers (11). It is beneficial to characterize the frequency of occurrence and variability of immune phenotypes within and among various cancer types, so as to understand the immune status for those untreated cancers. Typically, this method has been applied in more than 9,000 expression data of TCGA-derived cancer genes (12). Therefore, a pan-cancer analysis helps to illustrate the patterns that are beneficial for developing the combination treatments and individualized therapies.

In this regard, taking advantage of the large data sets from TCGA, this study aimed to examine the expression profiles of CD274/PDCD1LG2 and the prognostic significance in human gastrointestinal tumors. In addition, the association between CD274/PDCD1LG2 and the tumor infiltration level, tumor mutation burden (TMB), microsatellite instability (MSI), mismatch repair (MMR), and DNA methyltransferase (DNMT) were analyzed in the different tumor types. Our study helps to understand the vital roles of CD274/PDCD1LG2 in gastrointestinal tumor-immune interactions.

Abbreviations: PD-1, programmed death 1; TCGA, The Cancer Genome Atlas; CCLE, Cancer Cell Line Encyclopedia; CIK, cytokine-induced killer; ESTIMATE, MAlignant Tumor tissues using the Expression data; TMB, tumor mutation burden; MSI, microsatellite instability; MMR, mismatch repair; DNMT, DNA methyltransferase; GTEx, Genotype-Tissue Expression; ROC, Receiver operating characteristic; KM, Kaplan–Meier; OS, overall survival; CHOL, cholangiocarcinoma; COAD, colon adenocarcinoma; ESCA, esophageal carcinoma; LIHC, liver hepatocellular carcinoma; PAAD, pancreatic adenocarcinoma; READ, rectum adenocarcinoma; STAD, stomach adenocarcinoma.

MATERIALS AND METHODS

Patient Data Sets and Processing

The Cancer Genome Atlas, a milestone of the cancer genomics project, characterizes thousands of primary cancer samples and matched the characterized samples with the adjacent non-carcinoma samples from seven types of cancers, including cholangiocarcinoma (CHOL, $N = 45$), colon adenocarcinoma (COAD, $N = 521$), esophageal carcinoma (ESCA, $N = 173$), liver hepatocellular carcinoma (LIHC, $N = 424$), pancreatic adenocarcinoma (PAAD, $N = 182$), rectum adenocarcinoma (READ, $N = 177$), and stomach adenocarcinoma (STAD, $N = 407$). In this study, the TCGA level three RNA sequencing processed data and the corresponding clinical annotations were acquired by using the University of California Santa Cruz (UCSC) cancer genome browser (https://tcga.xenahubs.net, accessed April 2020). The gene expression data of healthy samples from the Genotype-Tissue Expression (GTEx) database (https://gtexportal.org/home/) was also downloaded for a comparison. The CCLE public project is established through a comprehensive characterization of tremendous human tumor models at both genetic and pharmacological levels. To examine the differential gene expression in cancers at a larger scale, the CCLE database containing the RNA-sequencing data sets for over 1,000 cell lines (https://portals.broadinstitute.org/ccle) was used in this study. Meanwhile, the approval from the Ethics Committee was exempted since only the open-access data were used. A total of 122 consecutive patients with LIHC receiving an adjuvant cytokine-induced killer (CIK) cell immunotherapy after a curative resection at our center were retrospectively enrolled, which were approved by the Ethics Committee of Sun Yat-sen University Cancer Center. A detailed treatment workflow is described in our previous study (13).

Gene Expression and Survival Analysis

To compare the gene expression levels between cancer and adjacent non-carcinoma samples, the data regarding the gene expression profiles of CD274 and PDCD1LG2 were extracted from the seven cancer types in TCGA to form an expression matrix. Thereafter, the formed expression matrix and clinical information were matched with a patient ID. Receiver operating characteristic (ROC) curve was drawn to evaluate the ability of CD274 and PDCD1LG2 to distinguish the tumor sample from the normal sample. Moreover, the Kaplan-Meier (KM) analysis was conducted to compare the overall survival (OS) of the patients with TCGA cancer stratified based on the gene expression level of CD274 and PDCD1LG2 using a log-rank test.

PD-1 Ligands and Tumor Immunity

The Estimation of STromal and Immune cells in MAlignant Tumor tissues using the Expression data (ESTIMATE) is an approach that uses gene expression profiles to predict the tumor purity and the infiltrating stromal cells/immunocytes in tumor tissues (14). The ESTIMATE algorithm produces three scores based on the gene set enrichment analysis (GSEA) of a single sample, including (1) stromal score, which determines stromal cells in tumor tissues, (2) immune score, which stands for the immunocyte infiltration level in tumor tissues, and (3) estimate score, which infers the tumor purity. In this study, we used the ESTIMATE algorithm to estimate the immune and stromal scores in tumor tissues according to the corresponding transcriptional data. Later, we calculated the correlation of these scores with the expression of CD274 and PDCD1LG2.

Additionally, we examined the association of the expression level of CD274 and PDCD1LG2 with the gene markers in the selected tumor-infiltrating immunocytes with reference to the previous research studies (15–17). The estimated statistical significance and the Spearman's correlation coefficient were generated through a correlation analysis. Thereafter, we plotted an expression heatmap between a pair of genes in a specific type of cancer.

Tumor mutation burden measures the number of mutations in a specific cancer genome. Numerous articles have been conducted to explore the significance of using the TMB status as a biomarker to predict the patients with the highest response to checkpoint inhibitors (18). In this study, the somatic mutation data of all patients with TCGA were downloaded (https://tcga.xenahubs.net), their TMB scores were calculated, and the correlation between TMB and CD274/PDCD1LG2 was determined. MSI is characterized by the widespread length polymorphisms of microsatellite sequences resulting from DNA polymerase slippage. Recently, it was suggested that the patients with high MSI cancers can gain benefits from immunotherapy, and MSI was used as the genetic instability index for cancer detection (19). In this study, we calculated the MSI score for each patient, followed by a correlation analysis between MSI and CD274/PDCD1LG2. Notably, MMR, also referred to

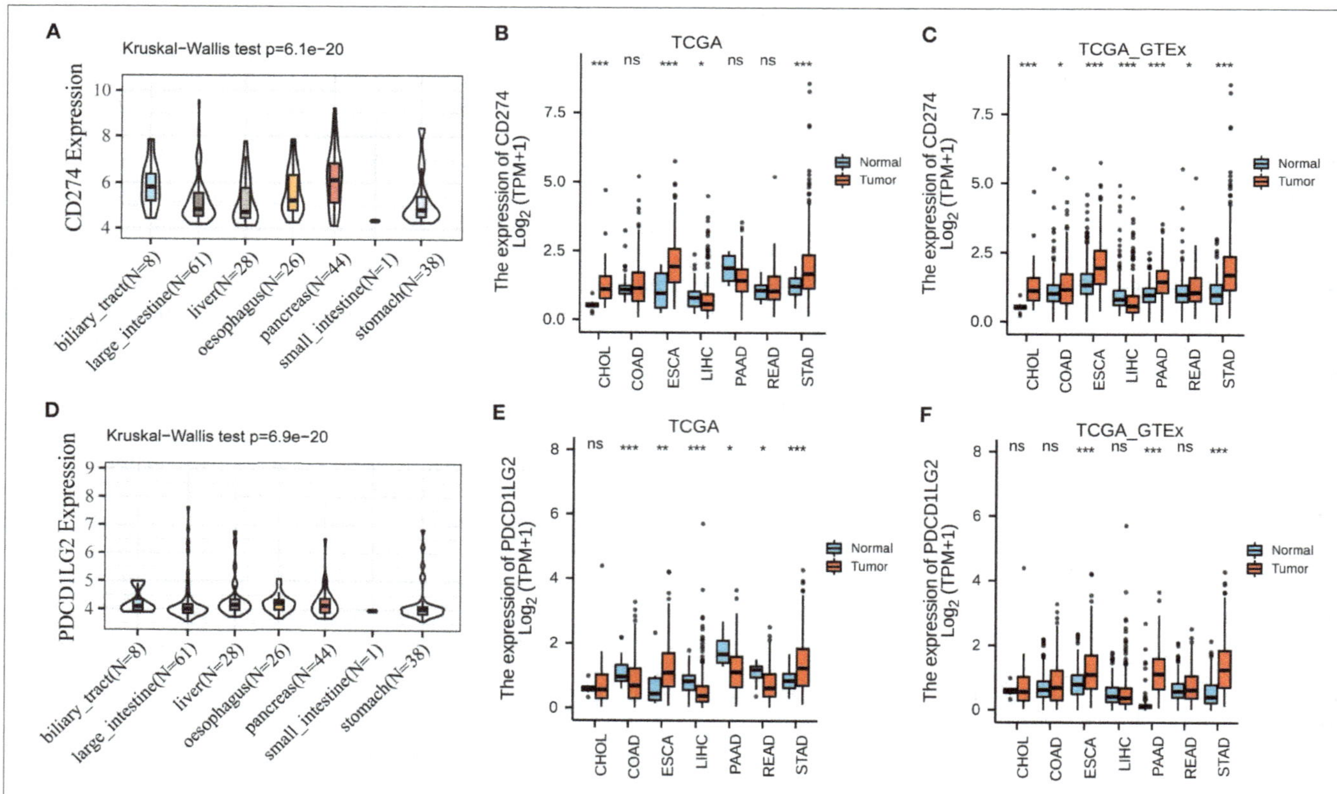

FIGURE 1 | CD274/PDCD1LG2 expression level in human pan-cancer. **(A)** The messenger RNA (mRNA) level of CD274 in Cancer Cell Line Encyclopedia (CCLE). **(B)** The mRNA level of CD274 in The Cancer Genome Atlas (TCGA). **(C)** CD274 mRNA level in TCGA and genotype-tissue expression (GTEx). **(D)** The mRNA level of PDCD1LG2 in CCLE. **(E)** The mRNA level of PDCD1LG2 in TCGA. **(F)** PDCD1LG2 mRNA level in TCGA and GTEx. $^{*}p < 0.05$; $^{**}p < 0.01$; $^{***}p < 0.001$; ns, not significant.

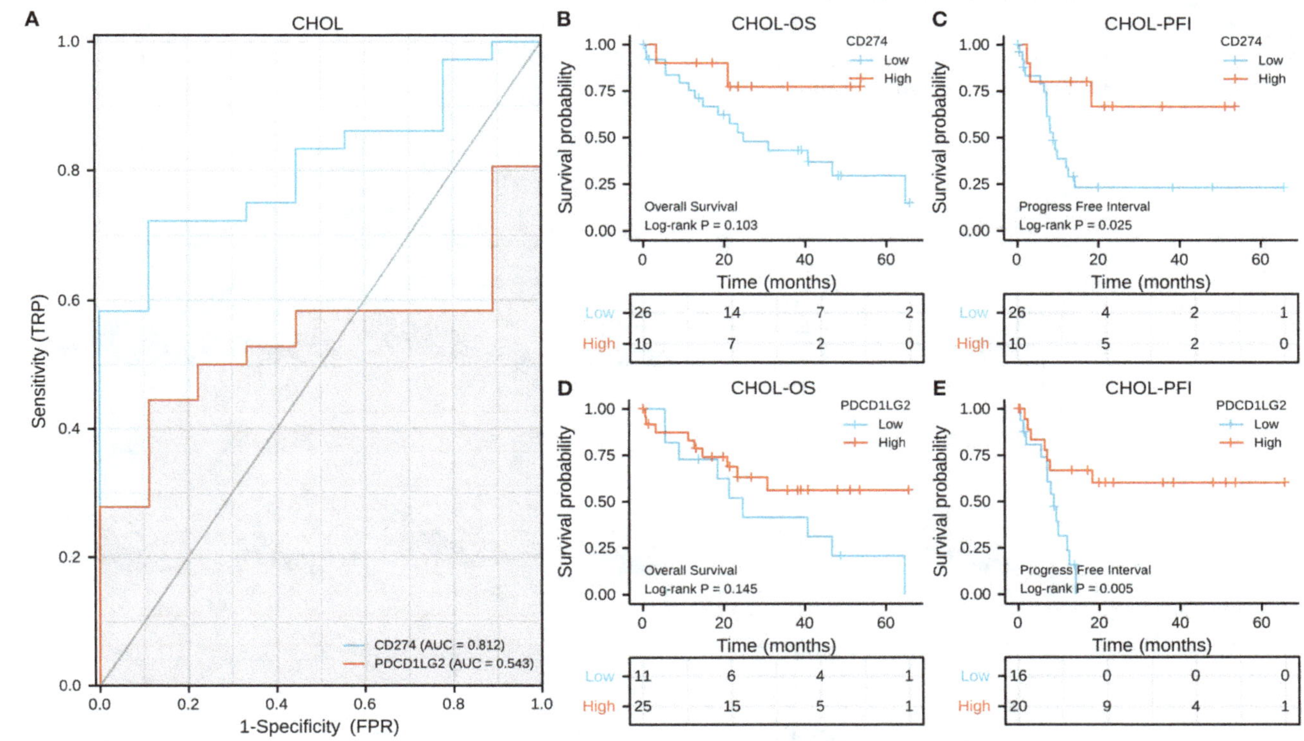

FIGURE 2 | CD274/PDCD1LG2 expression and its correlation with cholangiocarcinoma (CHOL) patient survival. **(A)** Receiver operating characteristic (ROC) curves CD274/PDCD1LG2 of distinguishing tumor from normal samples. **(B,C)** The Kaplan–Meier (KM) analysis shows the association between the CD274/PDCD1LG2 expression and overall survival (OS). **(D,E)** CD274/PDCD1LG2 expression and progression-free interval (PFI).

as the normal tissue DNA repair system, can correct errors in the process of DNA replication. However, due to the lack of MMR genes in tumor cells or the defects during the replication repair, the possibility of gene mutation has increased (19). Later, we performed a correlation analysis between MMR genes (including MLH1, MSH2, MSH6, PMS2, and EPCAM) and CD274/PDCD1LG2. DNMT participates in the process of tumorigenesis and development, whereas DNMT1, DNMT3A, and DNMT3B are the major key enzymes that catalyze DNMT (20). We also analyzed a correlation between DNMTs and CD274/PDCD1LG2.

Statistical Analysis

In the present work, the clinical survival types, including OS and progression-free interval (PFI), were selected for analysis. Generally, OS is deemed as the duration from the date of diagnosis to the date of death due to any cause, while PFI is defined as the disease progression or death from any cause.

The Wilcox log-rank test was adopted to determine the presence or absence of a markedly increased sum of the gene expression z-scores in cancer tissues compared with the adjacent normal tissues. The area under the ROC curve was calculated to evaluate the ability of CD274 and PDCD1LG2 in distinguishing the tumor sample from the normal sample. Meanwhile, the Kruskal-Wallis test was employed to compare the difference in the expression of CD274 and PDCD1LG2 in cell lines. Survival was analyzed by the KM curves and a log-rank test. The Spearman test was utilized for a correlation analysis. The R language (version 3.6.0; R Foundation) was used for all analyses. A two-sided difference of $p < 0.05$ indicated statistical significance.

RESULTS

Pan-Cancer Expression Landscape of CD274 and PDCD1LG2

According to the results of CCLE analysis, CD274 and PDCD1LG2 showed inconsistent gene expression levels among the diverse cancer cell lines (p = 6.1e-20 and 6.9e-20, **Figures 1A,D**), where pancreas cells had a relatively higher gene expression. Consistent with the different gene expression levels in CCLE, CD274, and PDCD1LG2 also displayed distinct expression in TCGA. For the seven TCGA-derived cancer types, we detected that ESCA, PAAD, and STAD showed a relatively higher gene expression. The expression landscapes of CD274 and PDCD1LG2 in TCGA cohorts are presented in **Figures 1B,E**, respectively. In addition, CD274 and PDCD1LG2 also exhibited a higher gene expression when more samples from GTEx were added **Figures 1C,F. Figure 2A** shows the AUC values of CD274 (0.812) and PDCD1LG2 (0.543) in the patients with CHOL, and the AUC results of the other six cancer types are presented in **Supplementary Figures 1–6**.

Screening of the Survival-Associated Cancers

In the OS analysis, KM analysis showed that the subjects with high CD274 levels had short OS compared with those with low CD274 levels in PAAD ($p = 0.012$, **Supplementary Figure 4B**) whereas those with an increased CD274 expression showed superior OS to those with a decreased CD274 expression in COAD ($p = 0.001$, **Supplementary Figure 1B**); the subjects

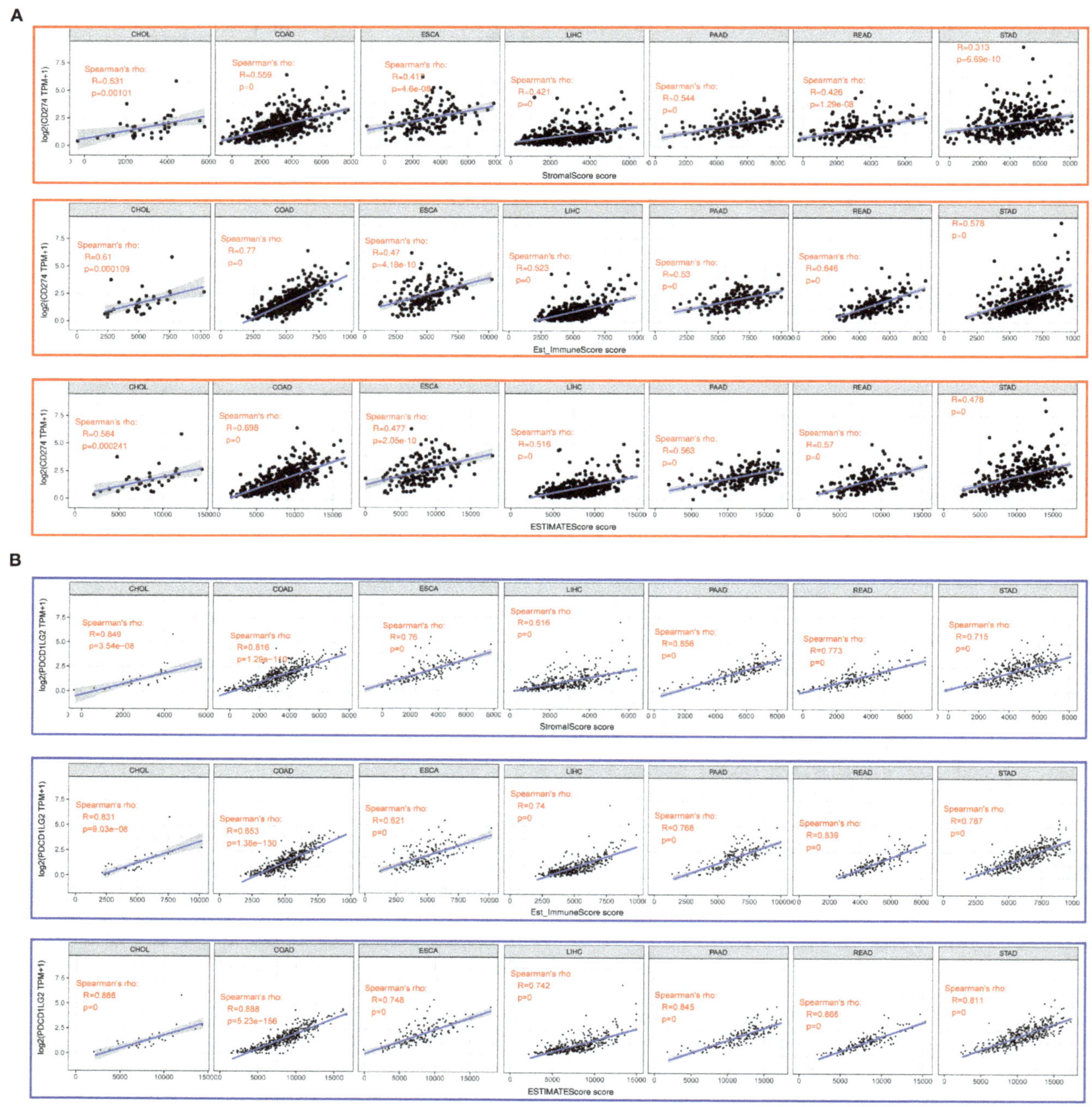

FIGURE 3 | CD274/PDCD1LG2 expression is correlated with cancer immunity in Estimation of STromal and Immune cells in MAlignant Tumor tissues using the Expression data (ESTIMATE). **(A)** ESTIMATE predicting CD274 expression is correlated with tumor immune infiltration level across seven cancer types. Top panel, stromal score; middle panel, immune score; and bottom panel, estimate score. **(B)** ESTIMATE predicting PDCD1LG2 expression is correlated with tumor immune infiltration level across seven cancer types. Top panel, stromal score; middle panel, immune score; and bottom panel, estimate score.

with a high PDCD1LG2 expression had poorer OS than those with a low PDCD1LG2 expression in STAD ($p = 0.025$, **Supplementary Figure 6D**) while the subjects with an increased PDCD1LG2 expression showed superior OS to those with a decreased PDCD1LG2 expression in ESCA ($p = 0.015$, **Supplementary Figure 2D**). In CHOL, no significant overall

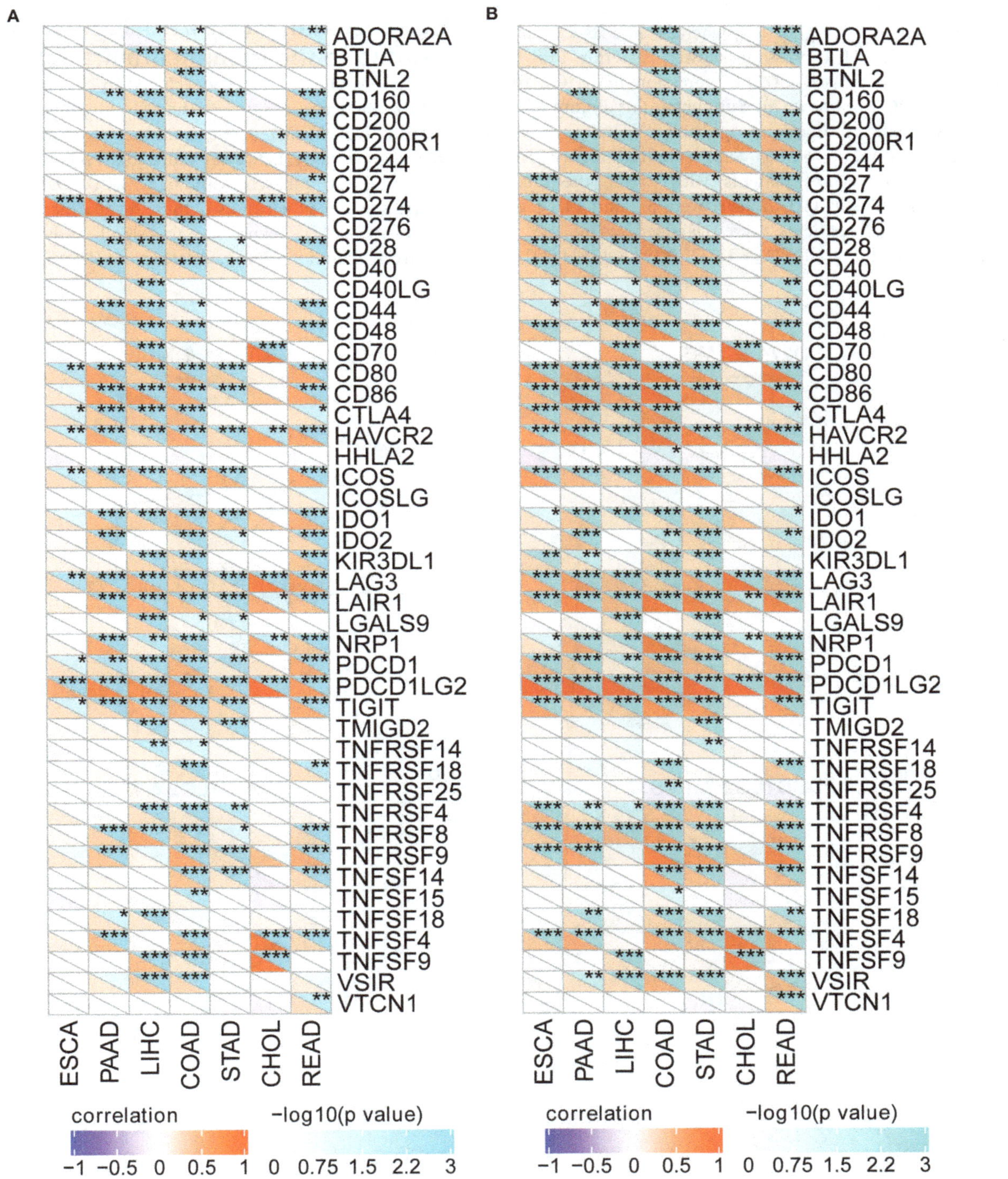

FIGURE 4 | CD274/PDCD1LG2 expression is correlated with immune markers. **(A)** Heatmap shows that the CD274 expression is correlated with the tumor immune marker level across seven cancers. For each pair, right top triangle is colored representing a *p*-value; left bottom is colored representing a correlation coefficient. **(B)** Heatmap shows that the PDCD1LG2 expression is correlated with the tumor immune marker level across seven cancers. $^{*}p < 0.05$; $^{**}p < 0.01$; $^{***}p < 0.001$.

survival difference was seen between high and low gene expression patients (both p values of CD274 and PDCD1LG2 were more than 0.05, **Figures 2B,D**).

In the PFI analysis, according to the results of KM analysis, the subjects with a high CD274 expression had poor PFI relative to those with a low CD274 expression in PAAD ($p = 0.027$, **Supplementary Figure 4C**); whereas the subjects having an increased CD274 expression showed superior PFI than those having a decreased CD274 expression in CHOL ($p = 0.025$, **Figure 2C**), as shown in **Supplementary Figure 3**; high PDCD1LG2 predicted superior prognosis for CHOL ($p = 0.005$, **Figure 2E**) and LIHC ($p = 0.003$, **Supplementary Figure 3E**).

In our cancer center patients with LIHC, the median serum CD274 and PDCD1LG2 level were 5.1 and 14.7 μg/μl, respectively. When patients were classified using the best statistical cutoff values (CD274 = 11.22 μg/μl and PDCD1LG2 = 27.67 μg/μl), survival analysis showed that the patients with LIHC with a high level of CD274 and PDCD1LG2 had worse disease-free survival after CIK immunotherapy (both $p < 0.01$, **Supplementary Figure 7**).

Expression of CD274/PDCD1LG2 Was Related to the Immune Infiltration Level

The ESTIMATE method is developed to calculate the immune and stromal scores of cancer tissues. By adopting the ESTIMATE method, we calculated the immune, stromal, and estimate scores, respectively. Later, we evaluated the relationships between the immune/stromal scores and CD274/PDCD1LG2 expression. **Figure 3** exhibits the results in these seven cancer types. Clearly, CD274/PDCD1LG2 expression was significantly correlated with the stromal, immune, and estimate scores (all values of $p < 0.05$).

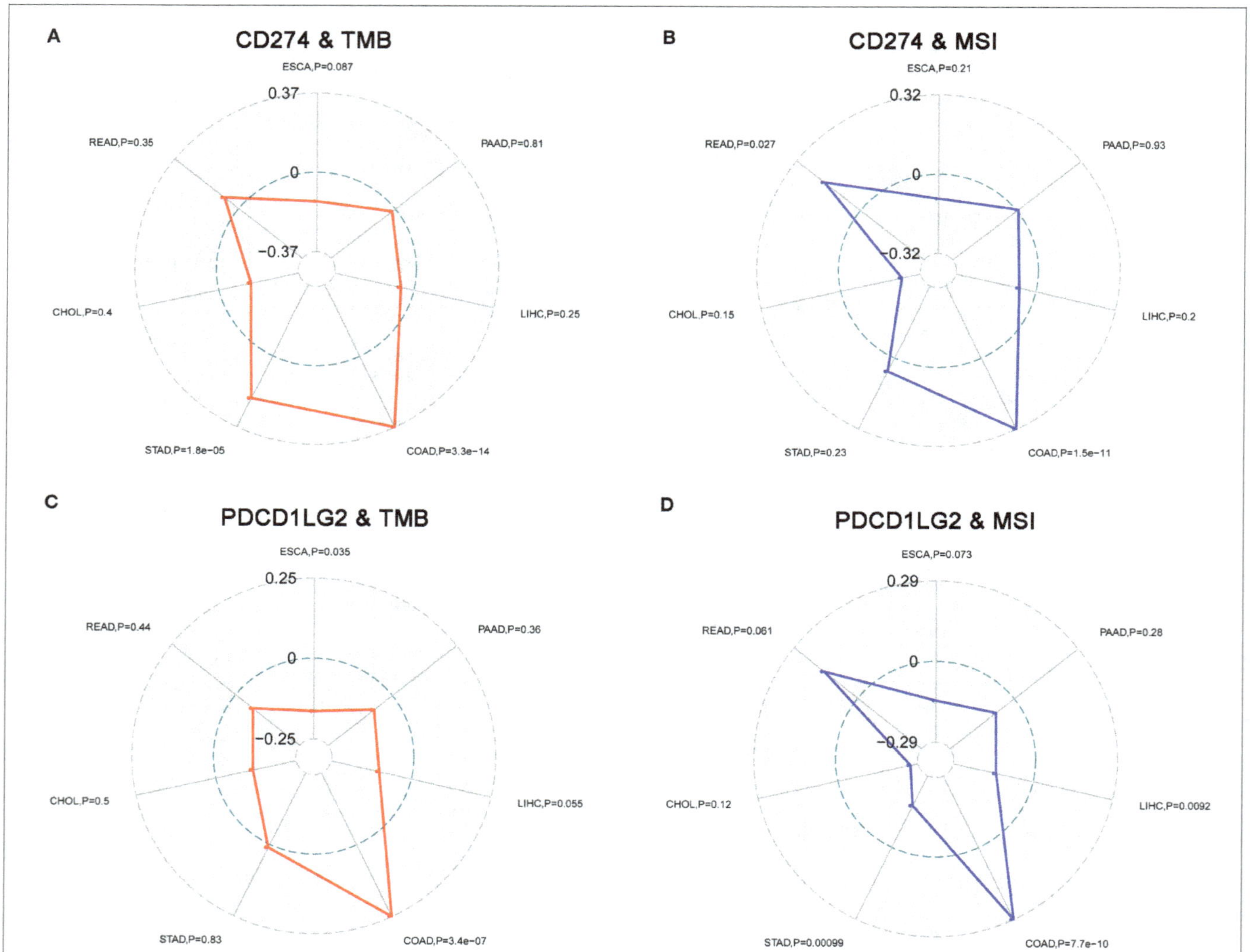

FIGURE 5 | CD274/PDCD1LG2 expression is correlated with tumor mutation burden (TMB) and microsatellite instability (MSI). **(A)** Radar chart displaying a correlation between CD274 and TMB across seven cancers. Red line representing the Spearman correlation coefficient. **(B)** Radar chart displaying a correlation between CD274 and MSI. Blue line representing the Spearman correlation coefficient. **(C)** PDCD1LG2 expression and TMB. **(D)** PDCD1LG2 and MSI.

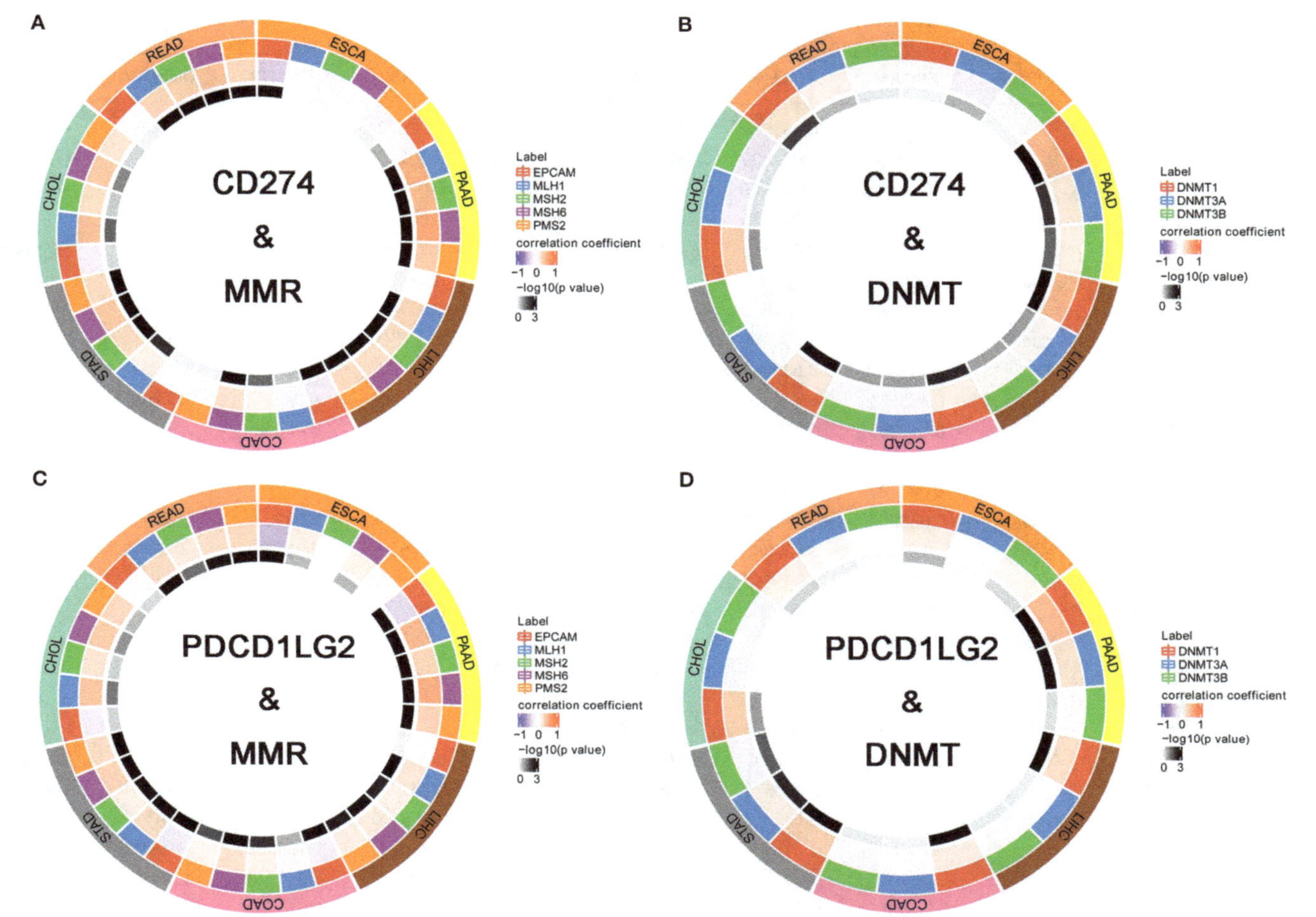

FIGURE 6 | CD274/PDCD1LG2 expression is correlated with mismatch repair (MMR) and DNA methyltransferase (DNMT). **(A)** Circle chart displaying the overlap between CD274 and MMR across seven cancers. The first outer ring representing cancer types; the second outer ring representing five MMR genes; the third outer ring representing a correlation coefficient; and the fourth outer ring is colored representing a *p*-value. **(B)** CD274 and DNMTs. **(C)** PDCD1LG2 and MMRs. **(D)** PDCD1LG2 and DNMTs.

To better investigate the association of CD274/PDCD1LG2 expression with different immune infiltrating cells, we analyzed the relationship of CD274/PDCD1LG2 expression with the gene markers in diverse immunocytes, as shown in **Figure 4**. Our results suggested that CD274/PDCD1LG2 expression was significantly correlated with many immune markers in diverse immunocytes and distinct T cells.

Correlation Analysis on TMB, MSI, MMR, and DNMT

Moreover, we evaluated the association of TMB/MSI with CD274/PDCD1LG2 expression as shown in **Figure 5**. We discovered that the CD274 expression was correlated with the TMB in STAD (p = 1.8e-5), and COAD (p = 3.3e-14); while PDCD1LG2 expression was correlated with the TMB in ESCA (p = 0.035), and COAD (p = 3.4e-7), as presented in **Figures 5A,C**. Moreover, CD274 expression was found to be related to the MSI in COAD (p = 1.5e-11), and READ (p = 0.027); whereas PDCD1LG2 expression was associated with the MSI in COAD (p = 7.7e-10), LIHC (p = 0.009), and STAD (p = 0.001), as displayed in **Figures 5B,D**.

Further, we performed a correlation analysis between MMR genes (MLH1, MSH2, MSH6, PMS2, and EPCAM) and CD274/PDCD1LG2 as shown in **Figures 6A,C**. In all seven cancer types, CD274/PDCD1LG2 was correlated with at least one MMR gene. Besides, we also conducted a correlation analysis between DNMT (DNMT1, DNMT2, DNMT3A, and DNMT3B) and CD274/PDCD1LG2. As a result, in all seven cancer types, CD274/PDCD1LG2 was correlated with at least one DNMT gene (**Figures 6B,D**). Detailed correlation results are summarized in **Table 1**.

DISCUSSION

The present work illustrated a comprehensive workflow for a pan-cancer analysis and thoroughly investigated the

TABLE 1 | Correlation analysis of CD274/PDCD1LG2 expression with mismatch repair (MMR) and DNA methyltransferase (DNMT).

	Tumor	Spearman	MMR					DNMT		
			EPCAM	MLH1	MSH2	MSH6	PMS2	DNMT1	DNMT3A	DNMT3B
CD274	CHOL	*R*	−0.18816	0.453539	0.289318	0.400772	0.235521	0.359917	−0.18746	−0.21202
	CHOL	*P*-value	0.333454	0.027339	0.260987	0.061694	0.333454	0.093221	0.4289	0.4289
	COAD	*R*	−0.17445	−0.07269	0.119258	0.249567	0.024473	0.144956	−0.0889	−0.08137
	COAD	*P*-value	0.000702	0.240673	0.031913	3.11E-07	0.601398	0.00561	0.114561	0.114561
	ESCA	*R*	−0.32706	0.009353	−0.08905	0.026681	−0.11629	0.041869	−0.148	−0.07887
	ESCA	*P*-value	0.000108	1	0.779336	1	0.56227	0.636896	0.180519	0.636896
	LIHC	*R*	−0.02565	0.323872	0.276122	0.268484	0.287001	0.490804	0.09953	0.08108
	LIHC	*P*-value	0.621419	7.39E-10	1.78E-07	2.81E-07	6.67E-08	1.57E-23	0.109575	0.117999
	PAAD	*R*	−0.10438	0.533641	0.48648	0.576787	0.36405	0.496813	0.213342	0.163804
	PAAD	*P*-value	0.165564	6.89E-14	1.74E-11	1.79E-16	1.17E-06	5.24E-12	0.008492	0.028903
	READ	*R*	0.042965	0.329019	0.355855	0.428334	0.300045	0.225528	0.128959	0.056493
	READ	*P*-value	0.581419	4.25E-05	9.46E-06	3.86E-08	0.000163	0.010155	0.193449	0.468364
	STAD	*R*	0.020888	0.151739	0.287854	0.392907	0.293081	0.183127	0.040141	−0.03326
	STAD	P-value	0.686804	0.006445	4.13E-08	1.36E-14	2.92E-08	0.001093	0.876637	0.876637
PDCD1LG2	CHOL	*R*	−0.21905	0.430888	0.248649	0.385328	0.306821	0.351351	−0.09472	−0.10579
	CHOL	*P*-value	0.287307	0.043513	0.287307	0.08119	0.206213	0.106864	1	1
	COAD	*R*	−0.17776	0.065562	0.142451	0.236716	0.122061	0.161801	0.021428	−0.05155
	COAD	*P*-value	0.000525	0.161284	0.006733	1.49E-06	0.017852	0.001526	0.647399	0.541866
	ESCA	*R*	−0.44693	0.157969	0.000631	0.148759	0.020448	0.146261	0.01071	0.105305
	ESCA	*P*-value	1.25E-08	0.17871	1	0.17871	1	0.189854	0.892398	0.36464
	LIHC	*R*	0.030398	0.231375	0.157928	0.181724	0.16655	0.273517	0.057927	0.053573
	LIHC	*P*-value	0.558383	3.17E-05	0.00444	0.001679	0.003735	2.4E-07	0.528893	0.528893
	PAAD	*R*	−0.32388	0.493875	0.324009	0.537676	0.331045	0.472252	0.249401	0.063617
	PAAD	*P*-value	2.05E-05	9.87E-12	2.05E-05	5.02E-14	1.91E-05	8.5E-11	0.001575	0.398879
	READ	*R*	−0.07558	0.287624	0.182248	0.258266	0.294101	0.125439	0.082768	0.01599
	READ	*P*-value	0.331687	0.000656	0.036821	0.002257	0.000572	0.318773	0.575208	0.837492
	STAD	*R*	−0.20015	0.279894	0.159715	0.333779	0.277346	0.350788	0.15516	−0.11656
	STAD	*P*-value	0.00019	1.41E-07	0.001919	1.64E-10	1.43E-07	8.03E-12	0.005175	0.023985

role of CD274/PDCD1LG2 in gastrointestinal cancers. The CD274/PDCD1LG2 expression among the different cancer cell lines was reported. It was found that most cancer types showed a CD274/PDCD1LG2 alteration frequency, and the abnormal expression served as a prognostic factor in some cancer types. Serum CD274/PDCD1LG2 levels could predict disease-free survival after the CIK cell therapy in patients with LIHC. More importantly, the CD274/PDCD1LG2 expression was associated with the cancer immunity. Furthermore, CD274/PDCD1LG2 was identified to be correlated with TMB, MSI, MMR, and DNMT.

It is significant to identify the abnormal gene expression among the different types of cancers. Also, it is of great significance to identify the tumor-specific targets or tumor-related features in individualized treatment, thus enhancing the possibility of curing among the patients with cancer (21). A pan-cancer analysis of CD274/PDCD1LG2 is valuable for identifying a differential expression and its role in many cancer types (22, 23). Using CCLE and TCGA databases, a large number of diverse types of cancers are obtained, which contributes to discovering the abnormal CD274/PDCD1LG2 expression among the different types of cancers. Besides, a thorough pan-cancer cellular analysis of gene expression can be performed through CCLE, which sheds light on the future cellular experiments. On the other hand, TCGA genomic and survival analyses may provide guidance for clinical practice and future studies.

In recent years, immunotherapy has achieved prominent efficacy in the treatment of tumors. Notably, the present work also demonstrated that the expression of CD274/PDCD1LG2 was related to cancer immunity. According to this study, the CD274/PDCD1LG2 level was related to the immune infiltration levels in cancers. ESTIMATE has been reported as a metric for the evaluation of the prognosis for the patients with cancer (24). Numerous recent studies have employed the ESTIMATE method to assess various tumors, and it has been successfully applied to the genome data. For instance, ESTIMATE is used to predict the outcomes among the patients with glioblastoma and cutaneous melanoma (25, 26). Using a TCGA cohort, the ESTIMATE method was utilized to generate the immune and stromal scores. As a result, CD274/PDCD1LG2 was correlated with the ESTIMATE scores. Furthermore, CD274/PDCD1LG2 was also detected to be correlated with the gene markers in infiltrating cells as observed from **Figure 4**.

Gene mutation is a major cause of cancer formation (27). Typically, mutations in some specific genes may predict the patient prognosis and treatment response (28, 29). An adaptive immune system can identify and detect cancers through the non-self neoantigens associated with somatic mutations. Therefore, TMB affects the possibility of generation of an immunogenic peptide, thus impacting the patient response to immune checkpoint inhibitors (30, 31). Consequently, it is of great significance to comprehensively investigate the association of the CD274/PDCD1LG2 expression with TMB levels among the patients with cancer, using the TCGA-derived high-quality matched data. Moreover, TMB and MSI also indicate the production of new antibodies. Noteworthily, a number of cases with high MSI (MSI-H) show increased TMB levels (32). Further, as discovered by Bonneville et al. (33), the MSI-H cervical squamous cell carcinoma and adrenocortical carcinoma showed abnormally high mutation frequencies. On the other hand, MSI is a vital index to predict the tumor genesis and development (19). The National Comprehensive Cancer Network (NCCN) guidelines have recommended an MSI testing for all READ subtypes, and the READ mortality can be reduced by the early detection of MSI (34). Some studies have shown that the MMR defect (dMMR) in cancer cells produces antigens that can be easily recognized by T cells, in this way, the PD-1 inhibitors are highly effective on the MSI-H solid tumors (35). In this regard, FDA has approved the use of Keytruda for the treatment of MSI-H/dMMR solid tumors (36). Therefore, TMB, MSI, and MMR can serve as a predicting factor for the efficacy of immunotherapy at present. We found in this study that the CD274/PDCD1LG2 expression was correlated with TMB and MSI in some cancer types. Moreover, the gene DNA methylation can regulate gene expression, while such a change can be utilized by tumor cells to destroy the immunogenicity and the immune recognition mechanisms, thus obtaining the immune escape phenotypes. Notably, the application of a methylase inhibitor in combination with an immunocheckpoint inhibitor has achieved initial advantages (20). An analysis between CD274/PDCD1LG2 and a methylase inhibitor is expected to inject a new vitality into the cancer treatment. Taken together, our findings provide clues for the association between CD274/PDCD1LG2 and cancer immunity, which require further experiment investigations to clarify.

Collectively, our comprehensive pan-cancer analysis has characterized CD274/PDCD1LG2 in different cancer cell lines and tissues of seven gastrointestinal cancer types. Our new integrative omics-based workflow might provide novel insights into the patients with gastrointestinal cancer regarding immunotherapy.

AUTHOR CONTRIBUTIONS

WL conceived of and designed the study, supervised the study, and reviewed the manuscript. LD and ZH performed the literature search, collected and analyzed the data, generated the figures and tables, and wrote the manuscript. All authors contributed to the article and approved the submitted version.

SUPPLEMENTARY MATERIAL

Supplementary Figure 1 | CD274/PDCD1LG2 expression and its correlation with colon adenocarcinoma (COAD) patient survival.

Supplementary Figure 2 | CD274/PDCD1LG2 expression and its correlation with esophageal carcinoma (ESCA) patient survival.

Supplementary Figure 3 | CD274/PDCD1LG2 expression and its correlation with liver hepatocellular carcinoma (LIHC) patient survival.

Supplementary Figure 4 | CD274/PDCD1LG2 expression and its correlation with pancreatic adenocarcinoma (PAAD) patient survival.

Supplementary Figure 5 | CD274/PDCD1LG2 expression and its correlation with rectum adenocarcinoma (READ) patient survival.

Supplementary Figure 6 | CD274/PDCD1LG2 expression and its correlation with stomach adenocarcinoma (STAD) patient survival.

Supplementary Figure 7 | Serum CD274/PDCD1LG2 level and its correlation with disease free survival in LIHC CIK patients. **(A)** Serum CD274 (PDL1) distribution and cutoff of PDL1 level. **(B)** Lower serum PDL1 level was associated with longer disease free survival. **(C,D)** PDCD1LG2 (PDL2).

REFERENCES

1. Bray F, Ferlay J, Soerjomataram I, Siegel RL, Torre LA, Jemal A. Global cancer statistics 2018: GLOBOCAN estimates of incidence and mortality worldwide for 36 cancers in 185 countries. *CA: A cancer J Clin.* (2018) 68:394–424. doi: 10.3322/caac.21492
2. Syn NL, Teng MWL, Mok TSK, Soo RA. De-novo and acquired resistance to immune checkpoint targeting. *Lancet Oncol.* (2017) 18:e731–41. doi: 10.1016/S1470-2045(17)30607-1
3. Charoentong P, Finotello F, Angelova M, Mayer C, Efremova M, Rieder D, et al. Pan-cancer immunogenomic analyses reveal genotype-immunophenotype relationships and predictors of response to checkpoint blockade. *Cell Rep.* (2017) 18:248–62. doi: 10.1016/j.celrep.2016.12.019
4. Liu JN, Kong XS, Huang T, Wang R, Li W, Chen QF. Clinical implications of aberrant PD-1 and CTLA4 expression for cancer immunity and prognosis: a pan-cancer study. *Front Immunol.* (2020) 11:2048. doi: 10.3389/fimmu.2020.02048
5. Cancer Genome Atlas Research N, Weinstein JN, Collisson EA, Mills GB, Shaw KR, Ozenberger BA, et al. The cancer genome atlas pan-cancer analysis project. *Nat Gene.* (2013) 45:1113–20. doi: 10.1038/ng.2764
6. Li W, Chen QF, Huang T, Shen L, Huang ZL, Wu P. Profiles of m(6)A RNA methylation regulators for the prognosis of hepatocellular carcinoma. *Oncol Lett.* (2020) 19:3296–306. doi: 10.3892/ol.2020.11435

7. Huang ZL, Li W, Chen QF, Wu PH, Shen LJ. Eight key long non-coding RNAs predict hepatitis virus positive hepatocellular carcinoma as prognostic targets. *World J Gastrointest Oncol.* (2019) 11:983–97. doi: 10.4251/wjgo.v11.i11.983
8. Cancer Cell Line Encyclopedia C, Genomics of Drug Sensitivity in Cancer C. Pharmacogenomic agreement between two cancer cell line data sets. *Nature.* (2015) 528:84–7. doi: 10.1038/nature15736
9. Ye Y, Hu Q, Chen H, Liang K, Yuan Y, Xiang Y, et al. Characterization of hypoxia-associated molecular features to aid hypoxia-targeted therapy. *Nat Metab.* (2019) 1:431–44. doi: 10.1038/s42255-019-0045-8
10. Barger CJ, Branick C, Chee L, Karpf AR. Pan-cancer analyses reveal genomic features of FOXM1 overexpression in cancer. *Cancers.* (2019) 11:251. doi: 10.3390/cancers11020251
11. Li Y, Li L, Wang Z, Pan T, Sahni N, Jin X, et al. LncMAP: Pan-cancer atlas of long noncoding RNA-mediated transcriptional network perturbations. *Nucleic Acids Res.* (2018) 46:1113–23. doi: 10.1093/nar/gkx1311
12. Danaher P, Warren S, Lu R, Samayoa J, Sullivan A, Pekker I, et al. Pan-cancer adaptive immune resistance as defined by the Tumor Inflammation Signature (TIS): results from The Cancer Genome Atlas (TCGA). *J Immunother Cancer.* (2018) 6:63. doi: 10.1186/s40425-018-0367-1
13. Chang B, Huang T, Wei H, Shen L, Zhu D, He W, et al. The correlation and prognostic value of serum levels of soluble programmed death protein 1 (sPD-1) and soluble programmed death-ligand 1 (sPD-L1) in patients with hepatocellular carcinoma. *Cancer Immunol Immunother.* (2019) 68:353–63. doi: 10.1007/s00262-018-2271-4
14. Yoshihara K, Shahmoradgoli M, Martinez E, Vegesna R, Kim H, Torres-Garcia W, et al. Inferring tumour purity and stromal and immune cell admixture from expression data. *Nat Commun.* (2013) 4:2612. doi: 10.1038/ncomms3612
15. Siemers NO, Holloway JL, Chang H, Chasalow SD, Ross-MacDonald PB, Voliva CF, et al. Genome-wide association analysis identifies genetic correlates of immune infiltrates in solid tumors. *PLoS ONE.* (2017) 12:e0179726. doi: 10.1371/journal.pone.0179726
16. Danaher P, Warren S, Dennis L, D'Amico L, White A, Disis ML, et al. Gene expression markers of tumor infiltrating leukocytes. *J Immunother Cancer.* (2017) 5:18. doi: 10.1186/s40425-017-0215-8
17. Pan JH, Zhou H, Cooper L, Huang JL, Zhu SB, Zhao XX, et al. LAYN is a prognostic biomarker and correlated with immune infiltrates in gastric and colon cancers. *Front Immunol.* (2019) 10:6. doi: 10.3389/fimmu.2019.00006
18. Krieger T, Pearson I, Bell J, Doherty J, Robbins P. Targeted literature review on use of tumor mutational burden status and programmed cell death ligand 1 expression to predict outcomes of checkpoint inhibitor treatment. *Diagnostic Pathol.* (2020) 15:6. doi: 10.1186/s13000-020-0927-9
19. Li K, Luo H, Huang L, Luo H, Zhu X. Microsatellite instability: a review of what the oncologist should know. *Cancer Cell Int.* (2020) 20:16. doi: 10.1186/s12935-019-1091-8
20. Dan H, Zhang S, Zhou Y, Guan Q. DNA methyltransferase inhibitors: catalysts for antitumour immune responses. *OncoTargets Ther.* (2019) 12:10903–16. doi: 10.2147/OTT.S217767
21. Andre F, Mardis E, Salm M, Soria JC, Siu LL, Swanton C. Prioritizing targets for precision cancer medicine. *Ann Oncol.* (2014) 25:2295–303. doi: 10.1093/annonc/mdu478
22. Cao Z, Zhang S. An integrative and comparative study of pan-cancer transcriptomes reveals distinct cancer common and specific signatures. *Sci Rep.* (2016) 6:33398. doi: 10.1038/srep33398
23. Cava C, Bertoli G, Colaprico A, Olsen C, Bontempi G, Castiglioni I. Integration of multiple networks and pathways identifies cancer driver genes in pan-cancer analysis. *BMC Genom.* (2018) 19:25. doi: 10.1186/s12864-017-4423-x
24. Liu W, Ye H, Liu YF, Xu CQ, Zhong YX, Tian T, et al. Transcriptome-derived stromal and immune scores infer clinical outcomes of patients with cancer. *Oncol Lett.* (2018) 15:4351–7. doi: 10.3892/ol.2018.7855
25. Jia D, Li S, Li D, Xue H, Yang D, Liu Y. Mining TCGA database for genes of prognostic value in glioblastoma microenvironment. *Aging.* (2018) 10:592–605. doi: 10.18632/aging.101415
26. Yang S, Liu T, Nan H, Wang Y, Chen H, Zhang X, et al. Comprehensive analysis of prognostic immune-related genes in the tumor microenvironment of cutaneous melanoma. *J Cell Physiol.* (2020) 235:1025–35. doi: 10.1002/jcp.29018
27. Martincorena I, Campbell PJ. Somatic mutation in cancer and normal cells. *Science.* (2015) 349:1483–9. doi: 10.1126/science.aab4082
28. Sanz-Garcia E, Argiles G, Elez E, Tabernero J. BRAF mutant colorectal cancer: prognosis, treatment, and new perspectives. *Ann Oncol.* (2017) 28:2648–57. doi: 10.1093/annonc/mdx401
29. Allegra CJ, Rumble RB, Hamilton SR, Mangu PB, Roach N, Hantel A, et al. Extended RAS gene mutation testing in metastatic colorectal carcinoma to predict response to anti-epidermal growth factor receptor monoclonal antibody therapy: American society of clinical oncology provisional clinical opinion update 2015. *J Clin Oncol.* (2016) 34:179–85. doi: 10.1200/JCO.2015.63.9674
30. Wu HX, Wang ZX, Zhao Q, Chen DL, He MM, Yang LP, et al. Tumor mutational and indel burden: a systematic pan-cancer evaluation as prognostic biomarkers. *Ann Translat Med.* (2019) 7:640. doi: 10.21037/atm.2019.10.116
31. Havel JJ, Chowell D, Chan TA. The evolving landscape of biomarkers for checkpoint inhibitor immunotherapy. *Nat Rev Cancer.* (2019) 19:133–50. doi: 10.1038/s41568-019-0116-x
32. Chalmers ZR, Connelly CF, Fabrizio D, Gay L, Ali SM, Ennis R, et al. Analysis of 100,000 human cancer genomes reveals the landscape of tumor mutational burden. *Genome Med.* (2017) 9:34. doi: 10.1186/s13073-017-0424-2
33. Bonneville R, Krook MA, Kautto EA, Miya J, Wing MR, Chen HZ, et al. Landscape of microsatellite instability across 39 cancer types. *JCO Precis Oncol.* (2017) PO.17.00073. doi: 10.1200/PO.17.00073
34. Benson AB III, Venook AP, Cederquist L, Chan E, Chen YJ, Cooper HS, et al. Colon cancer, version 1.2017, NCCN clinical practice guidelines in oncology. *J Natl Comprehen Cancer Netw: JNCCN.* (2017) 15:370–98. doi: 10.6004/jnccn.2017.0036
35. Diaz LA Jr, Le DT. PD-1 blockade in tumors with mismatch-repair deficiency. *N Engl J Med.* (2015) 373:1979. doi: 10.1056/NEJMc1510353
36. Yu Y. Molecular classification and precision therapy of cancer: immune checkpoint inhibitors. *Front Med.* (2018) 12:229–35. doi: 10.1007/s11684-017-0581-0

11

Circulating Serum Exosomal Long Non-Coding RNAs FOXD2-AS1, NRIR and XLOC_009459 as Diagnostic Biomarkers for Colorectal Cancer

*Miao Yu[1,2,4], Xing-guo Song[2], Ya-jing Zhao[2], Xiao-han Dong[2], Li-min Niu[2], Zhi-jun Zhang[5], Xiao-ling Shang[2], You-yong Tang[2], Xian-rang Song[2,3] and Li Xie[2]**

[1] Shandong Provincial Third Hospital, Cheeloo College of Medicine, Shandong University, Jinan, China, [2] Department of Clinical Laboratory, Shandong Cancer Hospital and Institute, Shandong First Medical University and Shandong Academy of Medical Sciences, Jinan, China, [3] Shandong Provincial Key Laboratory of Radiation Oncology, Shandong Cancer Hospital and Institute, Shandong First Medical University and Shandong Academy of Medical Sciences, Jinan, China, [4] Department of Clinical Laboratory, Jinan Qilu Medical Inspection Co., Ltd., Jinan, China, [5] Department of Clinical Laboratory, Tai'an City Central Hospital, Tai'an, China

***Correspondence:**
Li Xie
l_xie2001@126.com

Background: Exosomes derived from cancer cells encapsulate various kinds of tumor-specific molecules and thus can interact with adjacent or distant cells to mediate information exchange. Long non-coding RNAs (lncRNAs) in exosomes have the potential as diagnostic and prognostic biomarkers in different types of cancers. The current study was aimed to identify circulating exosomal lncRNAs for the diagnosis of colorectal cancer (CRC).

Methods: Exosomes were isolated from the serum by ultracentrifugation and verified by transmission electron microscope (TEM), qNano, and immunoblotting. Exosomal lncRNAs FOXD2-AS1, NRIR, and XLOC_009459 were selected by lncRNA microarray and validated by qPCR in 203 CRC patients and 201 healthy donors. The receiver operating characteristic curve (ROC) was used to assess the diagnostic efficiency of serum exosomal lncRNAs.

Results: Exosomal FOXD2-AS1, NRIR, and XLOC_009459 (TCONS_00020073) levels were significantly upregulated in 203 CRC patients and 80 early-stage CRC patients compared to 201 healthy donors, possessing the area under the curve (AUC) of 0.728, 0.660, and 0.682 for CRC, as well as 0.743, 0.660, and 0.689 for early-stage CRC, respectively. Notably, their combination demonstrated the markedly elevated AUC of 0.736 for CRC and 0.758 for early-stage CRC, indicating their potential as diagnostic biomarkers for CRC.

Conclusions: Our data suggested that exosomal lncRNAs FOXD2-AS1, NRIR, and XLOC_009459 act as the promising biomarkers for the diagnostics of CRC and early-stage CRC.

Keywords: exosomes, lncRNA, CRC, diagnosis, biomarker

INTRODUCTION

Colorectal cancer (CRC) remains one of the most common cancers worldwide, ranking third in men and second in women overall (1, 2). Early detection of CRC provides the best chances to prevent deaths from CRC, since the 5-year survival rate is 90% after surgical removal of localized tumor when diagnosed early, but dramatically decreases to 10% once it has metastasized (2, 3). Therefore, it is extremely important to find new non-invasive biomarkers with high sensitivity and specificity to improve different aspects of CRC management, just as fluid biopsy based on blood contents including cell-free DNA, circulating tumor cells, and exosomes.

Exosomes are extracellular vesicles with a diameter of approximately 30–100 nm (4). They can be secreted into the body fluid by many cells, including tumor and normal cells (5, 6). Exosomes derived from cancer cells encapsulate various kinds of tumor-specific molecules, such as nucleic acid and proteins (7, 8). Therefore, they can reflect biological characteristics of parental cells and interact with adjacent or distant cells to mediate information exchange (9–12). Recently, a number of studies have revealed that long noncoding RNAs (lncRNAs) are enriched and more stable in exosome, playing the crucial role in tumorigenesis and tumor development.

LncRNAs with a length of more than 200 base pairs do not encode proteins due to a lack of open reading frames. They can exert regulatory functions at different gene expression levels, including chromatin modification, transcription, and post-transcription. It can weaken the inhibitory or promotion effect of microRNAs on their downstream target genes by competitive binding, and thus affect their expression and function (13). Aberration expression of lncRNAs is observed in many cancers and plays a crucial role in tumorigenesis and tumor development. More importantly, lncRNAs seem to be measurable in body fluids, including the plasma, serum, and urine, empowering their potential as the non-invasive biomarkers for diagnostics of malignancies. For example, lncRNA XLOC_009167 can serve as a novel diagnostic biomarker for distinguishing lung cancer from benign lung disease and healthy controls (14); LINC00310, upregulated in breast tumors, is detected in the serum of breast cancer patients and serves as a promising diagnostic biomarker (15).

Accumulating evidence suggests that exosomal lncRNAs have an essential role in growth, metastasis, and invasion (16, 17). For example, a recent study has shown that exosomal lnc-Sox2ot acts as a ceRNA (competing endogenous RNA) by competitively binding to the miR-200 family to regulate the expression of Sox2 in pancreatic ductal adenocarcinoma (PDAC), promoting EMT, metastasis, and stem cell-like features of PDAC cells (18); Shujun et al. investigated the stability of exosomal lncRNAs. He revealed that expression levels of exosomal lncRNAs remained unchanged upon RNase A treatment and room temperature incubation test (19). Lin et al. confirmed that exosomal lncUEGC1 might be used as sensitive and stable circulating biomarkers for early-stage gastric cancer (20). Consequently, exosomal lncRNAs have potential as novel biomarkers for cancers (21–23).

In the present study, we aimed to identify circulating exosomal lncRNAs for CRC diagnosis. Exosomal lncRNAs FOXD2-AS1, NRIR, and XLOC_009459 were selected by lncRNA microarray and validated by qPCR in 203 CRC patients and 201 healthy donors. Our data demonstrated they were significantly upregulated in CRC and early-stage CRC with the favorable diagnostic efficiency, thus acting as the promising biomarkers for the diagnostics of CRC and early-stage CRC.

MATERIALS AND METHODS

Patients and Healthy Donors

A total of 207 CRC patients, 203 healthy donors, and 20 patients with benign intestinal diseases (BIDs) admitted to Shandong Cancer Hospital and Institute between February 2018 and September 2019 were enrolled in the current study. All patients didn't receive any anti-tumor treatment before sampling, or suffer from any other endocrine, immune, or metabolic diseases. Healthy donors did not present any disease. TNM classification was estimated according to the AJCC Cancer Staging Handbook of the American Joint Committee on Cancer 2010. This study was approved by Ethics Committee of Shandong Cancer Hospital affiliated to Shandong First Medical University and Shandong Academy of Medical Sciences. Informed consent was obtained from all individuals.

LncRNA Sequence Data Sets and Analysis

Arraystar Human LncRNA Microarray V4.0 (KangCheng, Shanghai, China) was used for lncRNA microarray analysis. Total RNA was extracted from serum exosomes of 4 CRC patients and 2 healthy volunteers. RNA quantity and quality were measured by NanoDrop ND-1000 (Agilent Technology, California, USA), followed by Sample labeling using Arraystar RNA Flash Labeling Kit (Agilent Technology) as well as array hybridization using Agilent SureHyb (Agilent Technology). Agilent Gene GX v12.1 software was used to perform chip standardization and screen out differential lncRNAs.

Exosomes Isolation

Exosomes were extracted from 1 mL human serum using ultracentrifugation as previously described (24, 25). In brief, the serum was centrifuged at 10,000×g for 30 min at 4°C to remove the cellular debris, followed by ultracentrifugation (Beckman Coulter, Brea, CA, USA) at 100,000×g for 2 h at 4° C, after which exosomal pellets were re-suspended in PBS for further analysis.

Transmission Electron Microscopy (TEM)

The extracted exosomal samples were dissolved in 100 μL PBS, instantaneously centrifuged, after which 15 μL specimen was pipetted on copper wire for 1 min (copper tweezers were used to

Abbreviations: LncRNAs, Long non-coding RNAs; CRC, colorectal cancer; TEM, transmission electron microscope; qRT-PCR, Quantitative real-time polymerase chain reaction; BIDs, benign intestinal diseases; ΔCt, Comparative cycle threshold; ROC, Receiving operating characteristic; AUC, Area under the curve; CEA, Carcinoembryonic antigen.

lightly clamp the copper mesh and to prevent it from breaking). The specimen was dried with filter paper and stained using 15 μL of 2% uranyl acetate for 1 minute at room temperature. The stained samples were dried and roasted under the lamp for 10 minutes. The morphology of isolated exosomes was visualized by transmission electron microscopy (Tecnai, Oregon State, USA).

qNano

Isolated exosomes were diluted with PBS and thoroughly mixed. The exosomes' size and particle concentration were analyzed by qNano (Izon Science Ltd, Christchurch, New Zealand). Particle concentration was standardized by calibration beads of 1.0×10^{13} particles/mL. Data were analyzed using Izon Control Suite v.3.3.2.2000 (Izon Science Ltd).

Immunoblotting

Total exosomal and cellular proteins were separated using 12% SDS-PAGE and transferred onto a PVDF membrane (Millipore, Billerica, MA, USA). The membranes were blocked with 5% evaporated skimmed milk in TBST (50 mmol/L Tris-HCl, pH 7.5, 150mmol/L NaCl) containing 0.1% Tween-20 for 1 hour. Samples were then incubated overnight at 4°C with the appropriate primary antibodies, including antibodies against CD9, TSG101, and GM130 (Cell Signaling Technology, USA), followed by incubation with HRP-coupled secondary antibodies (Proteintech Group, China) for 1 hour at room temperature. Furthermore, the protein bands were visualized on photographic film using ECL blotting detection reagents (Bio-Rad, USA).

RNAs Extraction and qRT-PCR

Total RNA was extracted from exosomes using Trizol reagent (Thermo Fisher Scientific, Carlsbad, CA, USA) according to the manufacturer's protocol. The extracted RNA was reverse-transcribed into cDNA using the PrimeScript™ RT reagent Kit (Takara Bio, Kusatsu, Japan) according to the manufacturer's instructions. qRT-PCR was performed using TB-Green Premix Ex Taq II Reagent (TaKaRa Bio) on an LC480 (Roche Diagnostics, Germany) according to the manufacturer's instructions. ACTB was used as an internal control. Each sample was analyzed in duplicate. The relative expression levels of exosomal lncRNAs were normalized to ACTB using the ΔCT method (Ct^{lncRNA}-Ct^{ACTB}) as previously described (26). The primers (Biosune biotechnology, Shanghai) sequences used in this study are shown in **Table 1**.

Statistical Analysis

Graphpad prism version 6.0 (Graphpad, San Diego, CA, USA) and SPSS 22.0 software (IBM, Ehningen, Germany) were used for statistical analysis. The Shapiro-Wilk test was used to verify the distribution characteristics of the experimental data. Levene's test was used to verify the homogeneity of variance. Unpaired t-test, ANOVA analysis, and paired t-test were used for data that followed normal distribution and homogeneity of variance; numerical results were expressed in mean and interquartile range. For data with non-normal distribution, the Mann-Whitney test was used between two groups; the Wilcoxon rank-test was used between two paired groups of data; the Kruskal-Wallis test was used among multiple groups; numerical results are expressed in median and interquartile range. The area under the curve (AUC) was calculated according to the receiver operating characteristic (ROC) curves to determine the efficiency of the diagnostic. P-value < 0.05 was considered as statistically significant difference, and all tests were set as double-tailed.

TABLE 1 | Sequence Information of the primers for qRT-PCR.

lncRNA	Forward primer	Reverse primer
FOXD2-AS1	GCCCAGAACAATTGGGAGGA	AAGAGAGGGAGAGACGACCC
NRIR	CCTTGGCAACTGCTCACGAT	AGGAGGTTAGAGGTGTCTGCT
XLOC_009459	GGTGGGATACGTGCCTCTTC	AGACAGTGCTGTGTGAGACG
ACTB	TTAGTTGCGTTACACCCTTTC	GCTGTCACCTTCACCGTTC

RESULTS

Identification of the Differential Exosomal lncRNAs

First, the isolated exosomes were verified by TEM, qNano, and western blot analysis. As shown in **Figures 1A, B** they displayed special vesicles with double-layer membrane structure under transmission electron microscopy and measured 50–150 nm in diameter by qNano. The expressions of exosomal specific markers (CD9 and TSG101) were verified in the exosomes but were not detected in the cell lysis, whereas GM130 (the negative control) was only expressed in the cell lysis but not in exosomes (**Figure 1C**). In general, these results suggested that exosomes were successfully isolated by ultracentrifugation.

To explore the differential lncRNAs, exosomes isolated from 4 CRC primary patients and 2 healthy donors were subjected to microarray analysis. As show in **Figures 1D, E**, 1,131 upregulated and 808 downregulated lncRNAs with significantly different expression (fold change≥2.0 and P<0.05) were screened out. Among them, 16 lncRNAs with the most significance were selected including 7 upregulated genes (FOXD2-AS1, NRIR, XLOC_009459, MIAT, LINC001481, AP000892.4, FAM197Y9) and 9 downregulated genes (DICER1-AS1, LINC00570, MIRLET7BHG, LINC00885, HOTAIR, AC012456.3, DSCAM-AS1, MIR503HG, POC1B), then subjected to primer design and specificity verification, and 8 of them were excluded due to poor primer specificity; others were subjected to a cohort with 48 healthy people and 48 CRC patients, and 5 of them were excluded due to no difference. Finally, FOXD2-AS1 and NRIR and XLOC_009459 were identified and then subjected to a more expanded cohort for future validation (**Figure S1**).

Stability of Exosomal lncRNAs FOXD2-AS1, NRIR, and XLOC_009459

To prove the stability of exosomal lncRNAs, the isolated exosomes were incubated with RNase A and stored at room temperature. As shown in **Figures 2A–D** the expression levels of FOXD2-AS1 and NRIR and XLOC_009459 confirmed that exosomes could protect its contained lncRNAs from degradation by RNase A, as well as room temperature incubation for 0, 6, 12, 18, and 24 hours, indicating the exosomal membrane could maintain the stability of lncRNAs.

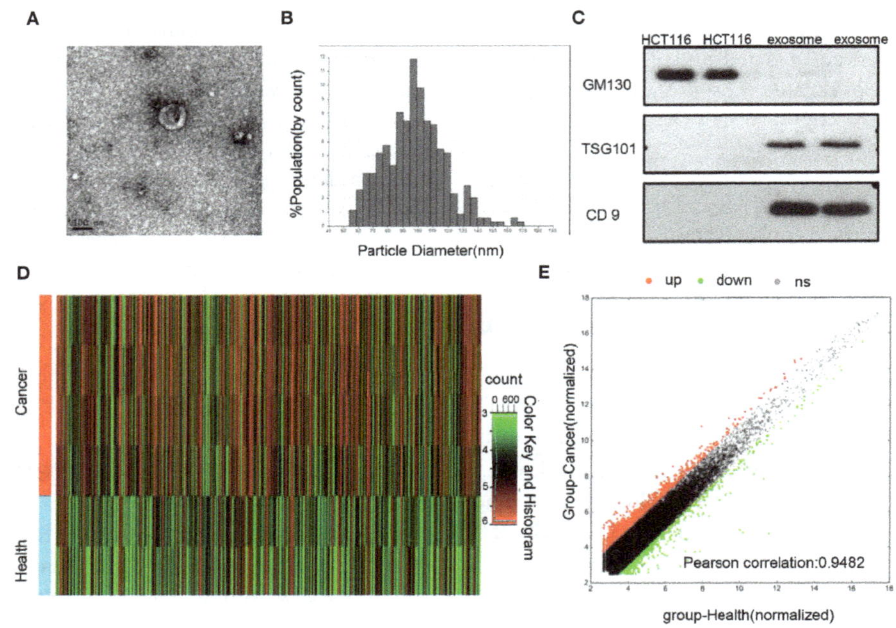

FIGURE 1 | Identification of the differential exosomal lncRNAs **(A)** TEM images showed that exosomes were oval or bowl-shaped capsules without the nucleus. **(B)** QNano results suggested that the isolated exosome enriched from serum was about 50–150 nm in diameter. **(C)** Exosome markers TSG101 and CD9 were detected in the exosomes isolated from the serum; GM130, a negative marker of the exosome, was absent in our isolated exosome. **(D)** Hierarchical clustering analysis of differentially expressed lncRNAs among CRC patients and healthy donors using lncRNAs microarray. **(E)** Differential expression analysis between CRC patients and healthy donors were expressed with hybridization signals. The red dot represents upregulated lncRNAs expression in colorectal cancer, and the green dot represents downregulated lncRNAs expression.

Exosomal lncRNAs FOXD2-AS1, NRIR, and XLOC_009459 Were Upregulated in CRC Patients

We then analyzed the expression levels of serum exosomal FOXD2-AS1, NRIR, and XLOC_009459 in 203 CRC patients, 201 healthy donors, and 20 BIDs. As shown in **Figures 3A–C**, they were significantly upregulated in CRC patients compared with those in the healthy donors or in BIDs ($P<0.0001$, respectively). Nevertheless, no significant differences of their expression were observed between healthy donors and BIDs. The correlation between these three exosomal LncRNAs expression and clinicopathological characteristics was also evaluated. As shown in **Table 2**, exosomal XLOC_009459 was obviously associated with age but not with others.

The differential expression of exosomal FOXD2-AS1, NRIR, and XLOC_009459 was also analyzed between 80 early-stage CRC patients (TNM stage I+II) and 201 healthy donors or 20 BIDs. Consistently, all of them were significantly higher in early-stage CRC patients than those in healthy donors or BIDs (**Figures 3D–F**). Moreover, exosomal FOXD2-AS1 and NRIR and XLOC_009459 expression seemed irrelated with clinicopathological characteristics of 80 early-stage CRC patients including age, gender, drinking status, history of diabetes mellitus, tumor position, histological type, lymph node metastasis status, and TNM stage as shown in **Table 3**.

Moreover, we also searched and analyzed the expression of lncRNAs FOXD2-AS1 and NRIR in cancer and paracancerous tissues in the TCGA database. As shown in **Figure S2**, FOXD2-AS1

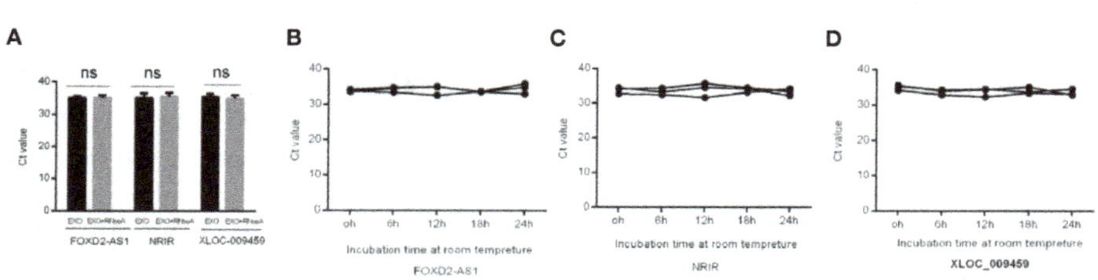

FIGURE 2 | Stability of Exosomal lncRNAs FOXD2-AS1 and NRIR and XLOC_009459. **(A)** qRT-PCR analysis of the three lncRNAs in the exosomes or exosomes deleted with Rnase A **(B–D)** The expressions of the three serum exosomal lncRNAs when incubated at room temperature (ns, not significant).

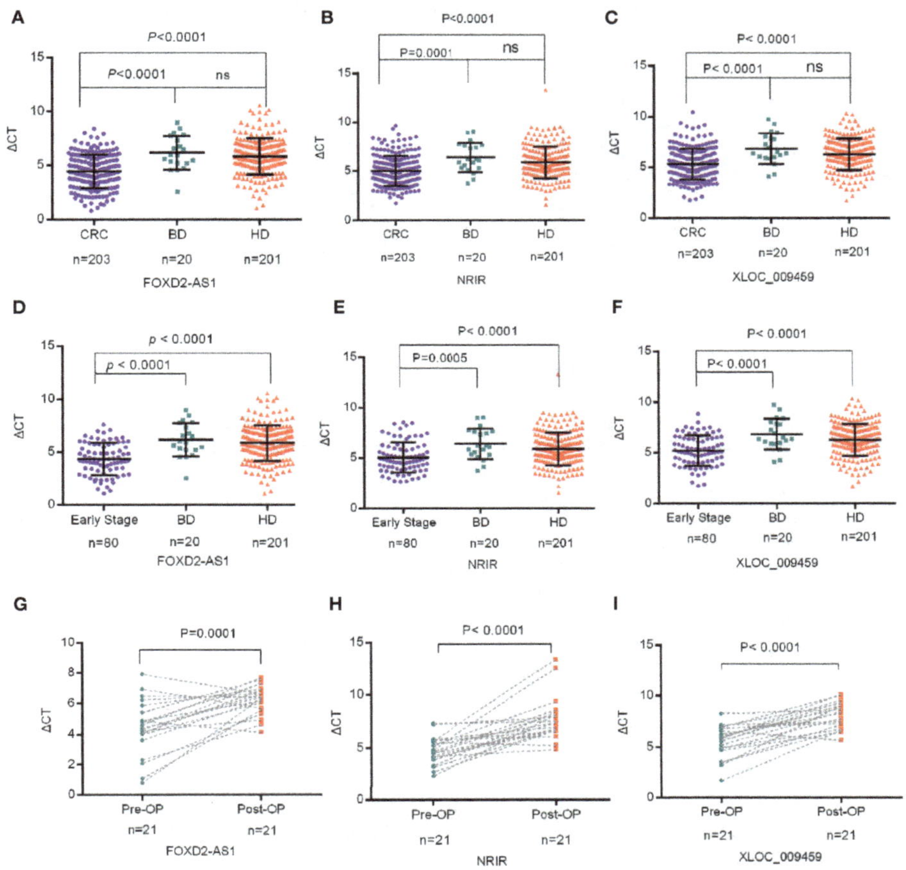

FIGURE 3 | Exosomal lncRNAs FOXD2-AS1, NRIR, and XLOC_009459 were upregulated in CRC patients **(A–F)** Mann-Whitney U test indicated that the expression levels of serum exosomal FOXD2-AS1 and NRIR and XLOC_009459 were significantly upregulated in CRC patients (n=203) and early CRC patients (n=80) as compared to healthy donors (n=201) and benign intestinal diseases (BIDs) (n=20). The expression levels of FOXD2-AS1, NRIR, and XLOC_009459 showed no difference between benign intestinal diseases (BIDs) (n=20) and healthy donors (n=201). **(G–I)** The expression levels of exosomal FOXD2-AS1 and NRIR and XLOC_009459 were significantly different in 21 preoperative (Pre-OP) patients and paired postoperative (Post-OP) patients. ns, no significance.

was upregulated in CRC tissues compared with the paracancerous, whereas NRIR had no difference in CRC and paracancerous tissues. However, the data of XLOC_009459 was absent in TCGA database since it was newly identified.

Finally, we studied the relationship between exosomal lncRNAs expression and tumor occupying *via* detecting the differences of these three lncRNAs expression pre- and post-operation of CRC. The expression levels of exosomal FOXD2-AS1 and NRIR and XLOC_009459 were significantly decreased after resection of the primary tumor (**Figures 3G–I**), suggesting that tumor burden may have an impact on the expression level of exosomal FOXD2-AS1 and NRIR and XLOC_009459.

Exosomal lncRNAs FOXD2-AS1 and NRIR and XLOC_009459 as Diagnostics Biomarker for CRC

To evaluate diagnostic performance of exosomal FOXD2-AS1 and NRIR and XLOC_009459 for CRC, a ROC curve was calculated *via* comparing the 203 CRC patients and 201 healthy donors. The AUC of exosomal FOXD2-AS1 and NRIR and XLOC_009459 were 0.728 with 72.6% sensitivity and 62.3% specificity, 0.660 with 77.1% sensitivity and 69.2% specificity, and 0.682 with 76.1% sensitivity and 67.2% specificity, respectively (**Figures 4A–C**). We also calculated diagnostics accuracy of their combination, possessing the most powerful efficiency with an AUC of up to 0.736 with 61.2% sensitivity and 75% specificity (**Figure 4D**), indicating that these three exosomal lncRNAs potentially act as the non-invasive circulating biomarkers for CRC.

ROC curves were also employed to evaluate diagnostic performance for early-stage CRC. As shown in **Figures 4E–G**, the AUC of serum exosomal FOXD2-AS1 and NRIR and XLOC_009459 were 0.743 with 70.6% sensitivity and 59.4% specificity; 0.660 with 68.7% sensitivity and 70.1% specificity; and 0.689 with 73.1% sensitivity and 65.6% specificity. Besides, the diagnostics accuracy of their combination possessed an AUC of up to 0.758 with 67.2% sensitivity and 73.8% specificity (**Figure 4H**).

TABLE 2 | Correlation between exosomal FOXD2-AS1, NRIR and XLOC_009459 expression and clinicopathologic characteristics of CRC patients.

Factor		Cases	FOXD2-AS1	P value	NRIR	P value	XLOC_009459	P value
Age(years)	<61	99	4.6288(4.3403-4.9173)	0.088	4.9500(4.8695-5.4966)	0.133	5.5448(5.2163-5.8734)	**0.024**
	≥61	104	4.2642(3.9568-4.5716)		4.6600(4.5715-5.1481)		5.0606(4.7906-5.3305)	
Gender	Male	135	4.4459(4.1947-4.6970)	0.96	4.7700(4.7349-5.2492)	0.831	5.3349(5.0655-5.6043)	0.619
	Female	68	4.4344(4.0406-4.8283)		4.7800(4.6847-5.4509)		5.2210(4.8709-5.5711)	
Drinking	No	155	4.3970(4.1393-4.6548)	0.368	4.80(4.7799-5.2776)	0.751	5.2370(4.9914-5.4826)	0.146
	Yes	48	4.5873(4.2553-4.9193)		4.7250(4.5678-5.3939)		5.6015(5.1991-6.0038)	
Diabetes	No	181	4.3878(4.1594-4.6162)	0.146	4.9654(4.7398-5.1910)	0.131	5.2598(5.0309-5.4888)	0.327
	Yes	22	4.8882(4.3778-5.3986)		5.4459(4.8079-6.0839)		5.6005(5.0253-6.1756)	
Tumor position	Rectum	128	4.3080(4.0432-4.5727)	0.102	4.7650(4.6437-5.1555)	0.256	5.1481(4.8920-5.4043)	0.072
	Colon	55	4.6708(4.3202-5.0214)		4.85(4.8429-5.5942)		5.5504(5.1757-5.9251)	
	unknown	20						
Histological	poor	23	4.4848 (3.7876-5.1819)	0.51	5.1478(4.4490-5.8466)	0.471	5.1243(4.4066-5.8421)	0.258
	moderate	97	4.3439 (4.0420-4.6458)		4.8905(4.5974-5.1836)		5.1755(4.8937-5.4572)	
	well	4	5.21 (3.4654-6.9546)		5.6725(3.8635-7.4815)		6.3725(4.8988-7.8462)	
	unknown	79						
Tumor size	≥26	65	4.2760 (3.8519-4.7001)	0.244	4.69(4.4716-5.2228)	0.465	5.3538(4.9286-5.7791)	0.969
	<26	65	4.5923 (4.2574-4.9273)		4.95(4.7235-5.45689)		5.3429(4.9798-5.7061)	
	unknown	73						
LN metastasis	No	80	4.3544(4.0289-4.6798)	0.505	4.8450(4.0289-4.6798)	0.755	5.28(4.9068-5.5602)	0.924
	Yes	119	4.5008(4.2193-4.7822)		4.5008(4.2193-4.7822)		5.11(5.0605-5.6372)	
	unknown	4						
Distant metastasis	No	144	4.3793(4.1229-4.6357)	0.452	4.7950(4.7576-5.2586)	0.767	5.1050(4.9961-5.508)	0.783
	Yes	54	4.5607(4.1876-4.9339)		4.6(4.5228-5.3709)		5.2550(4.9908-5.8062)	
	unknown	5						
TNM stage	I	20	4.38(3.535-5.225)	0.716	5.1430(4.2657-6.0203)	0.999	5.4370(4.5109-6.3631)	0.696
	II	60	4.3158(3.9571-4.6746)		4.7250(4.6704-5.3726)		5.1167(4.7763-5.4570)	
	III	60	4.4875(4.0604-4.9146)		4.9885(4.5887-5.3883)		5.4007(4.9776-5.8237)	
	IV	54	4.6385(4.2595-5.0175)		4.6450(4.6112-5.5088)		5.2850(5.0364-5.8555)	
	unknown	9						

Bold value: P < 0.05.

DISCUSSION

CRC is the third most common cancer and the third leading cause of cancer-related death worldwide, particularly in China (27). The discovery of new biomarkers for detecting CRC with high sensitivity and specificity might improve different aspects of CRC management. In the current study, our result demonstrated that exosomal FOXD2-AS1, NRIR, and XLOC_009459 were significantly upregulated in CRC and early CRC, thus revealing their potential as diagnostic biomarkers for CRC.

FOXD2-AS1, a 2527 bp lncRNA located on chromosome 1p33, is a promising candidate among all tumor-related lncRNAs (28). Related studies have shown that FOXD2-AS1 is upregulated in various malignancies, including gastric, lung, bladder, colorectal, etc., thus contributing to proliferation, migration, and invasion of tumor cells in various pathways (29),

TABLE 3 | Correlation between exosomal FOXD2-AS1 and NRIR and XLOC_009459 expression and clinicopathologic characteristics of early-stage CRC patients.

Factor		Cases	FOXD2-AS1	P value	NRIR	P value	XLOC_009459	P value
Age(years)	<60	38	4.2508(3.7927-4.7089)	0.282	4.64(4.5142-5.5532)	0.686	5.3234(4.7959-5.851)	0.477
	≥60	42	4.4052(3.9103-4.9002)		4.925(4.6236-5.513)		5.0821(4.6418-5.5225)	
Gender	Male	58	4.3184(3.9410-4.6959)	0.897	4.73(4.5894-5.3482)	0.484	5.2043(4.8116-5.5970)	0.942
	Female	22	4.3673(3.6287-5.1059)		4.98(4.5480-5.9939)		5.1768(4.4846-5.8691)	
Drinking	No	56	4.2995(3.8589-4.7400)	0.730	4.8(4.6826-5.4995)	0.741	5.1346(4.7337-5.5356)	0.576
	Yes	24	4.4075(3.9520-4.8630)		4.91(4.3522-5.5686)		5.3417(4.6924-5.9909)	
Diabetes	No	72	4.2738(3.9209-4.6266)	0.299	4.7250(4.6404-5.3435)	0.248	5.1715(4.8149-5.5282)	0.655
	Yes	8	4.8550(3.7015-6.0085)		5.3650(4.3895-6.7930)		5.4238(4.2261-6.6214)	
Tumor position	Rectum	42	4.3869(3.8502-4.9237)	0.871	4.9095(4.4319-5.3871)	0.590	5.1448(4.6107-5.6788)	0.764
	Colon	25	4.3216(3.7747-4.8685)		5.1188(4.4875-5.7501)		5.2668(4.6938-5.8398)	
	unknown	13						
Histological	poor	7	4.4984(4.0449-4.9520)	0.155	4.0943(2.9914-5.1972)	0.612	4.0943(2.9914-5.1972)	0.099
	moderate	51	4.99(1.9347-8.0453)		4.85(4.6849-5.5637)		5.2753(4.8366-5.7144)	
	well	3	4.99(1.9347-8.0453)		5.63(2.1808-9.0792)		6.23(3.5491-8.9109)	
	unknown	19						
Tumor size	<22.5	32	4.7403(4.2139-5.2668)	0.085	5.3841(4.7815-5.9867)	0.059	5.4719(4.8648-6.0789)	0.211
	≥22.5	33	4.0764(3.5116-4.6411)		4.6679(4.2022-5.1335)		4.9736(4.4453-5.5020)	
	unknown	15						

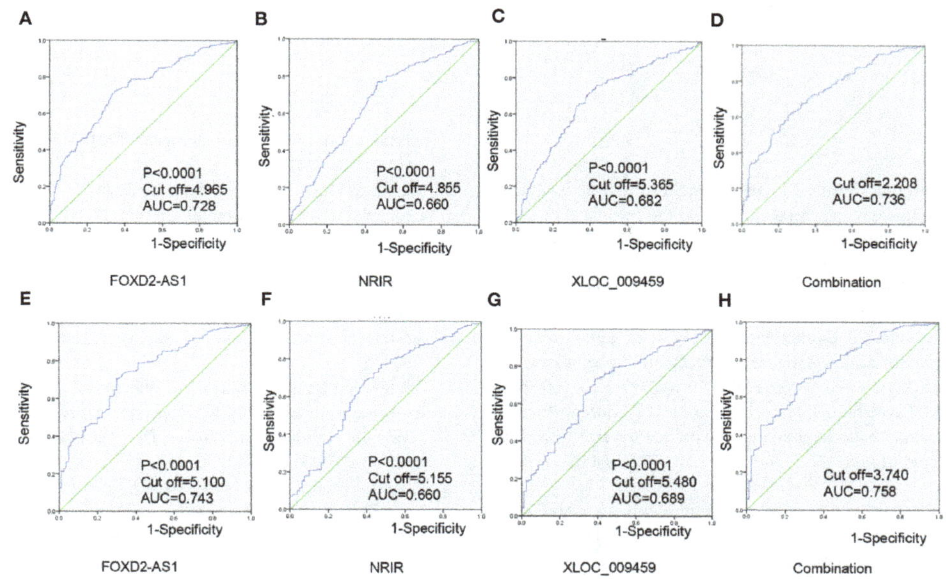

FIGURE 4 | Exosomal lncRNAs FOXD2-AS1 and NRIR and XLOC_009459 as diagnostics biomarker for CRC **(A–D)** Individual and combined diagnosis value of serum exosomal FOXD2-AS1 and NRIR and XLOC_009459 in 203 CRC patients and 201 healthy donors. **(E–H)** An individual and combined diagnosis value of exosomal FOXD2-AS1 and NRIR and XLOC_009459 in 80 early-stage CRC patients and 201 healthy donors.

such as through their interaction with microRNA-185-5p (30); NRIR, also known as lncRNA-CMPK2, is a spliced, polyadenylated nuclear transcript induced by IFN in diverse cell types from human and mouse. It was upregulated in CRC tissues and positively correlated with clinical stages (31), as well as differentially expressed in hepatocellular carcinoma (HCC) patients with or without fibrosis and effectively predicted survival in HCC patients with or without fibrosis (32); XLOC_009459, a 607 bp lncRNA located on chromosome 11q13.1, was recently identified (33); nevertheless, its role and functions in cancer still remain undefined.

In the current study, several lines of evidence validated that exosomal lncRNAs FOXD2-AS1, NRIR, and XLOC_009459 acted as diagnostic biomarkers for CRC. First, three exosomal lncRNAs were significantly upregulated in CRC patients and early-stage CRC patients compared with healthy donors. Besides, they were significantly decreased after surgery, indicating they were closely correlated with tumor occupying. Second, these three exosomal LncRNAs possessed rather high diagnostic efficiency, not only for CRC but also for early CRC. Finally, this study also confirmed that exosomes could protect lncRNAs from degradation caused by RNase A and make lncRNAs stable in serum, thus suggesting that exosomal lncRNAs FOXD2-AS1, NRIR, and XLOC_009459 could serve as non-invasive tumor markers for CRC diagnosis and early-stage CRC patients.

However, there are several limitations in the present study that should be pointed out. First, our study included 207 CRC patients, 201 healthy donors, and 20 BIDs, thus the total sample size was small and short of statistically vigorous power. In addition, the roles of FOXD2-AS1, NRIR, and XLOC_009459 in the prognosis evaluation of CRC were not analyzed as we lacked long-term clinical follow-up data. Second, we failed to analyze the combined diagnosis efficacy of the three exosomal lncRNAs with the common tumor biomarker, such as CEA, because the relative information was missing in the healthy donor cohort. In the future, we plan to investigate the mechanisms and prognostic value of these three serum exosomal lncRNAs in CRC.

In summary, we found that serum exosomal FOXD2-AS1, NRIR, and XLOC_009459 were significantly upregulated in 203 CRC patients and 80 early-stage CRC patients compared to 201 healthy donors, showing higher upregulation with favorable diagnostic efficiency. Also, the relative lncRNAs expression was significantly decreased postoperatively as compared to the baseline levels determined before surgery, thus providing evidence that exosomal FOXD2-AS1, NRIR, and XLOC_009459 could be used as biomarkers for diagnosis of patients with CRC.

ETHICS STATEMENT

This study was approved by the responsible committee for human experimentation of Shandong Cancer Hospital affiliated to Shandong First Medical University and Shandong Academy of Medical Sciences. Informed consent was obtained for all individuals.

AUTHOR CONTRIBUTIONS

LX designed experiments. MY carried out experiments. MY and X-GS wrote the manuscript and prepared figures. Y-JZ and X-HD provided the blood samples. L-MN, Z-JZ, X-LS, YT, and X-RS contributed to analysis the experimental data. All authors reviewed the manuscript. All authors contributed to the article and approved the submitted version.

REFERENCES

1. Grizzi F, Basso G, Borroni EM, Cavalleri T, Bianchi P, Stifter S, et al. Evolving notions on immune response in colorectal cancer and their implications for biomarker development. *Inflammation Res* (2018) 67(5):375–89. doi: 10.1007/s00011-017-1128-1
2. Siegel RL, Miller KD, Jemal A. Cancer statistics, 2020. *CA Cancer J Clin* (2020) 70(1):7–30. doi: 10.3322/caac.21590
3. Corbo C, Cevenini A, Salvatore F. Biomarker discovery by proteomics-based approaches for early detection and personalized medicine in colorectal cancer. *Proteomics Clin Appl* (2017) 11(5-6):1600072. doi: 10.1002/prca.201600072
4. Peinado H, Aleckovic M, Lavotshkin S, Matei I, Costa-Silva B, Moreno-Bueno G, et al. Melanoma exosomes educate bone marrow progenitor cells toward a pro-metastatic phenotype through MET. *Nat Med* (2012) 18(6):883–91. doi: 10.1038/nm.2753
5. Raposo G, Stoorvogel W. Extracellular vesicles: exosomes, microvesicles, and friends. *J Cell Biol* (2013) 200(4):373–83. doi: 10.1083/jcb.201211138
6. Conlan RS, Pisano S, Oliveira MI, Ferrari M, Mendes Pinto I, et al. Exosomes as Reconfigurable Therapeutic Systems. *Trends Mol Med* (2017) 23(7):636–50. doi: 10.1016/j.molmed.2017.05.003
7. Matsumura T, Sugimachi K, Iinuma H, Takahashi Y, Kurashige J, Sawada G, et al. Exosomal microRNA in serum is a novel biomarker of recurrence in human colorectal cancer. *Br J Cancer* (2015) 113(2):275–81. doi: 10.1038/bjc.2015.201
8. Ogata-Kawata H, Izumiya M, Kurioka D, Honma Y, Yamada Y, Furuta K, et al. Circulating exosomal microRNAs as biomarkers of colon cancer. *PloS One* (2014) 9(4):e92921. doi: 10.1371/journal.pone.0092921
9. Mashouri L, Yousefi H, Aref AR, Ahadi AM, Molaei F, Alahari SK. Exosomes: composition, biogenesis, and mechanisms in cancer metastasis and drug resistance. *Mol Cancer* (2019) 18(1):75. doi: 10.1186/s12943-019-0991-5
10. Maziveyi M, Dong S, Baranwal S, Mehrnezhad A, Rathinam R, Huckaba TM, et al. Exosomes from Nischarin-Expressing Cells Reduce Breast Cancer Cell Motility and Tumor Growth. *Cancer Res* (2019) 79(9):2152–66. doi: 10.1158/0008-5472.CAN-18-0842
11. Yang F, Liao X, Tian Y, Li G. Exosome separation using microfluidic systems: size-based, immunoaffinity-based and dynamic methodologies. *Biotechnol J* (2017) 12(4). doi: 10.1002/biot.201600699
12. Boukouris S, Mathivanan S. Exosomes in bodily fluids are a highly stable resource of disease biomarkers. *Proteomics Clin Appl* (2015) 9(3-4):358–67. doi: 10.1002/prca.201400114
13. Wang L, Cho KB, Li Y, Tao G, Xie Z, Guo B. Long Noncoding RNA (lncRNA)-Mediated Competing Endogenous RNA Networks Provide Novel Potential Biomarkers and Therapeutic Targets for Colorectal Cancer. *Int J Mol Sci* (2019) 20(22). doi: 10.3390/ijms20225758
14. Jiang N, Meng X, Mi H, Chi Y, Li S, Jin Z, et al. Circulating lncRNA XLOC_009167 serves as a diagnostic biomarker to predict lung cancer. *Clin Chim Acta* (2018) 486:26–33. doi: 10.1016/j.cca.2018.07.026
15. Li J, Peng W, Du L, Yang Q, Mo YY. The oncogenic potentials and diagnostic significance of long non-coding RNA LINC00310 in breast cancer. *J Cell Mol Med* (2018) 22(9):4486–95. doi: 10.1111/jcmm.13750
16. Chen HS, Tong HS, Zhao Y, Hong CY, Bin JP, Su L. Differential Expression Pattern of Exosome Long Non-Coding RNAs (lncRNAs) and MicroRNAs (miRNAs) in Vascular Endothelial Cells Under Heat Stroke. *Med Sci Monit* (2018) 24:7965–74. doi: 10.12659/MSM.909983
17. Wu DM, Deng SH, Liu T, Han R, Zhang T, Xu Y. TGF-beta-mediated exosomal lnc-MMP2-2 regulates migration and invasion of lung cancer cells to the vasculature by promoting MMP2 expression. *Cancer Med* (2018) 7 (10):5118–29. doi: 10.1002/cam4.1758
18. Li Z, Jiang P, Li J, Peng M, Zhao X, Zhang X, et al. Tumor-derived exosomal lnc-Sox2ot promotes EMT and stemness by acting as a ceRNA in pancreatic ductal adenocarcinoma. *Oncogene* (2018) 37(28):3822–38. doi: 10.1038/s41388-018-0237-9
19. Zhang S, Du L, Wang L, Jiang X, Zhan Y, Li J, et al. Evaluation of serum exosomal LncRNA-based biomarker panel for diagnosis and recurrence prediction of bladder cancer. *J Cell Mol Med* (2019) 23(2):1396–405. doi: 10.1111/jcmm.14042
20. Lin LY, Yang L, Zeng Q, Wang L, Chen ML, Zhao ZH, et al. Tumor-originated exosomal lncUEGC1 as a circulating biomarker for early-stage gastric cancer. *Mol Cancer* (2018) 17(1):84. doi: 10.1186/s12943-018-0834-9
21. Shah S, Wittmann S, Kilchert C, Vasiljeva L. lncRNA recruits RNAi and the exosome to dynamically regulate pho1 expression in response to phosphate levels in fission yeast. *Genes Dev* (2014) 28(3):231–44. doi: 10.1101/gad.230177.113
22. Zhang W, Cai X, Yu J, Lu X, Qian Q, Qian W. Exosome-mediated transfer of lncRNA RP11838N2.4 promotes erlotinib resistance in non-small cell lung cancer. *Int J Oncol* (2018) 53(2):527–38. doi: 10.3892/ijo.2018.4412
23. Gao T, Liu X, He B, Nie Z, Zhu C, Zhang P, et al. Exosomal lncRNA 91H is associated with poor development in colorectal cancer by modifying HNRNPK expression. *Cancer Cell Int* (2018) 18:11. doi: 10.1186/s12935-018-0506-2
24. Zhao YJ, Song X, Niu L, Tang Y, Song X, Xie L. Circulating Exosomal miR-150-5p and miR-99b-5p as Diagnostic Biomarkers for Colorectal Cancer. *Front Oncol* (2019) 9:1129. doi: 10.3389/fonc.2019.01129
25. Wang N, Song X, Liu L, Niu L, Wang X, Song X, et al. Circulating exosomes contain protein biomarkers of metastatic non-small-cell lung cancer. *Cancer Sci* (2018) 109(5):1701–9. doi: 10.1111/cas.13581
26. Sudhakar Reddy P, Dhaware MG, Srinivas Reddy D, Pradeep Reddy B, Divya K, Sharma KK, et al. Comprehensive evaluation of candidate reference genes for real-time quantitative PCR (RT-qPCR) data normalization in nutri-cereal finger millet [Eleusine Coracana (L.)]. *PloS One* (2018) 13(10):e0205668. doi: 10.1371/journal.pone.0205668
27. Arnold M, Sierra MS, Laversanne M, Soerjomataram I, Jemal A, Bray F. Global patterns and trends in colorectal cancer incidence and mortality. *Gut* (2017) 66(4):683–91. doi: 10.1136/gutjnl-2015-310912
28. Hu Q, Tai S, Wang J. Oncogenicity of lncRNA FOXD2-AS1 and its molecular mechanisms in human cancers. *Pathol Res Pract* (2019) 215(5):843–8. doi: 10.1016/j.prp.2019.01.033
29. Zhang M, Jiang X, Jiang S, Guo Z, Zhou Q, He J. LncRNA FOXD2-AS1 Regulates miR-25-3p/Sema4c Axis To Promote The Invasion And Migration Of Colorectal Cancer Cells. *Cancer Manag Res* (2019) 11:10633–9. doi: 10.2147/CMAR.S228628
30. Zhu Y, Qiao L, Zhou Y, Ma N, Wang C, Zhou J. Long non-coding RNA FOXD2-AS1 contributes to colorectal cancer proliferation through its interaction with microRNA-185-5p. *Cancer Sci* (2018) 109(7):2235–42. doi: 10.1111/cas.13632
31. Gao Q, Zhou R, Meng Y, Duan R, Wu L, Li R, et al. Long noncoding RNA CMPK2 promotes colorectal cancer progression by activating the FUBP3-c-Myc axis. *Oncogene* (2020) 39(19):3926–38. doi: 10.1038/s41388-020-1266-8
32. Ye J, Wu S, Pan S, Huang J, Ge L. Risk scoring based on expression of long noncoding RNAs can effectively predict survival in hepatocellular carcinoma patients with or without fibrosis. *Oncol Rep* (2020) 43(5):1451–66. doi: 10.3892/or.2020.7528
33. Cabili MN, Trapnell C, Goff L, Koziol M, Tazon-Vega B, Regev A, et al. Integrative annotation of human large intergenic noncoding RNAs reveals global properties and specific subclasses. *Genes Dev* (2011) 25(18):1915–27. doi: 10.1101/gad.17446611

12

Expression and Prognostic Significance of Metastasis-Associated Protein 1 in Gastrointestinal Cancer

Pengping Li[1,2†], Wei Cao[1†], Rui Ding[1,3†], Mengqiu Cheng[1], Xin Xu[1], Sihan Chen[1], Bo Chen[1], Guodong Cao[1*] and Maoming Xiong[1*]*

[1] Department of General Surgery, First Affiliated Hospital of Anhui Medical University, Hefei, China, [2] Department of General Surgery, First People's Hospital of Xiaoshan, Hangzhou, China, [3] Department of Emergency, the Lu'an Affiliated Hospital of Anhui Medical University, Lu'an, China

***Correspondence:**
Bo Chen
chenbo831116@163.com
Guodong Cao
ayfycgd@163.com
Maoming Xiong
ayfyxmm@163.com

[†]These authors have contributed equally to this work

Background: Metastasis-associated protein 1 (MTA1) has been considered as a transcriptional regulator, which is significantly related to the prognosis in various types of tumors. However, whether MTA1 is a potential prognostic index of gastrointestinal cancer (GIC) remains controversial. The current meta-analysis was performed to evaluate the role of MTA1 expression in the prediction of the clinicopathological features and survival in GIC cases. And the results of gastric cancer were verified by immunohistochemistry (IHC).

Methods: Eligible studies assessing the relationship between MTA1 and GIC by IHC were searched in the PubMed, Cochrane, Ovid, Web of Science and CNKI databases by various search strategies. The STATA 16.0 software was applied to gather data and to analyze the potential relationship between MTA1 and GIC. The expression level of MTA1 was examined in 80 GC samples by IHC assay. SPSS 20.0 was applied for statistical analysis, and the survival curves were calculated by the Kaplan-Meier method. The data of 95% CI was displayed as "[a-b]".

Results: According to the meta-analysis, the expression level of MTA1 was tightly associated with the tumor size (OR=1.82 [1.16–2.84], *P*=0.009), tumor tissue differentiation (OR=1.71 [1.24–2.37], *P*=0.001), depth of invasion (OR=3.12 [2.55–3.83], *P*<0.001), lymphatic metastasis (OR=2.99 [2.02–4.43], *P*<0.001), distant metastasis (OR=4.66 [1.13–19.24], *P*=0.034), TNM stage (OR=4.28 [2.76–6.63], *P*<0.001). In addition, MTA1 played the negative effects in 1- (RR=2.48 [1.45–4.25], *P*=0.001), 3- (RR=1.66 [1.30–2.11], *P*<0.001) and 5-year (RR=1.73 [1.37–2.20], *P*<0.001). Study in subgroup, grouped by language and tumor type, we reached similar conclusions. Further validation by IHC yielded similar conclusions. Tumor size (*P*=0.008), lymph node metastasis (*P*=0.007) and distant metastasis (*P*=0.023) significantly accompanied with higher expression of MAT1 in GC cases. Besides, the expression level of MTA1 was statistically significantly correlated with OS in GC cases (HR=2.061 [1.066–3.986], *P*=0.032), which suggested that MTA1 might be an independent prognostic marker for GC. Finally, we verified the correlation between the expression level of MTA1 and prognosis of GC in 80 GC samples.

Conclusions: MTA1 is tightly associated with metastasis-related factors and may constitute a promising prognostic factor of GIC.

Keywords: gastrointestinal cancer, metastasis-associated protein 1 (MTA1), prognosis, meta-analysis, immunohistochemistry

BACKGROUND

Gastrointestinal cancer (GIC) is a group of malignant tumors, including esophageal squamous cell carcinoma (ESCC), gastric cancer (GC) and colorectal cancer (CRC), which account for more than 27% of the total newly diagnosed tumors worldwide, and account for about 37% of tumor-related death events among all types of tumors (1, 2). ESCC is one of the most common tumors in the world, and its 5-year overall survival rate is less than 30% (3, 4). Gastric cancer (GC) is also one of the most common malignant tumors, the incidence of which at the 6th position reported by the "2012 Global Cancer Statistics" (1). In Europe, CRC is the second most common malignant tumor and the second most common cause of cancer death (5). As we all know, the occult distant metastasis of gastrointestinal tumors is one of the important reasons for tumor recurrence post-surgical resection, as well as one of the important reasons for the low quality of life and high mortality of tumor patients. Nevertheless, current assessment methods for tumor prognosis cannot meet our needs, to find out the patients who may have a high risk of tumor recurrent and disease progression. Therefore, the work of finding the new biomarkers for gastrointestinal tumor prognosis prediction is necessary.

GIC is always associated with a high risk of metastasis, with its occurrence accompanied by lymphatic metastases and distant metastases. The evaluations of lymph node, distant metastasis and tumor size are taken into consideration both in clinical and pathological diseases staging, among which the first two indexes are considered as the pivotal indicators for predicting clinical outcomes. Nevertheless, developed evidences imply that current staging criteria are weakening in differentiating the prognostic features of GIC cases. Metastasis is not a one-step process, which contains the dissemination of primary cancer cells into surrounding tissues and cycle system, and colonization at distant metastatic sites (6). These contribute to morbidity and mortality in cancer cases. So, further understanding the bimolecular procedure of metastasis and developing new prevention strategies may improve clinical treatment effect.

Various kinds of factors (miRNA, LncR NA, DNA and protein) are associated with prognosis in cancer, some of which are involved in the regulation of cancer invasion and metastasis. Metastasis-associated proteins (MTAs) playing prominent roles in that, especially MTA1. MTAs are consisting of MTA1, MTA2, and MTA3, all of which can directly bind with the nucleosome remodeling and histone deacetylation (NuRD) complex, which plays a transcriptional regulatory role *via* histone deacetylation and chromatin remodeling (7). MTA1 is firstly found at a higher level in metastatic rat breast adenocarcinoma cell lines as compared with poorly metastatic counterparts, and is considered a tumor invasion and metastasis-related gene for its over-expression is positively associated with tumor invasion and metastasis (8). Toh et al. (9) demonstrated that the higher expression level of mRNA of MTA1 was tightly associated with the depth of tumor invasion and lymphatic metastasis, especially for lymph node metastasis. Song et al. (10) pointed out that the expression level of MTA1 was an independent risk factor in cancer prognosis. Indeed, a higher expression level of MTA1 accompanies with worse disease-free survival and 5-year survival rate in cancer patients.

To our knowledge that few reports summarized the prognostic significance of MTA1 in solid tumors by meta-analysis, and the role of MTA1 in the evaluation of GIC prognosis remains inconclusive and unclear. Thus, this meta-analysis was a necessity to assess the MTA1 expression for patterns and associations with prognosis and survival in patients with GIC. Similar results were also obtained through further validation by IHC.

METHODS

Search Strategy

The method of this meta-analysis refers to an article published before (11), and the specific analysis process is as follows. Relevant articles were searched by two researchers independently in the PubMed, Cochrane, Ovid, Web of Science and CNKI databases, from inception to Oct 2020.The search strategies included ("MTA1" OR "Metastasis-associated protein 1") AND ("esophagus" OR "esophageal" OR "esophagus" OR "gastric" OR "stomach" OR "cardia" OR "colon" OR "colorectal" OR "gastrointestinal" OR "sigmoid" OR "sigmoidal" OR "rectal" OR "anal" OR "rectum" OR "digestive tract") AND ("carcinoma" OR "cancer" OR "tumor" OR "neoplasm" OR "tumor" OR "malignancy"). Full texts were reviewed to assess whether the reports met the inclusion criteria.

Inclusion and Exclusion Criteria

Studies were considered to be relevant if they met the following criteria (1): GIC diagnosis (2); immunohistochemistry (IHC) as evaluation method (3); association of MTA1 with GIC assessed (4); English and Chinese as publication language. Exclusion criteria were (1): data repetition (2); reviews (3); case reports (4); evaluation method not IHC (5); erroneous data.

Data Extraction and Quality Evaluation

According to the above selection criteria, all selected data in each study were rigorously extracted independently by two researchers (Pengping Li and Wei Cao). All disagreement has got consensus by a team discussion. The extracted data included 1st author's name, the time of publication, count of patient, clinical and pathological parameters, and survival status. Two investigators independently evaluated the quality of eligible studies by the Newcastle- Ottawa scale (12).

Gastric Cancer Sample Preparation

The whole work in this paper was approved by The No.1 Affiliated Hospital of Anhui Medical University (AMU) Review Board and the Ethics Committees of AMU. Eighty matched gastric cancer paraffin-embedded sections and three paired fresh-frozen samples of gastric cancer were collected. All samples came from the patients, whoever got gastrectomy at the No.1 Affiliated Hospital of AMU from 2013 to 2015. Each of the above gastric cancer samples got a consistent pathological diagnosis by at least two pathologists. Clinical outcome was evaluated and recorded from the surgical treatment day to that of an event (i.e. patient death or tumor recurrence) or withdrawal.

Immunohistochemistry

Simply put, as in our previous work. GC tissues were washed by pre-cooling phosphate-buffered saline (PBS) (1X) to remove the blood and any other impurities. Then these issues were fixed in formalin (10%) for 30 min and followed by being embedded in paraffin for making eligible sections. Next, these sections were de-paraffinized and hydrated by xylene and serially diluted ethanol under the protocol. The endogenous peroxidase was inactivated by being treated with H_2O_2 (3%) for 10 min. Following, a citrate solution was applied for antigen retrieval with a microwave oven. And then, these sections were incubated with the required primary antibody for an appropriate time (12h to 16h) at 4°C. Then, these sections were treated with three 5-min mild washing in PBS (1X), followed by 20-min-treatment of secondary antibody. Finally, diaminobenzidine tetrahydrochloride (DAB) was applied before counterstaining with hematoxylin.

Evaluation of Immunohistochemistry

Two independent pathologists evaluated the expression intensity of MTA1 in IHC staining sections, basing on a semiquantitative grading system (includes the proportion of stained cells and the staining intensity). Staining intensity was scored in four degrees as: 0 (negative,-), 1 (weak, +), 2 (moderate, ++), and 3 (strong, +++). The proportion of positive epithelial cells was scored in four degrees as: 0 (no staining, -), 1(<1/3 staining, +), 2 (1/3 to 2/3 staining, ++), and 3 (>2/3 staining, +++). And the histological score was performed basing on the above results. Finally, 3–4 score is defined as positive expression, while the 0–2 score is defined as a negative expression.

Statistical Analysis

In this paper, the meta-analysis was carried out with the help of STATA software (version 16.0, StataCorp LP, College Station, TX, USA). Two parameters as Crude odds ratios (ORs) and 95% confidence intervals (CIs) were applied to evaluate the strength of the correlation between the expression level of MTA1 and clinic-pathological indexes in GC cases. Both risk ratios (RRs) and 95% CIs were carried out in estimating the potential correlation between MTA1 status and overall survival (OS). The I^2 index was applied to assess statistical heterogeneity across the studies. A random-effects model was applied in case with significant heterogeneity (I^2>50% or P<0.1); otherwise, a fixed-effects model was employed. To estimate the potential publication bias, Begg's rank correlation test and Egger's weighted regression method were applied, with P<0.05 indicating statistically significant publication bias.

SPSS 16.0 (USA) was applied for any other statistical analysis. All experimental data are displayed as the mean ± SD. Chi-square (χ^2) test was also performed for the data without normal distribution. Survival curves were performed by the Kaplan–Meier method, and the statistical significance was evaluated *via* the log-rank test. Statistical significance was defined as P< 0.05.

RESULTS

Research Characteristics

The results of searching contained 356 eligible studies that can evaluate the potential relationship between the expression level of MTA1 and disease characteristics of GICs. After primary evaluation with titles, 60 reports were retained. Then, according to the description in abstracts and full texts, we found 15 studies assessed MTA1 and ESCC (10, 13–26), 6 evaluated MTA1 and GC (27–32), and 6 analyzed MTA1 and CRC (33–38), and all of which met the inclusion criteria (**Figure 1**). The included studies are described in detail in **Supplementary Table 1**. Antibodies (used for IHC) and assessment methods (MTA1 expression in IHC) in the eligible studies are displayed in **Supplementary Table 2**. MTA1 expression in 2,952 GIC patients was determined, and the sample size ranged from 44 to 436 in the 27 included reports. All of the above eligible studies applied IHC biotechnology to explore the relationship between the MTA1 of GIC. The overall positive expression rate of MTA1 in GIC samples was 57.5% (1,490/2,952), in which 51.8% (798/1,541) of ESCC samples with over-expression of MTA1, 43.8% (389/889) of GC specimens with over-expression of MTA1, and 58.0% (303/522) of CRC samples with over-expression of MTA1.

Associations of MTA1 Expression With Clinicopathological Parameters in Gastrointestinal Cancer Patients

The expression of MTA1 was statistically significantly related to some metastasis-associated clinical indexes. As displayed in **Table 1**, over-expression of MTA1 was close to tumor size (OR=1.82 [1.16–2.84], P=0.009, **Figure 2A**), tumor tissue differentiation (OR=1.71 [1.24–2.37], P=0.001, **Figure 2B**), depth of invasion (OR=3.12 [2.55–3.83], P<0.001, **Figure 2C**), lymph node metastasis (OR=2.99 [2.02–4.43], P<0.001, **Figure 2D**), distant metastasis (OR=4.66 [1.13–19.24], P=0.034, **Figure 2E**) and TNM stage (OR=4.28 [2.76–6.63], P<0.001, **Figure 2F**).

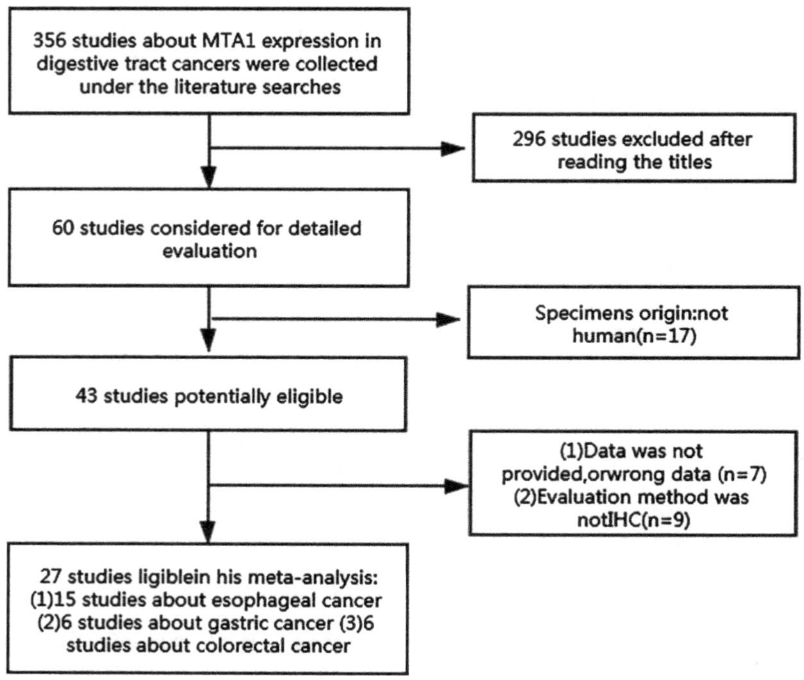

FIGURE 1 | Flow diagram of the study selection procedure.

TABLE 1 | Meta-analysis of a putative association between clinicopathological parameters and MTA1 expression in gastrointestinal cancer.

Parameters	Number of studies	Number of patients	Heterogeneity		Model	OR(95%CI)	*P* value
			I^2 (%)	*P* value			
Sex (male/female)	24	2,751	22	0.17	FE	0.91(0.77, 1.08)	0.279
Age (>60/<60)	10	960	0	0.94	FE	0.83(0.64, 1.10)	0.184
Tumor size (>5cm/<5cm)	10	1,428	70	0	RE	1.82(1.16, 2.84)	**0.009**
Differentiation (poor/well)	22	2,550	58	0	RE	1.71(1.24, 2.37)	**0.001**
Depth of invasion (T3+T4/T1+T2)	15	1,988	20	0.23	FE	3.12(2.55, 3.83)	**<0.001**
LN metastasis (positive/negative)	21	2,386	76	0	RE	2.99(2.02, 4.43)	**<0.001**
Metastasis (positive/negative)	3	564	83	< 0.01	RE	4.66(1.13, 19.24)	**0.034**
Tumor stage (III+IV/I+II)	15	1778	70	0	RE	4.28(2.76, 6.63)	**<0.001**
Vascular invasion (positive/negative)	6	983	92	0	RE	1.55(0.51, 4.78)	0.441

TNM stages are based on tumor-node-metastasis classification advocated by International Union against Cancer.
LN metastasis, lymph node metastasis; OR, odds ratio; CI, confidence interval; FE, fixed-effect model; RE, random-effect model.
Bold fonts are used for all tables when the P value is less than 0.05.

These results demonstrated that the higher expression level of MTA1 conferred the higher risk of digestive tract wall invasion, lymphatic metastasis and distant metastasis, which lead to advancing TNM stage. However, other clinicopathological variables had no associations with MTA1 expression, including gender, age, and vascular invasion.

Associations of MTA1 Over-Expression With Survival

Survival datum was extracted from Kaplan-Meier survival curves by the Engauge Digitizer software. In the current study, the expression level of MTA1 was significantly associated with OS in ESCC, GC, CRC and GIC cases (**Table 2**). GIC patients with positive expression of MTA1 all showed worse OS; indeed, MTA1 was significantly associated with 1- (RR=2.48 [1.45–4.25], *P*=0.001, **Figure 3A**), 3- (RR=1.66 [1.30–2.11], *P*<0.001, **Figure 3B**) and 5-year (RR=1.73 [1.37–2.20], *P*<0.001, **Figure 3C**) OS.

In the ESCC subgroup, MTA1 was also associated with 1- (RR=1.48 [1.11–1.95], *P*=0.007, **Figure 4A**), 3- (RR=1.60 [1.12–2.28], *P*=0.009, **Figure 4B**) and 5-year (RR=1.55 [1.14–2.11], *P*=0.006, **Figure 4C**) OS. In the GC subgroup, MTA1 was also associated with 1- (RR=7.30 [3.14–16.99], *P*<0.001, **Table 2**),

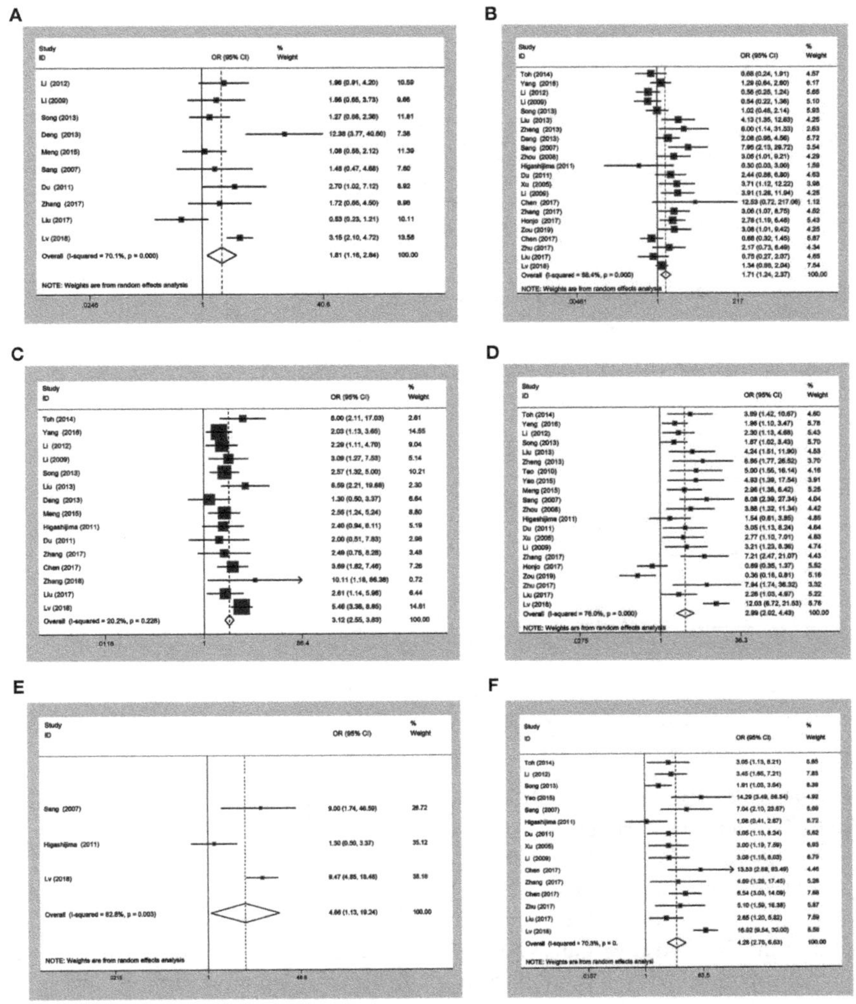

FIGURE 2 | Forest plots of odds ratios for associations of metastasis-associated protein 1 (MTA1) with tumor size **(A)** and differentiation **(B)**, depth of invasion **(C)**, lymph node metastasis **(D)**, distant metastasis **(E)** and TNM stage **(F)**.

TABLE 2 | Meta-analysis of a putative association between OS and metastasis-associated protein 1 (MTA1) expression in gastrointestinal cancer.

Tumor type	OS	Number of studies	Number of patients	Heterogeneity I^2 (%)P value	Model	RR(95%CI)	*P* value
Gastrointestinal cancers	1-year OS	13	1,766	56 0.01	RE	2.48(1.45, 4.25)	**0.001**
	3-year OS	13	1,766	70 <0.01	RE	1.66(1.30, 2.11)	**<0.001**
	5-year OS	11	1,508	83 <0.01	RE	1.73(1.37, 2.20)	**<0.001**
Esophageal cancer	1-year OS	8	983	33 0.17	FE	1.48 (1.11, 1.95)	**0.007**
	3-year OS	8	983	76<0.01	RE	1.60(1.12, 2.28)	**0.009**
	5-year OS	7	786	82<0.01	RE	1.55(1.14, 2.11)	**0.006**
Stomach cancer	1-year OS	3	608	0 0.98	FE	7.30(3.14, 16.99)	**<0.001**
	3-year OS	3	608	92<0.01	RE	3.23(1.12, 9.34)	**0.030**
	5-year OS	2	547	0 0.53	FE	2.08(1.80, 2.41)	**<0.001**
Colorectum cancer	1-year OS	2	175	0 0.88	FE	2.56(0.71, 9.25)	0.152
	3-year OS	2	175	0 0.84	FE	2.04(1.29, 3.22)	**0.002**
	5-year OS	2	175	0 0.65	FE	2.01(1.39, 2.92)	**<0.001**

OS, overall survival; RR, risk ratio; CI, confidence interval; FE, fixed-effect model; RE, random-effect model.
Bold fonts are used for all tables when the P value is less than 0.05.

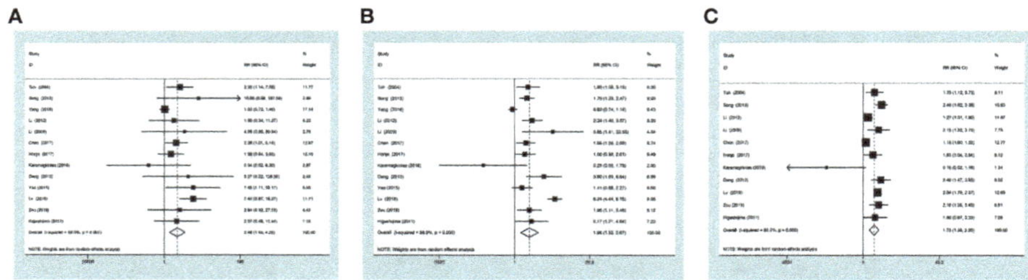

FIGURE 3 | Forest plots of risk ratios for associations of metastasis-associated protein 1 (MTA1) with 1-year overall survival (OS) **(A)**, 3-yearOS **(B)** and 5-yearOS **(C)** in the gastrointestinal cancer (GIC) patients.

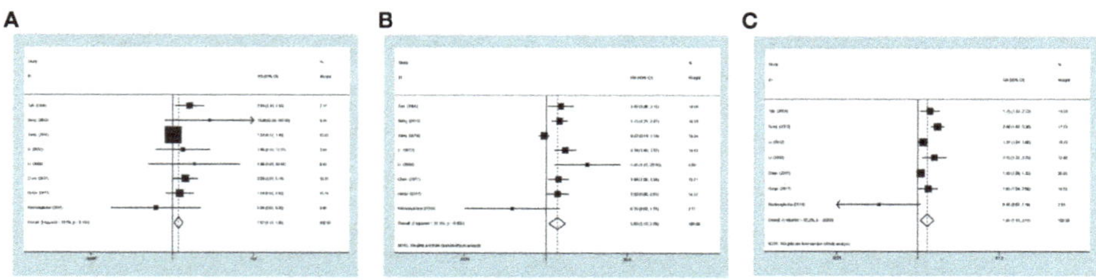

FIGURE 4 | Forest plots of risk ratios for associations of metastasis-associated protein 1 (MTA1) with 1-year overall survival (OS) **(A)**, 3-year OS **(B)**, and 5-year OS **(C)** in the esophageal squamous cell carcinoma (ESCC) subgroup patients.

3-(RR=3.23 [1.12–9.34], *P*=0.03, **Table 2**) and 5-year (RR=2.08 [1.80–2.41], *P*<0.001, **Table 2**) OS. In the CRC subgroup, MTA1 was also associated with 3- (RR=2.037 [1.29–3.22], *P*=0.002, **Table 2**) and 5-year (RR=2.01 [1.39–2.92], *P*<0.001, **Table 2**) OS.

A meta-analysis was considered to explore the potential correlation between MTA1 and the OS, and it was analyzed by the pooled HRs and their corresponded 95% CIs from each eligible study. The results of pooled HRs and 95% CIs were displayed with details in **Table 3**. Among the 27 eligible studies, the terrible prognosis of GIC cases was showed in the pooled HR estimate (HR=1.81 [1.36–2.39], *P*<0.001, **Figure 5**). A significant association was observed in univariate analysis (HR=1.82 [1.35–2.45], *P*<0.001, **Table 3**), but not in the multivariate analysis (HR=1.89 [0.98–3.64], *P*=0.059, **Table 3**). Moreover, the relationship between MTA1 and OS vary in the different cancer types subgroup. As displayed in **Table 3**, MTA1 was related to prognosis of ESCC (HR=1.56 [1.04–2.33], *P*=0.03, **Table 3**), GC (HR=2.30 [1.61–3.27], *P*<0.001, **Table 3**) and CRC patients (HR=2.11 [1.34–3.30], *P*=0.001, **Table 3**). A significant association was observed in the more than 100 patients subgroup (HR=1.83 [1.35–2.47], *P*<0.001, **Table 3**), but not in the less than 100 patients subgroup.

Subgroup Analysis

To further assess the correlation between the expression of MTA1 and prognosis of GIC patients, the selected studies were rigorously divided into subgroups based on language and tumor types. In these subgroups, MTA1 expression was meticulously assessed by different language (SCI articles and CNKI articles) groups and patients with ESCC, CRC and GC (**Supplementary Table 3**).

Among the articles in SCI and CNKI subgroups, the positive expression of MTA1 was close to clinical parameters. In the SCI articles subgroup, over-expression of MTA1 was tightly related to tumor size (OR=1.87 [1.10–3.18], *P*=0.021, **Supplementary Table 3**), depth of tumor invasion (OR=2.95 [2.36–3.68], *P*<0.001, **Supplementary Table 3**), lymphatic metastasis (OR=2.59 [1.57–4.27], *P*<0.001, **Supplementary Table 3**), and TNM stage (OR=4.14 [2.10–8.18], *P*<0.001, **Supplementary Table 3**), vascular invasion (OR=3.44 [1.84–6.42], *P*<0.001, **Supplementary Table 3**). A similar conclusion can be seen in the CNKI articles subgroup.

In the ESCC subgroup, higher expression of MTA1 conferred a higher risk of depth of invasion (OR=2.96 [2.28–3.84], *P*<0.001, **Supplementary Table 3**), increased odds of lymphatic metastasis (OR=2.79 [1.82–4.27], *P*<0.001, **Supplementary Table 3**) and advanced tumor stage (OR=3.30 [2.42–4.51], *P*<0.001, **Supplementary Table 3**). However, the expression of MTA1 showed no association with the remaining clinical parameters.

The expression of MTA1 was also close to clinical metastatic variables in patients with GC. MTA1 showed close associations with tumor tissue differentiation (OR=2.37 [1.21–4.64], *P*=0.012, **Supplementary Table 3**), depth of invasion (OR=2.84 [1.25–6.44], *P*=0.013, **Supplementary Table 3**), lymphatic metastasis (OR=5.80 [3.05–11.01], *P*<0.001, **Supplementary Table 3**), distant metastasis (OR=9.40 [5.06–17.46], *P*<0.001, **Supplementary Table 3**) and TNM stage (OR=14.69 [9.06–23.84], *P*<0.001, **Supplementary Table 3**) in GC.

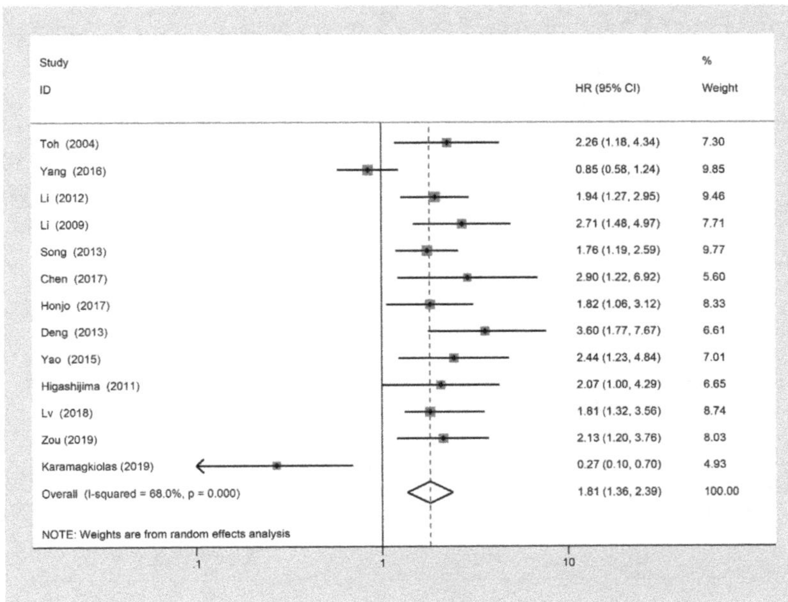

FIGURE 5 | Forest plot of the association between metastasis-associated protein 1 (MTA1) over-expression and the overall survival (OS) which analyzed by the pooled HRs and their corresponded 95% confidence intervals (CIs) from each eligible studies.

TABLE 3 | A meta-analysis of the pooled HRs to investigate the association between MTA1 expression and OS in patients with gastrointestinal cancer.

Categories	Subgroup	Studies	No of patients	HR	95% CI	I^2(%)	*P* value
Overall survival	Overall	13	1,800	1.81	(1.36, 2.39)	68	**<0.001**
Analysis of variable	Multivariate	4	834	1.89	(0.98, 3.64)	84	0.059
	Univariate	9	966	1.82	(1.35, 2.45)	54	**<0.001**
Cancer type	Esophagus	8	1,017	1.56	(1.04, 2.33)	77	**0.030**
	Stomach	3	608	2.30	(1.01, 3.27)	15	**<0.001**
	Colorectum	2	175	2.11	(1.34, 3.30)	0	**0.001**
Sample size	<100	5	364	1.64	(0.84, 3.20)	77	0.147
	>100	8	1,436	1.83	(1.35, 2.47)	64	**<0.001**

Bold fonts are used for all tables when the P value is less than 0.05.

Moreover, MTA1 expression was significantly related to metastasis-related clinical parameters in CRC patients. Indeed, high MTA1 expression always resulted in poor differentiation (OR=3.05[1.84–5.07, *P*<0.001, **Supplementary Table 3**), deep invasion (OR=2.25[1.04–4.89, *P*=0.04, **Supplementary Table 3**), increased odds of lymphatic metastasis (OR=2.51[1.57–4.02, *P*<0.001, **Supplementary Table 3**), and advanced tumor stage (OR=2.91[1.87–4.53, *P*<0.001, **Supplementary Table 3**).

Sensibility Analysis

In the main studies which held heterogeneity, sensitivity analysis was used to determine whether the conclusions were stable. After deleting any of the studies, there was no significant change in the combined indicators of the remaining studies. It can be concluded that associations of MTA1 expression with tumor size (**Figure 6A**), differentiation (**Figure 6B**), lymph node metastasis (**Figure 6C**), TNM stage (**Figure 6D**), 1- (**Figure 6E**), 3- (**Figure 6F**), 5-year (**Figure 6G**) OS, HR (**Figure 6H**) are stable.

Publication Bias

Both of the *Begg's Rank Correlation* test and *Egger's Weighted Regression* method were simultaneously applied to statistically assess publication bias. The *Begg's* (*P*=0.980) and *Egger's* (*P*=0.796) test gave out clear evidence of publication bias. These above results showed the credibility of the findings reported in this meta-analysis.

MTA1 Expression and Prognosis in Gastric Cancer Patients Through Immunohistochemistry

The potential relationships between the expression level of MTA1 and clinicopathological parameters were displayed in **Table 4**. In this paper, we found that the expression level of MTA1 was significantly higher in GC samples than it in adjacent non-tumor samples through analyzing 80 paired IHC-treated paraffin-embedded sections of GC samples. Here no statistical difference of MTA1 expression was found in some clinical parameters, such as

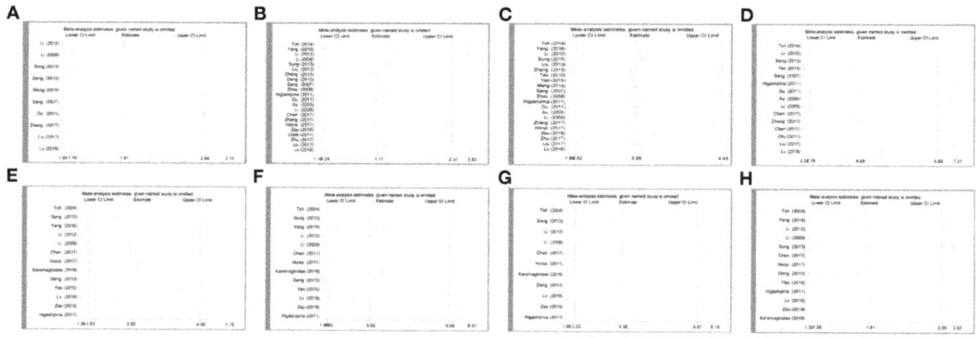

FIGURE 6 | Sensibility analysis of metastasis-associated protein 1 (MTA1) expression with tumor size **(A)**, differentiation **(B)**, lymph node metastasis **(C)**, TNM stage **(D)**, 1-year **(E)** overall survival (OS), 3-year **(F)** OS, 5-year **(G)** OS, HR **(H)** in the gastrointestinal cancer (GIC) patients.

TABLE 4 | The correlations between MTA1 protein over-expression and clinicopathological parameters in GC.

Parameters	Cases	MTA1 expression		X^2	*P* value
		High	Low		
Gender				1.528	0.216
Male	46	24	22		
Female	34	13	21		
Age (years)				0.030	0.861
≥60	62	29	33		
<60	18	8	10		
Tumor size (cm)				7.011	**0.008**
≥5	37	23	14		
<5	43	14	29		
Differentiation				0.775	0.379
Well + moderate	41	17	24		
Poor	39	20	19		
LN metastasis				7.242	**0.007**
Yes	55	31	24		
No	25	6	19		
Distant metastasis				5.144	**0.023**
Yes	17	12	5		
No	63	25	38		

GC, gastric cancer; LN metastasis, lymph node metastasis.
Bold fonts are used for all tables when the P value is less than 0.05.

gender (*P*=0.216, **Table 4**), age (*P*=0.861, **Table 4**) and tissue differentiation grade (*P*=0.379, **Table 4**). However, as **Table 4** showed, higher expression of MTA1 accompanied with larger tumor size (*P*=0.008, **Table 4**), higher rate of lymph node metastasis (*P*=0.007, **Table 4**), and higher rate of distant metastasis (*P*=0.023, **Table 4**). According to the IHC staining results, increased expression of MTA1 was accompanied by the worse tumor TNM stage (**Figure 7**). Furthermore, Kaplan-Meier analysis of 80 GC samples, grouped by the MTA1 expression, which measured by IHC, showed that higher expression of MTA1 with worse prognosis in GC patients (*P*<0.01, **Figure 7**).

Univariate and Multivariate Analysis of Overall Survival

The potential interaction, which determined GC prognosis, between the expression level of MTA1 and clinical factors was assessed with the help of univariate and multivariate analysis, respectively. In the results of univariate analysis, tumor size (HR = 1.922 [1.119–3.548], *P*= 0.019, **Table 5**), lymph node metastasis (HR = 1.927 [1.054–3.523], *P* = 0.033, **Table 5**), distant metastasis (HR = 5.572 [2.660–11.671], *P*< 0.001, **Table 5**) and MTA1 expression (HR = 2.778 [1.550–4.977], *P* = 0.001, **Table 5**) were associated with OS in GC patients. The multivariate Cox proportional hazard model showed that distance metastasis (HR = 4.077 [1.835–9.058], *P* = 0.001, **Table 5**) and MTA1 expression (HR = 2.061 [1.066–3.986], *P* = 0.032, **Table 5**) were tightly close to the OS in GC patients, which suggested that the expression of MTA1 might be an independent prognostic factor for gastric cancer.

DISCUSSION

The depth of tumor invasion (T), lymphatic metastasis (N), distant metastasis (M) stages and TNM stage are wildly considered the pivotal important prognostic index of GIC, including GC (39). Although patients undergo the complete

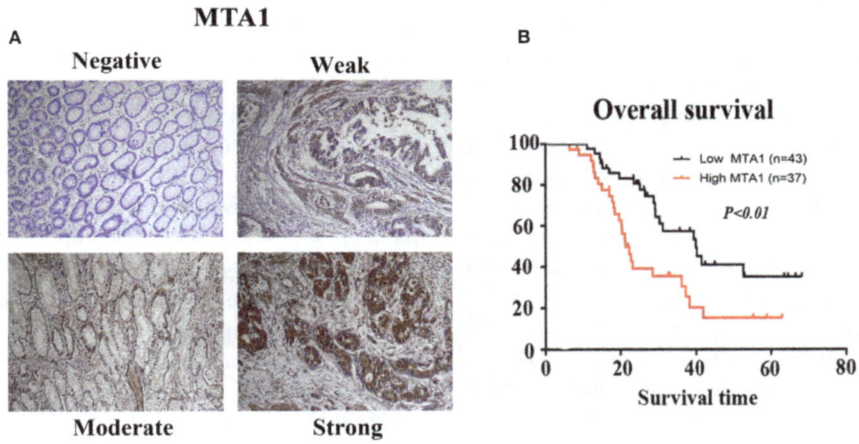

FIGURE 7 | The results of immunohistochemistry (IHC) staining confirmed the expression of metastasis-associated protein 1 (MAT1) is correlated with the TNM stage **(A)** and overall survival OS **(B)** of gastrointestinal cancer (GC) patients.

TABLE 5 | Univariate and multivariate analysis of clinicopathological variables and MTA1 expression associated with overall survival.

Parameters	Univariate analysis		Multivariate analysis	
	HR (95% CI)	*P*-value	HR (95% CI)	*P*-value
Gender	0.807(0.459–1.420)	0.458		
Age (years)	1.403(0.699–2.817)	0.341		
Tumor size (cm)	1.992(1.119–3.548)	**0.019**	1.172(0.588–2.334)	0.652
Differentiation	1.183(0.668–2.093)	0.564		
LN metastasis	1.927(1.054–3.523)	**0.033**	1.291(0.659–2.526)	0.456
Distant metastasis	5.572(2.660–11.671)	**<0.001**	4.077(1.835–9.058)	**0.001**
MTA1 expression	2.778(1.550–4.977)	**0.001**	2.061(1.066–3.986)	**0.032**

Bold fonts are used for all tables when the P value is less than 0.05.

surgical resection whose postoperative pathologic stage of GIC are same, clinical evidence demonstrates that survival is different among them, which indicates that the current tumor evaluation system misses the accurate prediction of prognosis. Prognosis of GIC patients is usually predicted by TNM staging in the clinic, although low sensitivity is sometimes encountered. To our knowledge that different digestive tract cancers show a high risk of tumor recurrence and metastasis. And even accepted with complete surgical resection or targeted therapy, lots of GIC patients still meet death events caused by local recurrence and/or distant metastasis. So, finding new predictors with good prognostic value that can timely find out the patients who may hold poor survival is urgently needed.

The members of the MTA family hold pivotal roles in both pathological and physiological processes, especially in cancer progression (such as invasion and distant metastasis), and their role as master regulators has been reported. Proteins of the MTA family are involved in metastasis regulation and comprise MTA1, MTA2, and MTA3, which are found in different isoforms such as MTA1, MTA1s, MTA2, MTA3, MTA3L, and MTA-ZG29p (40, 41). The primary founding of MTA1 was in rat metastatic tumors, and it is considered as a metastasis-associated gene (42). Since then, abnormal expression level of MTA1 has been wildly reported in various types of cancers. Nevertheless, its biomolecular roles in the carcinogenic process remain unclear until it is identified as an integral component of the NuRD complex (43). Luo et al. (44) performed a meta-analysis to further carry out the functions of MTA1 in solid tumors and pointed out that the expression level of MTA1 was tightly close to the prognosis. In addition, Ning et al. (45) demonstrated that the expression level of MTA1 is close to tumor invasion and lymph node metastasis in GIC. However, the role of MTA1 in the prediction of prognosis is not yet well understood in GIC. Indeed, several studies have implied that MTA1 without worth in the evaluation of OS in cancers, such as in esophageal squamous cell carcinoma and breast cancer (14, 46).

In this study, IHC results showed that tumor size, lymph node metastasis and distant metastasis were associated with MTA1 expression in GC patients. The K-M curve showed that GC patients with high expression of MTA1 had lower OS. The multivariate Cox proportional hazard model showed that MTA1 expression may be an independent prognostic factor in gastric cancer. In addition to gastric cancer, we also obtained similar results in GIC in meta-analysis. However, there was no statistical correlation between differentiation and MTA1 expression in the results of IHC, contrary to the conclusion reached by meta-analysis. The contradiction between the two conclusions may be caused by too few IHC samples.

From a clinical perspective, the expression level of MTA1 holds close associations with depth of invasion, lymph node metastasis, distant metastasis and TNM stage, which are separate and independent but internally linked parameters. Tumor tissues with MTA1 expression shows increased invasion, which traverses the lymphatic network under the mucosa, with a higher possibility of vascular invasion; finally, the tumor stage becomes advanced, resulting in reduced OS. Furthermore, the following molecular mechanisms are obtained for MTA1. As shown in previous studies, MTA1 may act as a transcriptional regulator; in fact, MTA1 mediates transcription repression through interacting with NuRD which facilitates the association between repressor molecules and chromatin (41, 47, 48). For example, MTA1 can directly bind to HDAC1 (49); both of them are the main components of the NuRD complex, by which it contains histone deacetylase, and acts as a pivotal role in histone deacetylation, chromatin alteration and transcriptional control. Toh et al. (13) pointed out that MTA1 is close to H4 histone deacetylase activity in ESCC. Of note, tumor suppressor genes, including p53, p21, and the Bcl-2 family of proteins, are regulated by histone acetylation (50, 51).

In a meta-analysis conducted in 2017 (52), we have preliminarily confirmed that the expression of MTA1 is statistically related to clinicopathological features and survival rates in patients with GIC. However, only 13 articles were included in previous studies, which may lead to errors in the results. On the basis of the original study, 14 new articles (27 articles in total) were included in this study, and the original results were updated. We found that the tumor size, differentiation, distant metastasis and high expression of MTA1 in GIC patients had no statistical correlation in the previous study, but the updated data showed all of them had a statistical correlation. Meantime, we found that vascular invasion and high expression of MTA1 in GIC patients had a statistical correlation in the previous study, but the updated data showed no statistical correlation between the two. Previous studies and current studies have shown that high MTA1 expression indicates low OS in patients with GIC. In this study, we also concluded that high expression of MTA1 indicates low HR in patients with GIC, which provides the latest evidence for the above conclusion.

The limitations of this meta-analysis should be noted (1): some eligible non-English and non-Chinese publications may have been excluded (2); IHC assessments of MTA1 remain discordant. Meanwhile, this study has several advantages (1): it is the first available study that applies meta-analysis to evaluate associations between MTA1 and HRs in GIC (2); we updated the data from previous studies and draw more reliable conclusions (3). we detected the expression of MTA1 in gastric cancer and verified the prognostic value of MTA1.

In conclusion, the expression level of MTA1 is obviously associated with clinical and pathological parameters and OS in GIC patients. And, it may make contributions in predicting aggressive tumor behavior and poor prognosis as an independent factor. The results of this study also imply that MTA1 is a potential target for anticancer therapy. Further research is required to unveil the mechanisms underlying MTA1 function.

AUTHOR CONTRIBUTIONS

GC and PL conceptualized the study. BC, GC, PL, and WC contributed to the methodology. GC, WC, RD, and MC were in charge of the software. PL, WC, GC, and MC conducted the formal analysis. GC, BC, and SC conducted the investigation. GC, RD, XX, WC,and MC performed the data curation. BC and MX were in charge of the project administration. GC wrote and prepared the original draft. SC, BC, MX wrote, reviewed, and edited the manuscript. GC and XX conducted the visualization. BC and MX acquired the funding. All authors contributed to the article and approved the submitted version.

REFERENCES

1. Torre LA, Bray F, Siegel RL, Ferlay J, Lortet-Tieulent J, Jemal A. Global cancer statistics, 2012. *CA Cancer J Clin* (2015) 65:87–108. doi: 10.3322/caac.21262
2. Glade MJ. Food, nutrition, and the prevention of cancer: a global perspective. American Institute for Cancer Research/World Cancer Research Fund, American Institute for Cancer Research, 1997. *Nutrition* (1999) 15:523–6. doi: 10.1016/s0899-9007(99)00021-0
3. Sano A, Kato H, Sakurai S, Sakai M, Tanaka N, Inose T, et al. CD24 expression is a novel prognostic factor in esophageal squamous cell carcinoma. *Ann Surg Oncol* (2009) 16:506–14. doi: 10.1245/s10434-008-0252-0
4. Ren Y, Cao B, Law S, Xie Y, Lee PY, Cheung L, et al. Hepatocyte growth factor promotes cancer cell migration and angiogenic factors expression: a prognostic marker of human esophageal squamous cell carcinomas. *Clin Cancer Res* (2005) 11:6190–7. doi: 10.1158/1078-0432.CCR-04-2553
5. Siegel R, Ma J, Zou Z, Jemal A. Cancer statistics, 2014. *CA Cancer J Clin* (2014) 64:9–29. doi: 10.3322/caac.21208
6. Nguyen DX, Bos PD, Massagué J. Metastasis: from dissemination to organ-specific colonization. *Nat Rev Cancer* (2009) 9:274–84. doi: 10.1038/nrc2622
7. Toh Y, Nicolson GL. The role of the MTA family and their encoded proteins in human cancers: molecular functions and clinical implications. *Clin Exp Metastasis* (2009) 26:215–27. doi: 10.1007/s10585-008-9233-8
8. Toh Y, Pencil SD, Nicolson GL. Analysis of the complete sequence of the novel metastasis-associated candidate gene, mta1, differentially expressed in mammary adenocarcinoma and breast cancer cell lines. *Gene* (1995) 159:97–104. doi: 10.1016/0378-1119(94)00410-T
9. Toh Y, Kuwano H, Mori M, Nicolson GL, Sugimachi K. Over-expression of metastasis-associated MTA1 mRNA in invasive oesophageal carcinomas. *Br J Cancer* (1999) 79:1723–6. doi: 10.1038/sj.bjc.6690274
10. Song L, Wang Z, Liu X. MTA1: A Prognosis Indicator of Postoperative Patients with Esophageal Carcinoma. *Thorac Cardiovasc Surg* (2013) 61:479–85. doi: 10.1055/s-0032-1304545
11. Cao GD, Chen K, Xiong MM, Chen B. HER3, but Not HER4, Plays an Essential Role in the Clinicopathology and Prognosis of Gastric Cancer: A Meta-Analysis. *PloS One* (2016) 11(8):e0161219. doi: 10.1371/journal.pone.0161219
12. Stang A. Critical evaluation of the Newcastle–Ottawa scale for the assessment of the quality of nonrandomized studies in meta-analysis. *Eur J Epidemiol* (2010) 25:603–5. doi: 10.1007/s10654-010-9491-z
13. Toh Y, Ohga T, Endo K, Adachi E, Kusumoto H, Haraguchi M, et al. Expression of the metastasis-associated MTA1 protein and its relationship to deacetylation of the histone H4 in esophageal squamous cell carcinomas. *Int J Cancer* (2004) 110:362 7. doi: 10.1002/ijc.20154

14. Yang H, Xu L, Qian H, Niu X, Zhao D, Zhao Z, et al. Correlation between insulin–like growth factor binding protein 3 and metastasis–associated gene 1 protein in esophageal squamous cell carcinoma. *Mol Med Rep* (2016) 13:4143–50. doi: 10.3892/mmr.2016.5046
15. Li SH, Tian H, Yue WM, Li L, Gao C, Li WJ, et al. Metastasis-associated Protein 1 Nuclear Expression is Closely Associated with Tumor Progression and Angiogenesis in Patients with Esophageal Squamous Cell Cancer. *World J Surg* (2012) 36:623–31. doi: 10.1007/s00268-011-1421-z
16. Li SH, Wang Z, Liu XY. Metastasis-Associated Protein 1 (MTA1) Over-expression is Closely Associated with Shorter Disease-Free Interval After Complete Resection of Histologically Node-Negative Esophageal Cancer. *World J Surg* (2009) 33:1876–81. doi: 10.1007/s00268-009-0119-y
17. Liu XC, Zhou B. Expression and significance of MTA1 and FLIP in Esophageal Squamous Cell Cancer. *Shanxi Med J* (2013) 42:1299–301.
18. Zheng WF, Li YX, Chen KS, Wen HT. Expression of USP22, MTA1 and Ki-67 in esophageal squamous cell carcinoma. *World Chin J Gastroenterol* (2013) 21:2915–21. doi: 10.11569/wcjd.v21.i28.2915
19. Tao SB, Zhang L, Zhang YH, Gao DL, Zhao AH, Mao XY, et al. Expression and clinical pathological significance of MTA1, MMP-9 and MVD in human esophageal squamous cell cancer. *J Henan Univ* (2010) 29:29–33. doi: 10.15991/j.cnki.41-1361/r.2010.01.026
20. Honjo H, Toh Y, Sohda M, Suzuki S, Kaira K, Kanai Y, et al. Clinical Significance and Phenotype of MTA1 Expression in Esophageal Squamous Cell Carcinoma. *Anticancer Res* (2017) 37:4147–55. doi: 10.21873/anticanres.11802
21. Zhang Q, Wan T. Relationship of MTA expression with clinical features and prognosis in esophageal carcinoma. *J Clin Exp Med* (2017) 16:873–5.
22. Karamagkiolas S, Giotakis I, Kyrodimos E, Giotakis EI, Kataki A, Karagianni F, et al. Expression of vimentin (VIM) and metastasis-associated 1 (MTA1) protein in laryngeal squamous cell carcinoma are associated with prognostic outcome of patients. *Am J Otolaryng* (2019) 40(4):487–93. doi: 10.1016/j.amjoto.2019.04.002
23. Liu J, Xia J, Zhang Y, Fu M, Gong S, Guo Y. Associations between the expression of MTA1 and VEGF-C in esophageal squamous cell carcinoma with lymph angiogenesis and lymph node metastasis. *Oncol Lett* (2017) 14 (3):3275–81. doi: 10.3892/ol.2017.6530
24. Chen WY, GY L, Xin C, Fu YQ, Fu CZ. The Expression of MTA1 and SOX2 in Esophageal Cancer Tissues and the Relationship betweenMTA1, SOX2 and Prognosis.Chinese. *J Modern Operative Surg* (2017) 21(04):251–6. doi: 10.16260/j.cnki.1009-2188.2017.04.003
25. Zhang DS. MTA1 protein, AEG-1 expression and TNM staging in esophageal cancer patientsRelationship and clinical significance. *Henan Med Res* (2018) 27(06):1019–20.
26. Zhu GXP, Meng QJ, Wang BS. Relationship between MTA1 protein expression in esophageal cancer tissue with clinicopathological features and 3-year survival rate. *Chongqing Med* (2017) 46(31):4378–80.
27. Deng X, Du L, Wang C, Yang Y, Li J, Liu H, et al. Close Association of Metastasis-Associated Protein 1 Over-expression with Increased Angiogenesis and Poor Survival in Patients with Histologically Node-Negative Gastric Cancer. *World J Surg* (2013) 37:792–8. doi: 10.1007/s00268-012-1898-0
28. Yao Y, Feng S, Xiao M, Li Y, Yang L, Gong J. MTA1 promotes proliferation and invasion in human gastric cancer cells. *Onco Targets Ther* (2015) 8:1785–94. doi: 10.2147/OTT.S85383
29. Meng QB, Kang WM, Yu JC, Liu YQ, Ma ZQ, Zhou L, et al. Over-expression of Eukaryotic Translation Initiation Factor 5A2 (EIF5A2) Correlates with Cell Aggressiveness and Poor Survival in Gastric Cancer. *PloS One* (2015) 10: e0119229. doi: 10.1371/journal.pone.0119229
30. Sang HQ, Wang Q. Expression of metastasis associated gene 1, PTEN and E-cadherin in gastric carcinoma. *World Chin J Gastroenterol* (2007) 15:1096–102.
31. Zhou F. Expression and significance of MTA1 in gastric cancer. *Shandong Med J* (2008) 48:72–3.
32. Lv ZY, Zhao ZS, Ye ZY, Wang YY, Wang HJ, Yang Q. Metastasis-associated protein 1 (MTA1) in gastric cancer tissues is positively associated with poorer prognosis. *Pathol Res Pract* (2018) 214:536–41. doi: 10.1016/j.prp.2018.02.011
33. Higashijima J, Kurita N, Miyatani T, Yoshikawa K, Morimoto S, Nishioka M, et al. Expression of histone deacetylase 1 and metastasis-associated protein 1 as prognostic factors in colon cancer. *Oncol Rep* (2011) 26:343–8. doi: 10.3892/or.2011.1312
34. Du B, Yang ZY, Zhong XY, Fang M, Yan YR, Qi GL, et al. Metastasis-associated protein 1 induces VEGF-C and facilitates lymph angiogenesis in colorectal cancer. *World J Gastroenterol* (2011) 17:1219–26. doi: 10.3748/wjg.v17.i9.1219
35. Xu H, Zhou XL, Du B. Expression and significance of MTA1 in gastric cancer. *J Pract Med* (2005) 21:2148–9.
36. Li Y, Zhang T, Gao H, Wei D, Cheng P. Correlation between the expression of MTA1, VEGF-C and lymph node metastasis in colon cancer. *Modern Med J* (2009) 37:401–4.
37. Chen XL, Wu YJ, Lu Z, Zhao HM, Han BJ. Expression and significance of MTA1 and RECK in the carcinogenesis of colon adenoma. *J Clin Exp Pathol* (2017) 33:432–4. doi: 10.11569/wcjd.v24.i33.4514
38. Zou HM, Zhang LL, Cai YT, Wang BJ, Yu C, Zhu LM. Expression of metastasis-associated gene 1 in colorectal carcinoma tissues and correlation with clinicopathologic characteristics and prognosis. *Modern Oncol* (2019) 27 (21):3839–42.
39. Yamashita K, Sakuramoto S, Kikuchi S, Katada N, Kobayashi N, Watanabe M. Validation of staging systems for gastric cancer. *Gastric Cancer* (2008) 11:111–8. doi: 10.1007/s10120-008-0466-7
40. Fujita N, Jaye DL, Kajita M, Geigerman C, Moreno CS, Wade PA. MTA3, a Mi-2/NuRD complex subunit, regulates an invasive growth pathway in breast cancer. *Cell* (2003) 113:207–19. doi: 10.1016/S0092-8674(03)00234-4
41. Kumar R, Wang RA, Bagheri-Yarmand R. Emerging roles of MTA family members in human cancers. *Semin Oncol* (2003) 30:30–7. doi: 10.1053/j.seminoncol.2003.08.005
42. Toh Y, Pencil SD, Nicolson GL. A novel candidate metastasis-associated gene, mta1, differentially expressed in highly metastatic mammary adenocarcinoma cell lines. cDNA cloning, expression, and protein analyses. *J Biol Chem* (1994) 269:22958–63.
43. Xue Y, Wong J, Moreno GT, Young MK, Côté J, Wang W. NURD, a novel complex with both ATP-dependent chromatin-remodeling and histone deacetylase activities. *Mol Cell* (1998) 2:851–61. doi: 10.1016/S1097-2765 (00)80299-3
44. Luo H, Li H, Yao N, Hu L, He T. Metastasis-associated protein 1 as a new prognostic marker for solid tumors: a meta-analysis of cohort studies. *Tumour Biol* (2014) 35:5823–32. doi: 10.1007/s13277-014-1772-9
45. Ning Z, Gan J, Chen C, Zhang D, Zhang H. Molecular functions and significance of the MTA family in hormone-independent cancer. *Cancer Metastasis Rev* (2014) 33:901–19. doi: 10.1007/s10555-014-9517-1
46. Jang KS, Paik SS, Chung H, Oh YH, Kong G. MTA1 over-expression correlates significantly with tumor grade and angiogenesis in human breast cancers. *Cancer Sci* (2006) 97:374–9. doi: 10.1111/j.1349-7006.2006.00186.x
47. Nicolson GL, Nawa A, Toh Y, Taniguchi S, Nishimori K, Moustafa A. Tumor metastasis-associated human MTA1 gene and its MTA1 protein product: role in epithelial cancer cell invasion, proliferation and nuclear regulation. *Clin Exp Metastasis* (2003) 20:19–24. doi: 10.1023/a:1022534217769
48. Mazumdar A, Wang RA, Mishra SK, Adam L, Bagheri-Yarmand R, Mandal M, et al. Transcriptional repression of oestrogen receptor by metastasis-associated protein 1 corepressor. *Nat Cell Biol* (2001) 3:30–7. doi: 10.1038/35050532
49. Toh Y, Kuninaka S, Endo K, Oshiro T, Ikeda Y, Nakashima H, et al. Molecular analysis of a candidate metastasis-associated gene, MTA1: possible interaction with histone deacetylase 1. *J Exp Clin Cancer Res* (2000) 19:105–11.
50. Roy S, Packman K, Jeffrey R, Tenniswood M. Histone deacetylase inhibitors differentially stabilize acetylated p53 and induce cell cycle arrest or apoptosis in prostate cancer cells. *Cell Death Differ* (2005) 12:482–91. doi: 10.1038/sj.cdd.4401581
51. Mahoney MG, Simpson A, Jost M, Noé M, Kari C, Pepe D, et al. Metastasis-associated protein (MTA)1 enhances migration, invasion, and anchorage-independent survival of immortalized human keratinocytes. *Oncogene* (2002) 21:2161–70. doi: 10.1038/sj.onc.1205277
52. Cao GD, Chen B, Xiong MM. Role of metastasis-associated protein 1 in prognosis of patients with digestive tract cancers: A meta-analysis. *PloS One* (2017) 12(6):e0176431. doi: 10.1371/journal.pone.0176431

13

The Suppressing Effects of Dkk3 Expression on Aggressiveness and Tumorigenesis of Colorectal Cancer

Shuang Zhao [1], Chang-lai Hao [2], En-hong Zhao [3], Hua-mao Jiang [4] and Hua-chuan Zheng [1]*

[1] Department of Oncology and Experimental Center, The Affiliated Hospital of Chengde Medical University, Chengde, China, [2] Department of Hematology, The Affiliated Hospital of Chengde Medical University, Chengde, China, [3] Department of Surgery, The Affiliated Hospital of Chengde Medical University, Chengde, China, [4] Department of Urology, The First Affiliated Hospital of Jinzhou Medical University, Jinzhou, China

***Correspondence:**
Hua-chuan Zheng
zheng_huachuan@hotmail.com

Dkk3 has been discovered during comparison of immortalized and parental cells. Its expression has been shown to reduce colony formation and induce apoptosis of cancer cells, acting as a tumor suppressor. Herein, we demonstrate that Dkk3 overexpression or protein treatment may inhibit colorectal cancer cell proliferation, migration, and invasion and that they may promote apoptosis and G_2 phase arrest with hypoexpression of Bcl-2, cdc25B, cdc25c, N-cadherin, slug, and twist and hyperexpression of Bax and E-cadherin. This effect is consistent with that of recombinant Dkk3 exposure and blocked with anti-Dkk3 antibody. Dkk3 deletion in intestinal cells was not associated with the emergence of epithelial lesions; however, adenoma emerged after sodium desoxycholate treatment. At both mRNA and protein levels, Dkk3 expression was higher in normal than in cancer tissues ($p<0.05$). *Dkk3* mRNA expression was negatively associated with its promoter methylation, growth pattern, differentiation, and favorable prognosis in the patients with colorectal cancer ($p<0.05$). *Dkk3*-related signal pathways in colorectal cancer included those of cellular adhesion and migration, melanogenesis, chemokine, Hedgehog, JAK-STAT, TOLL-like receptor, TGF-β, MAPK, and calcium signaling ($p<0.05$). These findings indicate that Dkk3 expression levels can help assess cancer aggressiveness and patient prognosis. It might also suppress aggressive phenotypes and tumorigenesis as a molecular target in gene therapy.

Keywords: Dkk3, colorectal cancer, tumorigenesis, aggressive phenotypes, pathological behaviors, prognosis

INTRODUCTION

Dkk3 was discovered by representational difference PCR analysis; its mRNA expression has been shown as downregulated in immortalized cells compared to control (1). A homology alignment indicates that *Dkk3* is identical with reduced expression in immortalized cells (*REIC*). Dkk3 cDNA encodes a secreted glycoprotein with five potential N-glycosylation sites, an N-terminal signal peptide, two cysteine-rich domains, and two coiled-coil domains (2). TNF-α downregulated Dkk3 expression in normal skin keratinocytes and mouse skin and hair culture models, which was abrogated by anti-TNF-α antibody (3). In prostate cancer cells, Dkk3 expression inhibited cell proliferation and tumor growth, induced apoptosis, and sensitized cells to doxorubicin by c-JNK activation, mitochondrial redistribution of Bax, or by triggering Bcl-2 hypoexpression (4).

Previous studies have reported that Dkk3 induced JNK activation *via* endoplasmic reticulum (ER) stress and mitochondrial pathways (4–6). Takata et al. (7) demonstrated that DKK3 initiated apoptosis *via* mitochondrial and Fas death receptor pathways in mucinous ovarian carcinoma cells. Exogenous Dkk3 inhibited Wnt/β-catenin signaling and cell proliferation in kidney cancer cells (8), and the cysteine-rich core domain of Dkk3 was required for dendritic cell–like differentiation from monocytes and for tumor regression, where it activated phosphorylation of GSK-3β and stat (9). Meanwhile, adeno-Dkk3 virus has been shown to inhibit tumor growth and lymph node metastasis and prolong survival in nude mice with prostate cancer by inducing apoptosis, suppressing cell invasion and migration, and decreasing MMP-2 activity (10).

Dkk3 protein is expressed in the brain, heart, kidney, mammary gland, liver, pancreas, and lymph node (11). Its expression has been reported as downregulated in cancer cells, including in hepatocellular carcinoma, renal clear cell carcinoma, cervical squamous carcinoma, non-small cell lung cancer, and seminoma (12–17). In gastric cancer, Dkk3 overexpression or Dkk3 treatment decreased the karyoplasmic ratio, cell proliferation, migration, invasion, and lamellipodia formation and increased the likelihood of G_1 phase arrest and apoptosis, which were blocked by anti-Dkk3 antibody. Dkk3 knockdown caused the opposite effect in immortalized gastric epithelial cells. Immunohistochemically, the level of Dkk3 expression was inversely correlated with tumor size, lymph node involvement, cell dedifferentiation, and unfavorable prognosis in gastric cancer. Moreover, serum Dkk3 concentration has been reported as remarkably higher in age-matched controls than in gastric cancer patients, where it was inversely associated with tumor size (18).

Colorectal cancer is a type of cancer associated with high risk of mortality (19, 20). Although colorectal adenoma pathologically and genetically precedes adenocarcinoma, its molecular mechanisms remain elusive. Previously, we have shown that Dkk3 expression was remarkably downregulated in colorectal non-neoplastic mucosa, adenoma to adenocarcinoma, and negatively correlated with invasion depth, TNM stage, and colorectal cancer cell dedifferentiation rate (21). Herein, we observed *in vitro* and *in vivo* the effects of Dkk3 expression and recombinant Dkk3 treatment on aggressive phenotypes of colorectal cancer cells, aiming to clarify the molecular mechanisms involved. Additionally, we established a mouse model of conditional *Dkk3* knockout in intestinal epithelial cells, using villin promoter to initiate cre recombination. Finally, pathological and bioinformatics analyses were performed to explore clinicopathological or prognostic significances of Dkk3 expression.

MATERIALS AND METHODS

Cell Culture

Colorectal cancer cell lines (HCT-15 and HCT-116) were isolated from the same colorectal cancer patients with Duke's C and purchased from the Cell Bank of Chinese Academy of Sciences, Shanghai, China. They were cultured in RPMI 1640 medium containing FBS, penicillin, and streptomycin in 5% CO_2 at 37°C. Both kinds of cells were transfected with pCDNA3.1-*Dkk3* and pcDNA3.1 at 70% confluence 24 h after seeding on dishes according to the manufacturer's instructions (QIAGEN, USA). Both HCT-15 and HCT-116 were treated with recombinant Dkk3 (R&D Systems, 1118-DK, USA) in RPMI 1640 at a dose of 50, 100, 150, or 200 ng/mL or their Dkk3 transfectants were exposed to anti-Dkk3 antibody (R&D Systems) at a dose of 30 or 60 ng/mL. Nontreated HCT-15 and HCT-116 cells were considered as control and pcDNA3.1 transfectant as mock.

Immunofluorescence

Cells were attached to glass coverslips and fixed with 4% neutral formaldehyde and permeabilized with 0.2% Triton X-100. After washing with PBS, cells were incubated overnight at 4°C with goat anti-Dkk3 antibody (R&D system) and subsequently with antigoat IgG-FITC antibody (Santa Cruz) at room temperature and then stained with DAPI for nuclear labeling. Finally, we mounted coverslips with SlowFade® Gold antifade reagent (Invitrogen) and observed them using a laser confocal microscope.

ELISA Assay

Human Dkk-3 DuoSet ELISA Kit (R&D Systems) was employed to detect the Dkk3 level of cell culture supernatant and patient serum.

Proliferation Assay

We used cell counting kit-8 (CCK-8) to determine cell proliferation. In brief, 2.0×10^3 cells/well were cultured on a 96-well plate. After adhering to the plate, 10 μL of CCK-8 solution was added to each well at a different time point; absorbance was measured at 450 nm after 3 h incubation.

Cell Cycle Analysis

We trypsinized, collected, and fixed the cell line using ethanol for 2 h. After RNase treatment for 1 h, cells were pelleted and stained by propidium iodide (PI) for 30 min. Finally, flow cytometry was used to examine the PI signal.

Apoptosis Assay

FITC-labeled annexin V staining (BD Pharmingen) was employed to indicate phosphatidylserine externalization of early apoptosis. In brief, 1×10^6 cells were collected, washed with PBS, and pelleted. FITC-labeled annexin V (5 μL, final concentration: 1 ug/mL) and PI (5 μL, final concentration: 50 μg/mL) were added to cell suspension, mixed, incubated for 15 min, and examined by flow cytometry.

Mitochondiral Membrane Potential

We determined the mitochondrial membrane potential using JC-1 Mitochondrial Membrane Potential Assay Kit (Kagen, China). In brief, cells were stained by JC-1 (100 uL/mL) for 30 min and harvested for flow cytometry with JC-1 monomer (green, low concentration in cytosol) as FL1 channel and JC-1 aggregates (red, high concentration in mitochondria) as FL2 channel. In addition, the harvested cells were prepared as slides and observed under a fluorescence microscope.

Transwell Chamber Assay

To assess the extent of cell invasion, we cultured 2.0×10^5 cells in FBS-free medium in the matrigel-coated insert on the chamber top and added 10% FBS-containing medium to the chamber bottom as a chemoattractant. After 24 h incubation, the upper part of the insert was scrubbed, and the lower part was fixed in methanol, followed by Giemsa dye. To measure capacity for cell migration, we repeated this procedure without the membrane control insert.

Animals

We housed three mice per plastic cage, which included paper chips, standard rodent food, and water provided in pathogen-free and temperature-controlled conditions with a 12-h light/dark illumination cycle. All experiments involving mice were approved by the Committee on Animal Experimentation of the Affiliated Hospital of Chengde Medical University. We performed cre- mediated deletion of floxed alleles in a germline by mating *Dkk3* conditional mutants (kindly presented by Prof. Kumon) with villin (intestine-specific)-cre mice (Jax Lab). At least 5 mice were sacrificed at 9 months, and their intestines were histologically analyzed. To chemically induce colorectal tumor, we orally administrated sodium desoxycholate in 0.09% agarose suspension to male villin-cre/*Dkk3* (*n*=5, 16–18 g, age 8 weeks) and wild-type (WT, *n*=5, 16–18 g, age 8 weeks) mice for 6 weeks. After 40 weeks, these mice were sacrificed, and their colorectal tissues were subjected to pathological examination, RNA, and protein extraction.

Subjects

Colorectal cancer and paired normal mucosa (*n*=107) tissues were sampled from surgical resection specimens, acquired at the Affiliated Hospital of Chengde Medical University between 2017 and 2019. The patients with CRC were 59 men and 48 women (22~85 years, mean=62.9 years). Among them, 47 cases are accompanied with lymph node metastasis. These cases included well (*n*=19), moderately (*n*=60), and poorly (*n*=12) differentiated; mucinous (*n*=7); and other (*n*=9) adenocarcinomas. Serum samples were obtained before surgery from 13 patients with colorectal cancer and 40 healthy individuals attending Affiliated Hospital of Chengde Medical University. None of the patients had undergone chemotherapy, radiotherapy, or any other treatment before the operation. All participants provided comprehensive consent to participate in research and for their data to be used further. The study protocol was approved by the Ethics Committee of the Affiliated Hospital of Chengde Medical University.

DNA Analysis

DNA was extracted from mouse tail and intestine using the phenol-chloroform method. We performed genotyping by PCR. The PCR primer sequences were CSD-lacF: 5'-GCTACCATTAC CAGTTGGTCTGGTGTC-3', CSD-neoF: 5'-GGGATCTCA TGCTGGAGTTCTTCG-3', CSD- loxF:5'-GAGATGGCGCAA CGCAATTAATG-3', CSD-*Dkk3*-R:5'-AACAGGAGATTC CAGGT GTCAGAGG-3', CSD-*Dkk3*-ttR: 5'-GCCTGGCCAG CACTTTTATCTATCC-3', CSD-*Dkk3*-F: 5'-TCTGCTTTA GCCATACCTCTTGGGG-3', *Dkk3*-F: 5'-ACCAAAGGTG GCAATGGGACC ATCT-3', *Dkk3*-R: 5'-GGTGGAAAGC ACTCTAAGGCCCAGC-3', cre: 5'-GCCTGCATTACC GGTCGATGC-3' and 5'-CAGGGTGTTATAAGCAATCCC-3'. The presence of truncated *Dkk3* and cre was confirmed by tail DNA PCR. *Dkk3* deletion was confirmed by PCR amplification of intestinal mucosa DNA.

Real-Time RT-PCR

We extracted total RNA from cells and tissues using Trizol (Takara). Reverse transcription of 1 μg RNA was performed using random primers and AMV reverse transcriptase. PCR primers were designed according to the sequences provided by GenBank. The oligonucleotide primer forward sequence was 5'-ACAGCCACAGCCTGGTGTA-3'. The reversed primer sequences were 5'-CC TCCATGAAGCTGCCAAC-3' for *Dkk3* (120 bp), 5'-TAGAATTGGTAGTTCTTCAT-3' and 5'-A TTG CATCCCAGACAGTG-3' for N-cadherin (100 bp), and 5'-CAGGTCTCCTCATGGCTT-3' and 5'-CATCCTTAAATC TCACTCT -3' for E-cadherin (140 bp). For internal control, *GAPDH*, forward primer sequences were 5'-CAATGACCCCT TCATTGACC-3'; reversed sequences were 5'-TGGAAGATGG TGATGGGATT-3' (135 bp). SYBR Premix Ex Taq II kit (Takara) was used to amplify *GAPDH* as an internal control.

Western Blot

Protein was extracted in RIPA lysis buffer and identified by BCA assay. We separated denatured protein in SDS-polyacrylamide gel and transferred it to the Hybond membrane, which was blocked with 5% milk in TBST. For immunoblotting, the membrane was incubated for 1 h with mouse anti-Bax (Santa Cruz), rabbit anti-cdc25B (H-85, Santa Cruz), anti-cdc25C (C-20, Santa Cruz), anti-E-cadherin (Cell Signaling Technology), anti-N-cadherin (Cell Signaling Technology), anti-slug (Cell Signaling Technology), anti-twist1 (Cell Signaling Technology), or anti-GAPDH (Santa Cruz) antibody for 1 h in TBST at room temperature. Subsequently, these membranes were incubated with antimouse or antirabbit IgG conjugated to horseradish peroxidase (Dako) for 1 h at room temperature. Bands were visualized using ECL- Plus (Santa Cruz).

Histological Analysis

Tissues were subjected to routine pathological block preparation. Consecutive sections were deparaffinized, dehydrated, and subjected to immunostaining as previously described (18) or to the TUNEL procedure, using ApopTag Plus Peroxidase in Situ Apoptosis Detection Kit (Millipore) as recommended.

Bioinformatics Analysis

The differences in level of Dkk3 expression were examined between colorectal normal and colorectal cancer tissues using Oncomine (www.oncomine.com). Data on the rate of expression (RNA-seqV2) and methylation as well as data on clinicopathological characteristics of colorectal cancer patients were extracted from the TCGA database using TCGA-assembler in R software. We integrated our raw data and examined Dkk3 expression levels in colorectal cancer tissue, which were subsequently examined against patient clinicopathological and prognostic characteristics. The Kaplan-Meier method was used to examine the prognostic significance of Dkk3 mRNA expression. Moreover, we used these data to examine the rate of promoter methylation and to perform GSEA. Based on Dkk3 expression levels, the data were divided into high- and low-expression groups based on the median value of colorectal cancer patients. GSEA was performed with GSEA-3.0. The impact of *Dkk3* methylation and expression on survival rates was examined using methylation, clinical, and transcriptome data. Methylated and unmethylated signals were employed to calculate β-coefficients, which are a quantitative representation of DNA methylation levels. Cutoff values were defined as median values of β-coefficients and mRNA expression levels. Kaplan-Meier survival curves of *Dkk3* methylation were obtained as well.

Statistical Analyses

We repeated 3 different experiments to calculate mean and standard deviation. Statistical analysis was performed using Mann-Whitney U to differentiate the means and log-rank statistic to compare the survival rate. We used SPSS 10.0 for data analysis. *P*-values < 0.05 were considered indicative of statistical significance.

RESULTS

Dkk3 Expression and Aggressive Colorectal Cancer Cell Phenotype

After transfection with pcDNA3.1-*Dkk3*, HCT-15, and HCT-116 cells overexpressed Dkk3 protein by western blot using anti-Dkk3 or anti-His antibody (**Figure 1A**). In Dkk3 transfectants, mRNA levels increased 7- to 13-fold compared to those in the control cells (**Figure 1B**, $p<0.05$). Immunofluorescence testing showed higher levels of Dkk3 expression in the cytoplasm of transfectants than in that of control or mock cells (**Figure 1C**, $p<0.05$). The cell culture supernatant of Dkk3 tranfectants had a higher Dkk3 concentration than that of control or mock cells (**Figure 1D**, $p<0.05$). However, a higher level of Dkk3 expression was detected in the serum of colorectal cancer patients than in that of healthy controls regardless of age (**Figure 1E**, $p<0.05$). The rate of growth of Dkk3 transfectants was slower than that of control and mock cells (**Figure 1F**, $p<0.05$). Cell cycle analysis indicated G_2 phase arrest in the transfectants but not in the control or mock cells (**Figure 1G**, $p<0.05$). There was a high rate of apoptosis in HCT-15 and HCT-116 cells after *Dkk3* transfection (**Figure 1H**, $p<0.05$),. JC-1 staining demonstrated that Dkk3 expression significantly reduced mitochondrial membrane potential in these cells (**Figures 1I, J**). Compared with control and mock cells, Dkk3 overexpression suppressed migration and invasion capacities of both colorectal cancer cell types (**Figures 1K, L**, $p<0.05$). Finally, treatment of Dkk3 transfectants with anti-Dkk3 antibody resulted in blocked effects of Dkk3 overexpression on these phenotypes (**Figures 1F–L**, $p<0.05$).

Recombinant Dkk3 and Aggressive Colorectal Cancer Cell Phenotypes

Treatment with recombinant Dkk3 protein significantly suppressed the proliferation of HCT-15 and HCT-116 cells (**Figure 2A**, $p<0.05$). Exposure to Dkk3 protein resulted in G_2 phase arrest in HCT-15 and HCT-116 cells in a dose-dependent manner (**Figure 2B**, $p<0.05$). In addition, there was a higher level of apoptosis in HCT-15 and HCT-116 cells treated with Dkk3 protein (**Figure 2C**, $p<0.05$) than in the control cells. JC-1 staining also demonstrated that Dkk3 exposure significantly reduced the mitochondrial membrane potential of these cells (**Figures 2D, E**, $p<0.05$). In compare to control cells, Dkk3 protein exposure suppressed migration and invasion capacity of both colorectal cancer cell types (**Figures 2F, G**, $p<0.05$).

Dkk3 and Expression of Phenotype-Related Proteins in Colorectal Cancer Cells

As indicated in **Figure 3**, Dkk3 overexpression and treatment decreased the levels of expression of Bcl-2, cdc25B, cdc25c, N-cadherin, slug, and twist; in contrast, it increased the levels of expression of Bax and E-cadherin in HCT-15 and HCT-116 cells. Use of anti-Dkk3 antibody suppressed the effects of Dkk3 overexpression on these phenotype-related proteins.

The Effects of Dkk3 on Colorectal Carcinogenesis

We matched the conditional *Dkk3*-KO mice with villin-cre mice and designed primers to confirm deletion of Dkk3 using DNA from tail and intestinal mucosa (**Figure 4A**). Using PCR, we confirmed biallelic deletion of *Dkk3* in intestinal mucosa of *Dkk3*-villin-cre mice (**Figure 4B**). Expression levels of Dkk3 and E-cadherin were downregulated in intestinal mucosa of Dkk3-villin-cre at both mRNA and protein levels compared to WT mice; the reverse was observed for N-cadherin expression (**Figures 4C, D**). However, no remarkable lesions were observed in the intestinal mucosa of either mouse group (data not shown). A single case of colorectal adenoma was observed in villin-cre/Dkk3 mice after chemical induction, showing a higher level of expression of CDX1, ki-67, and c-erB2 than that observed in normal mucosa (**Figure 4E**).

Dkk3 Expression in Colorectal Cancer

Dkk3 mRNA expression was examined in colorectal cancer tissues using RT-PCR (**Figure 5A**). *Dkk3* mRNA expression levels were lower in cancer than in normal tissues (**Figure 5B**, $p<0.05$). Concurrently, they were higher in tubular than in

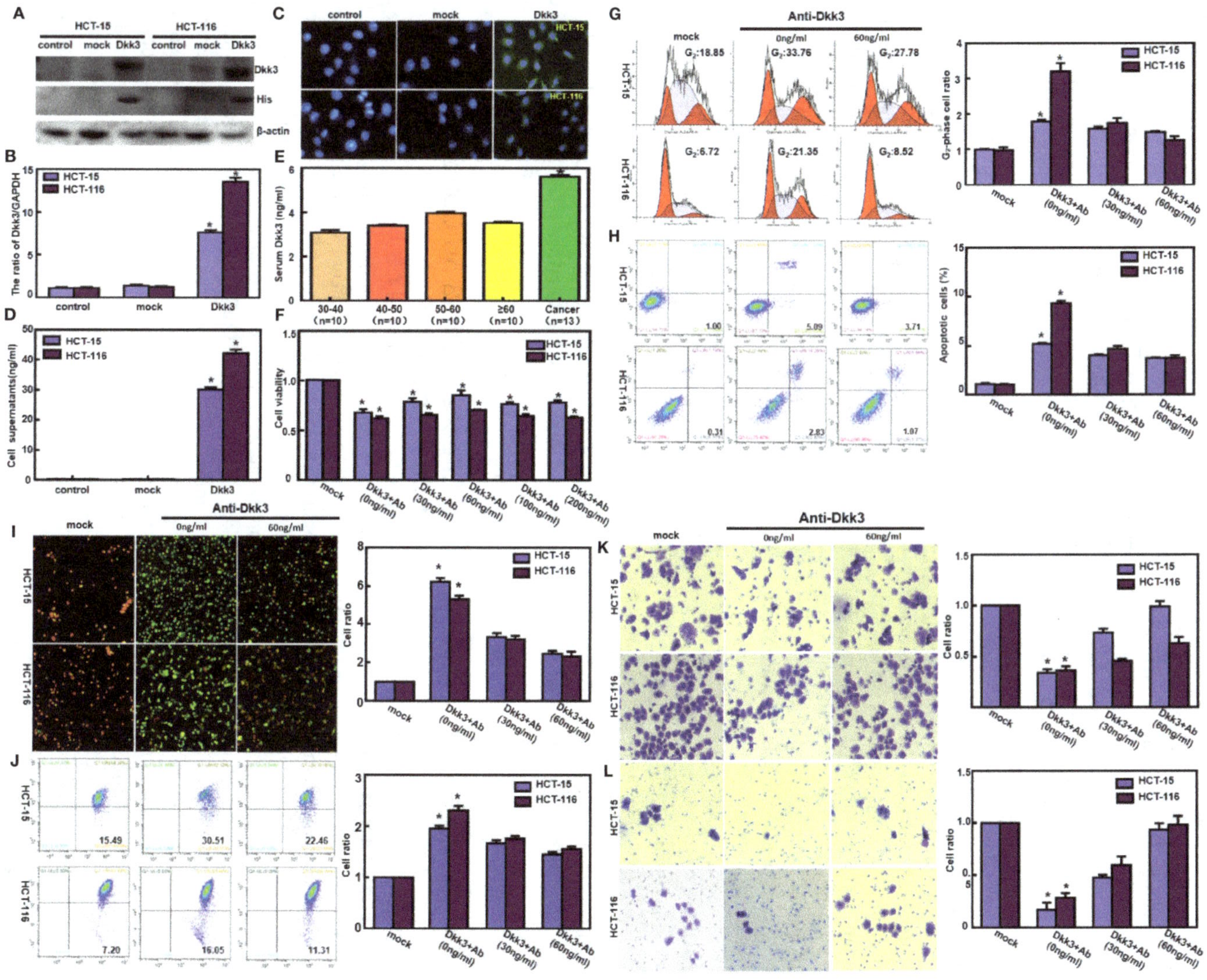

FIGURE 1 | Dkk3 overexpression suppressed the aggressive phenotypes of colorectal cancer cells. After transfection of pcDNA3.1-*Dkk3*, Dkk3 expression became strong in HCT-15 and HCT-116 cells using anti-Dkk3 and anti-His antibodies by Western blot **(A)**, real-time RT-PCR **(B)**, and immunofluorescence (**C**, green: positive for Dkk3, blue: DAPI for nuclei). The cell culture supernatant of Dkk3 transfectants showed a higher Dkk3 concentration in comparison with those of the control and mock **(D)**. Colorectal cancer patients showed a higher serum Dkk3 level than healthy individuals regardless of their age, evidenced by ELISA assay **(E)**. The transfectants showed a lower proliferation **(F)** and G_2 arrest **(G)** in comparison with the control and mock. There was an apoptosis-induced effect of Dkk3 overexpression in the transfectants of HCT-15 and HCT-116, evidenced by annexin V assay **(H)**. JC-1 staining displayed that the mitochondrial membrane potential was decreased in the abovementioned cells with Dkk3 overexpression by fluorescence **(I)** and flow cytometry **(J)**. Dkk3-overexpressing cells had a weaker ability to migrate **(K)** and invade **(L)**. We also treated the Dkk3 transfectants with anti-Dkk3 antibody (0, 30, and 60 ng/ml) and found that this antibody blocked the effects of Dkk3 overexpression on these phenotypes (**F–L**, $p < 0.05$). mock, cells transfected with pcDNA3.1 vector; *$P < 0.05$, compared with the control and treatment with anti-Dkk3 antibody.

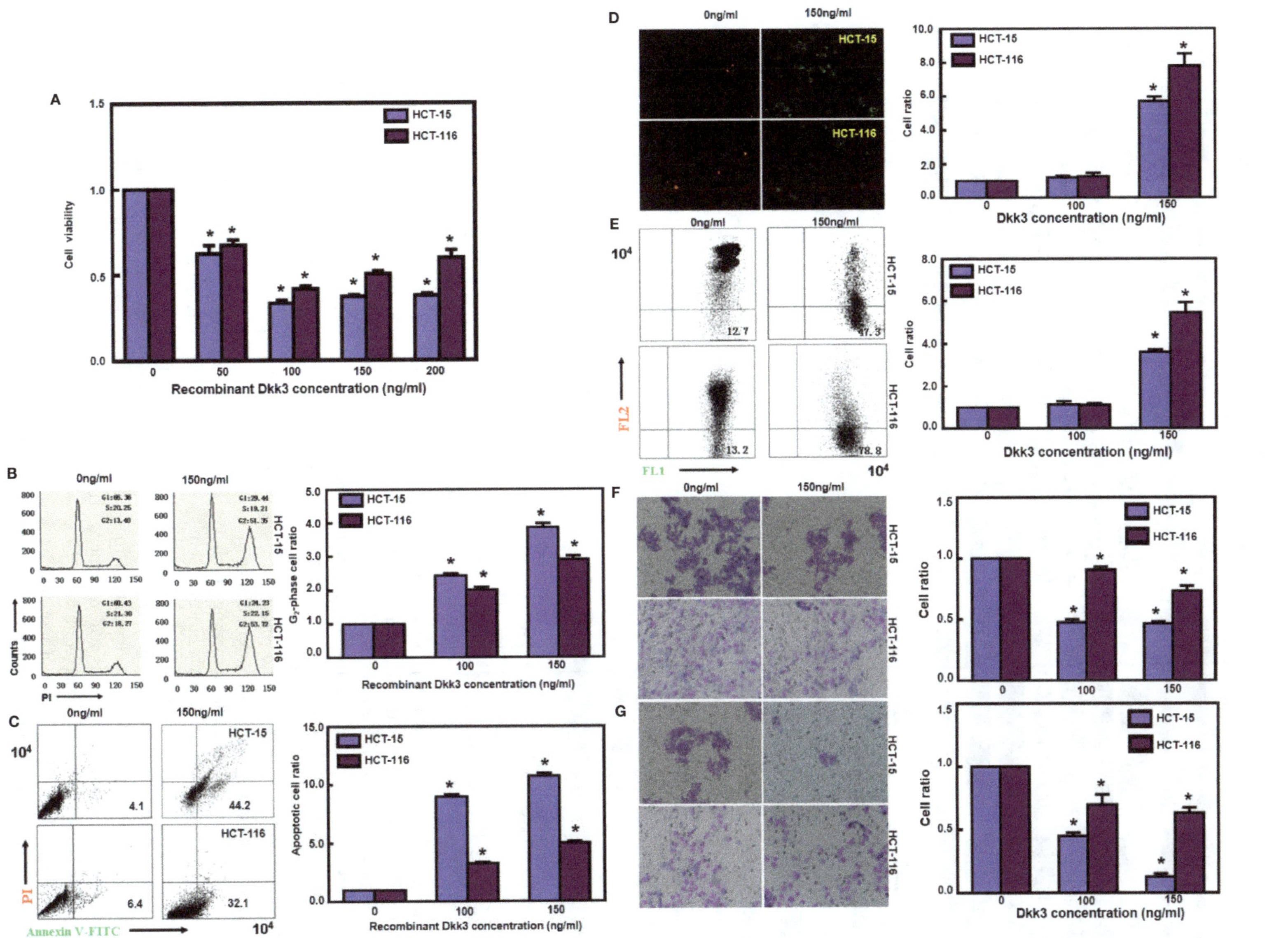

FIGURE 2 | Recombinant Dkk3 inhibited the aggressive phenotypes of colorectal cancer cells. Treatment with recombinant Dkk3 protein significantly suppressed the proliferation of HCT-15 and HCT-116, compared with the control cells **(A)**. Recombinant Dkk3 protein could induce G_2 arrest **(B)** and cell apoptosis **(C)** of both kinds of cells in a dose-dependent manner. JC-1 staining also demonstrated that recombinant Dkk3 exposure significantly reduced mitochondrial membrane potential of the abovementioned cells treated with 150 ng/mL recombinant protein by fluorescence **(D)** and flow cytometry **(E)**. After being exposed to recombinant Dkk3, both colorectal carcinoma cells exhibited a low ability to migrate **(F)** and invade **(G)**, compared with the control cells. *$P < 0.05$, compared with the control.

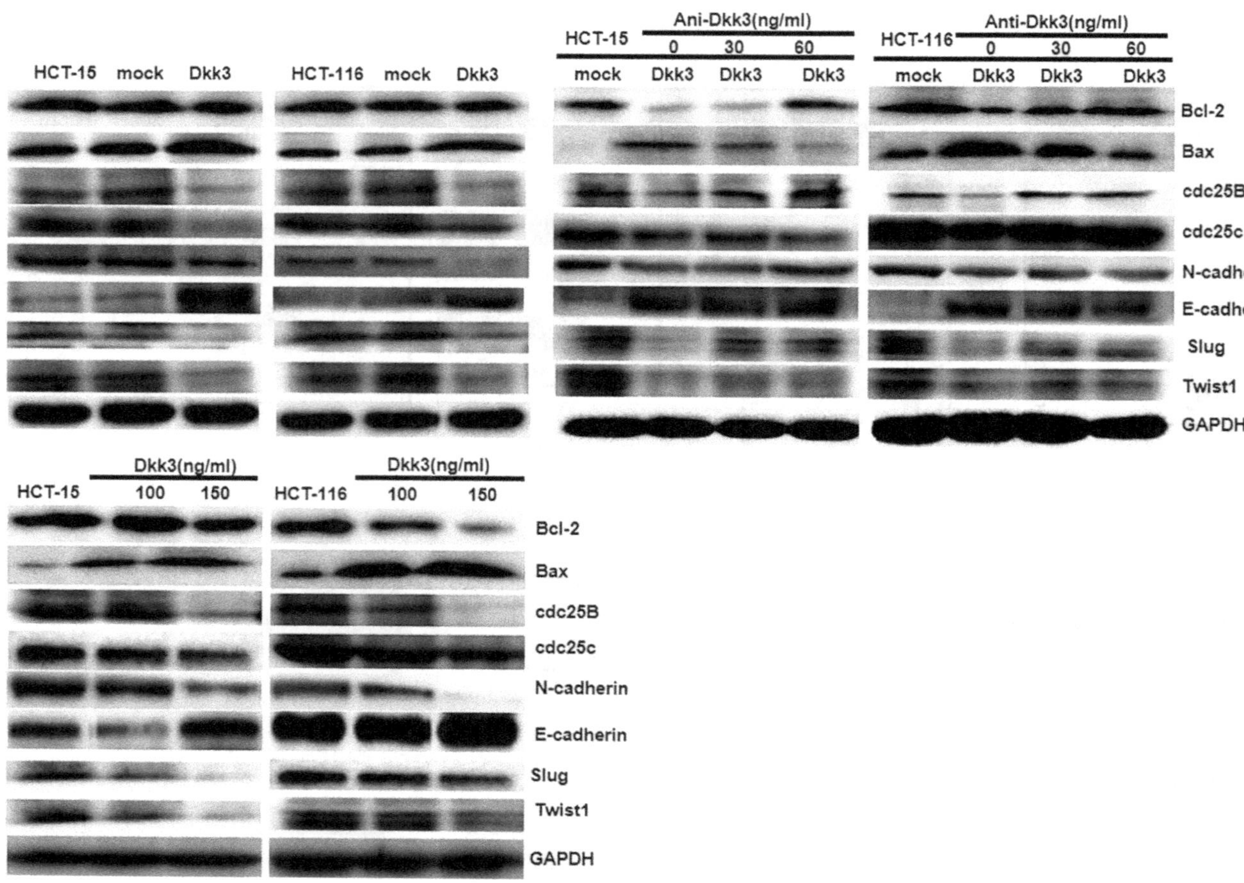

FIGURE 3 | The phenotype-related proteins were screened by Western blot. Dkk3 overexpression and treatment decreased the expression of Bcl-2, cdc25B, cdc25c, N-cadherin, Slug, and Twist and increased the expression of Bax and E-cadherin in HCT-15 and HCT-116 cells. The anti-Dkk3 antibody suppressed the effects of Dkk3 overexpression on the expression of the phenotype-related proteins.

mucinous adenocarcinoma (**Figure 5B**, $p<0.05$). Levels of Dkk3 expression were higher in nested than in infiltrative adenocarcinomas (**Figure 5B**, $p<0.05$). However, these levels of expression were not correlated with gender, age, cell differentiation, lymph node or distal metastasis status, peritoneal spread, lymphatic and venous invasion, or tumor size in colorectal cancer patients ($p>0.05$, data not shown).

Moreover, levels of *Dkk3* mRNA expression were higher in colorectal cancer than in normal mucosa according to the Skrzypczak and Gaedcke method (**Figure 6A**); however, no difference was detected in TCGA database analysis (**Figure 6B**). These levels were positively associated with lymph node metastasis status in colorectal cancer patients (**Figure 6B**). In addition, colorectal cancer-associated fibroblasts had a higher level of *Dkk3* expression compared to that observed in CD133+ or CD133- cancer cells (**Figure 6C**, $p<0.05$). There was no correlation between survival rate among colorectal cancer patients and *Dkk3* expression levels ($p>0.05$, data not shown). However, a negative relationship between *Dkk3* mRNA expression and prognosis was observed in patients with stage II or IV disease and in those with a high mutation burden (**Figure 6D**, $p<0.05$). Additionally, *Dkk3* mRNA expression levels were correlated negatively with the rate of promoter methylation ($p<0.05$, data not shown). There was no association between *Dkk3* promoter methylation and survival rates ($p>0.05$, data not shown).

Dkk3 protein expression levels were lower in cancer than in normal tissues (**Figure 7**, $p<0.05$). In addition, Dkk3 protein expression levels were lower in tubular than in mucinous adenocarcinomas ($p<0.05$); similarly, they were lower in nested than in infiltrative adenocarcinomas ($p<0.05$). However, Dkk3 protein expression levels did not correlate with gender, age, cell differentiation rate, lymph node or distal metastasis status, peritoneal spread, lymphatic and venous invasion, or tumor size in colorectal cancer patients ($p>0.05$).

Dkk3-Related Signal Pathways in Colorectal Cancer

In GSEA, enriched *Dkk3*-related signaling pathways in colorectal cancer tissue included those associated with cellular adhesion

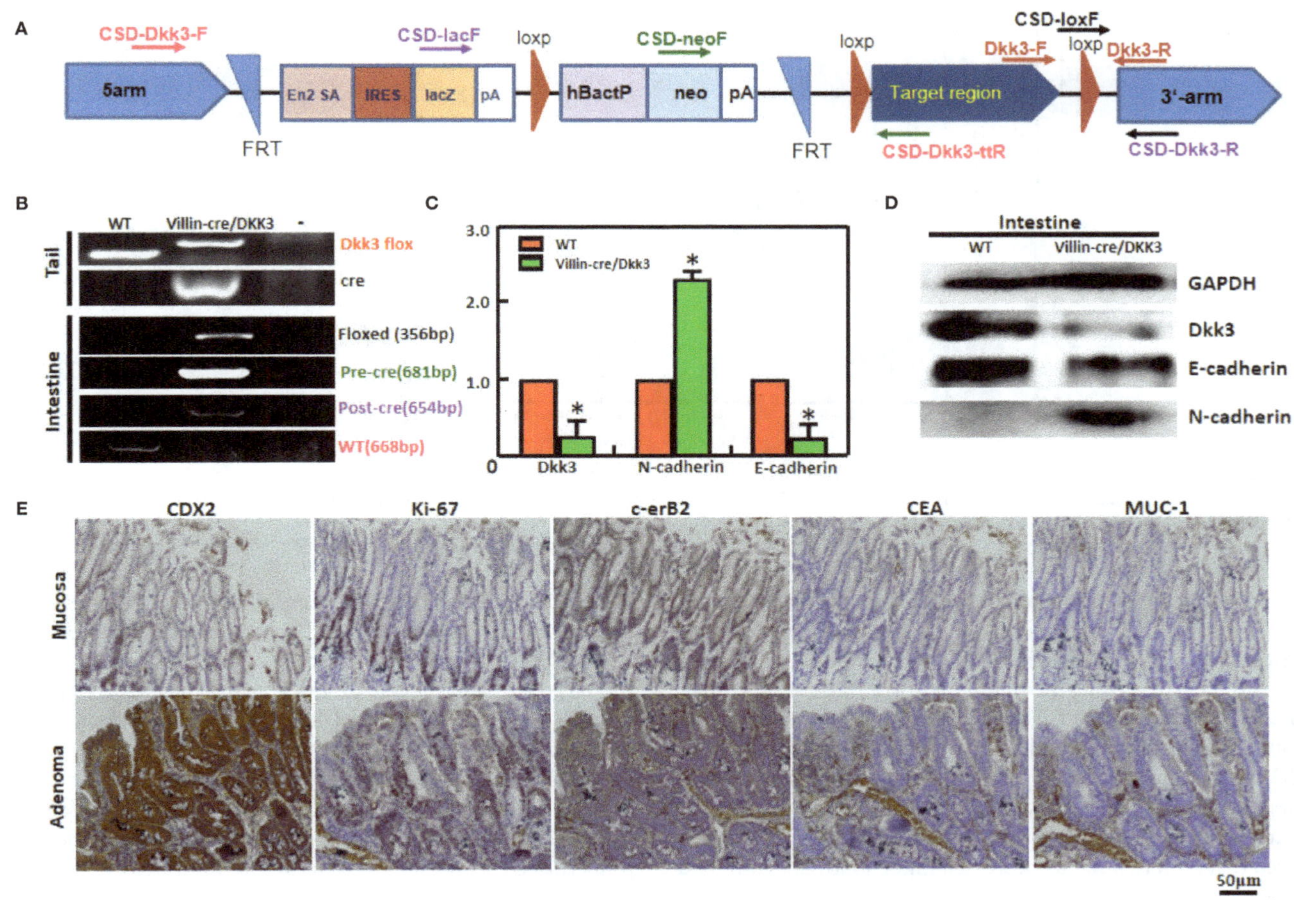

FIGURE 4 | The effects of Dkk3 on tumor growth and carcinogenesis of colorectal cancer. PCR primers were designed **(A)** and subjected to PCR of tail and stomach DNA **(B)** with the same color for the corresponding primers and products. Expression of Dkk3, N-cadherin, and E-cadherin was confirmed by real-time PCR **(C)** and Western blot **(D)**. Immunohistochemistry was employed to observe the maker proteins' expression in the intestinal adenoma of target villin-cre/Dkk3 knockout mice induced by sodium desoxycholate **(E)**. *$p < 0.05$, compared with the transfectant or knockout mice. WT, wild-type mice; VD, villin-cre +; Dkk3 -/-.

and migration, melanogenesis, chemokine, Hedgehog, JAK-STAT, TOLL-like receptor, TGF-β, MAPK, and calcium signaling (**Table 1**, $p<0.05$).

DISCUSSION

Shin et al. (22) reported that Dkk3 immunostaining was gradually downregulated from the epidermis in normal skin, actinic keratosis to squamous cell carcinoma (SCC). *Dkk3* mRNA expression level was lower in SCC than in normal skin. In the present study, expression of *Dkk3* mRNA and protein was downregulated in colorectal cancer cells, which is consistent with previous studies (12–17). A previous high-throughput study has shown a negative correlation between the level of *Dkk3* mRNA expression and its promoter methylation rate (18). These findings suggest that Dkk3 expression is downregulated in colorectal cancer due to Dkk3 promoter methylation. Our previous study of gastric and lung cancer cells treated with 5-Aza has shown a significantly negative association between Dkk3 promoter methylation and mRNA expression (18, 23). In a separate study, the rate of Dkk3 promoter methylation was higher in breast cancer than in normal tissue and was independently associated with adverse prognosis (24). Bioinformatics analysis has shown higher levels of *Dkk3* mRNA in colorectal cancer; however, this finding might be accounted by between-study differences in methods used (RT-PCR, Western blot, and tissue microarray vs. RNA sequencing). Herein, we have shown that colorectal adenoma occurred in chemical-exposed and Dkk3-deleted intestine, suggesting that Dkk3 abrogation might enhance chemically induced colorectal carcinogenesis.

Horikawa et al. (25) found that Dkk3 overexpression suppressed the proliferation of human bladder cancer cells by downregulating CD147 expression. Here, it was observed that both recombinant Dkk3 protein and Dkk3 overexpression might inhibit cell proliferation and trigger G_2 phase arrest in both colorectal

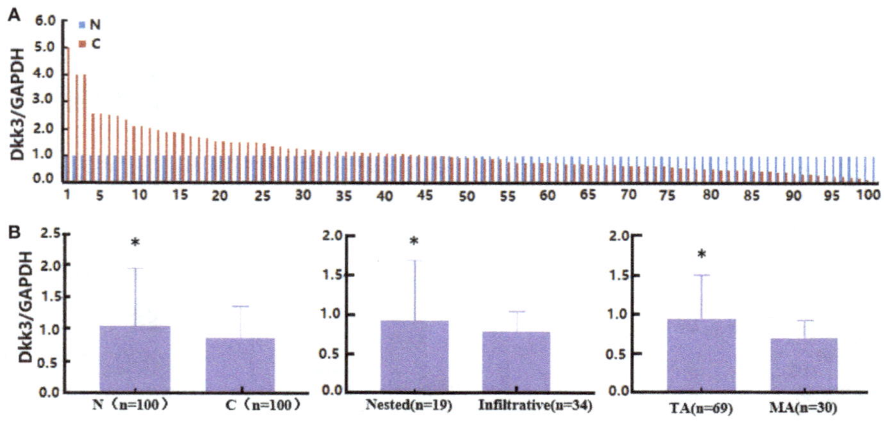

FIGURE 5 | The clinicopathological significance of *Dkk3* mRNA expression in colorectal cancer. Real-time RT-PCR was employed to detect *Dkk3* mRNA expression in colorectal cancer samples **(A)**. Its expression was compared with pathological behaviors of colorectal cancer **(B)**. N, normal; C, cancer, TA, tubular adenocarcinoma; MA, mucinous adenocarcinoma. $^{*}p < 0.05$.

cancer cell types. Previously, we observed that the presence of Dkk3 overexpression and recombinant Dkk3 triggered G_1 phase arrest in gastric cancer cells by downregulating Cyclin D2 and Cyclin E expression *via* the Wnt/β-catenin pathway (18). These data indicated that the effect of Dkk3 on the cell cycle depended on cell specificity. Additionally, a higher apoptosis rate was detected in both colorectal cancer cell types exposed to recombinant Dkk3 protein or transfected with Dkk3-expressing plasmid; this finding was consistent with that of our previous study (18). JC-1 staining showed that both treatments decreased mitochondrial membrane potential of colorectal cancer cells, suggesting both treatments induced colorectal cancer cell apoptosis *via* the mitochondrial pathway. Previously, we have reported on a positive relationship between Dkk3 and Caspase-3 expression in both colorectal and lung cancers (21, 23). It has been suggested that Dkk3 could cause c-JNK activation, mitochondrial translocation of Bax, and Bcl-2 under-expression in apoptotic induction (4). Shin et al. (22) have shown that Ad-Dkk3 induced JNK activation and subsequent apoptosis in lung cancer cells. It has been suggested that expression of cytosolic and secretory Dkk3 protein types might contribute to apoptotic induction of colorectal cancer cells *via* the mitochondrial pathway. Altogether, this evidence suggests that downregulated expression or loss of Dkk3 in colorectal cancer cells might disrupt the balance between apoptosis and proliferation.

In both gastric and colorectal cancers, Dkk3 expression was negatively correlated with the depth of invasion, lymph node involvement, and clinicopathological staging (18, 21); this finding was consistent with that of another study (26). Herein, the *Dkk3* mRNA expression level was higher in nested than in filtrated cancer tissue, and recombinant Dkk3 and ectopic Dkk3 expression seemed to attenuate the migrative and invasive capacities of colorectal cancer cells, indicating that both kinds of intervention might effectively inhibit the risk of invasion or metastasis in advanced colorectal cancer. Dkk3-related signal pathways included cellular adhesion and migration in colorectal cancer, supporting this hypothesis. Hoang et al. (27) have previously reported that Dkk3 can inhibit invasion and motility of osteosarcoma cells *via* the Wnt/β-catenin pathway. Meanwhile, adeno-Dkk3 gene delivery has been demonstrated to suppress tumor growth and the rate of invasion and metastasis of prostate cancer cells (10). Moreover, Dkk3 expression enhanced cellular adhesion and reduced the rate of cellular migration of melanoma cells (28). Than et al. (29) reported that intraperitoneal adeno-Dkk-3 administration suppressed peritoneal dissemination of scirrhous gastric cancer. These findings suggest that invasive and metastatic properties of malignancies might be due to decreased expression levels or loss of Dkk3.

Zenzmaier et al. (30) report that plasma Dkk3 level was increased among older adults and that it might serve as a marker of senescence. Concurrently, the serum level of Dkk-3 was significantly lower in ovarian, gastric, and colorectal cancer patients than in healthy controls (18, 31, 32). In contrast, serum Dkk3 concentration appeared higher in colorectal cancer patients than in healthy individuals; a similar finding was reported in a study of cervical cancer (32). In addition, we found higher supernatant Dkk3 level in Dkk3 transfectants of colorectal and gastric cancer cells (18). Dkk3 treatment caused the same results as Dkk3 overexpression in line with our data (18, 23), which could be blocked with anti-Dkk3 antibody (18). Zhang et al. (33) reported that soluble Dkk-3 protein levels were associated with prostate acinar growth. It has been proposed that soluble Dkk3 protein may bind to transmembrane co-receptor Lrp6 to suppress Wnt/β-catenin signaling (4, 34). As a result, we hypothesized that recombinant Dkk3 might bind to receptors to reverse aggressive phenotypes of gastrointestinal cancer cells in either an autocrine or a paracrine manner (17).

Dkk3 expression has been shown to induce β-catenin degradation by interacting with protoesome βTrCP, blocking the effect of nuclear β-catenin on TCF-4 activity, and suppressing the expression of TCF-4 targets (c-myc, VEGF and cylcin D) (17, 35). The human dynein light chain, Tctex-1, may interact with

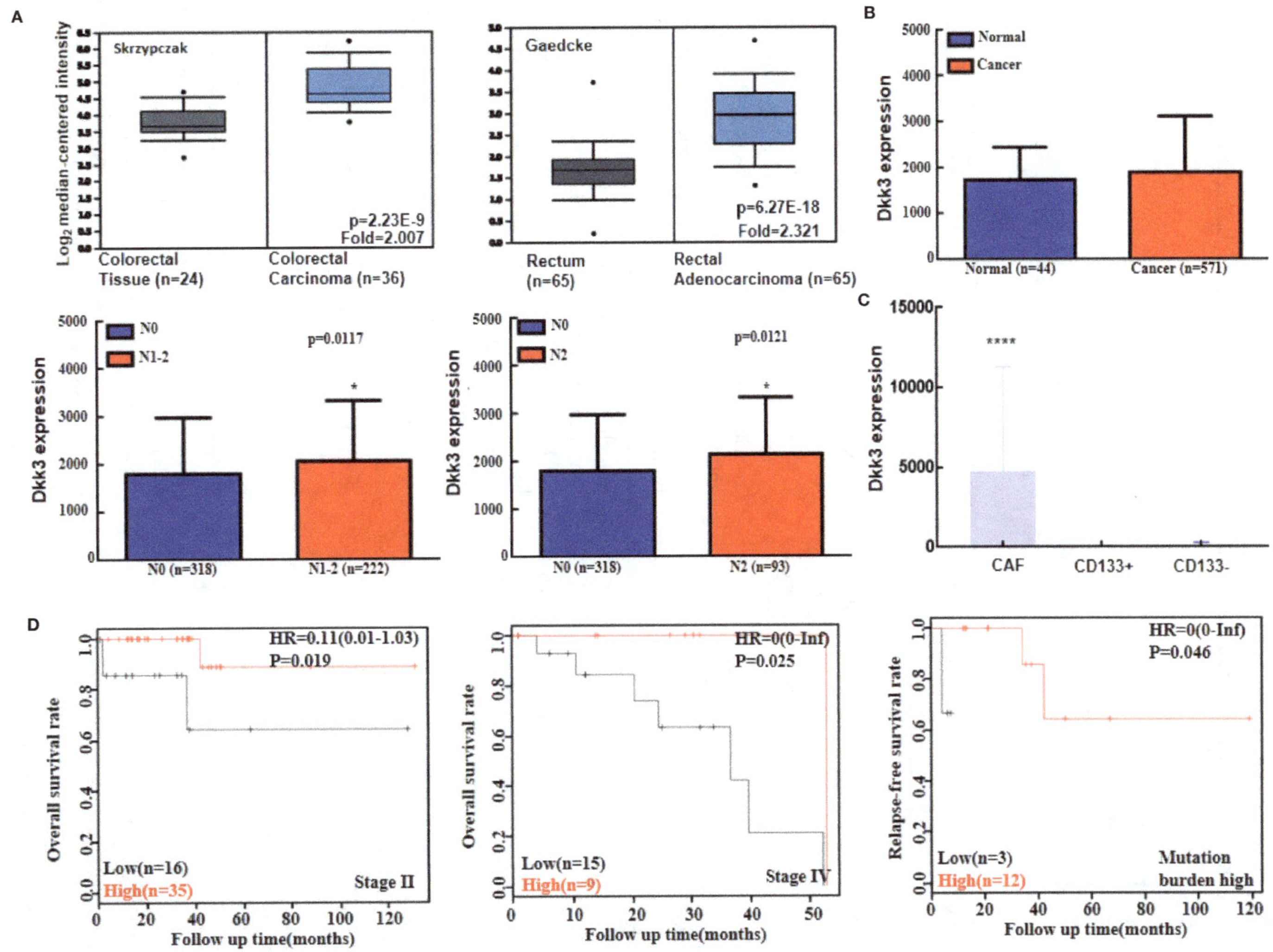

FIGURE 6 | The bioinformatics analysis of *Dkk3* mRNA expression in colorectal cancer. Oncomine **(A)** and TCGA **(B)** data sets were employed to analyze Dkk3 expression in colorectal cancer, and its expression was compared with pathological parameters of cancers. *Dkk3* mRNA expression was higher in cancer-associated fibroblasts (CAF) than CD133-positive (CD133+) and -negative (CD133-) colorectal cancer cells **(C)**. Kaplan-Meier curves were used to analyze the prognostic significance of *Dkk3* mRNA expression according to KM plotters **(D)**. HR, hazard ratio; N, lymph node metastasis. $^{*}p < 0.05$; $^{****}p < 0.001$.

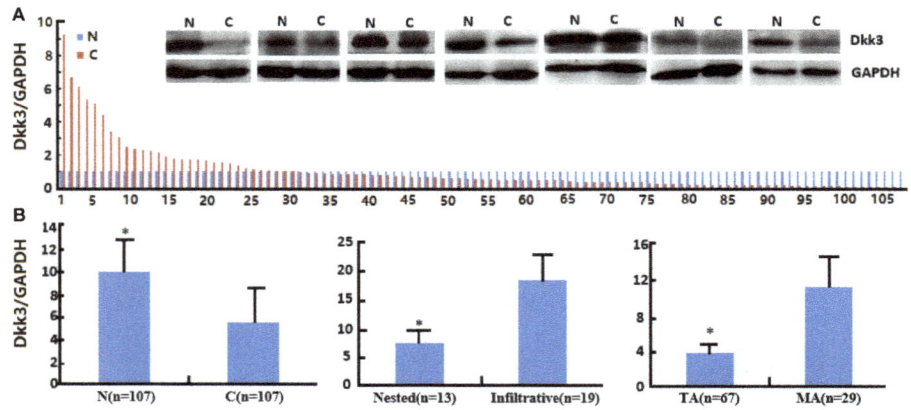

FIGURE 7 | The clinicopathological significance of Dkk3 protein expression in colorectal cancer. Western blot was employed to detect Dkk3 protein expression in colorectal cancer samples **(A)**. Its expression was compared with pathological behaviors of colorectal cancer **(B)**. N, normal; C, cancer, TA, tubular adenocarcinoma; MA, mucinous adenocarcinoma. *$p < 0.05$.

TABLE 1 | *Dkk3*-enriched signal pathway in colorectal cancer according KEGG analysis.

Pathway	Size	P value
Focal adhesion	197	<0.001
Gap junction	87	<0.001
Cytokine -cytokine receptor interaction	234	<0.001
Cell adhesion molecules CAMS	129	<0.001
Dilated cardiomyopathy	86	<0.001
Chemokine signaling pathway	183	<0.001
Hypertrophic cardiomyopathy	79	<0.001
Leukocyte transendothelial migration	111	<0.001
Hedgehog signaling pathway	54	<0.001
Regulation of actin cytoskeleton	207	<0.001
Melanogenesis	99	<0.001
ECM receptor interaction	83	<0.001
Axon guidance	127	<0.001
Pathways in cancer	322	<0.001
Basal cell carcinoma	54	<0.001
Arrhythmogenic right ventricular cardiomyopathy	71	0.001
Complement and coagulation cascades	64	0.001
Neuroactive ligand receptor interaction	231	0.001
JAK-STAT signaling pathway	130	0.001
Leishmania infection	70	0.005
TOLL-like receptor signaling pathway	87	0.006
Glycosaminoglycan biosynthesis chondroitin sulfate	22	0.006
Vascular smooth muscle contraction	113	0.006
Hematopoietic cell lineage	81	0.006
Calcium signaling pathway	169	0.007
TGF-β signaling pathway	85	0.009
MAPK signaling pathway	257	0.015
Glycosaminoglycan biosynthesis heparan sulfate	26	0.02
Melanoma	70	0.039

Dkk3, which might be involved in ER stress and intracellular dynein motor dynamics (36). However, a separate study has reported that Dkk3-carrying adenovirus infection of normal human fibroblasts induced interleukin-7 production, triggered by ER stress proteins (ASK1, p38, IRE1α and IRF-1) (37). The repressing effects of Dkk3 overexpression on aggressive colorectal cancer cell phenotypes might be due to a higher rate of secretion of its soluble form alongside interaction of its cytosolic and other types of protein.

In this study, hypoexpression of cdc25B and cdc25c was associated with the suppressing effects of Dkk3 on proliferation and tumor growth as cdc25B activates Cyclin-dependent kinase CDC2 required for mitosis progression; concurrently, cdc25C promotes Cyclin B-Cdk1 complex formation required for G_2/M phase transition (38). The presence of Bax-Bcl-2 complex on the mitochondrial membrane can lower the rate of apoptosis as Bax can open the mitochondrial anion channel to initiate apoptosis (39). Consequently, Bax hyperexpression and Bcl-2 hyperexpression may explain the inductive effect of Dkk3 in apoptosis of colorectal cancer cells. Slug and twist promoted epithelial-mesenchymal transition (EMT) alongside E-cadherin under-expression and N-cadherin hyperexpression (40); downregulated expression of N-cadherin and of slug and twist, and upregulation of E-cadherin might result in the inhibitory effects of Dkk3 in EMT of colorectal cancer cells.

It has been reported that Dkk3 might orchestrate concomitant activation of β-catenin and YAP/TAZ in cancer-associated fibroblasts (CAFs) by interfering with the Kremen negative regulator and increasing cell-surface levels of LRP6 as an HSF1 effector, required to promote tumor aggressiveness (41). Zhou et al. (42) demonstrated that Dkk3 was produced by pancreatic stellate cells and stimulated tumor growth, metastasis, and chemoresistance of pancreatic ductal adenocarcinoma in the paracrine and autocrine manner *via* the NF-κB pathway. Zenzmaier et al. (43) found that Dkk-3 promoted fibroblast proliferation and myofibroblast differentiation and regulated angiopoietin-1 expression in prostatic stroma potentially by enhancing PI3K/Akt signaling, which triggered angiogenesis in prostate cancer. Our bioinformatics data showed higher *Dkk3* expression in CAF than in CD133+ or in CD133- cancer cells, supporting the hypothesis that Dkk3 in cancer stromal cells might be involved in cancer progression.

Dkk3 was positively associated with survival rate among patients with nasopharyngeal carcinoma (26). Yang et al. (23) found that *Dkk3* mRNA overexpression positively correlated with overall, progression-free, and post-progression survival rates among lung cancer patients even when stratified by sex, histological subtyping, disease grade, TNM stage, chemotherapy and radiotherapy type, or smoking status. Herein, Kaplan-Meier analysis indicated that mRNA expression or promoter methylation of *Dkk3* was not linked to overall survival rate among colorectal cancer patients; this finding was consistent with that of our immunostaining tests (21). Moreover, Dkk3 expression had no prognostic significance in colorectal cancer at either mRNA or protein level. However, its mRNA expression was negatively correlated with poor prognosis among colorectal cancer patients with Stage II and IV disease and among those with a high mutation burden; these findings might provide guidance for clinical practice.

In conclusion, Dkk3 expression was downregulated in colorectal cancer tissue due to its promoter methylation; this finding can be used in assessing cancer aggressiveness. Recombinant Dkk3 protein and forced Dkk3 overexpression might suppress aggressive phenotypes of colorectal cancer cells. These findings indicate that Dkk3 might be a promising target for gene therapy in colorectal cancer if it can specifically be expressed in cancer cells. However, future studies need to elucidate Dkk3 receptor or partner and the associated signaling pathway.

ETHICS STATEMENT

The studies involving human participants were reviewed and approved by Affiliated Hospital of Chengde Medical University. The patients/participants provided their written informed consent to participate in this study. The animal study was reviewed and approved by Affiliated Hospital of Chengde Medical University. Written informed consent was obtained from the owners for the participation of their animals in this study.

AUTHOR CONTRIBUTIONS

SZ, C-lH, E-hZ, H-mJ, and H-cZ designed and carried out the experiment, and H-cZ wrote the manuscript. All authors contributed to the article and approved the submitted version.

ACKNOWLEDGMENTS

Conditional *Dkk3* knockout mice were kindly presented by Prof. Kumon, Department of Urology, Okayama University, Japan, and pCDNA3.1-*Dkk3* plasmid was kindly presented by Yoshifumi Mizobuchi, University of Tokushima, Japan.

REFERENCES

1. Tsuji T, Miyazaki M, Sakaguchi M, Inoue Y, Namba M. A Dkk3 gene shows down-regulation in human immortalized cells and human tumor-derived cell lines. *Biochem Biophys Res Commun* (2000) 268(1):20–4. doi: 10.1006/bbrc.1999.2067
2. Hsieh SY, Hsieh PS, Chiu CT, Chen WY. Dickkopf-3/REIC functions as a suppressor gene of tumor growth. *Oncogene* (2004) 23(57):9183–9. doi: 10.1038/sj.onc.1208138
3. Kataoka K, Maehara N, Ayabe Y, Murata H, Huh NH, Sakaguchi M. Tumor necrosis factor-α downregulates the REIC/Dkk-3 tumor suppressor gene in normal human skin keratinocytes. *Mol Med Rep* (2018) 17(5):6661–6. doi: 10.3892/mmr.2018.8676
4. Abarzua F, Sakaguchi M, Takaishi M, Nasu Y, Kurose K, Ebara S, et al. Adenovirus-mediated overexpression of REIC/Dkk-3 selectively induces apoptosis in human prostate cancer cells through activation of c-Jun-NH2-kinase. *Cancer Res* (2005) 65(21):9617–22. doi: 10.1158/0008-5472.CAN-05-0829
5. Tanimoto R, Sakaguchi M, Abarzua F, Kataoka K, Kurose K, Murata H, et al. Down-regulation of BiP/GRP78 sensitizes resistant prostate cancer cells to gene-therapeutic overexpression of REIC/Dkk-3. *Int J Cancer* (2010) 126 (7):1562–9. doi: 10.1002/ijc.24764
6. Abarzua F, Sakaguchi M, Tanimoto R, Sonegawa H, Li DW, Edamura K, et al. Heat shock proteins play a crucial role in tumor-specific apoptosis by REIC/Dkk-3. *Int J Mol Med* (2007) 20(1):37–43. doi: 10.3892/ijmm.20.1.37
7. Takata A, Terauchi M, Hiramitsu S, Uno M, Wakana K, Kubota T. Dkk-3 induces apoptosis through mitochondrial and Fas death receptor pathways in human mucinous ovarian cancer cells. *Int J Gynecol Cancer* (2015) 25(3):372–9. doi: 10.1097/IGC.0000000000000340
8. Xu J, Sadahira T, Kinoshita R, Li SA, Huang P, Wada K, et al. Exogenous DKK-3/REIC inhibits Wnt/β-catenin signaling and cell proliferation in human kidney cancer KPK1. *Oncol Lett* (2017) 14(5):5638–42. doi: 10.3892/ol.2017.6833
9. Kinoshita R, Watanabe M, Huang P, Li SA, Sakaguchi M, Kumon H, et al. The cysteine-rich core domain of REIC/Dkk-3 is critical for its effect on monocyte differentiation and tumor regression. *Oncol Rep* (2015) 33(6):2908–14. doi: 10.3892/or.2015.3885
10. Edamura K, Nasu Y, Takaishi M, Kobayashi T, Abarzua F, Sakaguchi M, et al. Adenovirus-mediated REIC/Dkk-3 gene transfer inhibits tumor growth and metastasis in an orthotopic prostate cancer model. *Cancer Gene Ther* (2007) 14(9):765–72. doi: 10.1038/sj.cgt.7701071
11. Kobayashi K, Ouchida M, Tsuji T, Hanafusa H, Miyazaki M, Namba M, et al. Reduced expression of the REIC/Dkk-3 gene by promoter-hypermethylation in human tumor cells. *Gene* (2002) 282(1-2):151–8. doi: 10.1016/S0378-1119 (01)00838-1
12. Kurose K, Sakaguchi M, Nasu Y, Ebara S, Kaku H, Kariyama R, et al. Decreased expression of REIC/Dkk-3 in human renal clear cell carcinoma. *J Urol* (2004) 171(3):1314–8. doi: 10.1097/01.ju.0000101047.64379.d4
13. Tsuji T, Nozaki I, Miyazaki M, Sakaguchi M, Pu H, Hamazaki Y, et al. Antiproliferative activity of REIC/Dkk-3 and its significant down-regulation in non-small-cell lung carcinomas. *Biochem Biophys Res Commun* (2001) 289 (1):257–63. doi: 10.1006/bbrc.2001.5972
14. Nozaki I, Tsuji T, Iijima O, Ohmura Y, Andou A, Miyazaki M, et al. Reduced expression of REIC/Dkk-3 gene in non-small cell lung cancer. *Int J Oncol* (2001) 19(1):117–21. doi: 10.3892/ijo.19.1.117
15. Tanimoto R, Abarzua F, Sakaguchi M, Takaishi M, Nasu Y, Kumon H, et al. REIC/ Dkk-3 as a potential gene therapeutic agent against human testicular cancer. *Int J Mol Med* (2007) 19(3):363–8. doi: 10.3892/ijmm.19.3.363
16. Ding Z, Qian YB, Zhu LX, Xiong QR. Promoter methylation and mRNA expression of DKK-3 and WIF-1 in hepatocellular carcinoma. *World J Gastroenterol* (2009) 15(21):2595–601. doi: 10.3748/wjg.15.2595
17. Lee EJ, Jo M, Rho SB, Park K, Yoo YN, Park J, et al. Dkk3, downregulated in cervical cancer, functions as a negative regulator of beta-catenin. *Int J Cancer* (2009) 124(2):287–97. doi: 10.1002/ijc.23913
18. Xu XY, Xia P, Yu M, Nie XC, Yang X, Xing YN, et al. The roles of Dkk3 gene and its encoding product in gastric carcinoma. *Cell Cycle* (2012) 11(7):1414–31. doi: 10.4161/cc.19823
19. Colorectal cancer facts and figures. *Am Cancer Soc* (2005).

20. Yoshida D, Kono S, Moore MA, Toyomura K, Nagano J, Mizoue T, et al. Colorectal polypectomy and risk of colorectal cancer by subsite: the Fukuoka Colorectal Cancer study. *Jpn J Clin Oncol* (2007) 37(8):597–602. doi: 10.1093/jjco/hym065
21. Wang W, Zhu W, Xu XY, Nie XC, Yang X, Xing YN, et al. The clinicopathological significance of Dkk3 expression in colorectal carcinomas. *Histol Histopathol* (2012) 27(6):735–43. doi: 10.14670/HH-27.735
22. Shin JM, Choi DK, Kang HY, Sohn KC, Lee Y, Kim CD, et al. The expression pattern and functional role of REIC/Dkk-3 in the development of cutaneous squamous cell carcinoma. *J Dermatol Sci* (2016) 84(1):88–96. doi: 10.1016/j.jdermsci.2016.06.006
23. Yang L, Zhao S, Xia P, Zheng HC. Down-regulated Dkk3expression in lung carcinogenesis: a molecular target for gene therapy. *Histol Histopathol* (2018) 33(7):691–704. doi: 10.14670/HH-11-964
24. Veeck J, Wild PJ, Fuchs T, Schüffler PJ, Hartmann A, Knüchel R, et al. Prognostic relevance of Wnt-inhibitory factor-1 (WIF1) and Dickkopf-3 (DKK3) promoter methylation in human breast cancer. *BMC Cancer* (2009) 9:217. doi: 10.1186/1471-2407-9-217
25. Horikawa Y, Watanabe M, Sadahira T, Ariyoshi Y, Kobayashi Y, Araki M, et al. Overexpression of REIC/Dkk-3 suppresses the expression of CD147 and inhibits the proliferation of human bladder cancer cells. *Oncol Lett* (2017) 14 (3):3223–8. doi: 10.3892/ol.2017.6548
26. Pang Q, Hu W, Zhang X, Pang M. Wnt/β-Catenin signaling pathway-related proteins (DKK-3, β-Catenin, and c-MYC) are involved in prognosis of nasopharyngeal carcinoma. *Cancer Biother Radiopharm* (2019) 34(7):436–43. doi: 10.1089/cbr.2019.2771
27. Hoang BH, Kubo T, Healey JH, Yang R, Nathan SS, Kolb EA, et al. Dickkopf 3 inhibits invasion and motility of Saos-2 osteosarcoma cells by modulating the Wnt-beta-catenin pathway. *Cancer Res* (2004) 64(8):2734–9. doi: 10.1158/0008-5472.CAN-03-1952
28. Kuphal S, Lodermeyer S, Bataille F, Schuierer M, Hoang BH, Bosserhoff AK. Expression of Dickkopf genes is strongly reduced in malignant melanoma. *Oncogene* (2006) 25(36):5027–36. doi: 10.1038/sj.onc.1209508
29. Than SS, Kataoka K, Sakaguchi M, Murata H, Abarzua F, Taketa C, et al. Intraperitoneal administration of an adenovirus vector carrying REIC/Dkk-3 suppresses peritoneal dissemination of scirrhous gastric carcinoma. *Oncol Rep* (2011) 25(4):989–95. doi: 10.3892/or.2011.1149
30. Zenzmaier C, Sklepos L, Berger P. Increase of Dkk-3 blood plasma levels in the elderly. *Exp Gerontol* (2008) 43(9):867–70. doi: 10.1016/j.exger.2008.05.012
31. Safari E, Mosayebi G, Khorram S. Dkk-3 as a potential biomarker for diagnosis and prognosis of colorectal cancer. *Med J Islam Repub Iran* (2018) 32:86. doi: 10.14196/mjiri.32.86
32. Jiang T, Huang L, Wang S, Zhang S. Clinical significance of serum Dkk-3 in patients with gynecological cancer. *J Obstet Gynaecol Res* (2010) 36(4):769–73. doi: 10.1111/j.1447-0756.2010.01234.x
33. Zhang K, Watanabe M, Kashiwakura Y, Li SA, Edamura K, Huang P, et al. Expression pattern of REIC/Dkk-3 in various cell types and the implications of the soluble form in prostatic acinar development. *Int J Oncol* (2010) 37 (6):1495–501. doi: 10.3892/ijo_00000802
34. Nakamura RE, Hackam AS. Analysis of Dickkopf3 interactions with Wnt signaling receptors. *Growth factors (Chur Switzerland)* (2010) 28(4):232–42. doi: 10.3109/08977191003738832
35. Yue W, Sun Q, Dacic S, Landreneau RJ, Siegfried JM, Yu J, et al. Downregulation of Dkk3 activates beta-catenin/TCF-4 signaling in lung cancer. *Carcinogenesis* (2008) 29(1):84–92. doi: 10.1093/carcin/bgm267
36. Ochiai K, Watanabe M, Ueki H, Huang P, Fujii Y, Nasu Y, et al. Tumor suppressor REIC/ Dkk-3 interacts with the dynein light chain, Tctex-1. *Biochem Biophys Res Commun* (2011) 412(2):391–5. doi: 10.1016/j.bbrc.2011.07.109
37. Sakaguchi M, Kataoka K, Abarzua F, Tanimoto R, Watanabe M, Murata H, et al. Overexpression of REIC/Dkk-3 in normal fibroblasts suppresses tumor growth via induction of interleukin-7. *J Biol Chem* (2009) 284(21):14236–44. doi: 10.1074/jbc.M808002200
38. Laphanuwat P, Jirawatnotai S. Immunomodulatory roles of cell cycle regulators. *Front Cell Dev Biol* (2019) 7:23. doi: 10.3389/fcell.2019.00023
39. D'Arcy MS. Cell death: a review of the major forms of apoptosis, necrosis and autophagy. *Cell Biol Int* (2019) 43(6):582 92. doi: 10.1002/cbin.11137
40. Aiello NM, Kang Y. Context-dependent EMT programs in cancer metastasis. *J Exp Med* (2019) 216(5):1016–26. doi: 10.1084/jem.20181827
41. Ferrari N, Ranftl R, Chicherova I, Slaven ND, Moeendarbary E, Farrugia AJ, et al. Dickkopf-3 links HSF1 and YAP/TAZ signalling to control aggressive behaviours in cancer-associated fibroblasts. *Nat Commun* (2019) 10:130. doi: 10.1038/s41467-018-07987-0
42. Zhou L, Husted H, Moore T, Lu M, Deng D, Liu Y, et al. Suppression of stromal-derived Dickkopf-3 (DKK3) inhibits tumor progression and prolongs survival in pancreatic ductal adenocarcinoma. *Sci Transl Med* (2018) 10 (464):3487. doi: 10.1126/scitranslmed.aat3487
43. Zenzmaier C, Sampson N, Plas E, Berger P. Dickkopf-related protein 3 promotes pathogenic stromal remodeling in benign prostatic hyperplasia and prostate cancer. *Prostate* (2013) 73(13):1441–52. doi: 10.1002/pros.22691

14

MiR-21-5p Induces Pyroptosis in Colorectal Cancer *via* TGFBI

Rilei Jiang[1†], Xiaolei Chen[1†], Shaohua Ge[2†], Qin Wang[3], Yichang Liu[2], Haijun Chen[2], Jiatuo Xu[1] and Jiang Wu[2*]*

[1] School of Basic Medicine Science, Shanghai University of Traditional Chinese Medicine, Shanghai, China, [2] Department of Oncology, Kunshan Hospital of Traditional Chinese Medicine Affiliated to Nanjing University of Chinese Medicine, Kunshan, China, [3] First Clinical Medical College, Nanjing Medical University, Nanjing, China

***Correspondence:**
Jiatuo Xu
xjt@fudan.edu.cn
Jiang Wu
wujiangkunshan@163.com

[†]These authors have contributed equally to this work

Pyroptosis is a distinct form of programmed cell death in eukaryotic cells that has garnered increasing attention in cancer-related research. Moreover, although miR-21 has been reported as abnormally expressed in colorectal cancer, due to a lack of in-depth research on the transcriptional regulation mechanisms of miR-21, its clinical usage remains limited. Our study is the first, to our knowledge, to compare the clinical manifestations and laboratory phenotypes associated with miR-21-3p and miR-21-5p. Morphologically, the transfection of miR-21-3p or miR-21-5p inhibitors, as well as miR-21-5p mimics into HCT-116 and HT-29 cell lines, induced cell death. Surprisingly, overexpression of miR-21-5p induced cell death more strongly than its knockdown. Mechanistic studies of miR-21-5p overexpression revealed that various inflammatory factors including IL-1β and IL-18 were released, while pyroptosis-associated mRNAs were upregulated and proteins were activated. Moreover, miR-21-5p was found to act as a downstream factor to significantly and directly regulate transforming growth factor beta-induced (*TGFB1*). Specifically, miR-21-5p overexpression caused downregulation of *TGFBI*, which may have led to pyroptosis. Collectively, we revealed that miR-21-5p induces pyroptosis in colorectal cancer *via TGFBI* regulation, thereby providing important mechanistic insights into its antitumor effects and expanding its potential for clinical applications.

Keywords: colorectal cancer, pyroptosis, programmed cell death, TGFBI, miR-21

INTRODUCTION

Colorectal cancer (CRC) was among the most common cancers diagnosed in men and women in 2019 (1); while the difficulties associated with its early detection, as well as its strong tendency for metastasis, and resistance to conventional therapies (2–4) makes its treatment challenging. In fact, in 2015, approximately 376,300 new CRC cases were reported with an estimated 191,000 associated mortalities in China alone (5).

Pyroptosis is recognised as a distinct form of programmed cell death in eukaryotic cells (6), and has recently become a new frontier in cancer-associated research (7). Pyroptosis is characterised by cell swelling with large bubbles emerging from the plasma membrane (8). In cells undergoing pyroptosis, mature caspase-1 cleaves a protein from the gasdermin family and activates inflammatory cytokines, such as IL-18 and IL-1β7, which recruit inflammatory cells and expand the inflammatory response (9).

Programmed cell death (PCD) depends on specific genes encoding proteins associated with various signalling pathways or functions (8). Regarding pyroptosis specifically, studies on its underlying mechanisms have primarily focused on non-coding RNAs (ncRNAs), such as long non-coding RNAs (lncRNAs) and microRNAs (miRNAs), that are upstream of both the canonical and noncanonical inflammasome pathways. For instance, knockdown of lncRNA RP1–85F18.6, which represents a tumour promoter in CRC, decreases the expression of ΔNp63 and inhibits tumour growth and metastases by inducing pyroptosis (10). Moreover, metformin has been reported to induce pyroptosis of oesophageal carcinoma cells through the miR-497/PELP1 axis (11). MiRNA-214 also induces pyroptosis in glioma cells by targeting caspase 1 (12). Although some studies have reported on the role of pyroptosis in various cancers, compared to the detailed mechanisms reported for other types of PCD, such as apoptosis, those related to pyroptosis are lacking with only the proverbial tip of the iceberg exposed. Hence, the detailed mechanism underlying pyroptosis in cancer requires further elucidation.

Generally, miRNAs repress the expression of target genes by binding to complementary sequences at the 3′UTR of mRNAs to prevent their translation (13). Since the discovery of miRNAs two decades ago, their biological functions have been extensively studied (14), particularly in the field of cancer. miR-21, specifically, has been extensively studied in various diseases, including renal fibrosis (15), hepatocellular carcinoma (16), atherogenesis (17), and cancer. In fact, miR-21 has been reported as overexpressed in many cancerous tissues compared to normal tissues and was briefly recognised as an onco-predictive biomarker (18, 19). However, due to a lack of in-depth understanding of miR-21 transcriptional regulatory mechanisms, target genes, and associated mechanisms, the clinical application of miR-21 is limited.

As a precursor, pre-miR-21 is processed by an RNase III complex to generate two mature miRNAs, namely, miR-21-3p and miR-21-5p (20). Currently, reports on CRC have primarily focused on miR-21-5p (guide strand), with the most commonly reporting pathways being those associated with the miR-21-5p/PTEN-regulatory networks which seem to intersect with the PI3K/Akt pathway (21, 22). However, minimal research has been undertaken on miR-21-3p in CRC or on the comparison of miR-21-3p and miR-21-5p networks in the context of CRC.

In this study, we first compared the clinical manifestations and laboratory phenotypes of miR-21-3p and miR-21-5p in CRC cells. The overexpression of miR-21-5p was found to induce cell death more strongly than its knockdown. Meanwhile, mechanistically, inflammatory factors were observed to be released, thereby activating pyroptosis. Downstream analysis further determined that miR-21-5p directly downregulates *TGFBI* leading to subsequent pyroptosis.

MATERIALS AND METHODS

Reagents, Cell Lines, and Clinical Tissues

HCT-116 and HT-29 cell lines were purchased from Shanghai Zhong Qiao Xin Zhou Biotechnology Co. Ltd. (Shanghai, China). The 293T cell line was provided by Stem Cell Bank, Chinese Academy of Sciences (Shanghai, China). Human colonic epithelial cells (HCECs) were kindly provided by the Traditional Chinese Medicine Hospital of Kunshan (Kuanshan, China). The HCECs, HCT-116 and 293T cells were cultured in DMEM-high glucose (HyClone, USA) supplemented with 10% foetal bovine serum (FBS; Gibco, South America) and 1% penicillin/streptomycin (P/S; Gibco, Australia). HT-29 cells were cultured in McCoy's 5A (Gibco, Australia) with 10% FBS and 1% P/S.

Five colon cancer patients were random selected from the Department of Oncology, Kunshan Hospital of Traditional Chinese Medicine Affiliated with Nanjing University of Chinese Medicine. Patient demographic information is provided in **Supplementary Table 6**. From each patient, tissues were obtained from colonic tumours as well as from adjacent normal tissue (2 cm away from tumour). All protocols were approved by the Ethics Review Committee of Kunshan Hospital of Traditional Chinese Medicine (Approval No: KZY2017-16).

Plasmid Construction and Cell Transfection

The mimics and inhibitors for hsa-miR-21-3p, hsa-miR-21-5p, and non-specific control (NC; **Supplementary Table 1**) were constructed by Genomeditech Co. (Shanghai, China). Three individual short hairpin RNA plasmids for *TGFB1* (sh-TGFBI-1, sh-TGFBI-2, and sh-TGFBI-3) and a negative control (sh-NC) (**Supplementary Table 2**) were purchased from Genomeditech Co. (Shanghai, China). The wild-type and mutant type dual-luciferase reporter plasmids (**Supplementary Table 3**), constructed using pmirGLO vector, were also purchased from Genomeditech Co. (Shanghai, China). The plasmids were transfected according to the manufacturer's instructions using Lipofectamine 2000 (Invitrogen, USA).

qRT-PCR

Total RNA was extracted using TRIzol reagent (Invitrogen). Next, miRNA quantification was performed using miRNA First Strand cDNA Synthesis (Stem-loop Method; Sangon Biotech, Shanghai, China) and the microRNA qPCR Kit (SYBR Green Method; Sangon Biotech, Shanghai, China). Quantification of mRNA was performed as previously described (23). The amount of cDNA template used in each reaction was between 20~200 ng (10 μl). The reaction conditions were as follows: denaturation at 95°C for 5 min (Hot-Start) followed by 40 cycles of amplification at 95°C for 10 s and 60°C for 30 s. Ct values between 20 and 30 were regarded as valid results. The primer sequences used are listed in **Supplementary Table 4**. The value of $2^{-\Delta\Delta CT}$ was used for analysis. *GAPDH* was used as internal control mRNA, U6 was used as an internal control for miRNA.

Western Blot Analysis

The proteins were isolated using a radio-immunoprecipitation assay (RIPA) protein extraction reagent (Beyotime, Shanghai, China) with 1% phenylmethanesulfonyl fluoride (PMSF, Beyotime). Next, proteins were suspended in 10%–15% SDS-PAGE gels (Beyotime) and transferred to PVDF membranes

(Invitrogen), followed by incubation with the following primary antibodies: Caspase-1 (1:1,000, #3866, CST, USA), cleaved Caspase-1 (1:1,000, #4199, CST, USA), GSDMD (1:1,000, #93709, CST, USA), cleaved GSDMD (1:1,000, #36425, CST, USA), interleukin (IL)-1β (1:1,000, #12703, CST, USA), cleaved IL-1β (1:1,000, #83186, CST, USA), TGFBI (1:500, 10188-1-AP, Proteintech, Wuhan, China), and β-actin (1:2,000, #4970, CST, USA).

Cell Counting Kit-8 Assay

The viability of CRC cells was assayed using the Cell Counting Kit-8 (CCK-8; Dojindo, Beijing, China) assay. After transfecting cells with mimics or inhibitors, 5×10^3 cells/well were seeded in a 96-well plate, with 100 μl of suspension in each well. After culturing for 24 h, the cells were stained with CCK-8 solution and incubated for 30 min. Cell viability was calculated after measuring the absorbance at 450 nm.

TUNEL Assay Analysis

Cells cultured in confocal dishes were fixed with 4% paraformaldehyde for 20 min and were subsequently stained with the TUNEL kit on ice followed the manufacturer's protocol (One-step TUNEL Detection Kit, Beyotime, Shanghai, China). TUNEL-positive cells were counted under a laser scanning confocal microscope (Leica, TCS SP5, Germany).

Flow Cytometric Analysis

The FITC-Annexin V apoptosis detection kit (MEILUN, Dalian, China) was used to detect the cell apoptosis ratio according to the manufacturer's protocol. In brief, the CRC cells were double-stained with propidium iodide (PI) and Annexin V for 30 min in the dark. The cell apoptosis ratio was then detected using a FACS ARIA II SORP Flow Cytometer (BD, USA).

ELISA Assays

IL-1β and IL-18 levels in the cell culture medium were detected by using a Human IL-1β High Sensitivity ELISA kit (EK101BHS-01, Multi Science, China) and Human IL-18 ELISA kit (EK118-01, Multi Science, China), according to the manufacturer's instructions. The optical density was measured at a wavelength of 450 nm, while measurement at 570 nm were screened as an internal control.

Immunofluorescence

Cells were treated with 4% buffered paraformaldehyde for 20 min at room temperature. Next, 1% BSA and 0.1% Triton-X were used to block the membrane for 2 h at room temperature. The membranes were then treated with primary antibodies against ASC/TMS1 (1:200, 10500-1-AP, Proteintech, Wuhan, China) or TGFBI (1:200, 10188-1-AP, Proteintech, Wuhan, China) at 4°C overnight. The secondary antibody (anti-rabbit IgG (H+L), F (ab')2 fragment (Alexa Fluor® 488 Conjugate, #4412, CST, US), or anti-rabbit IgG (H+L), F(ab')2 Fragment (Alexa Fluor® 594 Conjugate, #8889, CST, US) were added to the cells for 1 h at room temperature. Cells were incubated with Antifade Mounting Medium with 4',6-Diamidine-2'-phenylindole dihydrochloride (DAPI; Beyotime, Shanghai, China) to detect ASC specks or TGFBI expression and distribution using a laser scanning confocal microscope (Leica, TCS SP5, Germany).

Dual-Luciferase Reporter Assays

The fragments of wild-type and mutant type *TGFBI* were amplified by PCR and cloned into a pmirGLO Dual-Luciferase miRNA Target Expression Vector (Promega, USA) to generate pmirGLO-TGFBI-wt and pmirGLO-TGFBI-mut reporter vectors. The above vectors with miR-21-5p mimics and NC mimics were co-transfected into 293T, HCT-116, and HT-29 cells by Lipofectamine 2000 (Invitrogen, US). Finally, the cells were lysed using the Dual-Luciferase Reporter Assay System (Promega, USA) and luciferase activity was detected. Renilla luciferase activity was used as an internal control.

Statistical Analysis

Experimental groups were compared with controls using the Student unpaired, two-tailed *t*-test. Multiple groups were expressed as mean ± SD and analysed by Kruskal-Wallis analysis. $P < 0.05$ was considered as statistically significant. Graph Pad Prism 6.0 was used for statistical analysis.

RESULTS

miR-21-3p and miR-21-5p Expression in CRC and Model Establishment

By using clinical colon tissues from CRC patients' tumours (n = 5) and adjacent normal tissues (n = 5), we found that the expression of miR-21-3p did not differ significantly between the normal and tumour tissues, while miR-21-5p was more highly expressed in the tumours (**Figure 1A**). Similarly, the expression of miR-21-3p was low in the CRC cell lines while that of miR-21-5p showed a high expression trend in the HT29 and HCT116 cells by PCR (**Figure 1B**). To further investigate the roles of these miRNAs in CRC, we constructed miR-21-3p/miR-21-5p mimics and inhibitor vectors. After transfection of these vectors, the expression levels of the two miRNAs changed as expected, mimicking the results described above (**Figures 1C, D**).

Overexpression of miR-21-5p Induced Cell Death and Repressed Cell Viability in the CRC Cells Lines

In an attempt to identify the precise roles of miR-21-3p and miR-21-5p in CRC cells, we transfected the miR-21-3p/miR-21-5p mimics and inhibitor vectors into HCT-116 and HT-29 CRC cells. TUNEL staining showed that transfection of miR-21-3p inhibitors and miR-21-5p mimics induced nuclear fragmentation in both the HCT-116 and HT-29 cells, while other transfections did not have an effect (**Figure 2A**). Flow cytometric analysis also indicated that the death rate of CRC cells was upregulated in the treated with the miR-21-5p mimic (**Figures 2B, C**). Meanwhile, the cell counting kit-8 assay showed that the miR-21-5p mimic reduced the cell viability while the other groups had less of an impact on the CRC cells (**Figure 2D**).

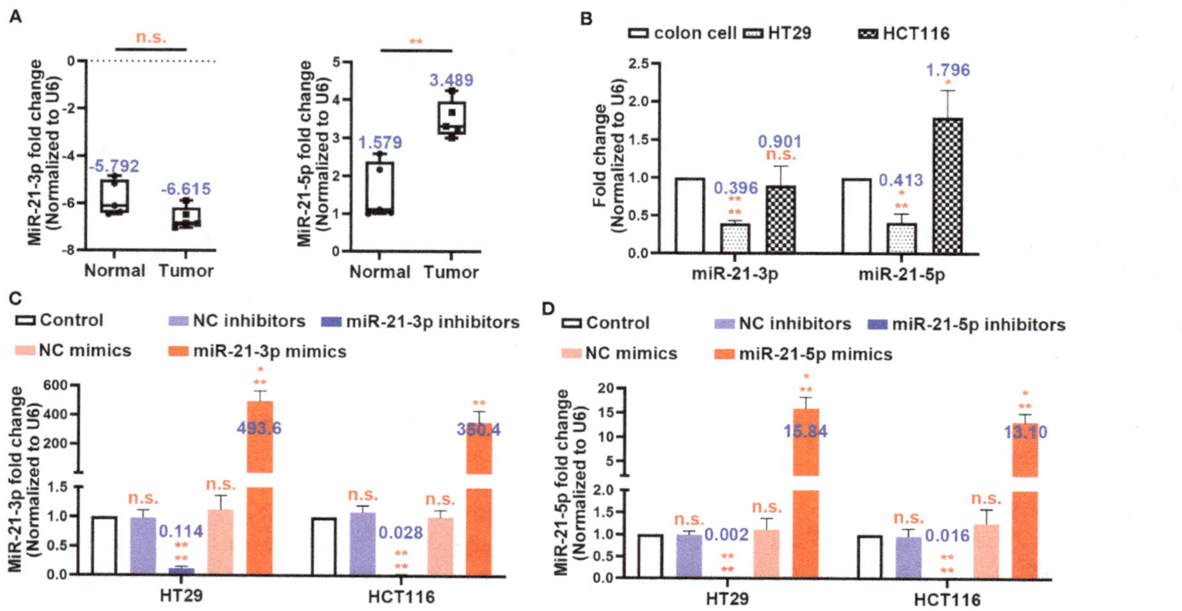

FIGURE 1 | MiR-21-3p and miR-21-5p expression in colorectal cancer (CRC) and model establishment. **(A)** The expression levels of miR-21-3p and miR-21-5p in CRC patients' tumours (n = 5) and normal tissues (n = 5). **(B)** The expression levels of miR-21-3p and miR-21-5p in normal colon cell, HT29, and HCT116. **(C, D)** Validation of miR-21-3p mimics/inhibitors **(C)** and miR-21-5p mimics/inhibitors **(D)** efficiency in HT29 and HCT116 cells as determined by qRT-PCR. The bars and error bars indicate the mean ± SD. n.s.p > 0.05, *p < 0.05, **p < 0.01, ***p < 0.005, ****p < 0.001.

Evidence that the miR-21-5p Pathway Induces Pyroptosis in CRC Cells

In an attempt to determine the mechanism of cell death, we assayed inflammation-related indicators in the cell culture medium. Interestingly, the levels of IL-1β and IL-18 were significantly upregulated in the cells transformed with the miR-21-5p mimic compared to the other plasmids in both the HT29 and HCT116 cell lines (**Figure 3A**). As pyroptosis was the most immune-related cell death method, we detected pyroptosis-associated mRNAs and proteins. As suspected, the mRNAs related to pyroptosis were upregulated in the miR-21-5p transformed cells (**Figure 3B**) as were the cleavage products of caspase 1, IL-1β, and GSDMD (**Figures 3C, D**), indicating that the pyroptosis signalling pathway was activated. Furthermore, ASC oligomerization, as detect by immunofluorescence was apparent as ASC specks in cells transfected with miR-21-5p mimic (**Figure 3E**). It provided the final piece of evidence to pyroptosis.

TGF-β1 Is a Potential Target of miR-21-5p

To further elucidate the molecular mechanism underlying how miR-21-5p exerts its effect on pyroptosis in CRC cells, we used bioinformatic tools to predict candidate downstream targets. After applying a target score ≥ 90, we identified 70 candidate targets (**Figure 4A**; **Supplementary Table 5**) and performed PCR to verify the target with the most potential using the more stringent inclusion criteria of a target score ≥ 98 in the HT29 and HCT116 cells (**Figure 4B**). The *TGFBI* mRNA was extremely changed following the variation tendency of complementary base pairing (**Figure 4B**). An analysis of data from the Cancer Genome Atlas (TCGA) demonstrated that higher *TGFBI* levels in CRC patients were always associated with poor overall survival and disease-free survival outcomes (**Figure 4C**). Moreover, western blotting analysis revealed that TGFBI expression increased as miR-21-5p decreased, and vice versa in the HT29 and HCT116 cells (**Figure 4D**). Meanwhile, immunofluorescence confirmed the western blot results (**Figure 4E**). Thus, we suspect that TGFBI is a potential target influenced by miR-21-5p.

Binding Sites Between miR-21-5p and TGFBI and the Function of TGFBI in Pyroptosis

With the rigorous bioinformatic prediction, we sub-cloned the wild-type (WT) or mutated-type (MUT) binding regions (predicted to have miR-21-5p binding sites; **Supplementary Table 3**) of *TGFBI* mRNA downstream of the firefly luciferase gene in the pmirGLO vector (**Figure 5A**). The evaluation of luciferase activity after co-transfection of cells with the miRNA mimics and luciferase plasmids revealed that overexpression of miR-21-5p significantly reduced the luciferase activity of pmirGLO-WT in the HT29, HCT116, and 293T cell lines (**Figure 5B**).

To further demonstrate the function of TGFBI, we constructed three short hairpin RNA plasmids to knockdown *TGFBI* (sequences are listed in **Supplementary Table 2**), and selected the knockdown efficiency of sh-TGFBI-3 as the best (**Figure 5C**). The qRT-PCR and western blot assays for HT29 and HCT116 cells with knockdown *TGFBI* revealed an

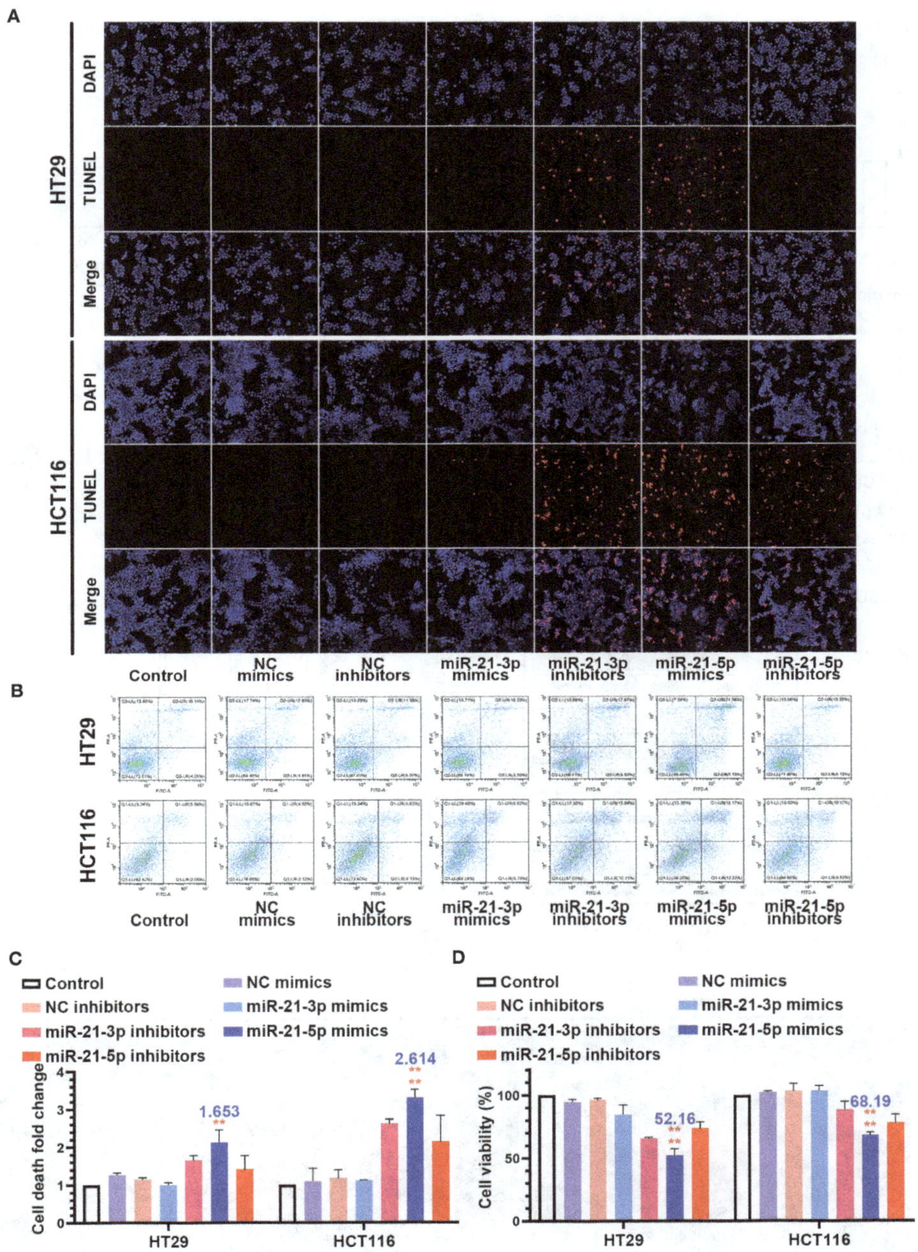

FIGURE 2 | Overexpression of miR-21-5p induced cell death and repress cell viability in colorectal cancer (CRC) cells lines. **(A)** HT29 and HCT116 cells were transferred by miR-21-3p/miR-21-5p mimics and inhibitors, and cell death was determined by TUNEL stain assay. **(B, C)** Annexin V and PI staining flow cytometric analysis of cell death in miR-21-3p/miR-21-5p mimic and inhibitor transfected HT29 and HCT116 cells. **(D)** CCK-8 assay of HT29 and HCT116 cell viability changes with miR-21-3p/miR-21-5p mimics and inhibitors transfection. The bars and error bars indicate the mean ± SD. **p < 0.01, ****p < 0.001.

overexpression of pyroptosis-associated mRNA (**Figure 5D**) and further cleavage of pyroptosis-related proteins (**Figures 5E, F**). Functionally, the TUNEL staining assay demonstrated that transfection of sh-TGFBI-3 exacerbated cell death (**Figure 5G**), while immunofluorescence of ASC specks demonstrated that cell death was primarily caused by pyroptosis (**Figure 5H**).

DISCUSSION

In this study, we compared miR-21-3p and miR-21-5p expression in CRC tissues and cell lines. The miR-21-5p levels in the patients' tissues and HCT116 cells were significantly higher when compared to the other groups, however, the same

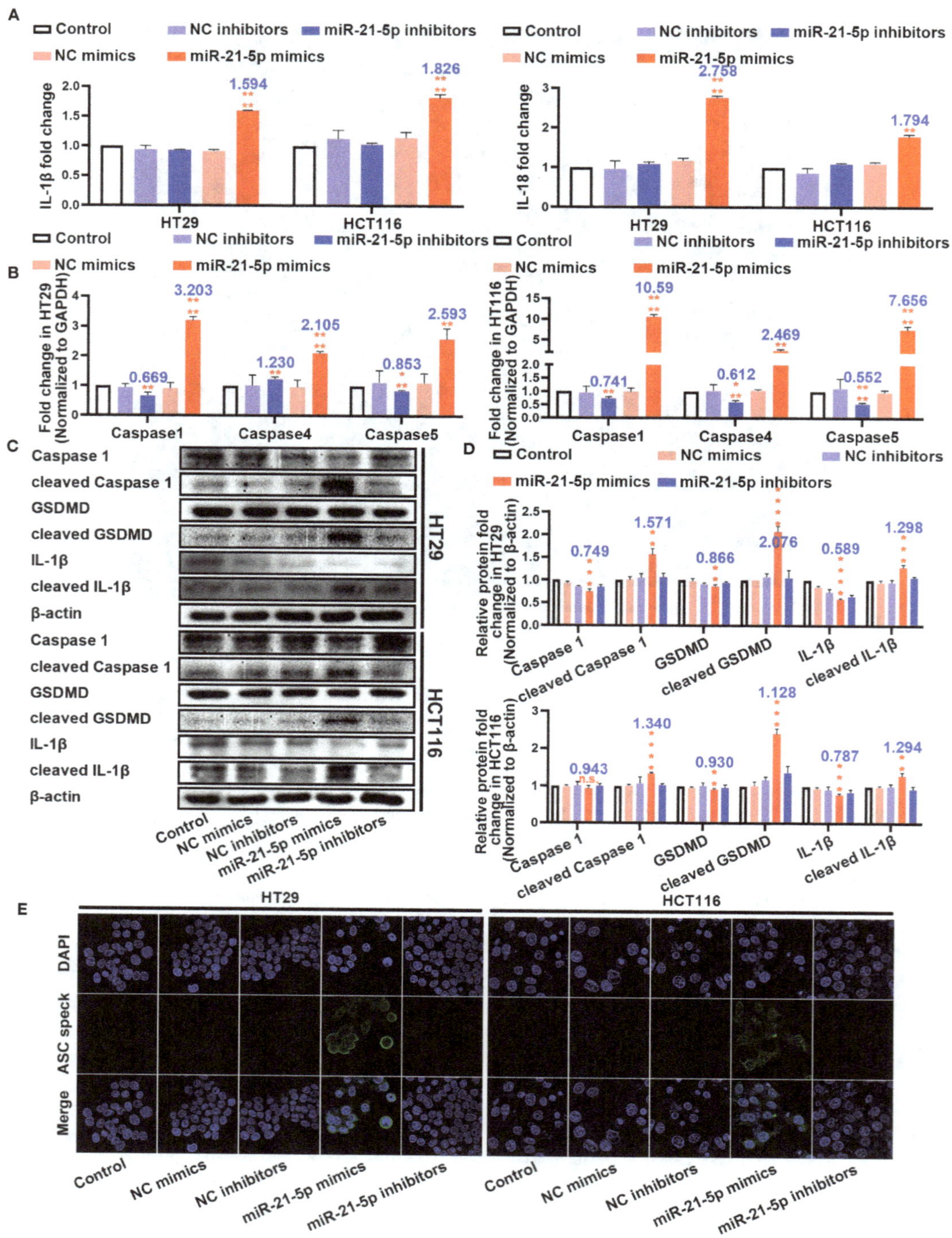

FIGURE 3 | Pathway evidence of miR-21-5p induced pyroptosis of colorectal cancer (CRC) cells. **(A)** ELISA assay tested the IL-1β and IL-18 which released in HT29 and HCT116 cell culture mediums by the transfection of miR-21-5p mimics and inhibitors. **(B)** Pyroptosis-associated mRNA levels in HT29 and HCT116 cells after miR-21-5p mimics and inhibitors transfection as determined by qRT-PCR. **(C, D)** Expression of Pyroptosis-associated proteins in HT29 and HCT116 cells after miR-21-5p mimics and inhibitors transfection as determined by western blot analysis. **(E)** Immunofluorescence staining of ASC specks expression in miR-21-5p mimics and inhibitors transfected HT29 and HCT116 cells. The bars and error bars indicate the mean ± SD. n.s.p > 0.05, **p < 0.01, ***p < 0.005, ****p < 0.001.

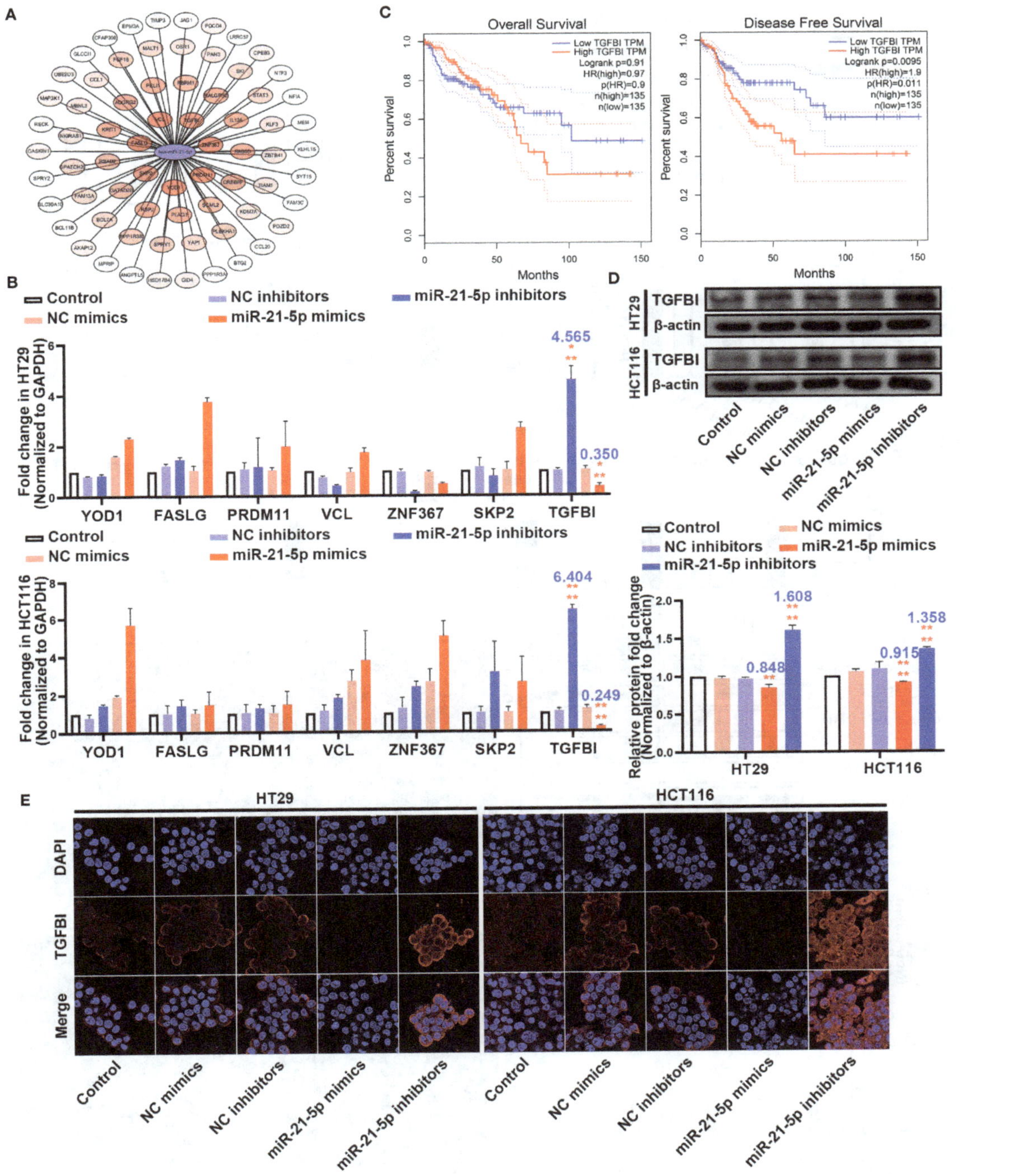

FIGURE 4 | TGFBI is a potential target of miR-21-5p. **(A)** Bioinformatic prediction for candidate downstream targets of miR-21-5p. **(B)** Verification of miR-21-5p downstream targets by qRT-PCR in HT29 and HCT116. **(C)** Association of TGFBI expression with colorectal cancer (CRC) patient disease-free survival and overall survival. The areas between the same colour dotted lines represent 95% confidence interval for low/high TGFBI. **(D)** TGFBI expression in miR-21-5p mimics and inhibitors transfected HT29 and HCT116 cells as determined by western blot analysis. **(E)** Immunofluorescence staining of TGFBI expression in miR-21-5p mimics and inhibitors transfected HT29 and HCT116 cells. The bars and error bars indicate the mean ± SD. n.s.p > 0.05, **p < 0.01, ***p < 0.005, ****p < 0.001.

effect was not observed in HT29 cells. This is consistent with the findings of a previous study (23). Surprisingly, we found that phenotypically CRC cell death was induced when the miR-21-3p inhibitor and miR-21-5p mimic/inhibitor were transfected into cells. In a previous CRC study, the apoptotic mechanism induced *via* inhibition of miR-21-3p was considered to be associated with multiple splicing through the Smad4/extra cellular signal-regulated protein kinase signalling pathway (24). There have

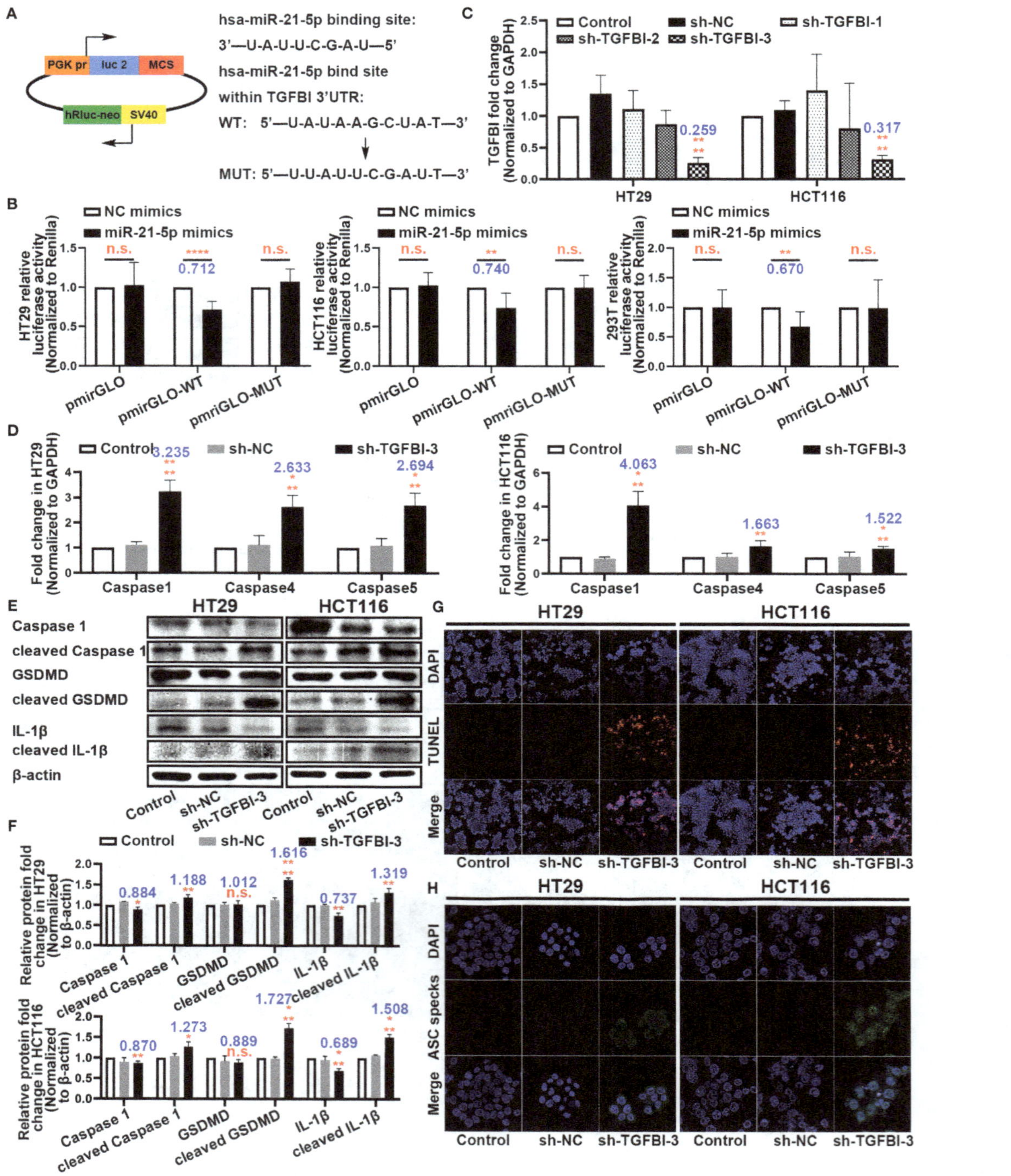

FIGURE 5 | Binding sites between miR-21-5p and TGFBI and function research of TGFBI in pyroptosis. **(A)** Predicted binding sites for miR-21-5p on TGFBI and a diagram depicting the construction of the wild-type (WT) and mutant type (MUT) pmirGLO plasmids. **(B)** 293T, HT29, and HCT116 cells were co-transfected with miR-21-5p/NC mimics and pmirGLO/pmirGLO-WT/pmirGLO-MUT plasmids. Luciferase activity was detected 24 h after transfection using a dual-luciferase assay. **(C)** Validation of TGFBI sh-RNA knockdown efficiency in HT29 and HCT116 cells as determined by qRT-PCR. **(D)** Pyroptosis-associated mRNA levels in HT29 and HCT116 cells after sh-TGFBI-3 transfection as determined by qRT-PCR. **(E–F)** Expression of Pyroptosis-associated proteins in HT29 and HCT116 cells after sh-TGFBI-3 transfection as determined by western blot analysis. **(G)** TUNEL stain assay of cell death in sh-TGFBI-3 transferred HT29 and HCT116 cells. **(H)** Immunofluorescence staining of ASC specks expression in sh-TGFBI-3 transfected HT29 and HCT116 cells.The bars and error bars indicate the mean ± SD. n.s. $p > 0.05$, *$p < 0.05$, **$p < 0.01$, ***$p < 0.005$, ****$p < 0.001$.

also been various studies on miR-21-5p (25–27), however, currently the consensus is that repressing miR-21-5p suppresses proliferation and promotes apoptosis by modulating the PTEN/PI3K/AKT pathway (21, 22). Surprisingly, the miR-21-5p mimic also induced cell death and had a stronger effect than the miR-21-5p inhibitor. We, therefore, designed subsequent experiments based on these observations.

Various types of cell death have been discovered in cancers. The immunogenicity of cancer cells is an emerging determinant of anticancer immunotherapy (28). Recently, investigators have focused on the immunobiology of dying cancer cells and attempted to determine their relevance for the success of anticancer therapies (29–31). To verify whether miR-21-5p activates the immune responses associated with cell death, we investigated the levels of IL-1β and IL-18 and found that only miR-21-5p mimic upregulated inflammatory factors, suggesting that miR-21-5p-induced cell death occurs *via* a completely different mechanism from the apoptosis induced by the inhibitors. Interestingly, qRT-PCR revealed that caspase 1, caspase 4, and caspase 5 mRNA were upregulated, while western blot analysis showed that the caspase 1, GSDMD, and IL-1β proteins were cleaved; both of which indicate activation of the pyroptosis pathway.

Pyroptosis was previously referred to as caspase-1-induced PCD process (32). The induction factors of pyroptosis were regarded as immunopathological, including a range of microbial infections and non-infectious stimuli, such as host factors (33). The question then became how miR-21-5p induces pyroptosis in CRC cells. Accordingly, we screened the potential targets of miR-21-5p and used qRT-PCR to identify the genes with a target score ≥ 98. TGFBI was found to strongly follow the miRNA regulatory mechanism. Previously, TGFBI was considered to be a high-risk factor for increased incidence of spontaneous tumours in gastrointestinal tract cancers (34). In addition, mechanistic studies have shown that TGFBI is strongly associated with chemotherapy in NSCLC (35) and ovarian cancer (36). Similarly, the data from TCGA showed high expression of TGFBI in CRC patients, often resulting in low survival. In addition, western blot and immunofluorescence showed a high degree of consistency with the TGFBI qRT-PCR results, while dual-luciferase reporter assays in three cell lines suggested direct binding between miR-21-5p and mRNA of TGFBI.

As the nomenclature implies, TGFBI was first identified as a TGF-β-inducible gene (37), which has since been reported to regulate the premetastatic activity of TGF-β in some cancers (38, 39). In breast cancer research, distant metastases tend to develop when TGFBI and CD44 were expressed at high levels (40), which verifies the relationship between TGFBI and immune responses. Moreover, a previous report on CRC highlighted that TGFBI promotes metastasis by enhancing cell extravasation (41). In our study, with the establishment of the TGFBI-knockdown model, pyroptosis-associated mRNAs were upregulated and showed high levels of cleavage; whereas, the TUNEL assay further corroborated the presence of pyroptosis cell death.

However, pyroptosis cannot occur without inflammasome sensors. Inflammasome complexes become assembled upon activation of certain nucleotide-binding domain, leucine-rich repeat-containing proteins (NLR), AIM2-like receptors, or pyrin. Of these, NLRP1, NLRP3, NLRC4, NLRP6, and AIM2 influence the pathogenesis of cancer using various mechanisms of action (42). Specifically, NLRP3, which assembles the NLRP3-ASC-Caspase-1 inflammasome complex, activates pyroptosis of CRC cells (43). Meanwhile, the NAIP-NLRC4 inflammasome complex can also induce caspase-1-dependent cleavage of IL-1β, IL-18, and the pore-forming protein, gasdermin, D, leading to pyroptosis (44). However, recent studies demonstrated that the regulation and suppression of NLRC4 is not always consistent between cancer models or even within the same CRC model (45, 46). Still further, AIM2 has been reported as exhibiting tumour-suppressive functions in colon cancer (47) by suppressing the PI3K/AKT pathways to inhibit proliferation of colonic stem cells and promote cell death (48, 49). In our study, various inflammatory indicators, including IL-1β and IL-18 were upregulated and ACS specks were observed. These results provide evidence for the activation of the NLRP3-ASC-Caspase-1 inflammasome complex; however, the precise inflammasome sensor that becomes activated by miR-21-5p requires further exploration.

The first reported research on miR-21 in CRC was 13 years ago (50). Several clinical researchers have since performed miRNA microarray expression analysis between colon adenocarcinoma and normal tissues, and have reported high levels of miR-21 to be associated with poor survival and poor therapeutic outcome (51). Even the precursory clinical statistics of prognostic and predictive value of a miRNA signature in stage II colon cancer declared that miR-21-5p is strongly relevant to CRC (52). However, the precise role of miR-21-5p remains to be characterised. In other words, it is necessary to determine if miR-21-5p is simply a characteristic of tumours, or if it promotes CRC as the malignancy grade of CRC has been found to be positively correlated with the level of miR-21-5p.

In conclusion, our data demonstrated that overexpression of miR-21-5p could induce pyroptosis in CRC cells. Moreover, TGFBI may serve as an intermediate of this biological process. But the further mechanism of TGFBI in pyroptosis still unknown. Especially, the inflammasome sensor of the biological progress is the next focus point in our study. Furthermore, the mechanism certification on animal model and even on clinic is the next step on our scheme.

Combined with previous studies, we believe that miR-21-5p plays a distinct role in CRC. The sensitivity of CRC cells to the level of miR-21-5p is highly expressed *in vitro*. Thus, it might be suggested that miR-21-5p has great potential as a therapeutic target in CRC, however, the mechanism requires further elucidation.

ETHICS STATEMENT

The studies involving human participants were reviewed and approved by Ethics Committee of Kunshan Hospital of Traditional Chinese Medicine. The patients/participants provided their written informed consent to participate in this study.

AUTHOR CONTRIBUTIONS

JX and JW conceived of the study and provided the project direction. RJ guided the experiments, analyzed the data, and wrote the manuscript. XC and SG completed the cell experiments. QW made contributions to the bioinformatics results. YL and HC read and revised the manuscript. All authors contributed to the article and approved the submitted version.

REFERENCES

1. Siegel RL, Miller KD, Jemal A. Cancer statistics, 2019. *CA Cancer J Clin* (2019) 69:7–34. doi: 10.3322/caac.21551
2. Levin B, Lieberman DA, McFarland B, Andrews KS, Brooks D, Bond J, et al. Screening and surveillance for the early detection of colorectal cancer and adenomatous polyps, 2008: a joint guideline from the American Cancer Society, the US Multi-Society Task Force on Colorectal Cancer, and the American College of Radiology. *Gastroenterology* (2008) 134:1570–95. doi: 10.1053/j.gastro.2008.02.002
3. Woolston A, Khan K, Spain G, Barber LJ, Griffiths B, Gonzalez-Exposito R, et al. Genomic and Transcriptomic Determinants of Therapy Resistance and Immune Landscape Evolution during Anti-EGFR Treatment in Colorectal Cancer. *Cancer Cell* (2019) 36:35–50.e9. doi: 10.1016/j.ccell.2019.05.013
4. Roper J, Tammela T, Cetinbas NM, Akkad A, Roghanian A, Rickelt S, et al. In vivo genome editing and organoid transplantation models of colorectal cancer and metastasis. *Nat Biotechnol* (2017) 35:569–76. doi: 10.1038/nbt.3836
5. Chen W, Zheng R, Baade PD, Zhang S, Zeng H, Bray F, et al. Cancer statistics in China, 2015. *CA Cancer J Clin* (2016) 66:115–32. doi: 10.3322/caac.21338
6. Bergsbaken T, Fink SL, Cookson BT. Pyroptosis: host cell death and inflammation. *Nat Rev Microbiol* (2009) 7:99–109. doi: 10.1038/nrmicro2070
7. Fang Y, Tian S, Pan Y, Li W, Wang Q, Tang Y, et al. Pyroptosis: A new frontier in cancer. *BioMed Pharmacother* (2020) 121:109595. doi: 10.1016/j.biopha.2019.109595
8. Yu J, Li S, Qi J, Chen Z, Wu Y, Guo J, et al. Cleavage of GSDME by caspase-3 determines lobaplatin-induced pyroptosis in colon cancer cells. *Cell Death Dis* (2019) 10:193. doi: 10.1038/s41419-019-1441-4
9. Shi J, Zhao Y, Wang K, Shi X, Wang Y, Huang H, et al. Cleavage of GSDMD by inflammatory caspases determines pyroptotic cell death. *Nature* (2015) 526:660–5. doi: 10.1038/nature15514
10. Ma Y, Chen Y, Lin C, Hu G. Biological functions and clinical significance of the newly identified long noncoding RNA RP185F18.6 in colorectal cancer. *Oncol Rep* (2018) 40:2648–58. doi: 10.3892/or.2018.6694
11. Wang L, Li K, Lin X, Yao Z, Wang S, Xiong X, et al. Metformin induces human esophageal carcinoma cell pyroptosis by targeting the miR-497/PELP1 axis. *Cancer Lett* (2019) 450:22–31. doi: 10.1016/j.canlet.2019.02.014
12. Jiang Z, Yao L, Ma H, Xu P, Li Z, Guo M, et al. miRNA-214 Inhibits Cellular Proliferation and Migration in Glioma Cells Targeting Caspase 1 Involved in Pyroptosis. *Oncol Res* (2017) 25:1009–19. doi: 10.3727/096504016X14813859905646
13. Bartel DP. MicroRNAs: genomics, biogenesis, mechanism, and function. *Cell* (2004) 116:281–97. doi: 10.1016/s0092-8674(04)00045-5
14. Lin S, Gregory RI. MicroRNA biogenesis pathways in cancer. *Nat Rev Cancer* (2015) 15:321–33. doi: 10.1038/nrc3932
15. Loboda A, Sobczak M, Jozkowicz A, Dulak J. TGF-beta1/Smads and miR-21 in Renal Fibrosis and Inflammation. *Mediators Inflamm* (2016) 2016:8319283. doi: 10.1155/2016/8319283
16. Cao LQ, Yang XW, Chen YB, Zhang DW, Jiang XF, Xue P. Exosomal miR-21 regulates the TETs/PTENp1/PTEN pathway to promote hepatocellular carcinoma growth. *Mol Cancer* (2019) 18:148. doi: 10.1186/s12943-019-1075-2
17. Canfran-Duque A, Rotllan N, Zhang X, Fernandez-Fuertes M, Ramirez-Hidalgo C, Araldi E, et al. Macrophage deficiency of miR-21 promotes apoptosis, plaque necrosis, and vascular inflammation during atherogenesis. *EMBO Mol Med* (2017) 9:1244–62. doi: 10.15252/emmm.201607492
18. Hao JP, Ma A. The ratio of miR-21/miR-24 as a promising diagnostic and poor prognosis biomarker in colorectal cancer. *Eur Rev Med Pharmacol Sci* (2018) 22:8649–56. doi: 10.26355/eurrev_201812_16629
19. Tsukamoto M, Iinuma H, Yagi T, Matsuda K, Hashiguchi Y. Circulating Exosomal MicroRNA-21 as a Biomarker in Each Tumor Stage of Colorectal Cancer. *Oncology* (2017) 92:360–70. doi: 10.1159/000463387
20. Jiao W, Leng X, Zhou Q, Wu Y, Sun L, Tan Y, et al. Different miR-21-3p isoforms and their different features in colorectal cancer. *Int J Cancer* (2017) 141:2103–11. doi: 10.1002/ijc.30902
21. Liu H, Wang J, Tao Y, Li X, Qin J, Bai Z, et al. Curcumol inhibits colorectal cancer proliferation by targeting miR-21 and modulated PTEN/PI3K/Akt pathways. *Life Sci* (2019) 221:354–61. doi: 10.1016/j.lfs.2019.02.049
22. Xiong B, Cheng Y, Ma L, Zhang C. MiR-21 regulates biological behavior through the PTEN/PI-3 K/Akt signaling pathway in human colorectal cancer cells. *Int J Oncol* (2013) 42:219–28. doi: 10.3892/ijo.2012.1707
23. Yu Y, Nangia-Makker P, Farhana L, GR S, Levi E, Majumdar AP. miR-21 and miR-145 cooperation in regulation of colon cancer stem cells. *Mol Cancer* (2015) 14:98. doi: 10.1186/s12943-015-0372-7
24. Hou N, Guo Z, Zhao G, Jia G, Luo B, Shen X, et al. Inhibition of microRNA-21-3p suppresses proliferation as well as invasion and induces apoptosis by targeting RNA-binding protein with multiple splicing through Smad4/extra cellular signal-regulated protein kinase signalling pathway in human colorectal cancer HCT116 cells. *Clin Exp Pharmacol Physiol* (2018) 45:729–41. doi: 10.1111/1440-1681.12931
25. Faltejskova P, Besse A, Sevcikova S, Kubiczkova L, Svoboda M, Smarda J, et al. Clinical correlations of miR-21 expression in colorectal cancer patients and effects of its inhibition on DLD1 colon cancer cells. *Int J Colorectal Dis* (2012) 27:1401–8. doi: 10.1007/s00384-012-1461-3
26. Jiang J, Chang W, Fu Y, Gao Y, Zhao C, Zhang X, et al. SAV1, regulated by microRNA-21, suppresses tumor growth in colorectal cancer. *Biochem Cell Biol* (2019) 97:91–9. doi: 10.1139/bcb-2018-0034
27. Liu M, Tang Q, Qiu M, Lang N, Li M, Zheng Y, et al. miR-21 targets the tumor suppressor RhoB and regulates proliferation, invasion and apoptosis in colorectal cancer cells. *FEBS Lett* (2011) 585:2998–3005. doi: 10.1016/j.febslet.2011.08.014
28. Garg AD, Agostinis P. Cell death and immunity in cancer: From danger signals to mimicry of pathogen defense responses. *Immunol Rev* (2017) 280:126–48. doi: 10.1111/imr.12574
29. Hu B, Jin C, Li HB, Tong J, Ouyang X, Cetinbas NM, et al. The DNA-sensing AIM2 inflammasome controls radiation-induced cell death and tissue injury. *Science* (2016) 354:765–8. doi: 10.1126/science.aaf7532
30. Johnson DC, Taabazuing CY, Okondo MC, Chui AJ, Rao SD, Brown FC, et al. DPP8/DPP9 inhibitor-induced pyroptosis for treatment of acute myeloid leukemia. *Nat Med* (2018) 24:1151–6. doi: 10.1038/s41591-018-0082-y
31. Paludan SR, Reinert LS, Hornung V. DNA-stimulated cell death: implications for host defence, inflammatory diseases and cancer. *Nat Rev Immunol* (2019) 19:141–53. doi: 10.1038/s41577-018-0117-0
32. Doitsh G, Galloway NL, Geng X, Yang Z, Monroe KM, Zepeda O, et al. Cell death by pyroptosis drives CD4 T-cell depletion in HIV-1 infection. *Nature* (2014) 505:509–14. doi: 10.1038/nature12940
33. Fantuzzi G, Dinarello CA. Interleukin-18 and interleukin-1 beta: two cytokine substrates for ICE (caspase-1). *J Clin Immunol* (1999) 19:1–11. doi: 10.1023/a:1020506300324
34. Han B, Cai H, Chen Y, Hu B, Luo H, Wu Y, et al. The role of TGFBI (betaig-H3) in gastrointestinal tract tumorigenesis. *Mol Cancer* (2015) 14:64. doi: 10.1186/s12943-015-0335-z
35. Irigoyen M, Pajares MJ, Agorreta J, Ponz-Sarvise M, Salvo E, Lozano MD, et al. TGFBI expression is associated with a better response to chemotherapy in NSCLC. *Mol Cancer* (2010) 9:130. doi: 10.1186/1476-4598-9-130
36. Tumbarello DA, Temple J, Brenton JD. ss3 integrin modulates transforming growth factor beta induced (TGFBI) function and paclitaxel response in ovarian cancer cells. *Mol Cancer* (2012) 11:36. doi: 10.1186/1476-4598-11-36

37. Skonier J, Neubauer M, Madisen L, Bennett K, Plowman GD, Purchio AF. cDNA cloning and sequence analysis of beta ig-h3, a novel gene induced in a human adenocarcinoma cell line after treatment with transforming growth factor-beta. *DNA Cell Biol* (1992) 11:511–22. doi: 10.1089/dna.1992.11.511
38. Kang Y, He W, Tulley S, Gupta GP, Serganova I, Chen CR, et al. Breast cancer bone metastasis mediated by the Smad tumor suppressor pathway. *Proc Natl Acad Sci USA* (2005) 102:13909–14. doi: 10.1073/pnas.0506517102
39. Bierie B, Moses HL. Tumour microenvironment: TGFbeta: the molecular Jekyll and Hyde of cancer. *Nat Rev Cancer* (2006) 6:506–20. doi: 10.1038/nrc1926
40. Shipitsin M, Campbell LL, Argani P, Weremowicz S, Bloushtain-Qimron N, Yao J, et al. Molecular definition of breast tumor heterogeneity. *Cancer Cell* (2007) 11:259–73. doi: 10.1016/j.ccr.2007.01.013
41. Ma C, Rong Y, Radiloff DR, Datto MB, Centeno B, Bao S, et al. Extracellular matrix protein betaig-h3/TGFBI promotes metastasis of colon cancer by enhancing cell extravasation. *Genes Dev* (2008) 22:308–21. doi: 10.1101/gad.1632008
42. Karki R, Man SM, Kanneganti TD. Inflammasomes and Cancer. *Cancer Immunol Res* (2017) 5:94–9. doi: 10.1158/2326-6066.CIR-16-0269
43. Tang Z, Ji L, Han M, Xie J, Zhong F, Zhang X, et al. Pyroptosis is involved in the inhibitory effect of FL118 on growth and metastasis in colorectal cancer. *Life Sci* (2020) 257:118065. doi: 10.1016/j.lfs.2020.118065
44. Kay C, Wang R, Kirkby M, Man SM. Molecular mechanisms activating the NAIP-NLRC4 inflammasome: Implications in infectious disease, autoinflammation, and cancer. *Immunol Rev* (2020) 297:67–82. doi: 10.1111/imr.12906
45. Hu B, Elinav E, Huber S, Booth CJ, Strowig T, Jin C, et al. Inflammation-induced tumorigenesis in the colon is regulated by caspase-1 and NLRC4. *Proc Natl Acad Sci USA* (2010) 107:21635–40. doi: 10.1073/pnas.1016814108
46. Allen IC, TeKippe EM, Woodford RM, Uronis JM, Holl EK, Rogers AB, et al. The NLRP3 inflammasome functions as a negative regulator of tumorigenesis during colitis-associated cancer. *J Exp Med* (2010) 207:1045–56. doi: 10.1084/jem.20100050
47. Karki R, Kanneganti TD. Diverging inflammasome signals in tumorigenesis and potential targeting. *Nat Rev Cancer* (2019) 19:197–214. doi: 10.1038/s41568-019-0123-y
48. Man SM, Zhu Q, Zhu L, Liu Z, Karki R, Malik A, et al. Critical Role for the DNA Sensor AIM2 in Stem Cell Proliferation and Cancer. *Cell* (2015) 162:45–58. doi: 10.1016/j.cell.2015.06.001
49. Wilson JE, Petrucelli AS, Chen L, Koblansky AA, Truax AD, Oyama Y, et al. Inflammasome-independent role of AIM2 in suppressing colon tumorigenesis via DNA-PK and Akt. *Nat Med* (2015) 21:906–13. doi: 10.1038/nm.3908
50. Rossi L, Bonmassar E, Faraoni I. Modification of miR gene expression pattern in human colon cancer cells following exposure to 5-fluorouracil in vitro. *Pharmacol Res* (2007) 56:248–53. doi: 10.1016/j.phrs.2007.07.001
51. Schetter AJ, Leung SY, Sohn JJ, Zanetti KA, Bowman ED, Yanaihara N, et al. MicroRNA expression profiles associated with prognosis and therapeutic outcome in colon adenocarcinoma. *JAMA* (2008) 299:425–36. doi: 10.1001/jama.299.4.425
52. Zhang JX, Song W, Chen ZH, Wei JH, Liao YJ, Lei J, et al. Prognostic and predictive value of a microRNA signature in stage II colon cancer: a microRNA expression analysis. *Lancet Oncol* (2013) 14:1295–306. doi: 10.1016/S1470-2045(13)70491-1

15

The Roles of Beclin 1 Expression in Gastric Cancer: A Marker for Carcinogenesis, Aggressive Behaviors and Favorable Prognosis and a Target of Gene Therapy

Hua-chuan Zheng [1], *Shuang Zhao* [1], *Hang Xue* [1], *En-hong Zhao* [2], *Hua-mao Jiang* [3] *and Chang-lai Hao* [4*]

[1] Department of Oncology and Experimental Center, The Affiliated Hospital of Chengde Medical University, Chengde, China, [2] Department of Surgery, The Affiliated Hospital of Chengde Medical University, Chengde, China, [3] Department of Urology, The First Affiliated Hospital of Jinzhou Medical University, Jinzhou, China, [4] Department of Hematology, The Affiliated Hospital of Chengde Medical University, Chengde, China

***Correspondence:**
Chang-lai Hao
haochanglai882@163.com

Beclin 1 is encoded by *Becn1*, and plays a role in tumorigenesis, neurodegeneration, apoptosis and autophagy. Here, the aggressive phenotypes and relevant proteins were examined after Beclin 1 expression was altered in gastric cancer cells. We also observed the effects of Beclin 1 on gastric carcinogenesis using *Becn1* knockout mice. Finally, clinicopathological significances of Beclin 1 expression were analyzed using meta- and bioinformatics analyses. *Becn1* overexpression was found to inhibit proliferation, glucose metabolism, migration and invasion of gastric cancer cells, whereas its knockdown caused the opposite effects. Beclin 1 suppressed the tumor growth by decreasing proliferation and increasing apoptosis. The heterozygous abrogation of *Becn1* in gastric pit, parietal and chief cells could not cause any epithelial lesion. Beclin 1-mediated chemoresistance was closely linked to the autophagy, Bax underexpression, and the overexpression of Bcl-2, LRP1, MDR1, and ING5. Bioinformatics analysis showed higher Becn1 mRNA expression in intestinal- than diffuse-type carcinomas ($P<0.05$), and in male than female gastric cancer patients ($P<0.05$). *Becn1* hyperexpression was positively associated with both overall and progression-free survival rates of the cancer patients ($P<0.05$). Meta-analysis showed that down-regulated Beclin 1 expression in gastric cancer was positively with lymph node metastasis, TNM staging, dedifferentiation and poor prognosis ($P<0.05$). *Becn1*-related signal pathways in gastric cancer included prostate, lung, renal, colorectal, endometrial and thyroid cancers, glioma, and leukemia, the metabolism of amino acid, lipid and sugar, and some signal pathways of insulin, MAPK, TRL, VEGF, JAK-STAT, chemokine, p53, lysosome, peroxidome and ubiquitin-mediated protein degradation ($P<0.05$). These suggested that Beclin 1 might be considered as a potential marker of gastric carcinogenesis, aggressiveness and prognostic prediction, and as a target of gene therapy in gastric cancer.

Keywords: Beclin 1, gastric cancer, gene therapy, carcinogenesis, aggressive behaviors, prognosis

INTRODUCTION

There are a worldwide decrease in morbidity and mortality and rapid development in diagnostic and operative techniques, but gastric cancer still challenges the human health. The clinical outcome and prognosis of gastric cancer are generally worse because it has often metastasized by the time of discovery and most cancer patients are elderly at presentation (1, 2). Therefore, deep clarification of molecular mechanisms about gastric carcinogenesis and subsequent progression may remarkably improve early finding, diagnosis and treatment.

Autophagy is a conserved intracellular degradation pathway *via* autophagosomes formation, essential for protein development, homeostasis and survival, and mainly mediated by Beclin 1 (3, 4). EHMT2/G9a hypoexpression reduced H3K9me2 level, and dissociation of EHMT2 with H3K9me2 from *Becn1* promoter, and epigenetically up-regulated *Becn1* transcription *via* a high ROS level and NF-κB activation (5). Additionally, Beclin 1 binds to Bcl-2, Bcl-w, and Bcl-xL *via* BH3 receptor domain by phosphorylation and ubiquitination of Beclin 1 (6). Beclin 1 is phosphorylated at ser-90 by PP2A and DAPK3 to control autophagy (7). The phosphorylated Beclin 1 at S409 by CK1 is essential for p300 binding and Beclin 1 acetylation at lysine 430 and 437 (8). RNF216 interacts with and ubiquitinates Beclin 1 at lysine 48, thereby contributing to Beclin 1 degradation, while SLC9A3R1 and USP19 blocks ubiquitin-dependent Beclin 1 degradation by interacting with Beclin 1 and removing the K11-linked ubiquitin respectively (9, 10). Liu et al. (11) found that Beclin 1, the core molecule of the Becn1-PIK3C3 complex, could be SUMO3-conjugated by PIAS3 predominantly at K380 and deSUMOylated by SENP3. Tang et al. (12) reported that 14-3-3ζ bound to and stabilized phospho- Beclin 1(S295), and induced autophagy and chemoresistance in hepatocellular carcinoma cells. Caspase 3-mediated hydrolysis of Beclin 1 suppresses autophagy or enhances apoptosis by translocating Bax to the mitochondria for the release of cytochrome c (13, 14), whereas ABHD5 directly competes with Caspase 3 for binding to Beclin 1, and consequently prevents Beclin 1 from cleavage (15).

Previously, Beclin 1 overexpression in ovarian cancer was reported to negatively correlate with the differentiation and higher cumulative and relapse-free survival rates (16). Either Beclin 1 mRNA or protein hyperexpression was seen in colorectal and gastric cancers in comparison to precancerous lesion or mucosa. Beclin 1 expression was inversely associated with liver metastasis and distant metastasis of colorectal cancer, or venous invasion, lymph node metastasis, TNM staging, dedifferentiation and favorable prognosis of gastric cancer (17, 18). In colorectal cancer cells, Beclin 1 inhibited cell viability, migration and invasion, lamellipodia formation, and tumor growth, induced autophagy and apoptosis (19). Reportedly, Beclin 1 overexpression augmented the apoptotic induction of cis-diamminedichloroplatinum *via* enhancing Caspase-9 activity in gastric cancer cells (18). Gao et al. (20) reported that radiotherapy also induced autophagy and increased Beclin-1 expression *via* p53 pathway. Biallelic loss of *Becn1* is embryonically lethal for knockout mice, and promotes spontaneous tumorigenesis of lymphomas, liver and lung cancers (21–24). Here, we analyzed the effects of Beclin 1 expression on the aggressive behaviors and phenotypes of gastric cancer cells, and clarified relevant mechanisms. To explore the role of *Becn1* knockout in gastric carcinogenesis, we established conditional *Becn1* knockout mice in gastric pit, parietal and chief cells using the Capn8, Atp4b and PGC promoter to initiate Cre recombination respectively. Finally, clinicopathological significances were analyzed using meta- and bioinformatics analyses.

MATERIALS AND METHODS

Cell Line and Culture

Gastric cancer cell lines (BGC-823 and MKN28) were kindly presented by Prof. Su of Jinzhou Medical University. These cells were grown in RPMI 1640 medium containing FBS, penicillin, and streptomycin in 5% CO_2 at 37°C. BGC-823 and MKN28 cells were subjected to pcDNA3.1-*Becn1* or pcDNA3.1 vector transfection, and selected by G418 with monoclone collection. The target sequences of sh-*Becn1* were 5'-CACCGGAATGGA ATGAGATTAATGCTTCAAGAGAGCATTAATCTCATT CCATTCCTTTTTTG-3' and 3'-CCTTACTTACTCT AATTACGAAGTTCTCTCGTAATTAGAGTAA GGTAAGGAAAAAACCTAG-5'. Additionally, we treated cells with MG132 (proteasome inhibitor), paclitaxel (mitotic inhibitor), or SAHA (histone deacetylase inhibitor).

Proliferation Assay

We used cell counting kit-8 (CCK-8) to determine cell proliferation. In brief, 2.0×10^3 cells/well were cultured on 96-well plate. After adhering to plate.10 μl of CCK-8 solution was added into each well of the plate at different time points, and the absorbance was measured at 450 nm after 3 h incubation.

Cell Cycle Analysis

We trypsinized, collected, and fixed the cell using ethanol for 2 h. After RNase treatment for 1 h, cells were pelleted and stained by propidium iodide (PI) for 30 min. At final, flow cytometry was used to examine PI signal.

Apoptosis Assay

FITC-labeled annexin V staining (Kagen, China) was employed to indicate phosphatidylserine externalization of early apoptosis in terms of manufacturer's instructions.

Measurement of Extracellular Acidification Rate and Oxygen Consumption Rate

We measured the metabolic parameters using wing discs of abxUbxFLPase of Seahorse metabolic flux analyzer. Discs were measured in bicarbonate-free Schneider medium with 12 mM glutamine and 11 mM glucose. The glycolysis can be indicated by extracellular acidification rate (ECAR), and the mitochrondrial respiration by oxygen consumption rate (OCR). We also normalized ECAR and OCR values using protein amount according to BCA assay.

Transwell Chamber Assay

To assess invasion, we cultured 2.0 × 10^5 cells in FBS-free medium in the matrigel-coated insert on the chamber top, and added 10%-FBS-containing medium to the chamber bottom as a chemoattractant. After 24-h incubation, the upper member of insert was scrubbed, and the lower portion fixed in methanol and followed by Giemsa dye. To measure migration, we repeated the above-mentioned protocol excluding membrane-control insert.

Animals

We housed three mice per plastic cage with paper chips, standard rodent food and water in pathogen-free and temperature-controlled condition with a 12-h light/dark illumination cycle. All animal experiments were conducted using protocols approved by the Committee on Animal Experimentation of The Affiliated Hospital of Chengde Medical University. Female 8-week Balb/c nude mice were used for subcutaneous implantation by injection of 2.0× 10^6 cells per mouse to axilla (n=10 mice/group). Finally, the mice were anesthetized, photographed, and killed for tissue sampling. The part of tumors was subjected to routine pathological block preparation, and the remaining was stored in liquid nitrogen until protein, RNA or protein extract. The tumor volume was calculated as width^2× length ×0.52.

Additionally, we performed cre-mediated deletion of floxed alleles by mating *Becn1* conditional mutant mice (Mouse Biology Program, University of California, Davis USA) with Capn8-cre, Atp4b-cre (kindly presented by Prof. Yang) or PGC-cre (prepared in our Lab., unpublished) transgenic mice. At least 5 mice were killed at 9 month, and their stomachs were analyzed.

DNA Analysis

DNA was extracted from mouse tail and stomach using phenol-chloroform method. We performed genotyping by PCR. The PCR primer sequences were CSD-lacF: 5'-CTACCATTA CCAGTTGGTCT GGTGTC-3', CSD-neoF: 5'-GGGATCTCA TGCTGGAGTTCTTCG-3', CSD-*Becn1* -F: 5'-TTGTAC CGTGATTTAGGGCGTTTGC-3', CSD-*Becn1*-R: 5'-CAGAGTGAGTTCCAAGACAGCCAGG-3', CSD-*Becn1*-ttR: 5'-CTCCCAAGTGCTGGGATTAAAGACG-3' and cre: 5'-GCCTGCATTACCGG TCGATGC-3' and 5'-CAGGGTGT TATAAGCAATCCC-3'. The truncated *Becn1* and cre were confirmed by the tail DNA PCR. The deletion of *Becn1* was confirmed by PCR amplification of gastric mucosa DNA.

Real-Time RT-PCR

We extracted total RNA from cells or tissues using Trizol (Takara). Reverse transcription of 1 μg RNA was performed using random primers and AMV reverse transcriptase. PCR primers were designed according to the sequences in GenBank. Oligonucleotide primers for PCR were 5'-TTACCACAGC CCAGGCGA-3' and 5'-GCCACCATCAGATGCCTC-3' for mouse *Becn1*, and 5'-ACATACTCAG CACCGGCCTC-3' and 5'-TATGACTCCACTCACGGCAAA-3' for mouse *GAPDH*. SYBR Premix Ex Taq II kit (Takara) was employed to amplify target cDNAs using *GAPDH* as an internal control.

Western Blot

Protein was extracted in RIPA lysis buffer and determined by BCA assay. We separated denatured protein in SDS-polyacrylamide gel and transferred to Hybond membrane. After blocked in 5% skim milk, the membranes were incubated with primary antibodies (**Table 1**) and then with anti-rabbit, or anti-mouse IgG conjugated to horseradish peroxidase (Dako). We visualized bands using ECL-Plus detection reagents.

Histological Analysis

Tissues block were sectioned and consecutive 5μm-thick sections were stained with HE, alcian blue, PAS and HID. Sections were deparaffinized, dehydrated, and subjected to immunostaining using primary antibodies (**Table 1**) as previously described (17), or TUNEL using ApopTag Plus Peroxidase In Situ Apoptosis Detection Kit (Millipore) as reported (19).

Identification of Eligible Studies

We searched the articles using BIOSIS, PubMed, SciFinder, and Web of Science until July 10, 2020. The following strategy was (*Becn1* OR Beclin 1) AND (stomach OR gastric) AND (adenocarcinoma OR carcinoma OR cancer). The articles were included to observe Beclin 1 immunostaining in gastric cancers and compare Beclin 1 expression with their pathobiological features and prognosis. We excluded the abstract, comment, review and meeting, and papers about Western blot, RT-PCR, cDNA chip, or transcriptomic data for Beclin 1 expression.

Data Extraction and Quality Score Assessment

Both reviewers independently collected useful information from all eligible articles, including first author, publication year,

TABLE 1 | The antibodies used in the present study.

Name	Source	Company
Beclin 1	Rabbit	Santa Cruz
β-actin	Mouse	Santa Cruz
GAPDH	Rabbit	Wanleibio
LC3B	Rabbit	Wanleibio
Bax (B-9)	Mouse	Santa Cruz
Bcl-2 (C-21)	Rabbit	Santa Cruz
Akt	Rabbit	Santa Cruz
PI3K	Rabbit	Abcam
p-p38	Rabbit	Santa Cruz
P38	Rabbit	Santa Cruz
NF-κB	Rabbit	CST
Cdk4(C-22)	Rabbit	Santa Cruz
E-cadherin	Mouse	Abcam
Twist1	Rabbit	Abcam
Zeb2(E-11)	Mouse	Santa Cruz
β-catenin	Rabbit	Abcam
MRP1	Mouse	Abcam
GSTπ	Rabbit	Abcam
MDR1	Rabbit	Abcam
FBXW7	Rabbit	Wanleibio
LRP1	Rabbit	Abcam
ING5	Rabbit	Proteintech
CD147	Rabbit	Abcam

ethnicity, country, histological subtypes, control source, antibody company, numbers of cases and controls, and survival times. Engauge Digitizer software was employed to mine information from Kaplan-Meier curves and calculate Hazard ratios. We discussed to resolve disagreement until consensus. Publication quality was evaluated according to Newcastle Ottawa Scale.

Bioinformatics Analysis

The transcriptomic and clinicopathological data of gastric cancer patients were downloaded from TCGA database by TCGA-assembler of R software. We analyzed Becn1 mRNA level between gastric normal and cancer tissues using Oncomine and TACGA data. *Becn1* expression was compared with clinicopathological and prognostic data of gastric cancer patients. GSEA was performed with GSEA-3.0. We used *Becn1* level as a phenotype label and analyzed pathway enrichment. Kaplan- Meier plotter was employed to analyze the prognostic significance of Becn1 mRNA.

Statistics Analysis

We used Revman software 5.3 to carry out Meta-analysis, and evaluated HWE using Chi-square test. If there was no significant heterogeneity, the fixed effect model would be employed. Experimental and TCGA data was handled with SPSS 10.0 software using t test or survival analysis. We regarded $P<0.05$ as statistically significant.

RESULTS

The Effects of Beclin 1 Overexpression on the Aggressiveness of Gastric Cancer Cells

Beclin 1 was successfully overexpressed in BGC-823 and MKN28 cells according to real-time RT-PCR and Western blot (**Figure 1A**, $P<0.05$). Beclin 1 overexpression suppressed the proliferation of both cancer cells, evidenced by CCK-8 (**Figure 1B**, $P<0.05$). *Becn1* transfectants showed the chemoresistance to MG132, paclitaxel and SAHA at both time- and dose-dependent manners (**Figure 1C**, $P<0.05$). After transfected with *Becn1*-expressing plasmid, the appearance of gastric cancer cells became irregular, vacuolar, polynucleate and protrudent (**Figure 1D**). Flow cytometry showed G_1 or S arrest, and apoptotic induction in *Becn1* transfectants of gastric cancer cells (**Figures 1E, F**, $P<0.05$). Beclin 1 overexpression decreased glycolysis and following mitochondrial oxidization, cell migration and invasion according to oxygen consumption and transwell assays respectively (**Figures 1G, H**, $P<0.05$). As shown in **Figure 1I**, *Becn1* overexpression up-regulated the expression of LC-3B, Bax, Akt, p-Akt, PI3K, p-PI3K, E-cadherin, GST-π, MDR1, LRP1, ING5 and CD147, but down-regulated the expression of Bcl-2, p38, p-p38, NF-κB, Twist, Zeb2 and β-catenin. There was no difference in the expression of Cdk4 and MRP1 between gastric cancer cells and their *Becn1* transfectants.

Becn1 was successfully silenced in SGC-7901 cells, evidenced by real-time RT-PCR (**Figure 2A**, $P<0.05$) and Western blot (**Figure 2B**, $P<0.05$). *Becn1* knockdown promoted the cell viability (**Figure 2C**, $P<0.05$) and the chemosensitivity against MG132, 5-FU, and SAHA (**Figure 2D**, $P<0.05$), induced S phase progression (**Figure 2E**, $P<0.05$), and inhibited the apoptosis (**Figure 2F**, $P<0.05$). Down-regulated *Becn1* expression promoted migration and invasion according to transwell chamber assay (**Figure 2G**). *Becn1* knockdown decreased the expression of p-Akt, p-PI3K, LC-3B, E-cadherin, MRP1, MDR1, LRP1 and ING5, but increased the expression of Bcl-2, Akt, PI3K, p-p38, Cdk4, Zeb2, and β-catenin. No alteration was observed in the expression of GST-π, NF-κB and CD147 (**Figure 2H**).

Moreover, Beclin 1 overexpression suppressed tumor growth of gastric cancer cells in nude mice (**Figure 3A**, $P<0.05$). There was a higher Beclin 1 expression, a stronger signal of TUNEL and a weaker ki-67 expression in tumors of *Becn1*-overexpressing BCG-823 (**Figures 3B, C**). Beclin 1 down-regulated the expression of VEGF, E-cadherin, Bcl-2, but up-regulated the expression of LC-3B, NF-κB, PI3K, Akt1/2/3 and MDR in xenograft tumor of gastric cancer cells (**Figure 3C**). Moreover, we matched the conditional *Becn1*-knockout (KO) mice with Atp4b-cre, Capn8-cre or PGC-cre mice, and designed the primers to confirm the monoallelic deletion of *Becn1* using DNA from tail and gastric mucosa (**Figure 4A**). According to PCR results, we obtained the monoallelic deletion of *Becn1* in gastric mucosa in *Becn1*-PGC-cre, *Becn1*-Capn8-cre and *Becn1*-Atp4b-cre mice (**Figure 4B**). There was a weaker expression of *Becn1* in gastric epithelium of *Becn1*-PGC-cre, *Becn1*-Capn8-cre and *Becn1*-Atp4b-cre than those of wild-type (WT) mice at both mRNA and protein levels (**Figure 4C, D**). However, no remarkable lesions were observed in the gastric mucosa of these three kinds of mice although weaker Beclin 1 was immunohistochemically observed in gastric chief, pit and parietal cells of *Becn1*-PGC-cre, *Becn1*-Capn8-cre, and *Becn1*-Atp4b-cre than those of WT mice (**Figures 4E–G**). Additionally, there were no differences in sialic acid, neutral and sulfuric acid mucus between conditional KO and WT mice according to alcian blue, PAS and HID staining (**Figure 4H**).

Characteristics of Eligible Studies

We retrieved fifteen articles about the relationship between Beclin 1 expression and cancer risk, clinicopathological or prognostic features of gastric cancer for meta-analysis (**Table 2**). Five pieces of paper had the samples of normal gastric mucosa and cancer (18, 28, 31, 35, 37). In 12 articles, Beclin1 expression was compared with age, invasive depth, lymph node involvement, TNM staging and Lauren's classification (18, 25–37). Ten pieces of paper described the prognostic significance of Beclin 1 expression (18, 25–27, 30–34, 36).

Association Between Beclin 1 Expression and Clinicopathological Parameters of Gastric Cancer

We collected 986 cancers and 786 controls and found down-regulated Beclin 1 expression in gastric cancer (**Figure 5A**, $P=0.02$). As shown in **Figure 5B**, there was no difference in Beclin 1 expression between age >60 year and <60 year cancer patients ($P>0.05$), between male and female ones (**Figure 5C**, $P>0.05$) or between T_{1-2} than T_{3-4} gastric cancer (**Figure 5D**, $P=0.19$). Beclin 1 expression was negatively associated with lymph

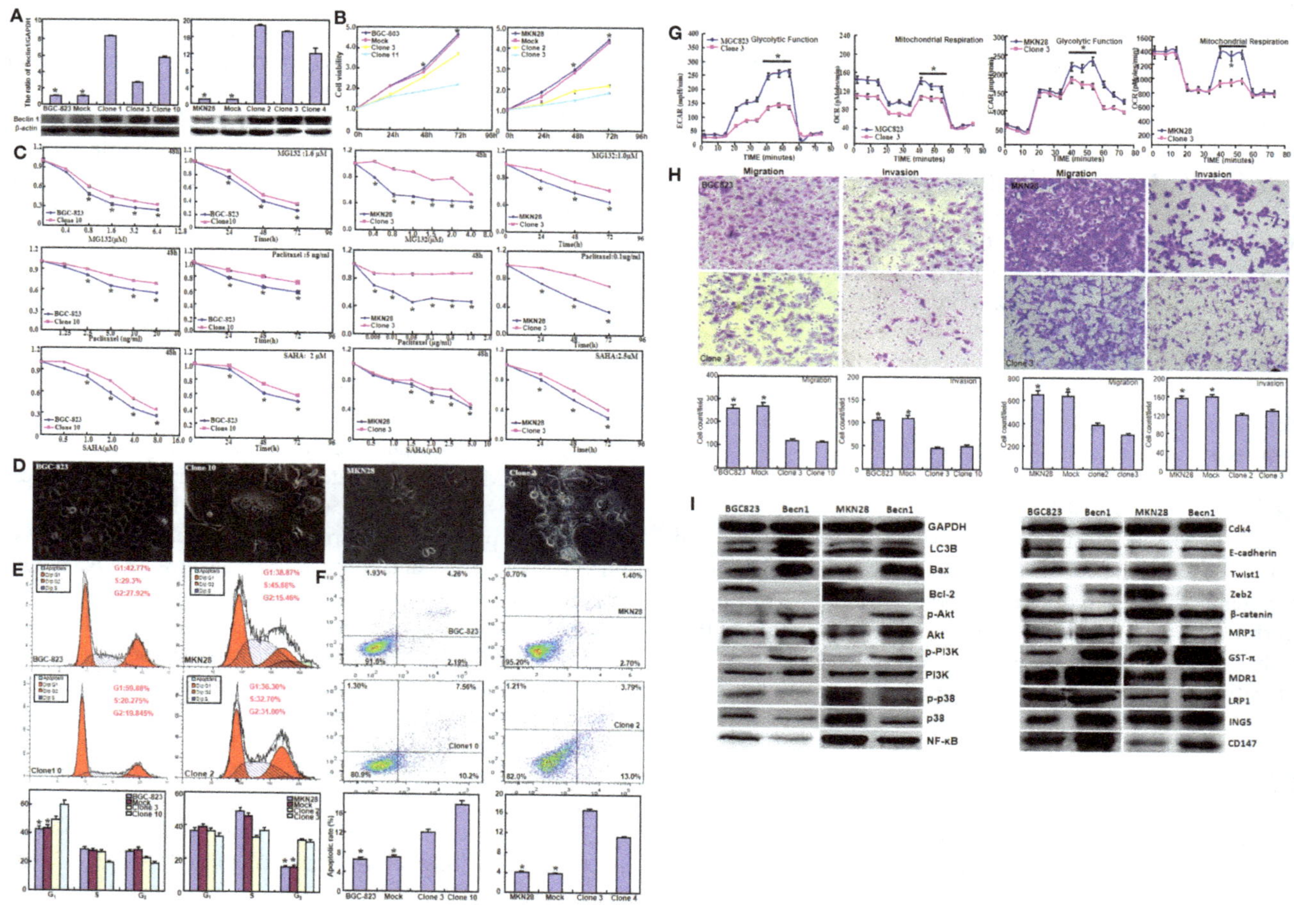

FIGURE 1 | The effects of Beclin 1 expression on aggressiveness of gastric cancer cells. Beclin 1 expression in BGC-823 and MKN28 cells was examined after transfection with pcDNA3.1-*Becn1* by real-time RT-PCR and Western blot **(A)**. The transfectants showed a decrease in growth **(B)** and chemosensitivity to MG132, Paclitaxel and SAHA **(C)** in comparison with the control or mock. After Becn1 was overexpressed, the morphological appearance was observed under microscope **(D)**. Flow cytometry showed that Beclin 1 expression induced the G_1 arrest of BGC-823 cells, but S arrest of MKN28 cells **(E)**. Apoptosis was increased by Beclin 1 overexpression, as evidenced by Annexin V assay **(F)**. Oxygen consumption and transwell assays were used to monitor the glucose metabolism, migration and invasion of gastric cancer cells respectively **(G, H)**. The phenotype-related proteins were screened by Western blot **(I)**. *$P < 0.05$, compared with the transfectants.

node involvement (**Figure 5E**, *P*=0.03), TNM staging (**Figure 5F**, *P*=0.03), and dedifferentiation (**Figure 5G**, *P*=0.01). Well-moderately adenocarcinoma had a higher Beclin 1 expression than the poorly-differentiated subtype (**Figure 5H**, *P*=0.0004). As indicated in **Figure 5I**, there was significant association between Beclin 1 expression and favorable overall survival in patients with gastric cancer (OR=1.34, 95% CI: 1.15–1.56, *P*=0.0002). Sensitivity analysis was performed to evaluate individual study's influence on the pooled results by deleting one single study (data not shown).

The Clinicopathological and Prognostic Significances of Becn1 Expression in Gastric Cancer

According to TCGA databases, Becn1 mRNA expression was found to be lower in gastric cancer than normal mucosa (**Figure 6A**, *P*<0.05). There was a higher Becn1 mRNA expression in intestinal- than diffuse-type adenocarcinoma according to DErricodata (**Figure 6B**, *P*<0.05). In TCGA data, Becn1 expression was higher in male than female cancer patients (**Figure 6C**, *P*<0.05). According to Kaplan-Meier plotter, Becn1 expression was found to positively correlate with overall and progression-free survival rates of all cancer patients (**Figure 6D**, *P*<0.05), even stratified by Lauren's classification, TNM staging and treatment (**Table 3**, *P*<0.05). Female, male, T2, T3, N1-N3, M1, M0 and Her-2-negative cancer patients with high Becn1 mRNA expression had a high overall survival rate than those with its low expression (*P*<0.05), while it was the same for progression-free survival rate in the male, T2, T4, N1-3, N1, M0, Her2-negative and -positive cancer patients (*P*<0.05).

Becn1-Related Signal Pathways in Gastric Cancer

As summarized in **Table 4**, we conducted a GSEA to analyze *Becn1*-related signal pathways in gastric cancer. The significant

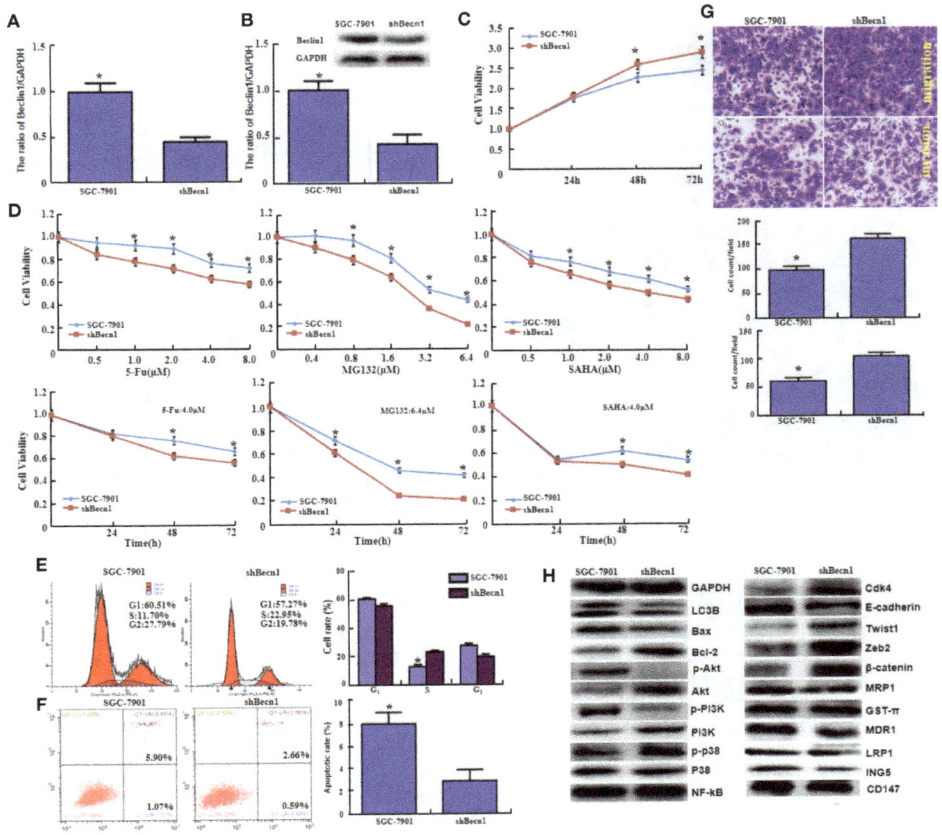

FIGURE 2 | The *in vitro* and *in vivo* effects of Beclin 1 silencing on aggressive phenotypes of gastric cancer cells. After transfection of shRNA-*Becn1*, its expression became weak in SGC-7901 cells by real-time RT-PCR **(A)** and Western blot **(B)**. The cell viability was measured in SGC-7901 cells and their sh*Becn1* transfectants using CCK-8 kit **(C)**, even treated with 5-FU, MG132, and SAHA **(D)**. Cell cycle and apoptosis were examined by propidium iodide (PI) **(E)** and Annexin-V **(F)** staining respectively. Both migration and invasion were determined in SGC-7901 and sh*Becn1* transfectants by transwell chamber assay **(G)**. The phenotype-associated proteins were screened by Western lot **(H)**. **P* < 0.05, compared with the transfectants.

enriched pathways included prostate, lung, renal, colorectal, endometrial, thyroid cancers, glioma, and leukemia, the metabolism of amino acid, lipid and sugar, and some signal pathways of insulin, MAPK, TRL, VEGF, JAK-STAT, chemokine and p53, lysosome, peroxidome and ubiquitin-mediated protein degradation ($P<0.05$).

DISCUSSION

Beclin 1 expression was reported to cause apoptosis *via* Bax activation and Bcl-2 suppression in HeLa cells, inhibited proliferation and increased the chemosensitivity to Taxol (38). In lung cancer cells, Beclin 1 induced apoptosis and weakened invasion by up-regulating ECRG4 (39). In breast cancer cells, Beclin 1 overexpression improved cellular autophagy, inhibited cell proliferation, decreased cell apoptosis, mediated G_1 arrest and promoted epithelial-mesenchymal transition (EMT) *via* Wnt/β- catenin pathway (40), but *Becn1* knockdown induced EMT by *via* posttranscriptional up-regulation and stabilization of Zeb1 mRNA (41). RelA-mediated *Becn1* expression was essential for ROS-induced autophagy in oral cancer cells irradiated by laser (42). Hasan et al. (43) found that HSP90 inhibitor (Gedunin) suppressed interaction between Hsp90: Beclin-1:Bcl-2, finally to inhibit autophagosome formation (Beclin-1, Atg5-12 complex, and LC3). Hu et al. (44) observed that Becn1 knockdown markedly promoted motility and invasion of colorectal cancer cells with STAT3 phosphorylation *via* the interaction between STAT and JAK2. Cheng et al. (45) found that Beclin 1 increased the migration of non-small cell lung cancer cells *via* interaction with Vimentin, followed by its K48-linked ubiquitination *via* ubiquitin-specific peptidase 14. Here, Beclin 1 was demonstrated to suppress proliferation, migration, invasion and tumor growth, and induce cell cycle arrest, apoptosis, autophagy and chemoresistance in gastric cancer cells, whereas versa for *Becn1*-silencing cells, suggesting that Beclin 1 can be used as a gene therapy target of gastric cancer if its chemoresistant induction could be avoided or alleviated. Additionally, gastric lesions were not observed from monoallelic conditional KO mice of *Becn1* in pit, parietal and chief cells

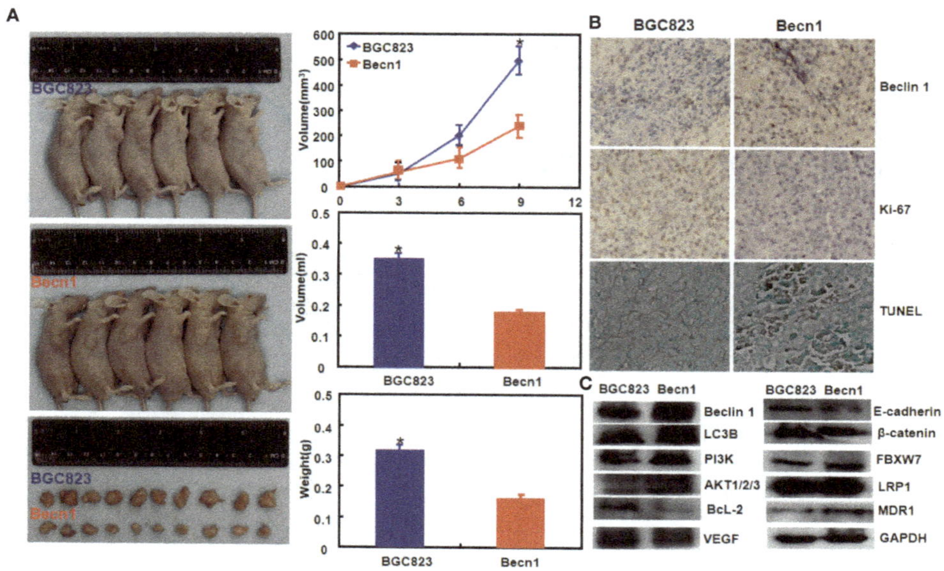

FIGURE 3 | The effects of *Becn1* expression on tumor growth of gastric cancer. The growth of gastric cancer cells was faster and heavier than their *Becn1* transfectants by gross appearance, and measuring tumor volume and weight [**(A)**, $P < 0.05$]. The transfectant cells showed stronger signals of Beclin 1 and apoptosis than the control in subcutaneous tumor, but versa for ki-67 immunoreactivity **(B)**. The phenotype-related proteins were screened using xenograft tumor tissues by Western blot **(C)**. $^{*}P < 0.05$, compared with the transfectant.

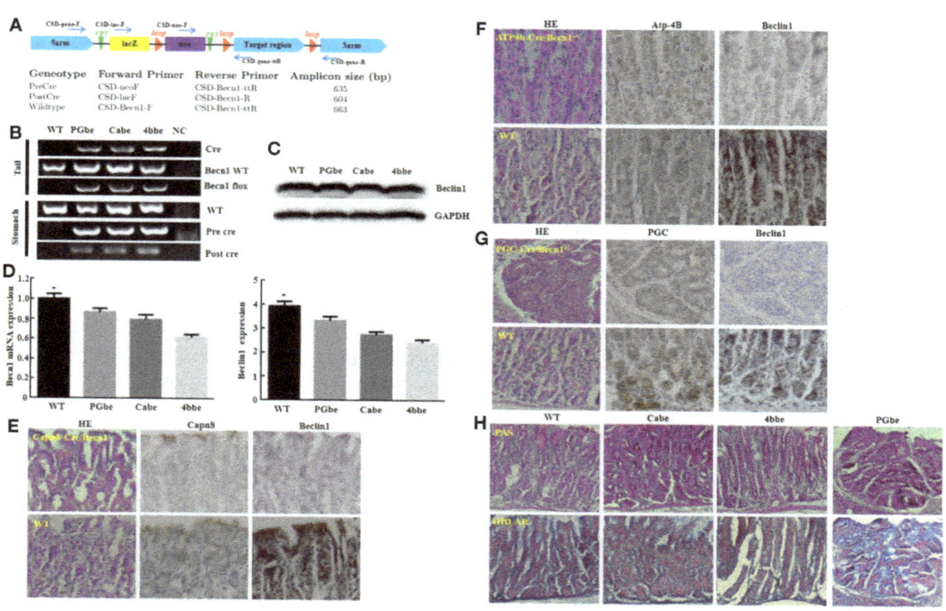

FIGURE 4 | The effects of *Becn1* expression on gastric carcinogenesis. PCR primers were designed **(A)** and subjected to PCR of tail and stomach DNA **(B)**. Monoallelic deletion of *Becn1* was confirmed by real-time PCR **(C)** and Western blot **(D)**, and couldn't cause any gastric lesions although Beclin 1 expression was reduced with Capn8, Atp-4B, and PGC immunoreactivity as control according to HE and immunohistochemistry **(E–G)**. There was no difference in alcian blue, PAS and HID staining between three conditional knock-out mice and wild-type mice **(H)**. $^{*}P < 0.05$, compared with the knockout mice. WT, wild-type mice; Cabe, Capn8-cre +; *Becn1* +/−; 4bbe, Atp-4b-cre +; *Becn1* +/−; PGbe, PGC-cre +; *Becn1* +/−.

TABLE 2 | Main characteristics of eligible studies.

First author	Year	Country	Ethnicity	Antibody Source	Cases	Ctr	Risk	Outcome	Quality
Won KY (25)	2015	Korea	Asian	Abcam	108		Down	Pos	8
Yu M (18)	2013	China	Asian	Sigma	565	586		Pos	9
Geng QR (26)	2012	China	Asian	Novus Biologicals	271		Up	Pos	8
Chen YB (27)	2012	China	Asian	Abcam	155	60	Up	Pos	9
Fei BY (28)	2016	China	Asian	Abcam	75	75			9
Qin WJ (29)	2015	China	Asian	Abcam	156				8
Zhou WH (30)	2012	China	Asian	Santa Cruz	153		Down	Pos	8
Yu SJ (31)	2016	China	Asian	Sigma	160	34	Down	Pos	9
Zhao Z (32)	2015	China	Asian	Abcam	113		Up	Neg	8
Qiu GL (33)	2016	China	Asian	Abcam	96	96	Up	Neg	9
Cao QH (34)	2016	China	Asian	Cell Signaling	352		Down	Pos	8
Huang JL (35)	2016	China	Asian	CST	120	120	Down		9
Hu YF (36)	2017	China	Asian	abcam	120	120	Up	Pos	9
Guo CQ (37)	2010	China	Asian	Santa cruz	62	36	Down		8

Crt, control; Down, down-regulated; Up, up-regulated; Pos, positive, Neg, negative.

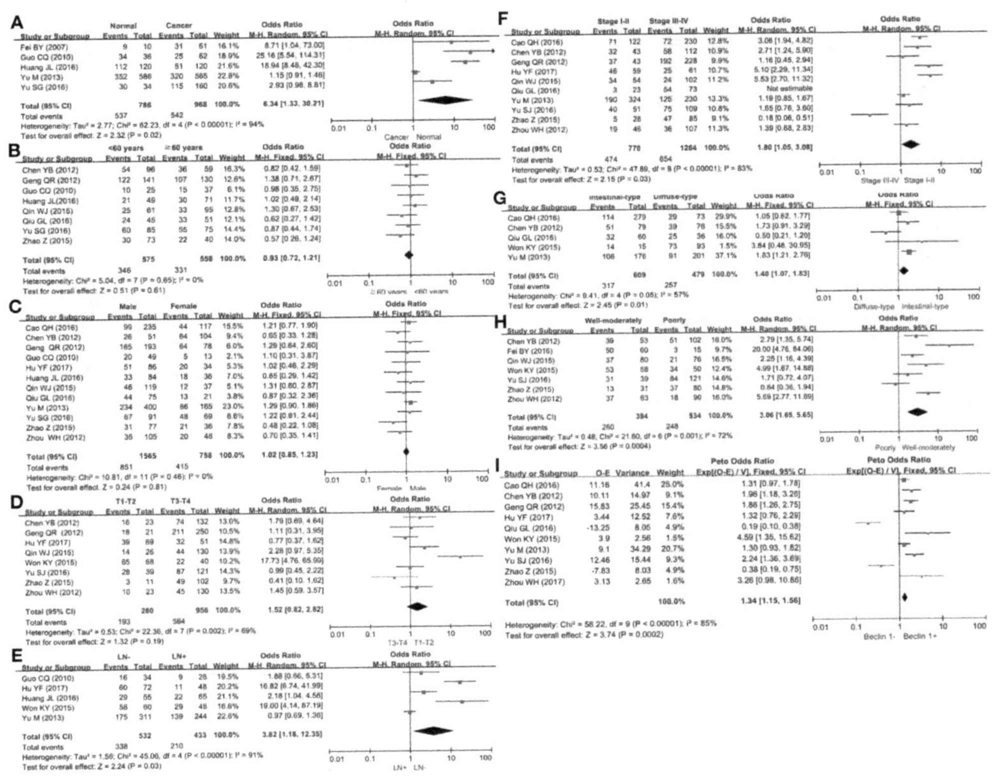

FIGURE 5 | Forest plot for the relationship between Beclin 1 expression and clinicopathological parameters of gastric cancer. **(A)** gastric carcinogenesis (cancer *vs* normal mucosa); **(B)** correlation between age and Beclin 1 expression (<60 years *vs* ≧60years); **(C)** correlation between gender and Beclin 1 expression (female *vs* male); **(D)** correlation between T staging and Beclin 1 expression (Tis-1 *vs* T2-4); **(E)** correlation between lymph node metastasis (LN) and Beclin 1 expression (LN- *vs* LN+); **(F)** correlation between TNM staging and Beclin 1 expression (stage I–II *vs* II–IV); **(G)** correlation between Lauren's classification and Beclin 1 expression (intestinal-type *vs* diffuse-type); **(H)** correlation between WHO' classification and Beclin 1 expression (Well-moderately differentiated *vs* poorly-differentiated); **(I)** correlation between prognosis and Beclin 1 expression (Beclin 1- *vs* Beclin 1+).

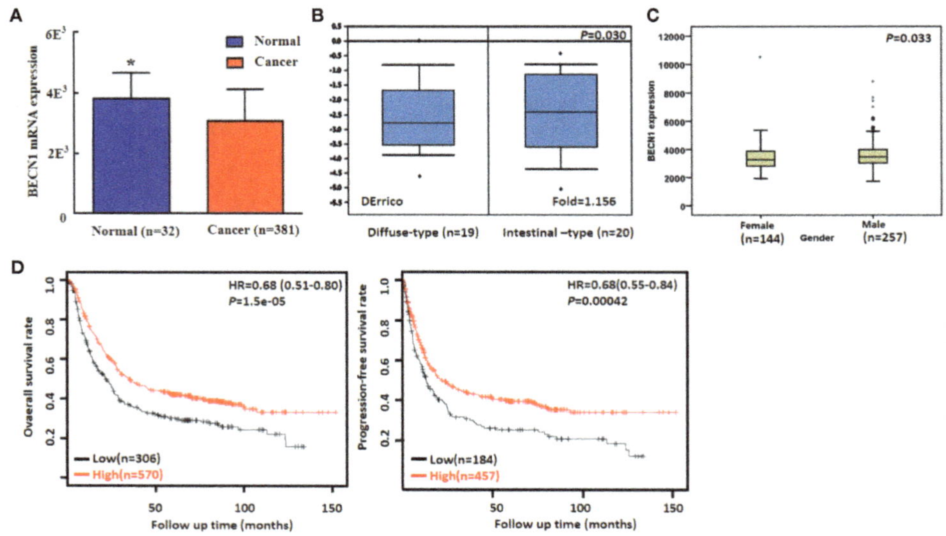

FIGURE 6 | *Becn1* mRNA expression in gastric carcinogenesis and subsequent progression. A lower *Becn1* mRNA expression was detectable in gastric cancer than that in normal gastric mucosa according TCGA data [**(A)**, $P < 0.05$]. There was *Becn1* overexpression in intestinal-type than diffuse-type carcinoma according to DErrico's database [**(B)**, $P < 0.05$]. TCGA database showed a higher *Becn1* mRNA expression in male than female patients with gastric cancer [**(C)**, $P < 0.05$]. According to the data from Kaplan-Meier plotter, *Becn1* mRNA expression was positively related to both overall and progression-free survival rates of the patients with gastric cancer [**(D)**, $P < 0.05$]. HR, hazard ratio. *P < 0.05, compared with the cancer.

TABLE 3 | The prognostic significance of *Becn1* mRNA in gastric cancer by Kaplan–Meier plotter.

Clinicopathological features	Overall survival		Progression-free survival	
	Hazard ratio	***P* value**	**Hazard ratio**	***P* value**
Sex				
Female	0.62(0.42–0.9)	0.012	0.72(0.47–1.09)	0.12
Male	0.61(0.49–0.75)	5.1e-06	0.61(0.48–0.77)	3.7e-05
T				
2	0.59(0.37–0.94)	0.025	0.59(0.38–0.92)	0.019
3	0.7(0.49–0.98)	0.039	0.87(0.62–1.21)	0.4
4	0.49(0.21–1.15)	0.094	0.43(0.2–0.93)	0.029
N				
0	1.73(0.73–4.1)	0.21	1.77(0.75–4.17)	0.19
1–3	0.53(0.4–0.69)	2e-06	0.6(0.46–0.78)	8.1e-05
1	0.35(0.22–0.55)	2.3e-06	0.38(0.25–0.59)	6.1e-06
2	0.52(0.33–0.82)	0.0047	0.66(0.42–1.03)	0.066
3	0.56(0.32–0.98)	0.039	0.61(0.36–1.06)	0.077
TNM staging				
I	0.33(0.12–0.88)	0.02	2.43(0.78–7.62)	0.12
II	0.46(0.24–0.86)	0.013	0.49(0.26–0.93)	0.025
III	0.57(0.42–0.76)	0.00011	0.61(0.41–0.91)	0.015
IV	0.68(0.46–1)	0.048	0.67(0.46–0.98)	0.04
Lauren's classification				
Intestinal-type	0.56(0.4–0.77)	0.00039	0.69(0.48–0.98)	0.04
Diffuse-type	0.55(0.38–0.79)	0.0011	0.57(0.4–0.83)	0.003
Her-2 positivity				
–	0.65(0.52–0.81)	0.00016	0.65(0.5–0.84)	0.00088
+	0.77(0.59–1)	0.051	0.7(0.5–0.99)	0.043
Treatment				
Surgery alone	0.66(0.48–0.91)	0.01	0.72(0.53–0.97)	0.03
5-FU-based adjuvant	1.68(1.18–2.39)	0.0034	1.66(1.17–2.35)	0.0044

TABLE 4 | *Becn1*-enriched signal pathway in gastric cancer according to the KEGG analysis.

Name	Size	*P* value
Phosphatidylinositol signaling system	76	<0.001
Inositol phosphate metabolism	54	<0.001
Endocytosis	178	<0.001
Amyotrophic lateral sclerosis	52	<0.001
Insulin signaling pathway	136	0.001
Lysosome	119	0.001
Endometrial cancer	52	0.001
Adipocytokine signaling pathway	67	0.001
Apoptosis	85	0.001
Fatty acid metabolism	42	0.001
Sphingolipid metabolism	36	0.001
Acute myeloid leukemia	57	0.001
mTOR signaling pathway	51	0.001
Prostate cancer	88	0.001
Pathways in cancer	324	0.001
ERBB signaling pathway	87	0.001
Chronic myeloid leukemia	73	0.001
Small cell lung cancer	84	0.002
Peroxisome	78	0.005
FC gamma r mediated phagocytosis	93	0.005
Neurotrophin signaling pathway	126	0.005
Non-small cell lung cancer	54	0.005
Vasopressin regulated water reabsorption	44	0.005
Colorectal cancer	62	0.005
Ubiquitin mediated proteolysis	134	0.005
Amino sugar and nucleotide sugar metabolism	44	0.005
MAPK signaling pathway	264	0.005
Vibrio cholerae infection	53	0.005
Fructose and mannose metabolism	34	0.007
Glycolysis gluconeogenesis	59	0.008
N-glycan biosynthesis	46	0.008
Snare interactions in vesicular transport	38	0.009
Renal cell carcinoma	70	0.009
Focal adhesion	199	0.01
Toll-like receptor signaling pathway	89	0.013
Regulation of actin cytoskeleton	210	0.013
Chemokine signaling pathway	185	0.014
Lysine degradation	41	0.014
Long term potentiation	69	0.014
Pancreatic cancer	70	0.014
Adherens junction	73	0.014
Wnt signaling pathway	149	0.014
Glycosaminoglycan degradation	21	0.014
VEGF signaling pathway	75	0.014
Valine leucine and isoleucine degradation	44	0.014
Epithelial cell signaling in helicobacter pylori infection	67	0.014
JAK-STAT signaling pathway	136	0.017
NOD-like receptor signaling pathway	61	0.019
Glioma	65	0.02
Galactose metabolism	25	0.02
Thyroid cancer	29	0.02
Axon guidance	128	0.022
FC epsilon RI signaling pathway	78	0.023
Selenoaminoacid metabolism	26	0.03
Betaalanine metabolism	22	0.032
GNRH signaling pathway	100	0.032
Glycerophospholipid metabolism	71	0.032
Propanoate metabolism	32	0.032
Aldosterone regulated sodium reabsorption	41	0.032
Progesterone mediated oocyte maturation	83	0.033
Glycerolipid metabolism	42	0.033
Tight junction	129	0.034
P53 signaling pathway	66	0.034
RIG I like receptor signaling pathway	56	0.034
O-glycan biosynthesis	27	0.037
Leukocyte transendothelial migration	115	0.039
Butanoate metabolism	33	0.043
Oocyte meiosis	109	0.046

respectively although spontaneous lymphomas, liver and lung cancers were detected in *Becn1*-/+ mice (23). Reportedly, microadenoma, macroadenoma to invasive well-differentiated adenocarcinoma were rapidly observed in the gastric Lgr5+ stem cells with the double deletion of Smad4 and PTEN using Lgr5-Cre mice (46). Our findings support the opinion that Becn-1-mediated gastric cancer might originate from local stem cells with genetic alteration, but not the differentiated cells. Additionally, *Becn1*-induced gastric carcinogenesis possibly needs the exposure to chemical carcinogen.

Bax can open the mitochondrial voltage-dependent anion channel during apoptosis, which is inhibited by interaction with Bcl-2 on the mitochondrial membrane (47). Consequently, Bax overexpression and Bcl-2 underexpression in gastric cancer cells may account for the inductive effect of Beclin 1 on apoptosis *via* mitochondrial pathway. Reportedly, activated p38 MAPK phosphorylates MAPKAP kinase 2 to phosphorylate the transcription factors (e.g. ATF2, Mac, and MEF2) and subsequently to mediate cell survival. PI3K/Akt activation results in drug resistance and cell proliferation. We observed p-p38 overexpression in *Becn1*-ovexpressing or silencing gastric cancer cells, but both p-PI3K and p-Akt hyperexpression was seen in *Becn1*-ovexpressing, but not *Becn1*-knockdown cells, suggesting that PI3K/Akt signal pathway might be involved in the effects of Beclin 1, but not p38. According to the literature, MDR1 and LRP1 are mainly responsible for drug resistance due to their ATP-dependent efflux pumping (47). ING5 overexpression also caused chemoresistance in neuroblastoma, glioma, gastric cancer, lung cancer, ovarian cancer and breast cancer cells (48–52). Cellular stress or increased metabolic demand activates autophagy, which can cause therapeutic resistance (47). Our results hinted that the Beclin 1-mediated chemoresistance might be due to autophagy and the hyperexpression of MDR1, LRP1, and ING5. *Becn1* overexpression was found to markedly attenuate the ability of gastric cancer cells to migrate and invade possibly due to VEGF hypoexpression because VEGF may promote mobility and proliferation of gastric cancer cells. In the study, E-cadherin hyperexpression, and Twist1 and Zeb2 hypoexpression in gastric Becn1 transfectants were closely linked to MET because Zeb2 and twist promote EMT process with E-cadherin underexpression. Therefore, the inhibitory of Beclin 1 on migration and invasion was dependent on MET in gastric cancer cells.

TGF-β1-induced autophagy linked β-catenin and Smad signaling to promote EMT of mouse kidney proximal tubular epithelial C1.1 (SV40 transformed) cells by disrupting E-cadherin/β-catenin- mediated cell-cell contact *via* ILK overexpression (53). SIRT1, SIRT6 and SPHK1 induced EMT by up-regulating autophagy-linked lysosomal degradation of E-cadherin in melanoma and hepatocellular cells *via* Beclin 1-E-cadherin cascade respectively (54–56). FSTL1 was demonstrated to induce EMT and airway remodeling by activating autophagy in asthma (57). HMGB1 also induced apoptosis and EMT in association with autophagy through the upregulated expression of DDR1 and the downregulation of the phosphorylation of mTOR following H/R injury in H9c2 cells (58). Persistent hypoxia induced autophage disorders, which could cause down-regulated E-cadherin and down-regulated MMP-9, thus promoting invasiveness of placenta trophoblasts (59). GRIM-19 suppressed hypoxia-triggered invasion and EMT by inhibiting hypoxia-induced autophagy through inactivation HIF-1α/STAT3 signaling axis (60). HIF-1α-mediated autophagy promoted EMT and metastatic ability of CD133+ pancreatic cancer stem-like cells during intermittent hypoxia (61). Endoplasmic reticulum stress induced EMT through autophagy *via* c-src kinase activation (62). In contrast, Catalano et al. (63) reported that autophagy induction impaired migration and invasion by reversing EMT in glioblastoma cells, in line with our inductive effects of Beclin 1 overexpression on E-cadherin expression in gastric cancer. In combination of these findings, we speculated that the regulatory correlation between Beclin 1 and E-cadherin depended on the cell types.

Reportedly, loss and down-regulation of Beclin 1 expression was immunohistochemically observed in esophageal adenocarcinoma (64), colorectal cancer (65), breast cancer (66), but versa in pancreatic cancer (67). Here, we performed meta-analysis and found that down-regulated Beclin 1 expression in gastric cancer was positively linked to lymph node metastasis, TNM staging, dedifferentiation and poor prognosis, in agreement with our bioinformatics findings. Reportedly, loss of Beclin-1 in cancer cells and Beclin 1 overexpression in stromal mesenchymal cells were closely linked to local recurrence and lymph node metastasis in breast cancer (68). Beclin-1 expression was related to HBV infection status and the grade of hepatocellular carcinoma (HCC) (69). In the hypoxic group, it was negatively correlated with high tumor grade, advanced stage, large size, and multifocal tumors of HCC, while positively with TNM stage and liver metastasis of gallbladder carcinoma (70), and with worse recurrence in intrahepatic cholangiocarcinoma (71). Beclin 1 expression was reported negatively correlate with tumor grade, lymph node involvement, TNM stage, tumor size, dedifferentiation, and recurrence of lung cancer (72). These findings indicated that its down-regulation contributed to gastric carcinogenesis and progression as a molecular marker.

Becn1 expression loss was demonstrated to act as a negative prognosticator in ovarian cancer patients receiving platinum-based chemotherapy (73). Tang et al. (74) found that low *Becn1* expression was associated with poor prognosis in breast cancer as an independent predictor, but the converse was true for breast cancer patients receiving tamoxifen treatment (75). Beclin 1 was considered as a dependent factor for favorable prognosis of the colorectal cancer patients (65). It was the same for ovarian clear cell carcinomas (76) and multiple myeloma (77). In contrast, Beclin 1 was significantly correlated with short disease-free survival and overall survival of pancreatic ductal adenocarcinoma (67). Here, meta- or bioinformatics analysis showed that either Beclin 1 protein or mRNA expression was positively linked to the favorable prognosis of the patients with gastric cancer. Taken together, Beclin 1 might be considered as a potential marker for the prognosis of the gastric cancer patients at either mRNA or protein level.

Down-regulated *Becn 1* expression in gastric cancer was positively correlated with aggressiveness and worse prognosis at either mRNA or protein level as a molecular marker. *Becn1* KO in pit, parietal or chief cells couldn't induce gastric carcinogenesis. It might be employed as a potential target for gene therapy of gastric cancer patients if its chemoresistant induction would be avoided and alleviated.

ETHICS STATEMENT

The animal study was reviewed and approved by The Affiliated Hospital of Chengde Medical University.

AUTHOR CONTRIBUTIONS

H-cZ, SZ, HX, E-hZ, H-mJ, and C-lH designed and carried out the experiments, and HZ wrote the draft. All authors read and approved the final manuscript. All authors contributed to the article and approved the submitted version.

ACKNOWLEDGMENT

Becn1 conditional mutants were kindly presented for research by Mouse Biology Program, University of California, Davis, USA. Atp-4b-cre and Capn8-cre mice were kindly presented by Prof. Yang from the Genetic Laboratory of Development and Diseases, State Key Laboratory of Proteomics, Institute of Biotechnology, Beijing, People's Republic of China.

REFERENCES

1. Venerito M, Link A, Rokkas T, Malfertheiner P. Gastric cancer - clinical and epidemiological aspects. *Helicobacter* (2016) 21(Suppl 1):39–44. doi: 10.1111/hel.12339
2. den Hoed CM, Kuipers EJ. Gastric cancer: how can we reduce the incidence of this disease? *Curr Gastroenterol Rep* (2016) 18(7):34. doi: 10.1007/s11894-016-0506-0
3. Sahni S, Merlot AM, Krishan S, Jansson PJ, Richardson DR. Gene of the month: BECN1. *J Clin Pathol* (2014) 67(8):656–60. doi: 10.1136/jclinpath-2014-202356
4. Hill SM, Wrobel L, Rubinsztein DC. Post-translational modifications of Beclin 1 provide multiple strategies for autophagy regulation. *Cell Death Differ* (2019) 26(4):617–29. doi: 10.1038/s41418-018-0254-9
5. Park SE, Yi HJ, Suh N, Park YY, Koh JY, Jeong SY, et al. Inhibition of EHMT2/G9a epigenetically increases the transcription of Beclin-1 via an increase in ROS and activation of NF-κB. *Oncotarget* (2016) 7(26):39796–808. doi: 10.18632/oncotarget.9290
6. Kang R, Zeh HJ, Lotze MT, Tang D. The Beclin 1 network regulates autophagy and apoptosis. *Cell Death Differ* (2011) 18(74):571–80. doi: 10.1038/cdd.2010.191
7. Fujiwara N, Usui T, Ohama T, Sato K. Regulation of Beclin 1 Protein Phosphorylation and Autophagy by Protein Phosphatase 2A (PP2A) and Death-associated Protein Kinase 3 (DAPK3). *J Biol Chem* (2016) 291 (20):10858–66. doi: 10.1074/jbc.M115.704908
8. Sun T, Li X, Zhang P, Chen WD, Zhang HL, Li DD, et al. Acetylation of Beclin 1 inhibits autophagosome maturation and promotes tumour growth. *Nat Commun* (2015) 6:7215. doi: 10.1038/ncomms8215
9. Liu H, Ma Y, He HW, Wang JP, Jiang JD, Shao RG. SLC9A3R1 stimulates autophagy via BECN1 stabilization in breast cancer cells. *Autophagy* (2015) 11(12):2323–34. doi: 10.1080/15548627.2015.1074372
10. Jin S, Tian S, Chen Y, Zhang C, Xie W, Xia X, et al. USP19 modulates autophagy and antiviral immune responses by deubiquitinating Beclin-1. *EMBO J* (2016) 35(8):866–80. doi: 10.15252/embj.201593596
11. Tang Y, Zhang Y, Liu S, Sun Z, Wang C, Li L, et al. 14-3-3ζ binds to and stabilizes phospho-beclin 1S295 and induces autophagy in hepatocellular carcinoma cells. *J Cell Mol Med* (2020) 24(1):954–64. doi: 10.1111/jcmm.14806
12. Liu K, Guo C, Lao Y, Yang J, Chen F, Zhao Y, et al. A fine-tuning mechanism underlying self-control for autophagy: deSUMOylation of BECN1 by SENP3. *Autophagy* (2020) 16(6):975–90. doi: 10.1080/15548627.2019.1647944
13. Zhu Y, Zhao L, Liu L, Gao P, Tian W, Wang X, et al. Beclin 1 cleavage by caspase-3 inactivates autophagy and promotes apoptosis. *Protein Cell* (2010) 1 (5):468–77. doi: 10.1007/s13238-010-0048-4
14. Siddiqui MA, Mukherjee S, Manivannan P, Malathi K. RNase L cleavage products promote switch from autophagy to apoptosis by Caspase-mediated cleavage of Beclin-1. *Int J Mol Sci* (2015) 16(8):17611–36. doi: 10.3390/ijms160817611
15. Peng Y, Miao H, Wu S, Yang W, Zhang Y, Xie G, et al. ABHD5 interacts with BECN1 to regulate autophagy and tumorigenesis of colon cancer independent of PNPLA2. *Autophagy* (2016) 12(11):2167–82. doi: 10.1080/15548627.2016.1217380
16. Zhao Y, Chen S, Gou WF, Xiao LJ, Takano Y, Zheng HC. Aberrant Beclin 1 expression is closely linked to carcinogenesis, differentiation, progression, and prognosis of ovarian epithelial carcinoma. *Tumour Biol* (2014) 35(3):1955–64. doi: 10.1007/s13277-013-1261-6
17. Zhang MY, Gou WF, Zhao S, Mao XY, Zheng ZH, Takano Y, et al. Beclin 1 expression is closely linked to colorectal carcinogenesis and distant metastasis of colorectal carcinoma. *Int J Mol Sci* (2014) 15(8):14372–85. doi: 10.3390/ijms150814372
18. Yu M, Gou WF, Zhao S, Xiao LJ, Mao XY, Xing YN, et al. Beclin 1 expression is an independent prognostic factor for gastric carcinomas. *Tumour Biol* (2013) 34(2):1071–83. doi: 10.1007/s13277-013-0648-8
19. Zhang MY, Wang LY, Zhao S, Guo XC, Xu YQ, Zheng ZH, et al. Effects of Beclin 1 overexpression on aggressive phenotypes of colon cancer cells. *OncolLett* (2019) 17(2):2441–50. doi: 10.3892/ol.2018.9817
20. Pickford F, Masliah E, Britschgi M, Lucin K, Narasimhan R, Jaeger PA, et al. The autophagy-related protein beclin 1 shows reduced expression in early Alzheimer disease and regulates amyloid beta accumulation in mice. *J Clin Invest* (2008) 118(6):2190–9. doi: 10.1172/JCI33585
21. Gao P, Hao F, Dong X, Qiu Y. The role of autophagy and Beclin-1 in radiotherapy-induced apoptosis in thyroid carcinoma cells. *Int J Clin Exp Pathol* (2019) 12(3):885–92.
22. Furuya D, Tsuji N, Yagihashi A, Watanabe N. Beclin 1 augmented cis-diamminedichloroplatinum induced apoptosis via enhancing caspase-9 activity. *Exp Cell Res* (2005) 307(1):26–40. doi: 10.1016/j.yexcr.2005.02.023
23. Qu X, Yu J, Bhagat G, Furuya N, Hibshoosh H, Troxel A, et al. Promotion of tumorigenesis by heterozygous disruption of the beclin 1 autophagy gene. *J Clin Invest* (2003) 112(12):1809–20. doi: 10.1172/JCI20039
24. Yue Z, Jin S, Yang C, Levine AJ, Heintz N. Beclin 1, an autophagy gene essential for early embryonic development, is a haploinsufficient tumor suppressor. *Proc Natl Acad Sci USA* (2003) 100(25):15077–82. doi: 10.1073/pnas.2436255100
25. Won KY, Kim GY, Lim SJ, Sung JY, Kim YW, Park YK, et al. Autophagy is related to the hedgehog signaling pathway in human gastric adenocarcinoma: prognostic significance of Beclin -1 and Gli2 expression in human gastric adenocarcinoma. *Pathol Res Pract* (2015) 211(4):308–15. doi: 10.1016/j.prp.2014.11.005
26. Geng QR, Xu DZ, He LJ, Lu JB, Zhou ZW, Zhan YQ, et al. Beclin-1 expression is a significant predictor of survival in patients with lymph node-positive gastric cancer. *PloS One* (2012) 7(9):e45968. doi: 10.1371/journal.pone.0045968
27. Chen YB, Hou JH, Feng XY, Chen S, Zhou ZW, Zhang XS, et al. Decreased expression of Beclin 1 correlates with a metastatic phenotypic feature and adverse prognosis of gastric carcinomas. *J Surg Oncol* (2012) 105(6):542–7. doi: 10.1002/jso.22151
28. Fei B, Ji F, Chen X, Liu Z, Li S, Mo Z, et al. Expression and clinical significance of Beclin-1 in gastric cancer tissues of various clinical stages. *Oncol Lett* (2016) 11(3):2271–7. doi: 10.3892/ol.2016.4183
29. Qin W, Li C, Zheng W, Guo Q, Zhang Y, Kang M, et al. Inhibition of autophagy promotes metastasis and glycolysis by inducing ROS in gastric cancer cells. *Oncotarget* (2015) 6(37):39839–54. doi: 10.18632/oncotarget.5674
30. Zhou WH, Tang F, Xu J, Wu X, Yang SB, Feng ZY, et al. Low expression of Beclin 1, associated with high Bcl-xL, predicts a malignant phenotype and poor prognosis of gastric cancer. *Autophagy* (2012) 8(3):389–400. doi: 10.4161/auto.18641
31. Yu S, Li G, Wang Z, Wang Z, Chen C, Cai S, et al. Low expression of MAP1LC3B, associated with low Beclin-1, predicts lymph node metastasis and poor prognosis of gastric cancer. *Tumour Biol* (2016) 37(11):15007–17. doi: 10.1007/s13277-016-5383-5
32. Zhao Z, Han F, Yang S, Wu J, Zhan W. Oxamate-mediated inhibition of lactate dehydrogenase induces protective autophagy in gastric cancer cells: involvement of the Akt-mTOR signaling pathway. *Cancer Lett* (2015) 358 (1):17–26. doi: 10.1016/j.canlet.2014.11.046
33. Qiu G, Li X, Wei C, Che X, He S, Lu J, et al. The prognostic role of SIRT1-autophagy axis in gastric cancer. *Dis Markers* (2016) 2016:6869415. doi: 10.1155/2016/6869415
34. Cao QH, Liu F, Yang ZL, Fu XH, Yang ZH, Liu Q, et al. Prognostic value of autophagy related proteins ULK1, Beclin 1, ATG3, ATG5, ATG7, ATG9, ATG10, ATG12, LC3B and p62/SQSTM1 in gastric cancer. *Am J Transl Res* (2016) 8(9):3831–47.
35. Huang JL, Zhong TM, Huang ZS, Li GZ, Zhou XH, He SG, et al. Correlation study of expression of autophagic factors Beclin 1 and LC3 and clinicopathological features in gastric cancer. *Pract J Cancer* (2016) 31:530–2.
36. Hu YF, Lei X, Zhao H, Yang WW, Feng XM, Yin XL, et al. The association of expressions of autophagy-related protein Beclin 1 and HP infection in gastric cancer. *Modern Oncol* (2017) 25:1093–6.
37. Guo CQ, Shao JH, Lu RL, Cao XG. Expression of Beclin 1 and PTEN proteins in gastric cancer tissues. *J Zhengzhou Univ (Med Sci)* (2010) 45(3):463–5.
38. Zhang Y, Lin S, Zhang Y, Chang S. Effect of beclin 1 expression on the biological behavior and chemotherapy sensitivity of cervical cancer cells. *Oncol Lett* (2016) 11(6):4089–94. doi: 10.3892/ol.2016.4542
39. Wang W, Fan H, Li X, Wu G, Zhao W, Zhang G, et al. Beclin 1 promotes apoptosis and decreases invasion by upregulating the expression of ECRG4 in A549 human lung adenocarcinoma cells. *Mol Med Rep* (2016) 14(1):355–60. doi: 10.3892/mmr.2016.5219
40. Wang MC, Wu AG, Huang YZ, Shao GL, Ji SF, Wang RW, et al. Autophagic regulation of cell growth by altered expression of Beclin 1 in triple-negative breast cancer. *Int J Clin Exp Med* (2015) 8(5):7049–58.
41. Li S, Zhang HY, Du ZX, Li C, An MX, Zong ZH, et al. Induction of epithelial-mesenchymal transition (EMT) by Beclin 1 knockdown via posttranscriptional upregulation of ZEB1 in thyroid cancer cells. *Oncotarget* (2016) 7(43):70364–77. doi: 10.18632/oncotarget.12217
42. Shu CW, Chang HT, Wu CS, Chen CH, Wu S, Chang HW, et al. RelA-mediated BECN1 expression is required for reactive oxygen species-induced autophagy in oral cancer cells exposed to low-power laser irradiation. *PloS One* (2016) 11(9):e0160586. doi: 10.1371/journal.pone.0160586

43. Hasan A, Haque E, Hameed R, Maier PN, Irfan S, Kamil M, et al. Hsp90 inhibitor gedunin causes apoptosis in A549 lung cancer cells by disrupting Hsp90: Beclin-1:Bcl-2 interaction and downregulating autophagy. *Life Sci* (2020) 256:118000. doi: 10.1016/j.lfs.2020.118000
44. Hu F, Li G, Huang C, Hou Z, Yang X, Luo X, et al. The autophagy-independent role of BECN1 in colorectal cancer metastasis through regulating STAT3 signaling pathway activation. *Cell Death Dis* (2020) 11 (5):304. doi: 10.1038/s41419-020-2467-3
45. Cheng Z, Xin H, Han T. BECN1 promotes the migration of NSCLC cells through regulating the ubiquitination of Vimentin. *Cell Adh Migr* (2019) 13 (1):249–59. doi: 10.1080/19336918.2019.1638690
46. Li XB, Yang G, Zhu L, Tang YL, Zhang C, Ju Z, et al. Gastric Lgr5(+) stem cells are the cellular origin of invasive intestinal-type gastric cancer in mice. *Cell Res* (2016) 26(7):838–49. doi: 10.1038/cr.2016.47
47. Zheng HC. The molecular mechanisms of chemoresistance in cancers. *Oncotarget* (2017) 8(35):59950–64. doi: 10.18632/oncotarget.19048
48. Zheng HC, Zhao S, Song Y, Ding XQ. The roles of ING5 expression in ovariancarcinogenesis and subsequent progression: a target of gene therapy. *Oncotarget* (2017) 8(61):103449–64. doi: 10.18632/oncotarget.21968
49. Wu JC, Jiang HM, Yang XH, Zheng HC. ING5-mediated antineuroblastoma effects ofsuberoyl- anilide hydroxamic acid. *Cancer Med* (2018) 7(9):4554–69. doi: 10.1002/cam4.1634
50. Ding XQ, Zhao S, Yang L, Zhao X, Zhao GF, Zhao SP, et al. The nucleocytoplasmic translocation and up-regulation of ING5 protein in breastcancer: a potential target for gene therapy. *Oncotarget* (2017) 8 (47):81953–66. doi: 10.18632/oncotarget.17918
51. Zhao S, Zhao ZJ, He HY, Wu JC, Ding XQ, Yang L, et al. The roles of ING5 in gliomas: a good marker for tumorigenesis and a potential target for gene therapy. *Oncotarget* (2017) 8(43):56558–68. doi: 10.18632/oncotarget.17802
52. Zhao S, Yang XF, Shen DF, Gao Y, Shi S, Wu JC, et al. The down-regulated ING5 expression in lung cancer: a potential target of genetherapy. *Oncotarget* (2016) 7(34):54596–615. doi: 10.18632/oncotarget.10519
53. Pang M, Wang H, Rao P, Zhao Y, Xie J, Cao Q, et al. Autophagy links β-catenin and Smad signaling to promote epithelial-mesenchymal transition via upregulation of integrin linked kinase. *Int J Biochem Cell Biol* (2016) 76:123–34. doi: 10.1016/j.biocel.2016.05.010
54. Sun T, Jiao L, Wang Y, Yu Y, Ming L. SIRT1 induces epithelial-mesenchymal transition by promoting autophagic degradation of E-cadherin in melanoma cells. *Cell Death Dis* (2018) 9(2):136. doi: 10.1038/s41419-017-0167-4
55. Han LL, Jia L, Wu F, Huang C. Sirtuin6 (SIRT6) promotes the EMT of hepatocellular carcinoma by stimulating autophagic degradation of E-cadherin. *Mol Cancer Res* (2019) 17(11):2267–80. doi: 10.1158/1541-7786.MCR-19-0321
56. Liu H, Ma Y, He HW, Zhao WL, Shao RG. SPHK1 (sphingosine kinase 1) induces epithelial- mesenchymal transition by promoting the autophagy-linked lysosomal degradation of CDH1/ E-cadherin in hepatoma cells. *Autophagy* (2017) 13(5):900–13. doi: 10.1080/15548627.2017.1291479
57. Liu T, Liu Y, Miller M, Cao L, Zhao J, Wu J, et al. Autophagy plays a role in FSTL1-induced epithelial mesenchymal transition and airway remodeling in asthma. *Am J Physiol Lung Cell Mol Physiol* (2017) 313(1):L27–40. doi: 10.1152/ajplung.00510.2016
58. Ouyang F, Huang H, Zhang M, Chen M, Huang H, Huang F, et al. HMGB1 induces apoptosis and EMT in association with increased autophagy following H/R injury in cardiomyocytes. *Int J Mol Med* (2016) 37(3):679–89. doi: 10.3892/ijmm.2016.2474
59. Chen Y, Wang L, Bao J, Sha X, Cui L, Huang Q, et al. Persistent hypoxia induced autophagy leading to invasiveness of trophoblasts in placenta accreta. *J Matern Fetal Neonatal Med* (2019) 3:1–7. doi: 10.1080/14767058.2019.1635582
60. Zhang J, Chu D, Kawamura T, Tanaka K, He S. GRIM-19 repressed hypoxia-induced invasion and EMT of colorectal cancer by repressing autophagy through inactivation of STAT3/HIF-1α signaling axis. *J Cell Physiol* (2019) 234(8):12800–808. doi: 10.1002/jcp.27914
61. Zhu H, Wang D, Zhang L, Xie X, Wu Y, Liu Y, et al. Upregulation of autophagy by hypoxia-inducible factor-1α promotes EMT and metastatic ability of CD133+ pancreatic cancer stem-like cells during intermittent hypoxia. *Oncol Rep* (2014) 32(3):935–42. doi: 10.3892/or.2014.3298
62. Moon SY, Kim HS, Nho KW, Jang YJ, Lee SK. Endoplasmic reticulum stress induces epithelial- mesenchymal transition through autophagy via activation of c-Src kinase. *Nephron Exp Nephrol* (2014) 126(3):127–40. doi: 10.1159/000362457
63. Catalano M, D'Alessandro G, Lepore F, Corazzari M, Caldarola S, Valacca C, et al. Autophagy induction impairs migration and invasion by reversing EMT in glioblastoma cells. *Mol Oncol* (2015) 9(8):1612–25. doi: 10.1016/j.molonc.2015.04.016
64. Weh KM, Howell AB, Kresty LA. Expression, modulation, and clinical correlates of the autophagy protein Beclin-1 in esophageal adenocarcinoma. *Mol Carcinog* (2016) 55(11):1876–85. doi: 10.1002/mc.22432
65. Liu L, Meng T, Wang QS, Jin HZ, Sun ZQ, Jin B, et al. Association of Beclin-1 and microRNA-30a expression with the severity and treatment response of colorectal cancer. *Genet Mol Res* (2016) 15(2):15027704. doi: 10.4238/gmr.15027704
66. Wu T, Li Y, Gong L, Lu JG, Du XL, Zhang WD, et al. Multi-step process of human breast carcinogenesis: a role for BRCA1, BECN1, CCND1, PTEN and UVRAG. *Mol Med Rep* (2012) 5(2):305–12. doi: 10.3892/mmr.2011.634
67. Song S, Wang B, Gu S, Li X, Sun S. Expression of Beclin 1 and Bcl-2 in pancreatic neoplasms and its effect on pancreatic ductal adenocarcinomaprognosis. *Oncol Lett* (2017) 14(6):7849–61. doi: 10.3892/ol.2017.7218
68. Morikawa A, Takeuchi T, Kito Y, Saigo C, Sakuratani T, Futamura M, et al. Expression of beclin-1 in the microenvironment of invasive ductal carcinoma of the breast: correlation with prognosis and the cancer-stromal interaction. *PloS One* (2015) 10(5):e0125762. doi: 10.1371/journal.pone.0125762
69. Qin Z, Yu X, Lin M, Wu J, Ma S, Wang N. Prognostic and clinicopathologicalvalue of Beclin-1 expression in hepatocellular carcinoma: a meta-analysis. *World J Surg Oncol* (2018) 1(1):170. doi: 10.1186/s12957-018-1465-8
70. Chen Y, Yan J, Yu S, Wang X, Zheng Q. Over-expression of beclin-1 in gallbladder carcinoma and its relationship with prognosis. *Contemp Oncol (Pozn)* (2014) 18(3):171–6. doi: 10.5114/wo.2014.41395
71. Bi C, Liu M, Rong W, Wu F, Zhang Y, Lin S, et al. High Beclin-1 and ARID1A expression corelates with poor survival and high recurrence in intrahepatic cholangiocarcinoma: a histopathological retrospective study. *BMC Cancer* (2019) 19:213. doi: 10.1186/s12885-019-5429-3
72. Zheng T, Li D, He Z, Feng S, Zhao S. Prognostic and clinicopathological significance of Beclin-1 in non-small-cell lung cancer: a meta-analysis. *OncoTargets Ther* (2018) 11:4167–75. doi: 10.2147/OTT.S164987
73. Minamoto T, Nakayama K, Nakamura K, Katagiri H, Sultana R, Ishibashi T, et al. Loss of beclin 1 expression in ovarian cancer: A potential biomarker for predicting unfavorable outcomes. *Oncol Lett* (2018) 15(1):1170–6. doi: 10.3892/ol.2017.7379
74. Tang H, Sebti S, Titone R, Zhou Y, Isidoro C, Ross TS, et al. Decreased BECN1 mRNA expression in human breast cancer is associated with estrogen receptor-negative subtypes and poor prognosis. *EbioMedicine* (2015) 2 (3):255–63. doi: 10.1016/j.ebiom.2015.01.008
75. Gu Y, Chen T, Li G, Xu C, Xu Z, Zhang J, et al. Lower Beclin 1 downregulates HER2 expression to enhance tamoxifen sensitivity and predicts a favorable outcome for ER positive breast cancer. *Oncotarget* (2016) 8(32):52156–77. doi: 10.18632/oncotarget.11044
76. Katagiri H, Nakayama K, Razia S, Nakamura K, Sato E, Ishibashi T, et al. Loss of autophagy-related protein Beclin 1 may define poor prognosis in ovarian clear cell carcinomas. *Int J Oncol* (2015) 47(6):2037–44. doi: 10.3892/ijo.2015.3191
77. Jung G, Roh J, Lee H, Gil M, Yoon DH, Suh C, et al. Autophagic markers BECLIN 1 and LC3 are associated with prognosis of multiple myeloma. *Acta Haematol* (2015) 134(1):17–24. doi: 10.1159/000368848

16

LINC00483 Has a Potential Tumor-Suppressor Role in Colorectal Cancer Through Multiple Molecular Axes

*Duilia Brex[1], Cristina Barbagallo[1], Federica Mirabella[1], Angela Caponnetto[1], Rosalia Battaglia[1], Davide Barbagallo[1], Rosario Caltabiano[2], Giuseppe Broggi[2], Lorenzo Memeo[3], Cinzia Di Pietro[1], Michele Purrello[1] and Marco Ragusa[1]**

[1] Department of Biomedical and Biotechnological Sciences – Section of Biology and Genetics "Giovanni Sichel," University of Catania, Catania, Italy, [2] Department of Medical, Surgical Sciences and Advanced Technologies G.F. Ingrassia, University of Catania, Catania, Italy, [3] Department of Experimental Oncology, Mediterranean Institute of Oncology (IOM), Catania, Italy

***Correspondence:**
Marco Ragusa
mragusa@unict.it

Long non-coding RNAs (lncRNAs) are the most heterogeneous class of non-protein-coding RNAs involved in a broad spectrum of molecular mechanisms controlling genome function, including the generation of complex networks of RNA-RNA competitive interactions. Accordingly, their dysregulation contributes to the onset of many tumors, including colorectal cancer (CRC). Through a combination of *in silico* approaches (statistical screening of expression datasets) and *in vitro* analyses (enforced expression, artificial inhibition, or activation of pathways), we identified LINC00483 as a potential tumor suppressor lncRNA in CRC. LINC00483 was downregulated in CRC biopsies and metastases and its decreased levels were associated with severe clinical features. Inhibition of the MAPK pathway and cell cycle arrest by starvation induced an upregulation of LINC00483, while the epithelial to mesenchymal transition activation by TGFβ-1 and IL-6 caused its down-modulation. Moreover, enforced expression of LINC00483 provoked a slowing down of cell migration rate without affecting cell proliferation. Since LINC00483 was predominantly cytoplasmic, we hypothesized a "miRNA sponge" role for it. Accordingly, we computationally reconstructed the LINC00483/miRNA/mRNA axes and evaluated the expression of mRNAs in different experimental conditions inducing LINC00483 alteration. By this approach, we identified a set of mRNAs sharing the miRNA response elements with LINC00483 and modulated in accordance with it. Moreover, we found that LINC00483 is potentially under negative control of transcription factor HNF4α. In conclusion, we propose that LINC00483 is a tumor suppressor in CRC that, through an RNA-RNA network, may control cell migration and participate in proliferation signaling.

Keywords: long non-coding RNAs, microRNAs, colorectal cancer, competing endogenous RNA, epithelial–mesenchymal transition, HNF4α, TGFβ-1, IL-6

INTRODUCTION

Colorectal cancer (CRC) is the most common malignancy in the digestive system and the fourth leading cause of cancer-related death around the world, mainly from tumor metastasis (1). Although modern oncology has made great efforts to shed light on the underlying molecular mechanisms of the development of CRC, much of it is still unclear. Accordingly, it is needed to explore new regulatory mechanisms of CRC onset and progression in order to improve diagnostics and the development of innovative therapeutic strategies. The Vogelstein's model, based on a sequence of molecular changes within protein-coding genes leading to cancer transformation, is now considered too simplistic to explain the complex heterogeneity of cancer, including and especially CRC (2, 3). Notably, only less than 2% of the human genome encodes proteins, while about 85% is pervasively transcribed in RNAs other than mRNAs, denominated non-coding RNAs (ncRNAs), including microRNAs (miRNAs) and long non-coding RNAs (lncRNAs) (4–6). LncRNAs are more than 200 nt in length with no or limited protein-coding power and account for a large part of the human genome (7). Although lncRNAs were initially considered as unfunctional transcriptional "noise," recent studies have revealed that they play a key regulatory role in multiple cellular processes, including stem cell pluripotency, apoptosis, cell differentiation, migration, genomic stability, and epithelial–mesenchymal transition (EMT) (8). Accordingly, it is not surprising that lncRNA dysregulation plays a very important role in tumorigenesis indeed, the oncogenic or tumor-suppressive action of lncRNAs has been largely demonstrated to participate in cancer transformation and progression (9, 10). Through binding DNA, RNAs, and proteins, lncRNAs exhibit a broad spectrum of molecular mechanisms by which they influence gene expression, such as chromatin modification, RNA transcription, pre-mRNA splicing, mRNA translation, and protein localization (11, 12). In the last few years, several pieces of evidence have been collected on the involvement of lncRNAs in CRC onset and progression. LncRNAs affect critical CRC signaling pathways by acting both as oncogenes and tumor suppressors through interactions with other regulatory molecules (13–15). Several lncRNAs have been reported to be dysregulated in CRC, suggesting promising potentiality for theranostic applications (16–18). However, the molecular mechanisms of action in CRC pathobiology were elucidated only for few of them, such as, CCAT1, CCAT2, H19, HOTAIR, MALAT1, and UCA1 (19–25). One of the most explored molecular mechanisms of lncRNAs in cytoplasm is their activity as miRNA sponges. The ability of lncRNAs to sequester miRNAs by sequence complementarity has important systemic effects on the RNA network inside cells. Indeed, the hypothesis of competing endogenous RNA (ceRNA) foresees that lncRNAs and mRNAs, sharing the same miRNA response elements (MREs), compete for binding to same miRNAs, regulating each other's expression (26, 27). According to the hypothesis that the expressions of lncRNAs and mRNAs with the same MREs would be positively and negatively correlated to each other and to miRNAs, respectively, in this paper we propose a combined approach of *in silico* and experimental biology to identify an lncRNA whose dysregulated expression is associated with CRC pathobiology. More specifically, based on the hypothesis that RNA-RNA network functioning is grounded on relative stoichiometric concentrations of interacting RNA molecules, our aim was the identification and characterization of a lncRNA whose expression was linearly related to that of mRNAs dysregulated in association with most serious clinical features of CRC patients. Following its computational identification, LINC00483 was experimentally analysed to understand its involvement in CRC and its associated molecular axes.

MATERIAL AND METHODS

Computational Analysis

We retrieved from "R2 Genomics" (https://hgserver1.amc.nl/cgi-bin/r2/main.cgi?&species=hs) datasets containing expression data on CRC (**Table S1**) in order to identify differentially expressed (DE) genes associated with the most severe features of the tumor phenotype (e.g., metastases, microsatellite instability, advanced tumor, node, metastasis [TNM] stage, KRAS, BRAF and TP53 mutations, CpG island methylator phenotype [CIMP] status). Results were filtered by p-value (≤ 0.01), using the ANOVA statistical test and the "false discovery rate" as correction criterion for multiple tests. From each dataset we recovered genes that were downregulated/upregulated in CRC, according to the above-mentioned clinical-pathological features.

By overlapping gene lists (downregulated/upregulated gene lists) retrieved from each dataset, we obtained a single list of genes showing the same type of dysregulation (i.e., up- or down-regulation) in at least 50% of consulted datasets. We employed these CRC deregulated genes as BGs to identify CRC related lncRNAs. More specifically, we selected those lncRNAs showing positive or negative correlation with BGs by calculating the Pearson coefficient (p-value < 0.01) between the expression values of the BGs and the expression values of all lncRNAs in each dataset previously analyzed. We compared the lists of lncRNAs associated with each BG for each dataset and selected only those lncRNAs shared by at least 50% of datasets.

Finally, we generated 4 lists of lncRNAs correlated with BGs associated with the most severe clinical-pathological features of CRC:

1. lncRNAs showing positive correlation with downregulated genes;
2. lncRNAs showing positive correlation with upregulated genes;
3. lncRNAs showing negative correlation with downregulated genes;
4. lncRNAs showing negative correlation with upregulated genes;

We overlapped lists 1–4, and lists 2–3, because we speculated that lncRNAs positively correlated with downregulated genes corresponded roughly with the list of lncRNAs negatively correlated with upregulated genes and, in the same way, lncRNAs positively correlated with upregulated genes were in the list of lncRNAs negatively correlated with downregulated genes. Therefore, lncRNAs shared by the two compared lists were selected. By this approach, we obtained i) a list of potential tumor-suppressor lncRNAs by overlapping of 1 and 4, and ii) a list of potential oncogene lncRNAs by overlapping of 2 and 3 (**Figure 1**).

Long Non-Coding RNA Target Identification

Since one of the most common functions of lncRNAs is that of "miRNA sponge," we identified miRNAs that could simultaneously bind the selected lncRNAs and the genes positively correlated with them. In this supposed "miRNA sponge" model, the lncRNA and mRNA should exhibit a mutual positive expression correlation, while the miRNA—acting as a "trait d'union" negative regulator RNA—should have a negative expression correlation with the same lncRNA and mRNA (**Figure S1**). To investigate this hypothesis, we retrieved miRNAs showing a negative correlation with the studied lncRNAs. MiRNA expression values were retrieved from TCGA colon cancer (COAD) (n=261), through UCSC XENA (https://xenabrowser.net/datapages/), and compared to lncRNA expression from the same dataset. We calculated the Pearson coefficient between miRNA and lncRNA expression values and selected miRNAs showing a negative correlation with the selected lncRNAs (p-value ≤0.001). We simultaneously retrieved miRNAs harboring binding sites for lncRNAs through LncBase (http://carolina.imis.athena-innovation.gr/diana_tools/web/index.php?r=lncbasev2%2Findex-experimental), miRcode (http://www.mircode.org/), and RNA22 v.2 tool (https://cm.jefferson.edu/rna22/Interactive/) and completed these outputs with those resulting from correlation analysis. To complete the molecular axis of the lncRNA-miRNA-mRNA interaction, we identified mRNAs targeted by these miRNAs. We interrogated the datasets selected in the early step of the study in order to identify those mRNAs that showed the strongest positive correlation with lncRNAs, as previously described. For these mRNAs were verified: a) the binding to miRNAs previously identified through TarBase v.8 (http://carolina.imis.athena-innovation.gr/diana_tools/web/index.php?r=tarbasev8%2Findex); b) their negative expression correlation with the same miRNAs (TCGA COAD). To make this analysis more effective and focused on our pathological model, it was performed just on those miRNAs showing an involvement in CRC by using mirCancer (http://mircancer.ecu.edu/) and mir2Disease (http://www.mir2disease.org/) databases.

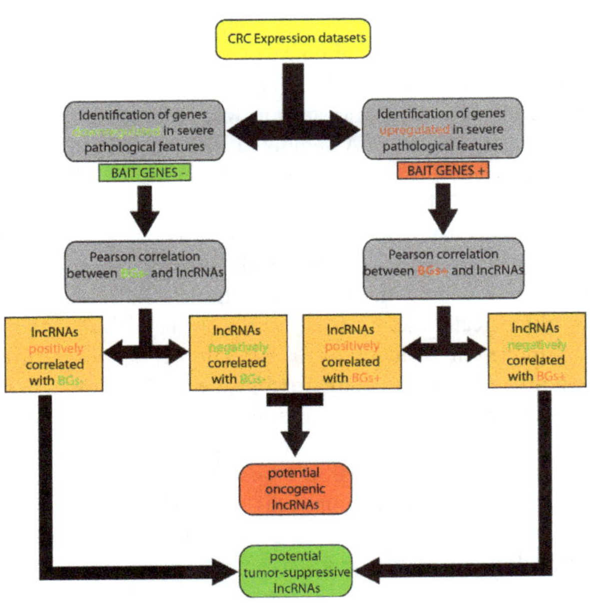

FIGURE 1 | Workflow of the computational approach followed to identify *long non-coding RNAs* (lncRNAs) associated to *colorectal cancer* (CRC).

Cell Lines

HCT-116 cell lines, derived from primary colon tumors, were obtained from the Interlab Cell Line Collection (ICLC), an "International Repository Authority" within the IRCCS Azienda Ospedaliera Universitaria San Martino-IST Istituto Nazionale per la Ricerca sul Cancro (Genova, Italia). HCT-116 cells were maintained in Roswell Park Memorial Institute-1640 (RPMI-1640) medium (Gibco), supplemented with 10% fetal bovine serum (FBS) (Gibco), 1% 2 mM L-glutammine (Lonza, Basel, Switzerland), and 1% penicillin/streptomycin (10,000 U/ml) (Gibco). Cells were cultured at 37°C and 5% CO2.

RNA Isolation From Cell Lines

Total RNA was extracted from cell lines with TRIzol® (Invitrogen, Carlsbad, CA, USA), according to the manufacturer's instructions, and quantified by GenQuant Pro Spectrophotometer (Biochrom) and Qubit fluorescence quantification system (Invitrogen). Isolated RNA was treated with DNase, according to the manufacturer's instructions. The RNA Subcellular Isolation Kit (Active Motif) was used to analyze lncRNA expression separately in the nucleus and cytoplasm of HCT-116 cells. The lncRNAs MALAT1 and TUG1 were used as markers of nuclear and cytoplasmic fractions, respectively.

RNA Isolation From Colorectal Cancer Formalin-Fixed, Paraffin-Embedded Samples

Twenty CRC patients were recruited from "Azienda Ospedaliero—Universitaria Policlinico Vittorio Emanuele" (Catania, Italy). Formalin-Fixed, Paraffin-Embedded (FFPE) tumor tissues and adjacent normal colon mucosa were isolated at the Section of Anatomic Pathology, Department G.F. Ingrassia, University of Catania (Catania, Italy) (**Table 1**). RNA was extracted from FFPE samples through the PureLink FFPE RNA Isolation Kit (Invitrogen), according to the manufacturer's instructions, and quantified by GenQuant pro spectrophotometer (Biochrom) and Qubit (Invitrogen).

TABLE 1 | Colorectal cancer (CRC) biopsies analyzed in this study.

Cohorts	Mean age (years ± Std Dev)	Sex		Grading		pT		pN		M	
		M	F	G1/G2	G3	T1/T2	T3/T4	N= 0	N > 0	M0	M1
OCT samples	68 ± 12	19	16	31	4	7	28	20	15	31	4
FFPE samples	69 ± 11	11	9	15	5	5	15	13	7	20	0

RNA Isolation From Colorectal Cancer Tissues Embedded in OCT and Fresh Biopsies

A second independent group of 35 CRC samples embedded in Optimal Cutting Temperature (OCT) were analyzed. All samples were provided from "Istituto Oncologico del Mediterraneo (IOM)" Viagrande (Catania, Italy) (**Table 1**). OCT tumor tissues were sliced with a cryostat at the Section of Anatomic Pathology, Department G.F. Ingrassia, University of Catania (Catania, Italy). Before RNA extraction, samples were treated to remove OCT as follows:

1. Wash OCT tissue samples three times with 500 µl DEPC H2O; centrifuge 4°C x 5 min at 11,000 g (Eppendorf Centrifuge 5424 R) and remove supernatant after each step;
2. Wash with 500 µl ETOH 25%; centrifuge 4°C x 5 min at 11,000 g (Eppendorf Centrifuge 5424 R) and remove supernatant.

Total RNA was extracted from OCT tissue samples and from fresh biopsies through the PureLink FFPE RNA Isolation Kit (Invitrogen) and TRIzol ® (Invitrogen, Carlsbad, CA, USA), respectively, according to the manufacturer's instructions. Isolated RNA was quantified by GenQuant pro spectrophotometer (Biochrom).

PCR Primer Design

We designed specific PCR primers for the selected lncRNAs and their target mRNAs by using the online tool Primer-Blast (http://www.ncbi.nlm.nih.gov/tools/primer-blast/). Specific PRC primers were also designed for the housekeeping gene PPIA (peptidylprolyl isomerase A), used for normalization. Primer pairs are shown in **Table S2**.

Expression Analysis by Real-Time PCR

We investigated the expression of the selected lncRNAs and mRNA axis in CRC cell lines and CRC patient tissues through Real Time PCR, by using Power SYBR Green RNA-to-CT 1-Step Kit (Applied Biosystems, Thermo Fisher Scientific, Waltham, MA, USA), according to the manufacturer's instructions. All reactions were performed on a 7900HT Fast Real-Time PCR System (Applied Biosystems). We used PPIA as reference gene, both for cell lines and CRC tissues. DE gene fold changes were calculated by applying the 2-ΔΔCt method. A paired T-test was used to compare FFPE sample ΔCts, while an unpaired T-test was used for evaluate all the other analyses. P-value ≤0.05 was established as statistically significance.

HCT-116 Transfection With LINC00483

We transfected the HCT-116 cell line with pcDNA3.1(+) expression vector to induce LINC00483 overexpression. The cDNA sequence of LINC00483 was cloned into pcDNA3.1(+) by EcoRV, consistent with the direction of the CMV promote. The empty pcDNA3.1(+) vector was used as a scramble molecule. Both constructs were synthesized and purchased from the GenScript company. Ten micrograms of plasmids were re-suspended in 40 µl TE buffer 1X. Cells (2 x 105 per well) were seeded in 24-well plates and transfected with 750 ng plasmid together with LipofectamineTM 2000 (Invitrogen) by using the direct transfection method, according to the manufacturer's instructions. Cells were harvested at 48 h after transfection and lysed with TRIzol for RNA extraction. Total RNA was used both to confirm transfection efficiency (>90%) and to evaluate the expression of axis's mRNAs by Real Time PCR. All experiments were performed in biological triplicates.

Functional Assays

The CCK-8 assay was performed to assess cellular viability/proliferation at 48 h AT, according to the manufacturer's instructions. Absorbance values were read with Varioskan™ LUX (Thermo Scientific™). We transfected HCT-116 cell lines with an expression vector and its respective scramble molecule by seeding 2.5 x 104 cells per well in 96-well plates and appropriately scaling the amount of transfection reagents. All experiments were performed in biological triplicates.

Migration rates after transfection were evaluated by OrisTM Universal Cell Migration Assembly kit (Platypus Technologies), according to the manufacturer's instructions. Briefly, we transfected HCT-116 cells with the expression vector and its scramble molecule by seeding 3.5 x 104 cells per well in 96-well plates—after insertion of Oris Cell Seeding Stoppers—and appropriately scaling the amount of transfection reagents. To create the detection zone at the center of the well, the stoppers were removed at 24 h AT (0 h). Detection zones for each well were photographed with a microscope, Leitz FLUOVERT (Leica Microsystems), at 0 h (premigration reference wells) and at 24, 48, 72, 96, and 144 h AT. Cells that migrated into the detection zone were quantified through the ImageJ software package. This analysis allowed us to quantify cells that had migrated into the detection zone for all the time points. All experiments were performed in biological triplicates.

TGFβ-1 Treatment

We performed an *in vitro* EMT by treatment with TGFβ-1, a cytokine secreted by tumor cells and stromal fibroblasts in the tumor microenvironment and considered a primary inducer of EMT (28). 5 x 104 cells per well were seeded in 24-well plates and maintained in serum starvation conditions (0.5% FBS) for 24 h. Successively, cells were treated with 20 ng/ml TGFβ-1 for 24 h. Control samples were maintained in RPMI-1640 medium (Gibco) supplemented with an equal volume of solvent. All experiments were performed in biological triplicates.

Interleukin-6 Treatment

We treated HCT-116 cell line with IL-6, a multifunctional cytokine whose signaling hyper-activation is associated with tumor onset and development. 3 x 104 cells per well were seeded in 24-well plates and maintained in serum starvation conditions (0.5% FBS) for 24 h. Successively, cells were treated with 200 ng/ml IL-6 and exposed for 24 and 48 h. Control samples were maintained in RPMI-1640 medium (Gibco) supplemented with an equal volume of solvent. All experiments were performed in biological triplicates.

Treatment With MAPK Inhibitor U0126

We performed a pharmacological inhibition of the MAPK pathway by treating the HCT-116 cell line with U0126, a highly selective ATP-non-competitive MEK1/2 inhibitor, which specifically prevents *in vitro* phosphorylation of MEK1/2 by binding to the inactive enzyme and blocking ERK recruitment. HCT-116 cells were seeded (3.2 x 104 per well) in 24-well plates and cultured in serum starvation conditions (no FBS) for 24 h; successively, cells were treated with 25 μM U0126 (MEK1/2 inhibitor, Merck, Darmstadt, Germany) and exposed to the drug for 12 and 24 h. Control samples were treated with an equivalent volume of DMSO (solvent of the drug used for treatment). All experiments were performed in biological triplicates.

Cell Cycle Arrest

To investigate if the expression of the selected lncRNAs is modulated during artificial cell cycle arrest, we evaluated HCT-116 response to serum starvation. 5 x 105 cells were seeded in 24-well plates. We separately treated two groups of samples: the first group of samples was exposed to serum starvation by maintaining cells in RPMI-1640 medium (Gibco) (no FBS) for 24 h. Control samples were maintained in RPMI-1640 (10% FBS). A second group of cells was synchronized by serum starvation (no FBS) for 24 h and subsequently incubated with fresh medium with 10% FBS for a further 24 h. Control samples were incubated with fresh RPMI-1640 without serum. All experiments were performed in biological triplicates.

Treatment With HNF4α Inhibitor BI6015

To verify the transcriptional regulation of LINC00483 by HNF4α, we treated the HCT-116 cell line with BI6015, a specific inhibitor of this transcription factor. 8 x 104 cell were seeded in 24-well plates and treated with 80 μM BI6015 (Focus Biomolecules) for 24 h. Control samples were treated with an equivalent volume of DMSO (solvent). All experiments were performed in biological triplicates.

Identification of Transcription Factor Binding Sites

Potential transcription factor binding sites (TFBSs) harbored on LINC00483 promoter and upstream regulatory region (1 kb) were retrieved from ENCODE tracks (i.e., transcription factor ChIP-seq clusters, DNaseI hypersensitivity clusters) and UCSC regulatory tracks (i.e., regulatory elements from ORegAnno, SwitchGear genomics transcription start sites) mapped on UCSC Genome Browser (https://genome.ucsc.edu/).

RESULTS

Screening of Colorectal Cancer Expression Datasets, Long Non-Coding RNA Selection

By following the approach reported in methods, we identified from each CRC expression dataset those genes that were downregulated/upregulated in CRC, according to the specified clinical-pathological features.

By overlapping gene lists (downregulated/upregulated gene lists) retrieved from each dataset, we obtained a single list of upregulated genes (CYP1B1, NPR3, RGL2, SLIT2, TSPAN2) and a single list of downregulated genes (ACOT7, AGPAT5, ATP5B, AURKAIP1, CASP1, CEP55, CXCL3, FUT4, GSR, HNRNPAB, IDO1, KIF11, MCM5, PBK, PIGR, RANBP1, SCO2, TOE1, TTLL12) showing the same trend of expression alteration in at least 50% of datasets.

These CRC deregulated genes were used as "bait genes" (BGs) to identify lncRNAs showing a statistically significant positive correlation (PC) or negative correlation (NC) of expression with BGs.

We compared the lists of lncRNAs associated with each BG from each dataset and selected only those lncRNAs shared by at least 50% of datasets.

Finally, we generated four lists of lncRNAs (**Table 2**) correlated with BGs:

1. lncRNAs showing PC with downregulated genes (**Table 2**, column A);
2. lncRNAs showing PC with upregulated genes (**Table 2**, column B);
3. lncRNAs showing NC with downregulated genes (**Table 2**, column C);
4. lncRNAs showing NC with upregulated genes (**Table 2**, column D);

Finally, as reported in methods, we overlapped these lists, in order to obtain a set of potential tumor-suppressor lncRNAs (i.e., DLEU1, LINC00261, LINC00483, LINC01207, MCF2L-AS1) and oncogene lncRNAs (MEG3, RUNX1-IT1, and TP73-AS1) to experimentally analyze.

The expression of the previously selected lncRNAs was investigated through real time PCR in 20 formalin-fixed, paraffin-embedded (FFPE) CRC biopsies and their normal adjacent tissues (NATs). The results showed a significantly

TABLE 2 | Long non-coding RNAs (LncRNAs) positively/negatively correlated with BGs.

Positive correlation (PC)		Negative correlation (NC)	
A	**B**	**C**	**D**
DLEU1	LINC00312	A2M-AS1	DLEU1
EP300-AS1	MEG3	ADAMTS9-AS2	LINC00261
HCP5	RUNX1-IT1	ASAP1-IT1	LINC00483
LINC00261	TP73-AS1	CCDC144NL-AS1	TMPO-AS1
LINC00483		CCDC18-AS1	LINC01207
LINC00675		DAPK1-IT1	MCF2L-AS1
LINC01207		DLEU2	
MCF2L-AS1		EGOT	
TFAP2A-AS1		HYMAI	
THAP9-AS1		KLF3-AS1	
TTC28-AS1		LINC00312	
USP30-AS1		LINC00622	
		LINC00623	
		LINC00663	
		LINC00702	
		LINC00865	
		LINC00869	
		LINC00893	
		LINC01138	
		LINC01279	
		LINC01410	
		LINC-PINT	
		MAGI2-AS3	
		MEG3	
		MIR99AHG	
		MLLT4-AS1	
		NR2F1-AS1	
		PSMA3-AS1	
		PSMD5-AS1	
		RUNX1-IT1	
		SERTAD4-AS1	
		STX17-AS1	
		TAPT1-AS1	
		TP53TG1	
		TP73-AS1	
		TUG1	
		ZNF561-AS1	
		ZNF667-AS1	

LncRNAs showing PC with downregulated BGs are shown in column A. LncRNAs showing PC with upregulated BGs are shown in column B. LncRNAs showing NC with downregulated BGs are shown in column C. LncRNAs showing NC with upregulated BGs are shown in column D.

differential expression of four lncRNAs. More specifically, MEG3, MCF2L-AS1, LINC00483, and TP73-AS1 were downregulated in CRC tumor tissues compared to NATs (**Figure 2**).

Long Non-Coding RNA Expression After TGFβ-Induced Epithelial–Mesenchymal Transition in HCT-116 Cells

To investigate the involvement of previously identified differentially expressed lncRNAs (DE lncRNAs) in cellular proliferation and metastases, we induced the EMT through TGFβ-1 (transforming growth factor beta 1). We investigated TGFβ-1 effects on HCT-116 cells analyzing the expression of DE lncRNAs 24 h after TGFβ-1 treatment. We assessed the expression of EMT gene markers (MMP7, VIM, and ZEB1) to verify the successful outcome of *in vitro* TGFβ-1 treatment. Results showed an increased expression of MMP7, VIM, and ZEB1 at 24 h after treatment (AT) (**Figure 3A**), in agreement with mesenchymal transformation. Moreover, the results showed that TGFβ-1 treatment significantly decreased the expression of lncRNA LINC00483 at 24 h AT, whereas the expression of two other lncRNAs (MCF2L-AS1, and TP73-AS1) increased, even if in a statistically non-significant way (**Figure 3A**).

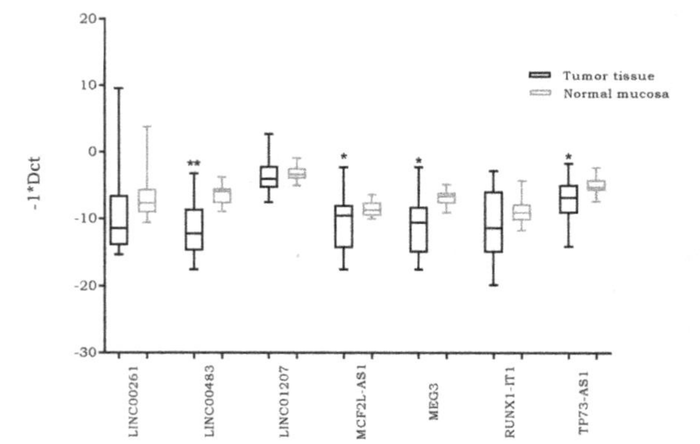

FIGURE 2 | Box plots showing differential expression of the selected long non-coding RNAs (lncRNAs) in 20 *formalin-fixed, paraffin-embedded* (FFPE) colorectal cancer *(*CRC) biopsies compared to normal adjacent tissues. Different primer pairs for DLEU1 did not produce any amplification. For this reason, DLEU1 data are not shown. *: p-value < 0.05; **: p-value < 0.001.

Inhibition of MAPKs Affects Long Non-Coding RNA Expression

We performed an *in vitro* inhibition of the MAPK pathway in order to investigate the involvement of previously identified DE lncRNAs in proliferative signaling. LncRNA expression was assessed in HCT-116 cells at 12 and 24 h AT with the MAPK inhibitor U0126. Results showed that the expression of DE lncRNAs was affected by the inhibition of the MAPK pathway (**Figures 3B, C**). More specifically, U0126 treatment did not alter the lncRNA expression after 12 h of treatment (**Figure 3B**), however, MCF2L-AS1, MEG3, and LINC00483 significantly increased their expression at 24 h AT, although the strongest upregulation was observed for LINC00483 (**Figure 3C**).

LINC00483 Affects Cell Migration but Not Cell Proliferation

As LINC00483 expression was altered by *in vitro* modulation of proliferation and EMT, we evaluated whether its enforced expression affected cellular migration and cell count. By OrisTM Universal Cell Migration Assembly kit (Platypus Technologies), we counted the cells migrated into the detection zone at different time points: 48, 72, 96, and 144 h after cell seeding stopper removal. Results showed a significant decrease of migration rate in LINC00483-transfected HCT-116 cells compared to negative controls (MOCK), at all specified time points, but the most statistically significant difference was observed at 96 h after transfection (**Figure 4A**). On the other

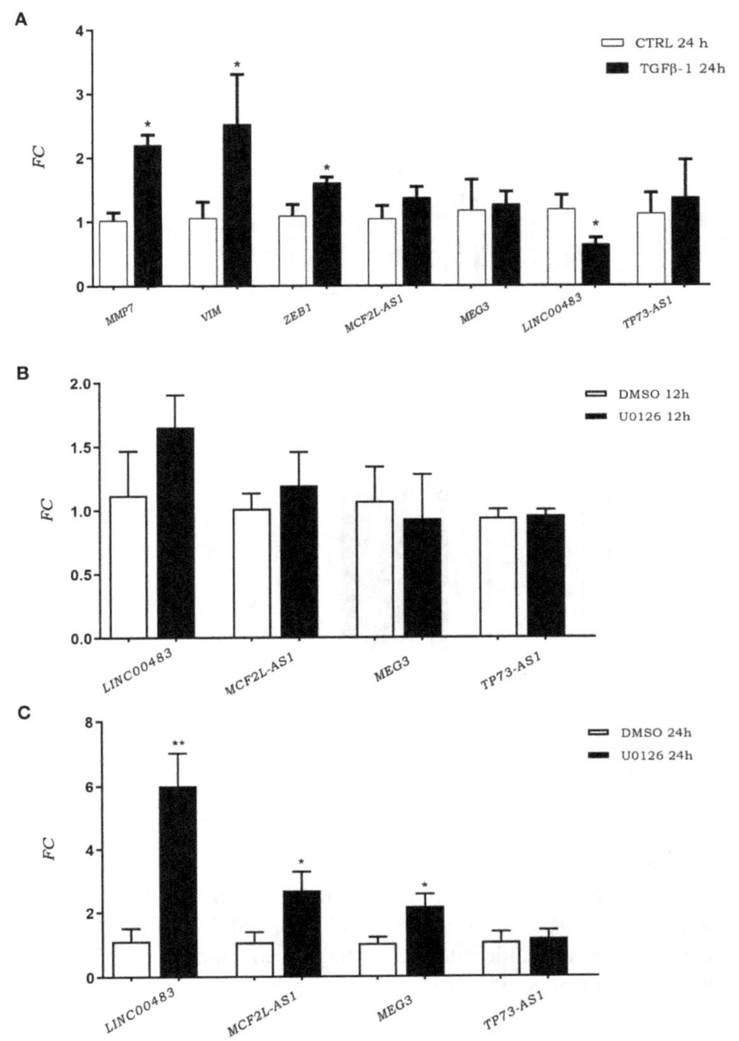

FIGURE 3 | **(A)** Expression of epithelial–mesenchymal transition (EMT) gene markers and DE long non-coding RNA (lncRNA) expression after TGFβ-1 treatment. **(B)** LncRNA expression in HCT-116 cell line post treatment with U0126 12 h and 24 h **(C)**. *p-value<0.05; **p-value<0.01.

hand, the cell viability/proliferation assay 48 h after LINC00483 transfection did not show any significant difference between transfected HCT-116 cells and their negative controls (**Figure 4B**). Taken together, the data on functional assays suggest that the upregulation of LINC00483 directly impaired cell migration but not cell viability/proliferation.

LINC00483 Molecular Axis Identification

Our previous results revealed a significant downregulation of LINC00483 in FFPE CRC biopsies compared to adjacent normal mucosa; furthermore, LINC00483 expression decreased in HCT-116 cells treated with TGFβ-1, while it increased when MAPK signaling was inhibited. Accordingly, we focused our next experimental analyses on LINC00483 due to its consistent data in biopsies and *in vitro* treatments. We screened all the datasets (1,313 datasets) deposited on R2 Genomics for LINC00483 dysregulation (**Table 3**) and found an almost specific downregulation of LINC00483 in CRC; moreover, its decreased expression was frequently associated with bad prognosis. Taken together all these data suggest a potential tumor suppressor role for LINC00483.

As the molecular functions of lncRNAs are strictly linked to their localization inside the cell, we first investigated the subcellular localization of LINC00483. We isolated RNA from the nuclear and cytoplasmic fractions of HCT-116 cells and analyzed LINC00483 in both, together with MALAT1, predominantly nuclear, and TUG1, preferentially located in the cytoplasm. Our data showed that LINC00483 is predominantly cytoplasmic (**Figure 5A**). Accordingly, we hypothesized a "miRNA sponge" role for LINC00483 and retrieved miRNAs that could simultaneously bind LINC00483 and the mRNAs showing a positive correlation of expression with LINC00483.

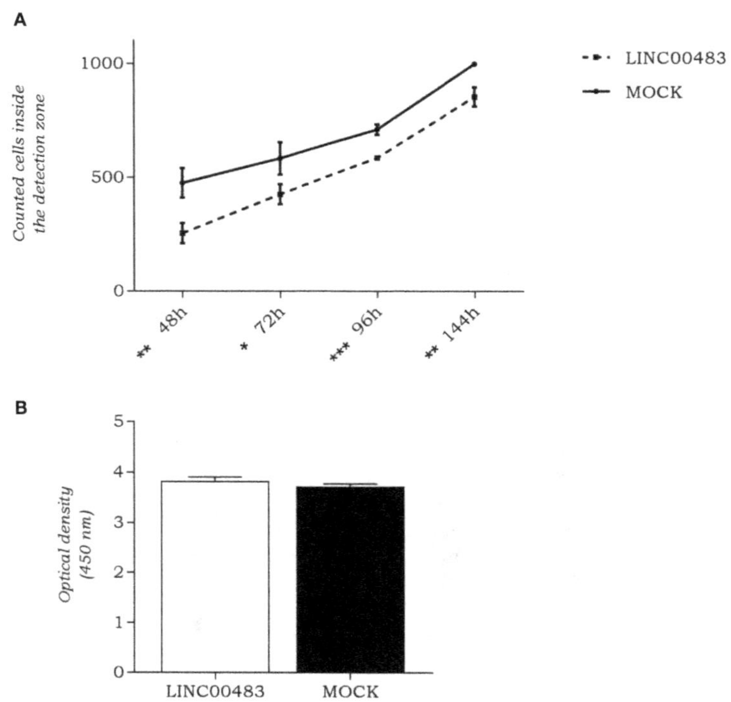

FIGURE 4 | LINC00483 functional assays. **(A)** Number of cells migrated into the detection zone in transfected HCT-116 cells compared to negative controls (MOCK), at 48, 72, 96, and 144 h after transfection. *p-value < 0.05; **p-value < 0.01; ***p-value < 0.001; **(B)** CCK-8 assay was performed to assess HCT-116 cell proliferation at 48 h after LINC00483 transfection.

More specifically, we selected miRNAs showing a negative correlation of expression with LINC00483 by using the TCGA COAD dataset (**Table S3**). We also retrieved miRNAs harboring binding sites for LINC00483 through LncBase, miRcode, and the RNA22 v.2 tool and overlapped these outputs with those resulting from correlation analysis (**Table S3**).

For each previously selected miRNA of **Table S3**, we identified the experimentally validated mRNA targets through TarBase v.8. This analysis did not produce any results for the following miRNAs: miR-4464, miR-4660, miR-4743-3p, and miR-7978, which were excluded from the next analyses. We also verified that the couples miRNA:mRNA target from TarBase showed a negative expression correlation (TCGA COAD). Moreover, to make this analysis more effective and focused on our cancer model, including a tumor-suppressor lncRNA, we considered just those miRNAs showing a potential involvement in CRC as oncomiRNAs by using mirCancer and mir2Disease databases. Finally, we filtered the list of miRNA targets with a set of mRNAs showing a positive correlation of expression with LINC00483 in several CRC datasets, as described in "*Material and Methods.*" By this approach, we obtained a list of potential LINC00483:miRNA:mRNA molecular axes. **Table 4** shows miRNAs harboring binding sites for LINC00483, which also show a negative expression correlation with LINC00483. For each miRNA, mRNA targets (positively correlated with LINC00483) are shown. The table has been filtered for mRNAs showing the highest R-values (ACVR1B, ADD3, ARL4A, CC2D1A, CD9, CTNNA1, DSP, EIF6, EPCAM, GALNT3, HIGD2A, MIER3, PLS1, PRKAA1, RNF43, SH3YL1, SRPK1, TPD52, USP7, VDR, and ZDHHC9). Data including all miRNA targets and their correlations with LINC00483 are reported in **Tables S4-S11**.

LINC00483 Expression in Colorectal Cancer Tissues Embedded in OCT and Fresh Biopsies

Our previous analysis on FFPE CRC biopsies showed a statically significant downregulation of LINC00483 in tumor tissues compared to normal mucosa. To corroborate these data and understand the potential LINC00483 association with clinical features of CRC patients, we assessed its expression on a second independent cohort of 35 CRC samples embedded in OCT (optimal cutting temperature). LINC00483 was significantly downregulated in metastatic CRCs compared to non-metastatic primary tumors (**Figure 5B**). We found no dysregulation of LINC00483 in association with other specific sub-groups of samples based on tumor and node staging and tumor grade.

Effects of Forced Expression of LINC00483 on the mRNA Axis

According to LINC00483 low expression in tumors tissues, we induced its *in vitro* overexpression by transfecting HCT-116 cells with the expression vector pcDNA3.1, including the LINC00483 cDNA sequence, in order to verify how the expression of mRNA

TABLE 3 | LINC00483 dysregulation in several expression datasets.

Dataset	Class	Expression	*P-value*
GSE3629 (121)	Class: colorectal cancer *vs.* non-neoplastic rectal mucosa	Down in tumor	1.50E−19
GSE3629 (121)	Group: sporadic ca *vs.* uc-nonca	Down in sporadic ca	1.50E−17
GSE21510 (148)	Tissue: cancer-lcm *vs.* normal-homogenized	Down in cancer	5.80E−16
GSE8671 (64)	Tissue: adenoma *vs.* normal	Down in adenoma	4.70E−10
GSE20916 (145)	Tissue: adenocarcinoma *vs.* normal_colon	Down in adenocarcinoma	1.20E−09
GSE3629 (121)	Group: sporadic ca *vs.* uc-ca	Down in sporadic ca	1.50E−09
GSE76124 (198)	tumor_grade: poorly_differentiated *vs.* well_differentiated	Down in poorly differentiated	5.70E−08
GSE20916 (145)	Malignancy: carcinoma vs distant_normal_colon	Down in carcinoma	4.50E−07
GSE8671 (64)	nt_size: 0.2_cm_(x3) *vs.* 2.0_cm	Down in 2 cm	4.60E−07
GSE35896 (62)	braf_mutation: n *vs.* y	Down in y	5.30E−07
GSE8671 (64)	nt_size: 0.2_cm_(x3) *vs.* 1.5_cm	Down 1.5 cm	8.60E−07
GSE2109 (315)	nt_pathological_grade: 2 *vs.* 3	Down in 3	3.10E−06
GSE39582 (566)	cimp_status: neg *vs.* pos	Down in pos	3.30E−06
GSE35896 (62)	braf_mutation: n *vs.* y	Down in y	7.50E−06
GSE20916 (145)	Tissue: carcinoma *vs.* normal_colon	Down in carcinoma	1.90E−05
GSE6791 (84)	sample_source: cervical normal *vs.*c head and neck cancer	Down in cancer	1.90E−05
GSE6791 (84)	Type: cervical normal *vs.* head and neck cancer	Down in cancer	1.90E−05
GSE4554 (84)	ms_status: msi *vs.* mss	Down in msi	2.00E−05
GSE8671 (64)	nt_location_tissue: sigmoid_colon_adenoma *vs.* sigmoid_colon_normal	Down in adenoma	2.60E−05
GSE76124 (198)	tumor_grade: moderately_differentiated *vs.* well_differentiated	Down in moderately differentiated	3.80E−05
GSE23878 (59)	Group: colon tumor *vs.* normal paired tissue	Down in colon tumor	4.70E−05
GSE29271 (210)	survival_time_(months): 35 *vs.* 9	Down in 35	5.60E−05
GSE20916 (145)	Malignancy: adenoma *vs.* carcinoma	Down in adenoma	6.10E−05
GSE13294 (155)	microsatellite_status: msi *vs.* mss	Down in msi	1.20E−04
GSE8671 (64)	nt_location_tissue: descending_colon_adenoma *vs.* rectum_normal	Down in adenoma	5.30E−04
GSE8671 (64)	nt_location_tissue: descending_colon_adenoma *vs.* descending_colon_normal	Down in adenoma	5.40E−04
GSE20916 (145)	Tissue: colon_tumor *vs.* norma_colon	Down in tumor	6.10E−04
GSE3629 (121)	Group: uc-associated ca *vs.* uc-nonca	Down in ca	6.90E−04
GSE41258 (390)	Tissue: normal colon *vs.* polyp	Down in polyp	2.20E−03
GSE17538 (232)	ajcc_stage: 2 *vs.* 4	Down in 2	4.20E−03
GSE35896 (62)	pten_mutation: n *vs.* y	Down in y	4.20E−03
GSE29271 (210)	survival_time_(months): 36 *vs.* 6	Down in 36	4.60E−03
GSE42363 (14)	tumor_grade: moderately *vs.* poorly	Down in poorly diffentiated	5.20E−03
GSE4183 (53)	Group: colon_adenoma *vs.* healthy_control	Down in adenoma	5.20E−03
GSE35896 (62)	pten_mutation: n *vs.* y	Down in y	5.40E−03
GSE50948 (156)	invasive_tumor_area_size: 15 *vs.* 6	Down in 15	5.80E−03
GSE33114 (108)	sample_descr: normal colon mucosa vs primary tumor resection	Down in tumor	8.30E−03
GSE33114 (108)	sample_source: normal colon mucosa *vs.* primary tumor resection	Down in tumor	8.30E−03
GSE33114 (108)	Type: normal *vs.* tumor	Down in tumor	8.30E−03
GSE21510 (148)	Tissue: cancer-homogenized *vs.* normal-homogenized	Down in cancer	8.30E−03
GSE4107 (22)	Tissue: mucosa_control *vs.* mucosa_patient	Down in patients	8.60E−03
GSE9891 (285)	Stagecode: ia *vs.* iii	Down in ia	9.50E−03
GSE35896 (62)	kras_mutation: n *vs.* y	Down in no	9.60E−03
GSE17538 (232)	ajcc_stage: 1 *vs.* 2	Down in 2	9.70E−03

In this table are reported 1) GEO ID (the sample number is shown in brackets); 2) class of comparison; 3) LINC00483 expression; 4) p-values of ANOVA test for each dataset.

nodes of the axes was modulated (**Figure 6**). The expression of 12 mRNAs statistically increased in HCT-116 cells transfected with LINC00483 compared to control samples, transfected with the scramble molecule (MOCK): ACVR1B, ARL4A, CTNNA1, EIF6, EPCAM, HIGD2A, MIER3, PLS1, SRPK1, TPD52, VDR, and ZDHHC9.

Inhibition of MAPKs Affected mRNA Expression of LINC00483 Axis

We previously observed that, after *in vitro* inhibition of the MAPK pathway, LINC00483 expression increased at 12 h AT, although a statistically significant variation was observed at 24 h AT. Accordingly, we evaluated if the expression of mRNAs showing increasing expression after LINC00483 enforced expression was altered by U0126 treatment. The expression of nine mRNAs statistically increased at 24 h AT: ACVR1B, ARL4A, CTNNA1, EIF6, EPCAM, HIGD2A, MIER3, PLS1, ZDHHC9 (**Figure 7**).The results would show that most of LIN00483-regulated mRNAs after MAPK blockage exhibited an expression modulation following that of LINC00483, thus suggesting the existence of a potential molecular relationship among these RNAs.

Expression of LINC00483 and the mRNA Axis After Cell Cycle Arrest

To investigate how the expression of LINC00483 and its target genes was modulated during artificial cell cycle arrest without chemical inhibitors, we exposed HCT-116 cells to serum starvation. More specifically, we assessed the expression of LINC00483 and mRNAs (ACVR1B, ARL4A, CTNNA1, EIF6,

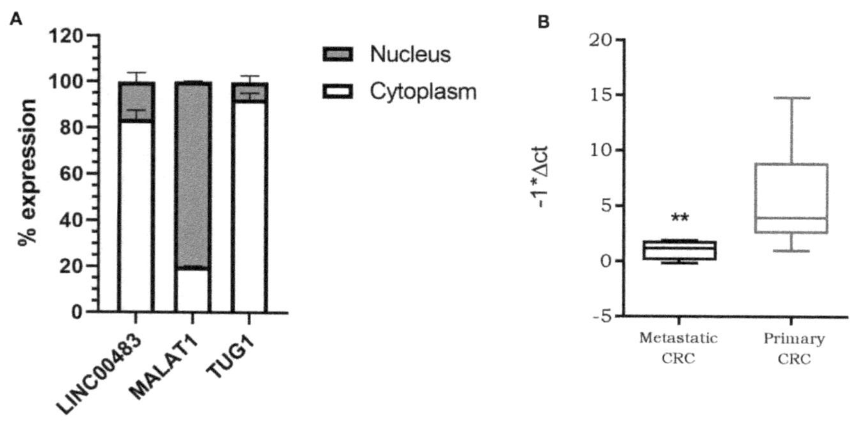

FIGURE 5 | **(A)** Nucleus/cytoplasm distribution of LINC00483. LncRNAs MALAT1 and TUG1 are analyzed as markers of nuclear and cytoplasmic localization, respectively; **(B)** Box plot showing LINC00483 expression in metastatic colorectal cancers (CRCs) compared to non-metastatic primary tumors. **p-value < 0.01.

TABLE 4 | Predicted LINC00483 molecular axes in *colorectal cancer* (CRC).

miRNA	miRNA expression (mirCancer/mir2Disease)	mRNA target	miRNA/mRNA correlation (panCancer)	LINC00483/mRNA correlation
miR-30a-5p	Downregulated	DSP	−0.11 (2.00E−02)	0.406 (2.68E−12)
		PLS1	−0.185 (7.57E−05)	0.569 (7.92E−26)
		TPD52	−0.271 (5.39E−09)	0.428 (1.02E−13)
miR-205-3p	Downregulated	PRKAA1	−0.098 (3.81E−02)	0.207 (2.27E−04)
miR-302c-3p	Downregulated	ARL4A	−0.087 (6.47E−02)	0.471 (7.75E−17)
		VDR	−0.072 (1.25E−01)	0.559 (1.61E−30)
miR-330-5p	Downregulated	ACVR1B	−0.106 (2.47E−02)	0.442 (1.14E−04)
		CC2D1A	−0.206 (1.09E−05)	0.32 (1.02E−07)
		HIGD2A	−0.158 (7.55E−04)	0.363 (5.07E−12)
		RNF43	−0.238 (3.37E−07)	0.451 (2.56E−15)
		ZDHHC9	−0.102 (2.98E−02)	0.389 (3.10E−11)
miR511-5p	Downregulated	SH3YL1	−0.084 (6.27E−01)	0.349 (3.84E−119
		USP7	−0.122 (9.56E−03)	0.372 (2.78E−10)
miR-544a	Upregulated	CD9	0.014 (7.73E−01)	0.391 (1.89E−10)
		DSP	−0.007 (8.80E−01)	0.406 (2.68E−12)
		EPCAM	−0.019 (6.95E−01)	0.479 (1.92E−17)
		GALNT3	0.041 (3.84E−01)	0.422 (2.66E−13)
		MIER3	0.015 (7.46E−01)	0.376 (1.53E−10)
miR-1231		CTNNA1	−0.238 (3.21E−07)	0.321 (2.00E−09)
		EIF6	−0.045 (3.45E−01)	0.44 (1.68E−14)
miR-3619-5p		ACVR1B	−0.133 (4.64E−03)	0.442 (1.14E−04)
		ADD3	−0.02 (6.76E−01)	0.437 (1.10E−17)
		SRPK1	−0.063 (1.81E−01)	0.38 (1.00E−10)

Expression in CRC, mRNA targets, mRNAs/miRNA correlations, mRNAs/LINC00483 correlations are reported for each miRNA negatively correlated with LINC00483 and harboring binding sites for it.

EPCAM, HIGD2A, MIER3, PLS1, SRPK1, TPD52, VDR, and ZDHHC9) in two different ways: 1) starved cells (0% FBS) *vs.* 10% FBS cells; 2) starved cells (0% FBS) *vs.* 10% FBS cells after cell synchronization obtained by 24 h of serum starvation. The expression of LINC00483 significantly increased after 24 h serum starvation, with and without cell synchronization. Interestingly, two mRNAs belonging to the LINC00483 axes (ARL4A and HIGD2A) showed statistically significant expression variations similar to LINC00483, while ZDHHC9 was upregulated only in starved cells compared to 10% FBS cells after cell synchronization (**Figure 8A**). These data would suggest again that, similar to MAPK inhibition, growth arrest induced by serum starvation

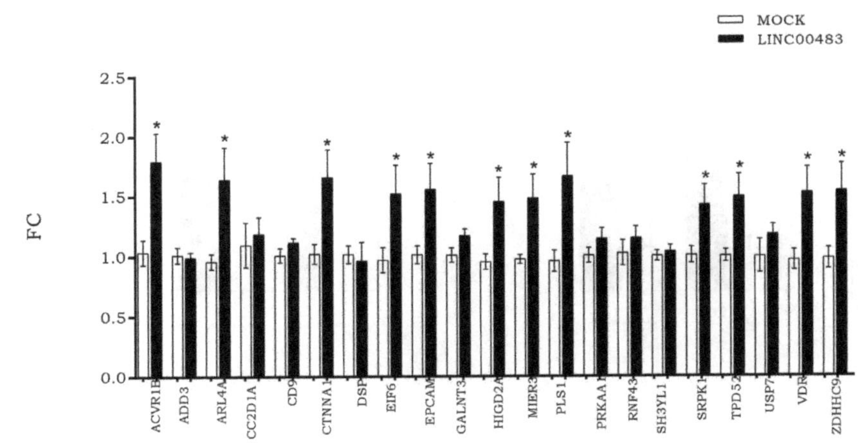

FIGURE 6 | The expression of messenger RNAs (mRNAs) selected as potentially involved in LINC00483 molecular axes after LINC00483 transfection in HCT-116 cells. *p-value < 0.05.

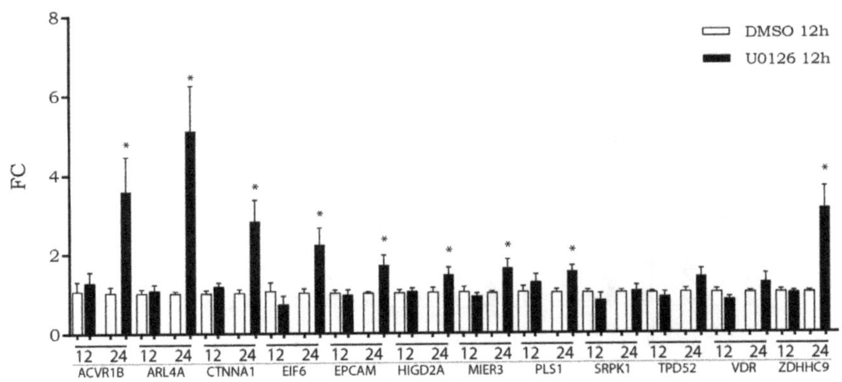

FIGURE 7 | Expression of messenger RNAs (mRNAs) of LINC00483 molecular axes in HCT-116 cells at 12 and 24 h after U0126 treatment. *p-value < 0.05.

activated the expression of LINC00483. However, in this specific cell condition only the expression of three mRNAs was induced, suggesting that the activation of LINC00483 axes depends on functioning of specific cellular pathways.

Expression of LINC00483 and Axes's mRNAs After In Vitro Epithelial–Mesenchymal Transition

To assess the involvement of LINC00483 and mRNAs potentially linked to it in metastasis-related mechanisms, we induced *in vitro* the EMT by treating HCT-116 cells with TGFβ-1 and IL-6 (interleukin-6). Both these treatments induced a downregulation of LINC00483 (**Figure 8B**). TGFβ-1 treatment showed a statistically significant downregulation for CTNNA1 and MIER3 while IL-6 provoked the downregulation of HIGD2A (**Figure 8B**). Notably, CTNNA1, HIGD2A, and MIER3 showed the same expression trends as LINC00483 in the same model of *in vitro* EMT. These data would show that two different signaling of EMT induction similarly repressed LINC00483. As previously observed, also in this case different cellular signaling could control different LINC00483 molecular axes.

HNF4α Transcription Factor Potentially Controls LINC00483 Expression

To get a better insight into transcriptional regulation of LINC00483, we screened the UCSC Genome Browser to find potential transcription factor binding sites (TFBSs). More specifically, by overlapping different tracks derived from ENCODE experiments to the UCSC Genome browser, we found TFBSs for HNF4α (hepatocyte nuclear factor 4α) about 180 nt upstream of the transcription start site (TSS) in correspondence with a DNase hypersensitive region (**Figure 9A**). Moreover, other HNF4α TFBSs were present about 1 kb upstream and downstream of TSS overlapping DNase

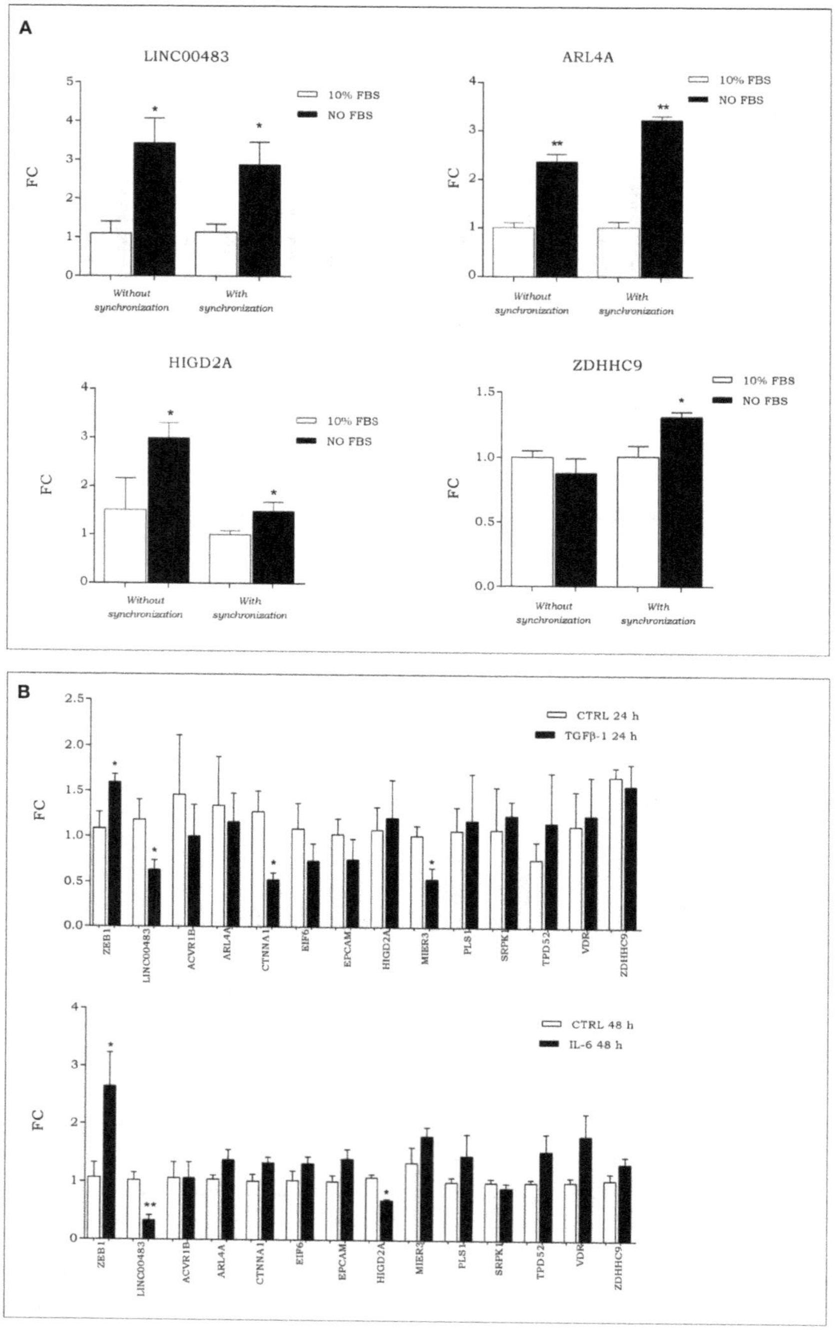

FIGURE 8 | **(A)** Expression of LINC00483 and messenger RNAs (mRNAs) associated with its molecular axes after 24 h serum starvation, with and without cell synchronization. To make this panel more readable, we reported just significant data. The complete panel of histograms is reported in **Figure S2**. **(B)** Expression of EMT marker ZEB1, LINC00483 and mRNAs potentially involved in the LINC00483 axes after TGFβ-1 and Il-6. *p-value ≤ 0.05; **p-value ≤ 0.01.

hypersensitive regions (**Figure 9A**). These data suggest that HNF4α could contribute to transcriptional regulation of LINC00483. Indeed, we treated CRC cells with BI6015, an HNF4α inhibitor, and evaluated the expression of LINC00483 and the axis's mRNAs. Chemical inhibition of HNF4α induced the significant upregulation of LINC00483 at 24 h after BI6015 treatment (**Figure 9B**), suggesting a potential negative control by HNF4α on LINC00483 transcription. Notably, the expression of all mRNAs strongly increased at 24 h after treatment (**Figure 9B**), corroborating our previous data concerning the positive

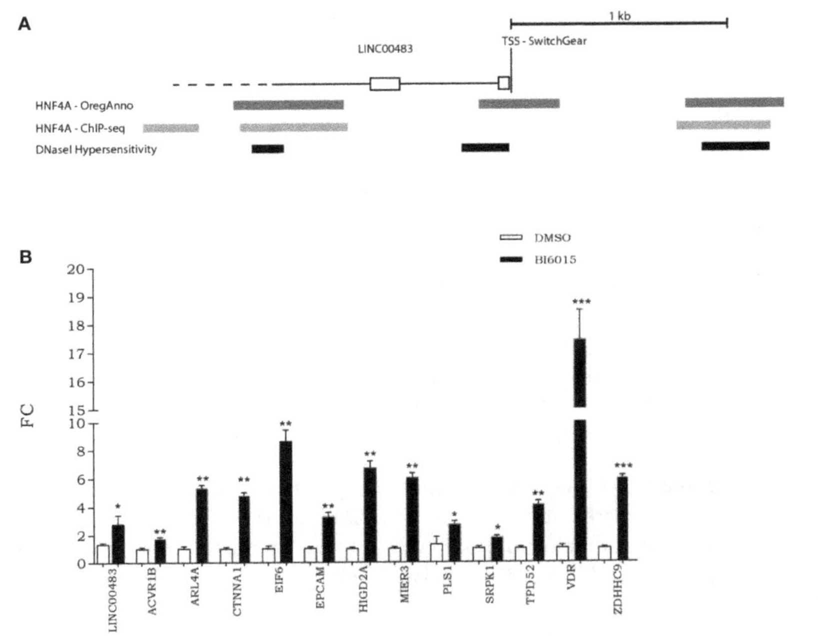

FIGURE 9 | Relationship between LINC00483 and the HNF4α transcription factor. **(A)** HNF4α binding sites and DNase hypersensitive regions upstream and downstream of the transcription start site (TSS) of LINC00483; **(B)** Expression of LINC00483 and messenger RNAs (mRNAs) potentially involved in LINC00483 axis at 24 h after treatment with BI6015, an HNF4α inhibitor. *p-value ≤ 0.05; **p-value ≤ 0.01; ***p-value ≤ 0.001.

expression association between LINC00483 and the mRNAs belonging to the LINC00483:miRNA:mRNA axes.

CTNNA1, HIGD2A, MIER3

As our data suggested a tighter association of expression between LINC00483 and CTNNA1, HIGD2A, and MIER3 with respect the other axis's mRNAs, we further analyzed them. We screened the expression of CTNNA1, HIGD2A, and MIER3 in all CRC datasets deposited on R2 genomics. The results showed their stable downregulation in CRC tumor tissues compared to controls, or, in most cases, in association with the severe features of the tumor (**Table S12**). We investigated CTNNA1, HIGD2A, and MIER3 expression in CRC biopsies compared to adjacent normal mucosa in order to confirm their downregulation in CRC observed by dataset screening: the three mRNAs showed a statistically significant downregulation in tumor tissues compared to normal mucosa (**Figure 10**). Moreover, we calculated the Pearson coefficients between the expression values of LINC00483 and CTNNA1, HIGD2A, and MIER3 in the same CRC samples, obtaining significant positive correlation of expression between LINC00483 and CTNNA1 (r-value: 0.47, p-value: 0.03), LINC00483 and HIGD2A (r-value: 0.41, p-value: 0.05), LINC00483 and MIER3 (r-value: 0.53, p-value: 0.01). Positive correlations between LINC00483 and CTNNA1, HIGD2A, and MIER3 was corroborated by the analysis of expression correlation performed on all CRC datasets previously studied. As shown in **Table S13**, the positive correlation between LINC00483 and CTNNA1, HIGD2A, and MIER3 represents a common feature of most CRC expression datasets.

DISCUSSION

In this work we identified LINC00483 as a long non-coding RNA with a potential role of tumor suppressor in CRC. By screening several CRC datasets, we found that LINC00483 expression correlated with several protein-coding genes whose dysregulation was associated with CRC. Expression analysis performed on CRC biopsies compared to normal adjacent tissues, revealed a statistically significant downregulation of LINC00483, as well as its low expression levels in metastatic CRCs compared to non-metastatic primary tumors. This reduced expression associated with CRC was corroborated by an additional screening of all cancer datasets deposited in the R2 genomics repository showing that LINC00483 was steadily and specifically downregulated in CRC specimens from most of the CRC datasets available. Interestingly, LINC00483 expression seems to be particularly conspicuous in the physiologic intestinal epithelium and almost absent in other tissues, according to Fagerberg et al. (29), as reported in BioProject PRJEB4337. This would suggest that LINC00483 could play a specific role in the normal intestinal epithelium. Notably, aberrant expression of LINC00483 was reported for other cancers for which this lncRNA is considered an oncogene (30–32).

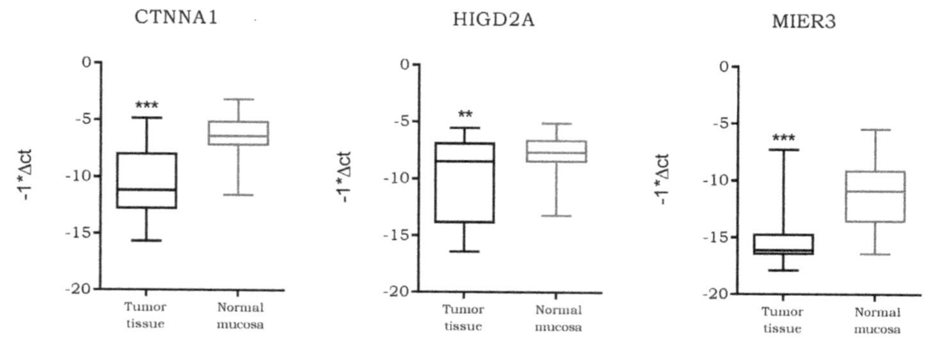

FIGURE 10 | Box plot showing the differential expression of CTNNA1, HIGD2A, and MIER3 in *colorectal cancer* (CRC) formalin-fixed, paraffin-embedded (FFPE) biopsies compared to normal adjacent mucosa. **p-value ≤0.01, ***p-value ≤0.001.

With the aim of understanding the functional involvement of LINC00483 in CRC biology, we evaluated its expression in CRC cells after the artificial block or induction of specific cancer related pathways. More specifically, LINC00483 levels increased after inhibition of MAPK signaling, which is usually overactivated in CRC cells and mainly responsible for cellular hyperproliferation (33). Notably, inhibition by U0126 treatment leads to G0/G1 arrest of cell cycle (34). Moreover, we observed an upregulation of LINC00483 also after serum starvation, an artificial experimental approach causing the exit of the cells from cell cycle (G0) and reducing the expression of genes responsible for cell cycle progression (e.g., HRAS, MYC), and components of the MAPK and PI3K pathways (35). These results would suggest that proliferative signals, including those mediated by ERK pathway, could transcriptionally or post-transcriptionally lower the amount of LINC00483. These considerations could explain the downregulation of LINC00483 in CRC biopsies (36, 37). When these signals were artificially inhibited, LINC00483 expression increased. Taken together, these data would suggest that LINC00483 could have a role in the G0/G1 cell cycle status of CRC cells, participating in a complex RNA-RNA network. Moreover, we don't exclude that LINC00483 could play a role in stress conditions that subsequently would lead to G0/G1 block. This consideration could also explain the unaffected proliferation after the ectopic expression of LINC00483. LINC00483 exhibited low levels of expression also in metastatic CRC compared to primary tumors. This observation suggested a potential involvement of this lncRNA in one of the pathways underlying the metastatic process. It is now commonly accepted that EMT is an essential process for distant metastases formation. Although the EMT program was originally described as part of morphogenesis in embryonic development, it was later observed in several pathogenic events, such as fibrosis, wound healing, tumor progression, and metastases (38, 39). According to the importance that EMT activation takes on CRC metastatic development, we artificially induced EMT in CRC cells by using TGFβ-1 and IL-6, two well-known inducers of EMT in CRC, through different molecular cascades (28, 40). As expected, EMT induction by TGFβ-1 and IL-6 caused a decrease of LINC00483 expression, suggesting that it could play a negative role in EMT activation.

We found that enforced expression of LINC00483 in CRC cells induced a slowing down of the cell migration rate, suggesting that this lncRNA may exert a negative regulation of the motile phenotype, which is a hallmark of EMT impairment. On the other hand, LINC00483 did not induce any modulation of cell proliferation. Based on the latter observation, the upregulation of LINC00483 after inhibition of proliferative signals could be the result of a joint RNA-RNA network. Accordingly, ectopic expression of LINC00483 may be functionally effective for cell proliferation under certain molecular conditions, such as specific stoichiometric concentrations of its direct or indirect interactors (9).

In the last few years there has been increasing evidence of lncRNA function as ceRNA (competitive endogenous RNA) (41–43). Since LINC00483 is predominantly cytoplasmic, we hypothesized a "miRNA sponge" role for it. According to this model, miRNAs are sponged by lncRNAs: this prevents their binding to targeted mRNAs and their subsequent degradation. According to the miRNA sponge hypothesis for LINC00483, we computationally retrieved miRNAs that could simultaneously bind LINC00483 and mRNAs showing a positive correlation of expression with LINC00483 itself. By this approach, we reconstructed potential LINC00483-miRNA-mRNA molecular axes and evaluated the expression of the latter in different experimental conditions provoking the alteration of LINC00483. We focused our analysis on those mRNAs whose expression increased after the enforced expression of LINC00483, according to the miRNA sponge model. A number of mRNAs were modulated similarly to LINC00483 in the different treatments (i.e., TGFβ-1, IL-6, U0126, serum starvation), confirming their mutual positive correlation of expression with LINC00483 during the block of proliferation and EMT induction. CTNNA1 (catenin alpha 1), HIGD2A (HIG1 hypoxia inducible domain family member 2a), and MIER3 (MIER family member 3) showed an upregulation after inhibition of the MAPK pathway and a downregulation after EMT induction, in the same way as LINC00483. Analysis of both our CRC cohort and R2 genomics expression datasets showed the downregulation of CTNNA1, HIGD2A and MIER3 (also in association with the severe features of the tumor), but also an evident positive correlation of expression with LINC00483. CTNNA1 and MIER3 have a well-known tumor suppressor function. MIER3 was downregulated in colorectal cancer tissue compared to healthy colon mucosa (44). Peng *et al.* reported that MIER3 was significantly reduced in human primary CRC and was associated with CRC metastasis and poor prognosis (45). Upregulation of MIER3 expression significantly inhibited CRC cell proliferation, migration, and invasion *in vitro* and repressed tumor growth and metastasis *in vivo*. Moreover, MIER3 suppressed colorectal cancer progression and inhibited epithelial-mesenchymal transition (45). Several studies have shown the tumor suppressor role of CTNNA1 in different tumors (46–48). CTNNA1 expression was markedly lower in CRC tissues compared to adjacent normal mucosa and its overexpression significantly inhibited proliferation and migration of CRC cells (49, 50). Moreover, ablation of CTNNA1 induced alterations in cell–cell adhesion and enhanced cell migration (51). HIGD2A function is not well known. However, Ameri *et al.*, showed that a member of the same family—HIGD1A (HIG1 hypoxia inducible domain family member 1A) interacts with the electron transport chain, modulating mitochondrial ROS production, oxygen consumption, and AMPK activity to promote survival during glucose starvation, while simultaneously decreasing tumor growth *in vivo* (52). HIGD1A may play an important role in tumor dormancy or recurrence mechanisms during tumor cell adaptation to extreme environments (52, 53). HIGD2A could play a similar role of tumor suppressor gene in CRC and be involved in tumor proliferation processes; however, its role in cancer biology remains to be elucidated. The other mRNA nodes of LINC00483 axes (ACVR1B, ARL4A, EIF6, EPCAM, PLS1, SRPK1, TPD52, VDR, ZDHHC9) could play a role in the regulation of the cell cycle, even if they were not modulated during artificial EMT induction. We suggest that the functional role of lncRNA molecular axes may not be ubiquitous but closely associated with specific molecular contexts (e.g., the interaction with other RNA molecules or proteins), which perturb the whole ceRNA network and, accordingly, the single lncRNA axis.

We identified HNF4α (hepatocyte nuclear factor 4 alpha) as a transcription factor that could potentially regulate LINC00483 expression. Indeed, by using a HNF4α inhibitor, we found that the expression levels of LINC00483 and all axis's mRNAs strongly increased. Thus, we could speculate that HNF4α negatively regulates this lncRNA. HNFAα regulates the expression of many genes involved in several processes, such as development, metabolism, and epithelial-mesenchymal transition (54–56). Through mechanisms not completely understood, transcription from P1 or P2 promoters, combined with alternative splicing, potentially generates 12 different transcripts and 12 HNFAα protein isoforms (57). Each isoform performs a distinct function to regulate a specific subset of genes in a tissue-dependent manner (58, 59). There are contradictory reports on whether HNF4α acts as an oncogene or a tumor suppressor in different cancer models, including CRC (60–66). The HNF4A locus is amplified in CRC tumors and its overexpression is associated with specific subtypes of colorectal cancer (64, 67). HNF4α is known to act as a transcriptional activator (68, 69). However, post-translational modifications can influence the recruitment of coactivators and corepressors in order to modify the transcriptional influence of HNF4α on its target genes (70, 71). Schwartz *et al.* investigated the putative role played by HNF4α in CRC by evaluating the effect of HNF4α antagonists and HNF4α small interfering RNA (siRNA) on CRC growth and proliferation in cultured CRC cells and xenotransplanted nude mice *in vivo*. These molecules are shown to inhibit growth and proliferation of HT29 and Caco2 CRC cells (61). Based on our data, we propose that HNF4α could exert an oncogenic role by inhibiting LINC00483 expression in CRC. Accordingly, a gain of function of oncogenic HNF4a may be involved in downregulation of LINC00483. Interestingly, a potential target of HNF4α is the well-known tumor suppressor PTEN (72), which counteracts the PI3K/Akt signaling cascade and controls cell proliferation/invasiveness (73–75). However, LINC00483 downregulation in CRC could be due also to different aberrant transcriptional or post-transcriptional regulations.

Finally, our data suggest that LINC00483 plays a role of a tumor suppressor in CRC and through the miRNA sponge mechanism potentially controls the levels of a heterogenous set of mRNAs, which, in turn, may directly or indirectly modulate cell cycle and migration.

AUTHOR CONTRIBUTIONS

MR and DuB designed and conceived the experiments with the critical collaboration of MP and CP. RC, GB, and LM obtained, characterized, and curated clinical data from patients' biopsies. DuB and CB performed the experiments. FM, AC, RB, and DaB contributed to the acquisition, analysis, and interpretation of data. MR and DuB wrote the paper. MP and CP reviewed and edited the final version of the manuscript. All authors contributed to the article and approved the submitted version.

ACKNOWLEDGMENTS

We wish to thank the Scientific Bureau of the University of Catania for language support. This study was supported by "linea intervento 3 Open Access Piano PIACERI 2020-2022" from University of Catania.

SUPPLEMENTARY MATERIAL

SUPPLEMENTARY FIGURE 1 | Schematic representation of lncRNA-miRNA-mRNA relationship based on the miRNA sponge model.

SUPPLEMENTARY FIGURE 2 | Expression of LINC00483 and mRNAs associated with its molecular axes after 24 h serum starvation, with and without cell synchronization (complete data).

REFERENCES

1. Rawla P, Sunkara T, Barsouk A. Epidemiology of colorectal cancer: incidence, mortality, survival, and risk factors. *Prz Gastroenterol* (2019) 14(2):89–103. doi: 10.5114/pg.2018.81072
2. Fearon ER, Vogelstein B. A genetic model for colorectal tumorigenesis. *Cell* (1990) 61(5):759–67. doi: 10.1016/0092-8674(90)90186-I
3. Arends JW. Molecular interactions in the Vogelstein model of colorectal carcinoma. *J Pathol* (2000) 190(4):412–6. doi: 10.1002/(SICI)1096-9896(200003)190:4<412::AID-PATH533>3.0.CO;2-P
4. Prasanth KV, Spector DL. Eukaryotic regulatory RNAs: an answer to the 'genome complexity' conundrum. *Genes Dev* (2007) 21(1):11–42. doi: 10.1101/gad.1484207
5. Hangauer MJ, Vaughn IW, McManus MT. Pervasive transcription of the human genome produces thousands of previously unidentified long intergenic noncoding RNAs. *PloS Genet* (2013) 9(6):e1003569. doi: 10.1371/journal.pgen.1003569
6. Jacquier A. The complex eukaryotic transcriptome: unexpected pervasive transcription and novel small RNAs. *Nat Rev Genet* (2009) 10(12):833–44. doi: 10.1038/nrg2683
7. Mattick JS. The State of Long Non-Coding RNA Biology. *Noncoding RNA* (2018) 4(3). doi: 10.3390/ncrna4030017
8. Yao RW, Wang Y, Chen LL. Cellular functions of long noncoding RNAs. *Nat Cell Biol* (2019) 21(5):542–51. doi: 10.1038/s41556-019-0311-8
9. Ragusa M, Barbagallo C, Brex D, Caponnetto A, Cirnigliaro M, Battaglia R, et al. Molecular Crosstalking among Noncoding RNAs: A New Network Layer of Genome Regulation in Cancer. *Int J Genomics* (2017) 2017:4723193. doi: 10.1155/2017/4723193
10. Ragusa M, Barbagallo C, Statello L, Condorelli AG, Battaglia R, Tamburello L, et al. Non-coding landscapes of colorectal cancer. *World J Gastroenterol* (2015) 21(41):11709–39. doi: 10.3748/wjg.v21.i41.11709
11. Hu G, Niu F, Humburg BA, Liao K, Bendi S, Callen S, et al. Molecular mechanisms of long noncoding RNAs and their role in disease pathogenesis. *Oncotarget* (2018) 9(26):18648–63. doi: 10.18632/oncotarget.24307
12. Wang KC, Chang HY. Molecular mechanisms of long noncoding RNAs. *Mol Cell* (2011) 43(6):904–14. doi: 10.1016/j.molcel.2011.08.018
13. Siddiqui H, Al-Ghafari A, Choudhry H, Al Doghaither H. Roles of long non-coding RNAs in colorectal cancer tumorigenesis: A Review. *Mol Clin Oncol* (2019) 11(2):167–72. doi: 10.3892/mco.2019.1872
14. Yang Y, Junjie P, Sanjun C, Ma Y. Long non-coding RNAs in Colorectal Cancer: Progression and Future Directions. *J Cancer* (2017) 8(16):3212–25. doi: 10.7150/jca.19794
15. He Q, Long J, Yin Y, Li Y, Lei X, Li Z, et al. Emerging Roles of lncRNAs in the Formation and Progression of Colorectal Cancer. *Front Oncol* (2019) 9:1542. doi: 10.3389/fonc.2019.01542
16. Dastmalchi N, Safaralizadeh R, Nargesi MM. LncRNAs: Potential Novel Prognostic and Diagnostic Biomarkers in Colorectal Cancer. *Curr Med Chem* (2019) 27(30):5067–77. doi: 10.2174/0929867326666190227230024
17. Saus E, Brunet-Vega A, Iraola-Guzman S, Pegueroles C, Gabaldon T, Pericay C. Long Non-Coding RNAs As Potential Novel Prognostic Biomarkers in Colorectal Cancer. *Front Genet* (2016) 7:54. doi: 10.3389/fgene.2016.00054
18. Jothimani G, Sriramulu S, Chabria Y, Sun XF, Banerjee A, Pathak S. A Review on Theragnostic Applications of Micrornas and Long Non- Coding RNAs in Colorectal Cancer. *Curr Top Med Chem* (2018) 18(30):2614–29. doi: 10.2174/1568026619666181221165344
19. Barbagallo C, Brex D, Caponnetto A, Cirnigliaro M, Scalia M, Magnano A, et al. LncRNA UCA1, Upregulated in CRC Biopsies and Downregulated in Serum Exosomes, Controls mRNA Expression by RNA-RNA Interactions. *Mol Ther Nucleic Acids* (2018) 12:229–41. doi: 10.1016/j.omtn.2018.05.009
20. Han Y, Yang YN, Yuan HH, Zhang TT, Sui H, Wei XL, et al. UCA1, a long non-coding RNA up-regulated in colorectal cancer influences cell proliferation, apoptosis and cell cycle distribution. *Pathology* (2014) 46(5):396–401. doi: 10.1097/PAT.0000000000000125
21. Yang MH, Hu ZY, Xu C, Xie LY, Wang XY, Chen SY, et al. MALAT1 promotes colorectal cancer cell proliferation/migration/invasion via PRKA kinase anchor protein 9. *Biochim Biophys Acta* (2015) 1852(1):166–74. doi: 10.1016/j.bbadis.2014.11.013
22. Svoboda M, Slyskova J, Schneiderova M, Makovicky P, Bielik L, Levy M, et al. HOTAIR long non-coding RNA is a negative prognostic factor not only in primary tumors, but also in the blood of colorectal cancer patients. *Carcinogenesis* (2014) 35(7):1510–5. doi: 10.1093/carcin/bgu055
23. Nissan A, Stojadinovic A, Mitrani-Rosenbaum S, Halle D, Grinbaum R, Roistacher M, et al. Colon cancer associated transcript-1: a novel RNA expressed in malignant and pre-malignant human tissues. *Int J Cancer* (2012) 130(7):1598–606. doi: 10.1002/ijc.26170
24. Ling H, Spizzo R, Atlasi Y, Nicoloso M, Shimizu M, Redis RS, et al. CCAT2, a novel noncoding RNA mapping to 8q24, underlies metastatic progression and chromosomal instability in colon cancer. *Genome Res* (2013) 23(9):1446–61. doi: 10.1101/gr.152942.112
25. Cui H, Onyango P, Brandenburg S, Wu Y, Hsieh CL, Feinberg AP. Loss of imprinting in colorectal cancer linked to hypomethylation of H19 and IGF2. *Cancer Res* (2002) 62(22):6442–6.
26. Zhang J, Liu L, Li J, Le TD. LncmiRSRN: identification and analysis of long non-coding RNA related miRNA sponge regulatory network in human cancer. *Bioinformatics* (2018) 34(24):4232–40. doi: 10.1093/bioinformatics/bty525
27. Tang X, Feng D, Li M, Zhou J, Li X, Zhao D, et al. Transcriptomic Analysis of mRNA-lncRNA-miRNA Interactions in Hepatocellular Carcinoma. *Sci Rep* (2019) 9(1):16096. doi: 10.1038/s41598-019-52559-x
28. Katsuno Y, Lamouille S, Derynck R. TGF-beta signaling and epithelial-mesenchymal transition in cancer progression. *Curr Opin Oncol* (2013) 25(1):76–84. doi: 10.1097/CCO.0b013e32835b6371
29. Fagerberg L, Hallstrom BM, Oksvold P, Kampf C, Djureinovic D, Odeberg J, et al. Analysis of the human tissue-specific expression by genome-wide integration of transcriptomics and antibody-based proteomics. *Mol Cell Proteomics* (2014) 13(2):397–406. doi: 10.1074/mcp.M113.035600
30. Li D, Yang M, Liao A, Zeng B, Liu D, Yao Y, et al. Linc00483 as ceRNA regulates proliferation and apoptosis through activating MAPKs in gastric cancer. *J Cell Mol Med* (2018) 22(8):3875–86. doi: 10.1111/jcmm.13661
31. Yang QS, Li B, Xu G, Yang SQ, Wang P, Tang HH, et al. Long noncoding RNA LINC00483/microRNA-144 regulates radiosensitivity and epithelial-mesenchymal transition in lung adenocarcinoma by interacting with HOXA10. *J Cell Physiol* (2019) 234(7):11805–21. doi: 10.1002/jcp.27886
32. Yan Y, Wang Z, Qin B. A novel long noncoding RNA, LINC00483 promotes proliferation and metastasis via modulating of FMNL2 in CRC. *Biochem Biophys Res Commun* (2019) 509(2):441–7. doi: 10.1016/j.bbrc.2018.12.090
33. Ragusa M, Statello L, Maugeri M, Majorana A, Barbagallo D, Salito L, et al. Specific alterations of the microRNA transcriptome and global network structure in colorectal cancer after treatment with MAPK/ERK inhibitors. *J Mol Med (Berl)* (2012) 90(12):1421–38. doi: 10.1007/s00109-012-0918-8
34. Beloueche-Babari M, Jackson LE, Al-Saffar NM, Workman P, Leach MO, Ronen SM. Magnetic resonance spectroscopy monitoring of mitogen-activated protein kinase signaling inhibition. *Cancer Res* (2005) 65(8):3356–63. doi: 10.1158/10.1158/0008-5472.CAN-03-2981
35. Wang F, Liang R, Soibam B, Yang J, Liu Y. Coregulatory long non-coding RNA and protein-coding genes in serum starved cells. *Biochim Biophys Acta Gene Regul Mech* (2019) 1862(1):84–95. doi: 10.1016/j.bbagrm.2018.11.004

36. Koveitypour Z, Panahi F, Vakilian M, Peymani M, Seyed Forootan F, Nasr Esfahani MH, et al. Signaling pathways involved in colorectal cancer progression. *Cell Biosci* (2019) 9:97. doi: 10.1186/s13578-019-0361-4
37. Urosevic J, Nebreda AR, Gomis RR. MAPK signaling control of colon cancer metastasis. *Cell Cycle* (2014) 13(17):2641–2. doi: 10.4161/15384101.2014.946374
38. Kalluri R, Weinberg RA. The basics of epithelial-mesenchymal transition. *J Clin Invest* (2009) 119(6):1420–8. doi: 10.1172/JCI39104
39. Thiery JP, Acloque H, Huang RY, Nieto MA. Epithelial-mesenchymal transitions in development and disease. *Cell* (2009) 139(5):871–90. doi: 10.1016/j.cell.2009.11.007
40. Mao L, Li Y, Zhao J, Li Q, Yang B, Wang Y, et al. Transforming growth factor-beta1 contributes to oxaliplatin resistance in colorectal cancer via epithelial to mesenchymal transition. *Oncol Lett* (2017) 14(1):647–54. doi: 10.3892/ol.2017.6209
41. Tang J, Zhuo H, Zhang X, Jiang R, Ji J, Deng L, et al. A novel biomarker Linc00974 interacting with KRT19 promotes proliferation and metastasis in hepatocellular carcinoma. *Cell Death Dis* (2014) 5:e1549. doi: 10.1038/cddis.2014.518
42. Yan S, Yue Y, Wang J, Li W, Sun M, Gu C, et al. LINC00668 promotes tumorigenesis and progression through sponging miR-188-5p and regulating USP47 in colorectal cancer. *Eur J Pharmacol* (2019) 858:172464. doi: 10.1016/j.ejphar.2019.172464
43. Yuan JH, Yang F, Wang F, Ma JZ, Guo YJ, Tao QF, et al. A long noncoding RNA activated by TGF-beta promotes the invasion-metastasis cascade in hepatocellular carcinoma. *Cancer Cell* (2014) 25(5):666–81. doi: 10.1016/j.ccr.2014.03.010
44. Pitule P, Vycital O, Bruha J, Novak P, Hosek P, Treska V, et al. Differential expression and prognostic role of selected genes in colorectal cancer patients. *Anticancer Res* (2013) 33(11):4855–65.
45. Peng M, Hu Y, Song W, Duan S, Xu Q, Ding Y, et al. MIER3 suppresses colorectal cancer progression by down-regulating Sp1, inhibiting epithelial-mesenchymal transition. *Sci Rep* (2017) 7(1):11000. doi: 10.1038/s41598-017-11374-y
46. Vite A, Li J, Radice GL. New functions for alpha-catenins in health and disease: from cancer to heart regeneration. *Cell Tissue Res* (2015) 360(3):773–83. doi: 10.1007/s00441-015-2123-x
47. Piao HL, Yuan Y, Wang M, Sun Y, Liang H, Ma L. alpha-catenin acts as a tumour suppressor in E-cadherin-negative basal-like breast cancer by inhibiting NF-kappaB signalling. *Nat Cell Biol* (2014) 16(3):245–54. doi: 10.1038/ncb2909
48. Zhou YN, Xu CP, Chen Y, Han B, Yang SM, Fang DC. Alpha-catenin expression is decreased in patients with gastric carcinoma. *World J Gastroenterol* (2005) 11(22):3468–72. doi: 10.3748/wjg.v11.i22.3468
49. Chen X, Zhu H, Wu X, Xie X, Huang G, Xu X, et al. Downregulated pseudogene CTNNAP1 promote tumor growth in human cancer by downregulating its cognate gene CTNNA1 expression. *Oncotarget* (2016) 7(34):55518–28. doi: 10.18632/oncotarget.10833
50. Vermeulen SJ, Nollet F, Teugels E, Vennekens KM, Malfait F, Philippe J, et al. The alphaE-catenin gene (CTNNA1) acts as an invasion-suppressor gene in human colon cancer cells. *Oncogene* (1999) 18(4):905–15. doi: 10.1038/sj.onc.1202348
51. Livshits G, Kobielak A, Fuchs E. Governing epidermal homeostasis by coupling cell-cell adhesion to integrin and growth factor signaling, proliferation, and apoptosis. *Proc Natl Acad Sci U S A* (2012) 109(13):4886–91. doi: 10.1073/pnas.1202120109
52. Ameri K, Jahangiri A, Rajah AM, Tormos KV, Nagarajan R, Pekmezci M, et al. HIGD1A Regulates Oxygen Consumption, ROS Production, and AMPK Activity during Glucose Deprivation to Modulate Cell Survival and Tumor Growth. *Cell Rep* (2015) 10(6):891–9. doi: 10.1016/j.celrep.2015.01.020
53. Chanrion M, Negre V, Fontaine H, Salvetat N, Bibeau F, Mac Grogan G, et al. A gene expression signature that can predict the recurrence of tamoxifen-treated primary breast cancer. *Clin Cancer Res* (2008) 14(6):1744–52. doi: 10.1158/1078-0432.CCR-07-1833
54. DeLaForest A, Nagaoka M, Si-Tayeb K, Noto FK, Konopka G, Battle MA, et al. HNF4A is essential for specification of hepatic progenitors from human pluripotent stem cells. *Development* (2011) 138(19):4143–53. doi: 10.1242/dev.062547
55. Xu Y, Zalzala M, Xu J, Li Y, Yin L, Zhang Y. A metabolic stress-inducible miR-34a-HNF4alpha pathway regulates lipid and lipoprotein metabolism. *Nat Commun* (2015) 6:7466. doi: 10.1038/ncomms8466
56. Santangelo L, Marchetti A, Cicchini C, Conigliaro A, Conti B, Mancone C, et al. The stable repression of mesenchymal program is required for hepatocyte identity: a novel role for hepatocyte nuclear factor 4alpha. *Hepatology* (2011) 53(6):2063–74. doi: 10.1002/hep.24280
57. Huang J, Levitsky LL, Rhoads DB. Novel P2 promoter-derived HNF4alpha isoforms with different N-terminus generated by alternate exon insertion. *Exp Cell Res* (2009) 315(7):1200–11. doi: 10.1016/j.yexcr.2009.01.004
58. Li K, Zhang H, Wang Y, Wang Y, Feng M. Differential expression of HNF4alpha isoforms in liver stem cells and hepatocytes. *J Cell Biochem* (2006) 99(2):558–64. doi: 10.1002/jcb.20939
59. Torres-Padilla ME, Weiss MC. Effects of interactions of hepatocyte nuclear factor 4alpha isoforms with coactivators and corepressors are promoter-specific. *FEBS Lett* (2003) 539(1-3):19–23. doi: 10.1016/S0014-5793(03)00174-1
60. Chellappa K, Robertson GR, Sladek FM. HNF4alpha: a new biomarker in colon cancer? *Biomark Med* (2012) 6(3):297–300. doi: 10.2217/bmm.12.23
61. Schwartz B, Algamas-Dimantov A, Hertz R, Nataf J, Kerman A, Peri I, et al. Inhibition of colorectal cancer by targeting hepatocyte nuclear factor-4alpha. *Int J Cancer* (2009) 124(5):1081–9. doi: 10.1002/ijc.24041
62. Consortium UIG, Barrett JC, Lee JC, Lees CW, Prescott NJ, Anderson CA, et al. Genome-wide association study of ulcerative colitis identifies three new susceptibility loci, including the HNF4A region. *Nat Genet* (2009) 41(12):1330–4. doi: 10.1038/ng.483
63. Chellappa K, Deol P, Evans JR, Vuong LM, Chen G, Briancon N, et al. Opposing roles of nuclear receptor HNF4alpha isoforms in colitis and colitis-associated colon cancer. *Elife* (2016) 5. doi: 10.7554/eLife.10903
64. Zhang B, Wang J, Wang X, Zhu J, Liu Q, Shi Z, et al. Proteogenomic characterization of human colon and rectal cancer. *Nature* (2014) 513(7518):382–7. doi: 10.1038/nature13438
65. Chang HR, Nam S, Kook MC, Kim KT, Liu X, Yao H, et al. HNF4alpha is a therapeutic target that links AMPK to WNT signalling in early-stage gastric cancer. *Gut* (2016) 65(1):19–32. doi: 10.1136/gutjnl-2014-307918
66. Kim JH, Eom HJ, Lim G, Park S, Lee J, Nam S, et al. Differential effects, on oncogenic pathway signalling, by derivatives of the HNF4 alpha inhibitor BI6015. *Br J Cancer* (2019) 120(5):488–98. doi: 10.1038/s41416-018-0374-5
67. Guinney J, Dienstmann R, Wang X, de Reynies A, Schlicker A, Soneson C, et al. The consensus molecular subtypes of colorectal cancer. *Nat Med* (2015) 21(11):1350–6. doi: 10.1038/nm.3967
68. Odom DT, Zizlsperger N, Gordon DB, Bell GW, Rinaldi NJ, Murray HL, et al. Control of pancreas and liver gene expression by HNF transcription factors. *Science* (2004) 303(5662):1378–81. doi: 10.1126/science.1089769
69. Eeckhoute J, Formstecher P, Laine B. Hepatocyte nuclear factor 4alpha enhances the hepatocyte nuclear factor 1alpha-mediated activation of transcription. *Nucleic Acids Res* (2004) 32(8):2586–93. doi: 10.1093/nar/gkh581
70. Ruse MDJr., Privalsky ML, Sladek FM. Competitive cofactor recruitment by orphan receptor hepatocyte nuclear factor 4alpha1: modulation by the F domain. *Mol Cell Biol* (2002) 22(6):1626–38. doi: 10.1128/MCB.22.6.1626-1638.2002
71. Ungaro P, Teperino R, Mirra P, Longo M, Ciccarelli M, Raciti GA, et al. Hepatocyte nuclear factor (HNF)-4alpha-driven epigenetic silencing of the human PED gene. *Diabetologia* (2010) 53(7):1482–92. doi: 10.1007/s00125-010-1732-x
72. Boyd M, Bressendorff S, Moller J, Olsen J, Troelsen JT. Mapping of HNF4alpha target genes in intestinal epithelial cells. *BMC Gastroenterol* (2009) 9:68. doi: 10.1186/1471-230X-9-68
73. Salvatore L, Calegari MA, Loupakis F, Fassan M, Di Stefano B, Bensi M, et al. PTEN in Colorectal Cancer: Shedding Light on Its Role as Predictor and Target. *Cancers (Basel)* (2019) 11(11). doi: 10.3390/cancers11111765
74. Furnari FB, Huang HJ, Cavenee WK. The phosphoinositol phosphatase activity of PTEN mediates a serum-sensitive G1 growth arrest in glioma cells. *Cancer Res* (1998) 58(22):5002–8.
75. Kotelevets L, van Hengel J, Bruyneel E, Mareel M, van Roy F, Chastre E. The lipid phosphatase activity of PTEN is critical for stabilizing intercellular

17

An Integrated Network, RNA Sequencing and Experiment Pharmacology Approach Reveals the Active Component, Potential Target and Mechanism of *Gelsemium elegans* in the Treatment of Colorectal Cancer

*Lin Wang, Hai-li Xu, Jing-wei Liang, Ying-ying Ding and Fan-hao Meng**

School of Pharmacy, China Medical University, Liaoning, China

Correspondence:
Fan-hao Meng
fhmeng@cmu.edu.cn

In this study, a combination of network pharmacology, bioinformatics analysis, molecular docking and transcriptomics was used to investigate the active ingredient and potential target of *Gelsemium elegans* in the treatment of colorectal cancer. Koumine was screened as the active component by targeting PDK1 through network pharmacology and reverse docking. RNA-Seq, enrichment analysis and validation experiment were then further employed to reveal koumine might function in inhibiting Akt/mTOR/HK2 pathway to regulate cell glycolysis and detachment of HK2 from mitochondria and VDAC-1 to activate cell apoptosis both *in vitro* and *in vivo.* In the present study, we provide a systematical approach for the identification of effective ingredient and potential target of herbal medicine. Our results have important implication for the intensive study of koumine as novel anticancer agents for colorectal cancer and could be supportive in its further structural modification.

Keywords: *Gelsemium elegans*, koumine, PDK1, Akt/mTOR/HK2, glycolysis

INTRODUCTION

Herbal medicine shows promising potential in clinic and plays an important role in disease prevention and treatment (1, 2). Various beneficial effects of herbal medicine have been reported for cancer prevention and treatment, such as extract of the aerial part of Scutellaria barbata BZL101 for patients with advanced breast cancer (3) and PHY906 (a pharmaceutical-grade formulation of four traditional Chinese herbs) in the treatment of advanced hepatocellular carcinoma (4). However, it is rather difficult to clarify the pharmacological effect of herbal medicine because it contains multiple chemical constituents. Therefore, the search for a targeted, effective ingredient is an urgent need.

Gelsemium elegans (Gardner&Champ.) Benth. (*G. elegans*) belonging to the Gelsemiaceae family is an extremely poisonous plant (5). It has attracted more attention for various therapeutic effects on anti-inflammatory, analgesic, anxiolytic and immunostimulatory activity (6–10). In recent years, a rich body of evidence has also demonstrated that *G. elegans* possesses anti-tumor effects *in vivo* and *in vitro* (11–13). Remarkably, it has also been applied in the treatment of colorectal cancer (CRC) in the folk for hundred years. Nevertheless, *G. elegans* has been greatly limited because of its toxicity and narrow therapeutic window. So far, almost 200 compounds have been separated from *G. elegans*, including alkaloids, iridoids, triterpenes, phenolic acids, steroids, coumarins, lignans, megastigmane glycosides, and other ingredients (14). Despite the extensive and rapid progress in active ingredient research, there is still an ever-growing need for efficient strategies to identify the effective ingredient and potential target of *G. elegans* for CRC treatment.

In the present study, an integrative pharmacology method including network, molecular docking, transcriptomics, bioinformatics analysis and immunoblot analysis was used to reveal the active component, potential target and mechanism of *G. elegans* on CRC. As a result, koumine (KM) which is the most abundant molecule among the alkaloids of *G. elegans* with relatively low toxicity was identified the active agent by targeting 3-phosphoinositide-dependent protein kinase-1 (PDK1). It inhibited glycolysis and interaction of hexokinase 2 (HK2) with voltage-dependent anion channel-1 (VDAC-1) on the mitochondria *via* suppressing its downstream Akt/mTOR/HK2 pathway. KM exhibited good lead compound properties and provide a great potential scaffold for future structure modification in developing highly efficient anti-CRC agents.

METHOD

Network Construction and Enrichment Analysis

The network construction and enrichment analysis was conducted according to our previous research method with minor improvements (15). A total of seven compounds (**Figure 1**) with significant pharmacological activities and high contents from *G. elegans* were selected. We imported the components' chemical structure into the public network server of the database PharmMapper (http://www.lilab-ecust.cn/pharmmapper/) which employs pharmacophore mapping strategy for the identification of the potential targets. The top 50 targets of each compound were selected for further study of the comprehensive network pharmacology analysis. The compound targets were imported into UniProt knowledgebase (https://www.uniprot.org/uploadlists/) to obtain official symbols for the following enrichment analysis.

The online database STRING (https://string-db.org/) was applied to construct the protein–protein interactions (PPI) analysis by importing the potent targets. The minimum required interaction score was set higher than 0.4. KEGG and GO enrichment analysis were carried out to identify the candidate targets. The cut-off criterion was set with the *P* values less than or equal 0.05 and the result of GO enrichment was only showed by the Biological Process terms.

Molecular Docking

The molecular docking study was conducted on Molecular Operating Environment package (MOE 2015.10). The structure of compounds was drawn and converted into 3D structure by ChemBio 3D Ultra 14.0 and the candidate targets crystal structure was extracted from the Protein Data Bank (http://www.rcsb.org/pdb/home/home.do). The ligand conformations were generated with the bond rotation method. The placement and refinement were set as "Triangle matcher" and "Induced Fit" respectively. The best docking conformation was selected from 30 predicted poses with the best binding affinity according to their E-strain and the London dG score was applied to evaluate ligand binding capacity to the receptor.

Cell Culture

The human CRC cell lines including HCT116 and HT29 were obtained from American Type Culture Collection (ATCC, Mansassas, VA, USA). All cells were grown in culture utilizing RPMI-1640 medium supplemented with 10% fetal bovine serum (Gibico; Thermo Fisher Scientific, Inc.), 100 μg/ml streptomycin and 100 U/ml penicillin (Sigma Aldrich, St. Louis, MO, USA). Cells were maintained in a humidified atmosphere with 5% CO_2 at 37°C.

MTT Assay

(4,5-dimethylthiazol-2-yl)-2,5-diphenyltetrazolium bromide (MTT) assay was carried out to evaluate the viability of HCT116 and HT29 cells. Cells in log phase was seeded in a 96-well plate at a density of 3×10^3 cells/well in 100 μl of complete culture medium and incubated in the presence of KM with increasing concentrations (0, 5, 10, 25, 50, 75, 100, 125 μM) at 37°C for 24 h, respectively. After incubation, MTT solution (10 μl of 5 mg/ml) (Boster Biotechnology Limited Company, Wuhan, China) was added to each well and maintained at 37°C for additional 4 h. Subsequently, the supernatant was removed and 100 μl dimethylsulfoxide (DMSO) was added to dissolve the formazan crystal. The optical density (OD) at 490 nm was measured on microplate reader (Bio-Rad Laboratories, Inc., Hercules, CA, USA).

Flow Cytometry Analysis of Apoptosis

HCT116 and HT29 cells were seeded in six-well plates overnight, and then treated with different concentration of KM (0, 25, 75, and 125 μM) for 24 h. The cells were harvested, washed twice with ice-cold PBS, and evaluated for apoptosis by double staining with 5 μl Annexin-V FITC (Promega Corporation, Madison, WI, USA) and 5 μl propidium iodide (Promega Corporation, Madison, WI, USA) in 500 μl binding buffer for 15 min in the dark. Stained cells were analyzed by flow cytometer (BD Biosciences, CA, USA).

PDK1 Kinase Assay

Different concentration of KM in 50 μl kinase reaction buffer (50 mM HEPES, pH 7.5, 10 mM $MgCl_2$, 0.1 mg/ml BSA, 2 mM DTT, 1% DMSO) were incubated with 5 ng/ml human recombinant PDK1 kinase (Invitrogen Corporation, Carlsbad, USA). The reaction was subsequently initiated by the addition of 5 μM

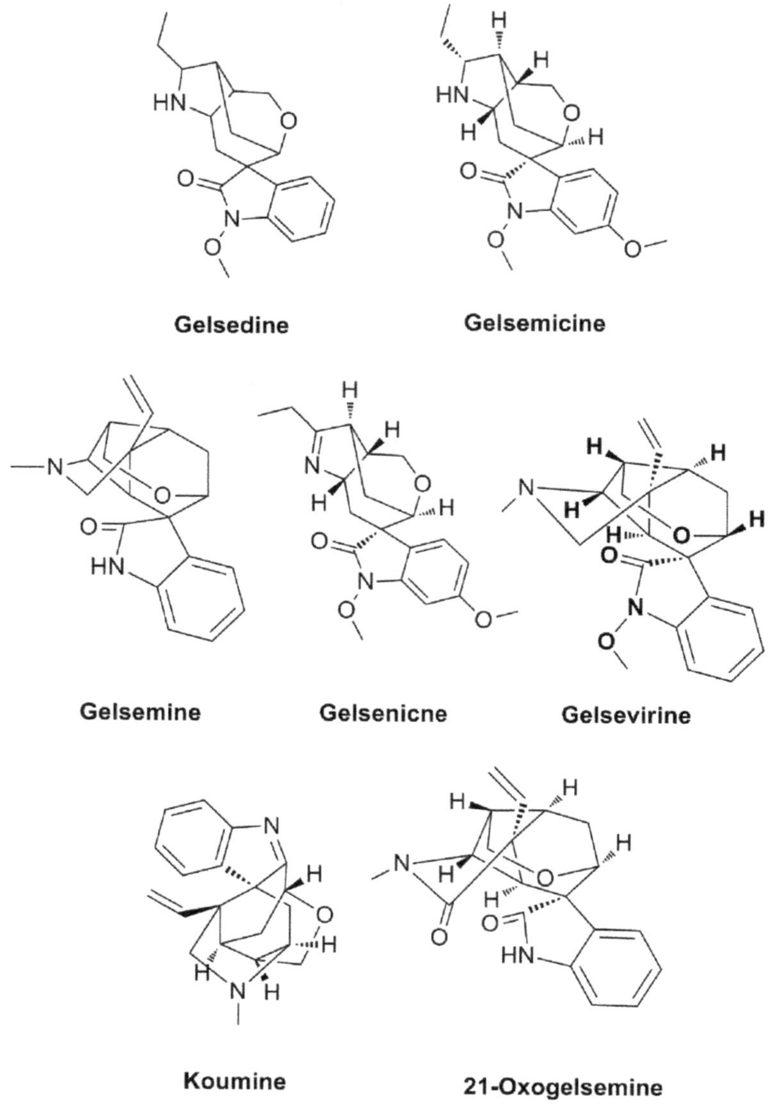

FIGURE 1 | Seven effective components of *G. elegans*.

ATP and 50 μM PDKtide substrate with the sequence: KTFCG TPEYL APEVR REPRI LSEEE QEMFR DFDYI ADWC. Kinase-Lumi™ Luminescent Kinase Assay Kit (Beyotime Biotechnology Company, Shanghai, China) was used for the PDK1 inhibitory activity as described in the manufacturer's protocol. After incubation for 30 min at room temperature, the luminescence value was measured by chemiluminescence module of a full-wavelength multi-function microplate reader (PerkinElmer, Singapore). The amount of luminescence from each reaction is inversely correlated with PDK1 kinase activity.

RNA Sequencing

After DMSO or KM treatment, HCT116 cells were collected and washed with cold PBS for twice. A total of six samples were available, including three samples of KM group and three sample of control group. Total RNA was extracted by TRIzol reagent following the manufacturer's instructions (Takara, Dalian, China). Library construction and mRNA sequencing were carried out by Personal Gene Technology Company (Nanjing, China). mRNA was enriched from total RNA by Oligo (dT) beads. The enriched mRNA underwent fragmentation and was reverse transcribed into cDNA. Then the cDNA fragments were purified with AmPure XP system (Beckman coulter, Beverly Hills, California, USA) and poly-A was added and ligated to Illumina sequencing adapters. The ligation products were evaluated using the Agilent 2100 Bioanalyzer (Agilent, Palo Alto, CA, USA) and sequenced on Illumina Hiseq Xten platform.

The differentially expressed genes (DEGs) were calculated by DESeq (version 1.30.0). The *P*-value was adjusted by the false discovery rate (FDR). P-value <0.05 and the fold change

≥2 were set to be statistically significant. Gene ontology (GO) functional enrichment and Kyoto Encyclopedia of Genes and Genomes (KEGG) pathway analyses were performed for the bioinformatics analysis.

Details of reverse transcription-quantitative polymerase chain reaction (RT-*q*PCR) are given in **Supplementary Materials**.

Glucose Uptake Level and ATP Production Assay

The cells were incubated in 6-well plates at a density of 70–80% and treated with various concentrations of KM for 24 h. The glucose level in the medium was measured by glucose assay kit (Nanjing Jiancheng Bioengineering Institute, Nanjing, China) according to the manufacturer's instructions. Then the concentrations of glucose uptake in each sample were calculated. Intracellular ATP level was estimated using an ATP assay kit (Nanjing Jiancheng Bioengineering Institute, Nanjing, China), strictly following the manufacturer's instructions. The relative glucose consumption rate and ATP production were normalized by the cell counts and protein concentration of samples, respectively. All experiments were performed for three times.

Western Blotting Analysis

Cells were harvested in RIPA lysis buffer (Thermo, MA, USA) containing protease and phosphatase inhibitors at 4°C. Protein extract was prepared according to the instruction of extraction kit (Beyotime Biotechnology Company, Shanghai, China). BCA protein assay kit (Beyotime Biotechnology Company, Shanghai, China) was used to quantify the protein. Then equal total amounts of proteins were separated by sodium dodecyl sulfate-poly-acrylamide gel electrophoresis and transferred onto the PVDF membrane (Bio-Rad Company, USA). After blocking with 5% non-fat milk, the membranes were incubated with specific primary antibodies against the indicated protein overnight at 4°C, and washed with PBST, followed by HRP-conjugated secondary antibodies for 1 h at room temperature. Protein bands were developed using the enhanced chemiluminescence reagent and scanned by the Bio-Rad Gel Doc 2000 gel imaging system with *β*-actin band as the reference.

Immunofluorescence Staining

Cells cultured on glass coverslips were washed with PBS, fixed in 4% paraformaldehyde for 30 min and permeabilized with 0.5% Triton X-100 for 20 min. Then cells were washed twice with PBS and blocked with 3% BSA for 30 min at room temperature, followed by incubation with primary antibody overnight at 4°C. After washing three times for 5 min, the cells were stained with FITC/Texas Red-conjugated secondary antibodies (1:200 dilution; Proteintech, Chicago, IL, USA) for 1 h in the dark. The mitochondria of the cells were exposed to Mitotracker Red (Molecular Probes, Inc., Eugene, OR) at a final concentration of 150 nM for 10 min at 37°C prior to fixation in the dark. After washing three times for 5 min, cells were counterstained with DAPI for 5 min in the dark and examined under confocal fluorescence microscopy (C2; Nikon, Tokyo, Japan).

Tumor Xenograft Model

All the experimentation for animals was complied with the approval and guidelines of the China Medical University Institutional Animal Care and Use Committee. BALB/c nude mice (six-week-old, male) were obtained from Huafukang Bioscience. CO. Inc (Beijing, China). HCT116 cells in 200 μl (5×10^7 cells/ml) were implanted subcutaneously into the left axillary of each nude mice. When the tumor volume reached about 100 mm^3, the mice were randomly divided into two groups (n = 8) and intraperitoneally injected with vehicle control (saline) or KM (2 mg/kg) every two days for 3 weeks. The body weight and tumor sizes were measured every other day. The tumor volume was determined by measuring length (L) and width (W) and calculated by the formula: tumor volume (mm^3) $=L*W^2/2$. After the experiment, mice were sacrificed and the tumors were weighed and photographed. The freezing tissues were fixed with 4% paraformaldehyde in 4°C in the purpose of preparing for subsequent immunohistochemical studies.

Immunohistochemistry Assay

After fixation, dehydration, and transparency, the tumor was embedded in paraffin and cut into 5 um thick sections. Tumor tissue sections were dewaxed in xylene, hydrated with gradient alcohol, 3% hydrogen peroxide blocked endogenous peroxidase and then 0.01 M citrate buffer solution (pH6.0) was used for antigen retrieval. Next, the sections were blocked with 3% fetal bovine serum, and incubated the primary antibody at 4°C overnight. After washed and incubated with the biotinylated secondary antibodies for 1 h at 37°C, the sections were added the horseradish peroxidase-labeled streptomycin avidin working solution to incubate at 37°C for 30 min. Then sections were washed with PBS, developed with diaminobenzidine (DAB), counterstained with hematoxylin, and finally imaged with a light microscope (ECLIPSE E600; Nikon, Tokyo, Japan).

Statistical Analysis

All statistical analysis was performed by SPSS20.0 software. All the presented data and results were confirmed in at least three independent experiments and expressed as mean ± SD. Statistical analysis of data was made by the student's t-test or one way ANOVA. $P < 0.05$ is considered statistically significant.

RESULTS

Acquisition of Potential Active Component and Target of *G. elegans*

After overlapping the results of seven ingredients from the PharmMapper database, structure of 289 predicted targets were downloaded from the PDB database by employing the Retrieve/ID mapping. As shown in **Figure 2A**, a total of 244 nodes, and 678 edges were mapped in the PPI network of the target genes.

GO analysis was performed to understand the relationship between functional units and their underlying significance in biological system networks. According to the GO enrichment analysis, 561 gene ontology terms were significantly associated

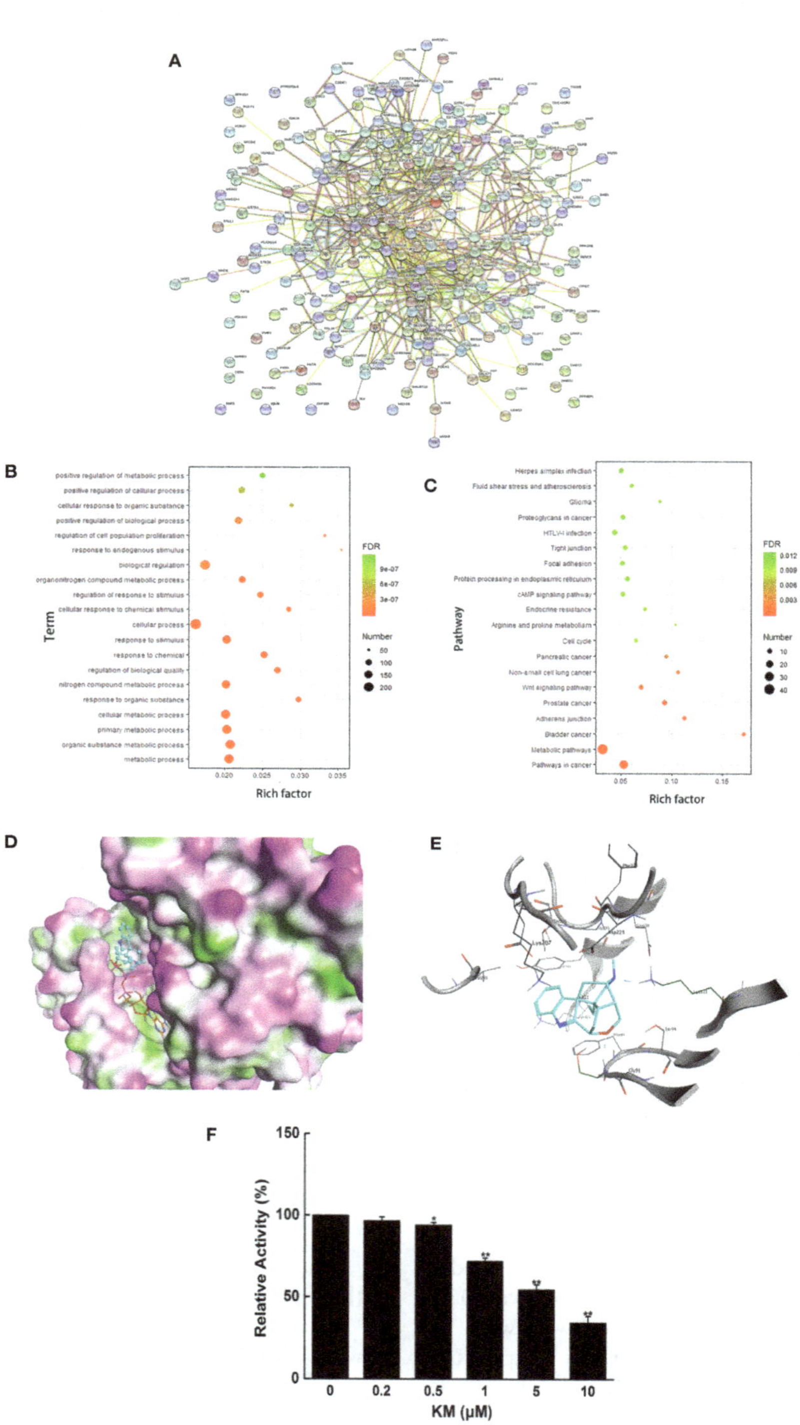

FIGURE 2 | **(A)** Clusters of screened PPI networks **(B)** The 20 representative terms with the lowest *P* value of biological process (BP) gene ontology enrichment. **(C)** The top 20 pathways with *P* <0.05 of KEGG pathway enrichment. **(D)** Molecular interaction of KM with PDK1. **(E)** The 2D representation of KM docking pose with PDK1. **(F)** The effect of KM on PDK1 kinase activity. Data were shown as mean ± SD (n = 3); significance: $^{*}P < 0.05$, $^{**}P < 0.01$ *vs* control.

with a large number of biological processes (**Supplementary Materials Table 1**), the 20 representative terms with the lowest *P* value in biological process groups was exhibited in **Figure 2B**. The results revealed that the target genes were mainly enriched in the biological process related to the metabolism including metabolic process, organic substance metabolic process and cellular metabolic process. Moreover, through KEGG analysis constructed on *P* value less than 0.05 (**Supplementary Materials Table 2**), top 20 pathways were also obtained (**Figure 2C**), which were associated with metabolic pathways, pathways in cancer and so on. After integrating the results of GO and KEGG analysis, the genes TP53 and PDK1 enriched in the above signaling pathway and closely related to metabolism were picked as candidate targets for further docking research.

The docking results of seven compounds from *G. elegans* were screened out by sorting the docking scores in descending order (**Supplementary Materials Table 3**). KM exhibited adequate spatial orientation in the active site and superior binding capacity to PDK1 with the score −9.1004. It is apparent KM formed hydrogen bond with the backbone of Lys111 and Glu130 located in the kinase domain (**Figures 2D, E**). The kinase activity assay also validated KM possessed the potential inhibitory effect on PDK1 (**Figure 2F**). These results provided great support that KM contributes to the potential anti-CRC effect *via* targeting PDK1.

KM Induced Apoptosis of CRC Cells

The MTT assay was performed to validate the effect of KM on cell viability. KM treatment exhibited loss of cell viability to HCT116 and HT29 cells with IC_{50} value of 70.56 and 62.82 μM, respectively (**Supplementary Materials Figure 1**). The cells were evaluated by V-FITC and PI double labeling for apoptosis evaluation. Significant increase in the rate of apoptosis was observed from 8.1% (control group) to 33.0% for HCT116 cells after treatment with KM at 125 μM. The effect exhibited a concentration-dependent increase. Similar results were obtained for another CRC cell line HT29 (**Figure 3A**).

In order to confirm this cell death was apoptotic, apoptosis-related proteins were assessed by western blotting with the absence or presence of KM. The results showed the hallmark protein of apoptosis, including Bax, CytC and Caspase-3 expressed a significantly dose-dependent increase. Moreover, Bcl-2, known as a cell survival protein, remarkably decreased depending on the concentration of KM (**Figure 3B**). These results showed that KM activated the apoptotic pathway *via* decreasing Bcl-2 expression associated with an increase in Bax, CytC and Caspase-3.

KM Suppressed Glycolysis of CRC Cells

The total gene expression was analyzed by RNA-Seq of HCT116 cells. The genes and pathways changed in response to KM treatment were revealed by this high-throughput method. A total of 306 differential expression genes (DEGs) were identified, including 153 downregulated genes and 153 upregulated genes (using twofold as the cut off value, **Supplementary Materials Tables 4** and **5**). The volcano plot map showed significant genes expressed in the KM treated group compared to the control group (**Figure 4A**). The heatmap used for hierarchical clustering analysis (HCA) exhibited distinct gene expression between control and treated group (**Figure 4B**).

GO functional enrichment was performed to explore the potential molecular or biological functions affected by KM treatment. All the DEGs were categorized into three major categories: cellular components, molecular functions, and biological process. The significantly enriched GO biological processes by the KM treatment included sterol, steroid and cholesterol metabolic and biosynthetic process (**Figure 4C**). Treatment with KM also altered glycometabolism by regulating key genes involved in glucose binding and fructose-bisphosphate aldolase activity like HKDC1, HK2, ALDOA and ALDOB. These results suggested KM might function in regulating the cell energy metabolism. These findings were further confirmed by KEGG pathway analysis. The top 20 pathways of KEGG assignments are listed in **Figure 4D**. At the transcriptomic level, 17 pathways were significantly ($P < 0.05$) enriched for gene expression in the KM treated and control group comparisons which showed that glycolysis/gluconeogenesis, fructose and mannose metabolism and steroid biosynthesis were highly enriched among the DEGs resulting from KM treatment. To confirm the DEGs identified by RNA-Seq, *q*RT-PCR validation was performed on the representative genes in metabolism pathway. The mRNA

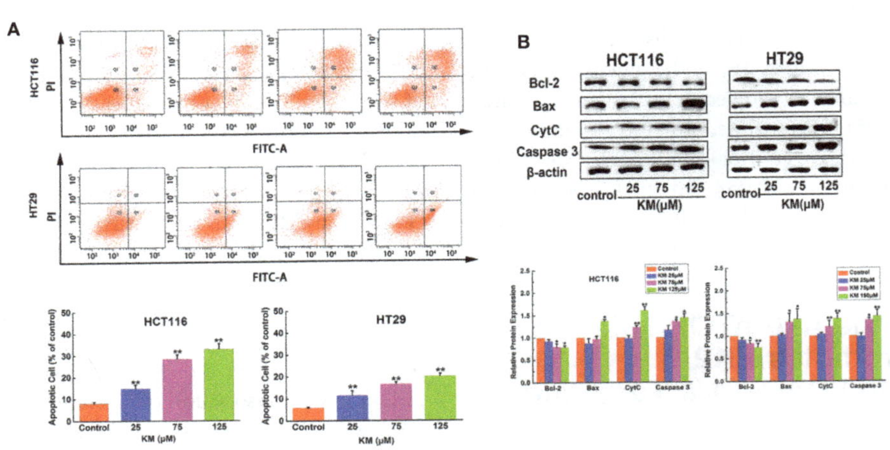

FIGURE 3 | KM promoted CRC cells apoptosis in a dose-dependent manner. **(A)** Flow cytometric analysis of HCT116 and HT29 cell apoptosis after incubation with KM for 24 h. **(B)** Western blot and quantification of proteins associated with apoptosis (Bcl-2, Bax, Cyt-C and caspase 3) in HCT116 and HT29 cells after incubation with KM for 24 h. Data were presented as mean ± SD (n = 3); significance: *$P < 0.05$, **$P < 0.01$ *vs* control.

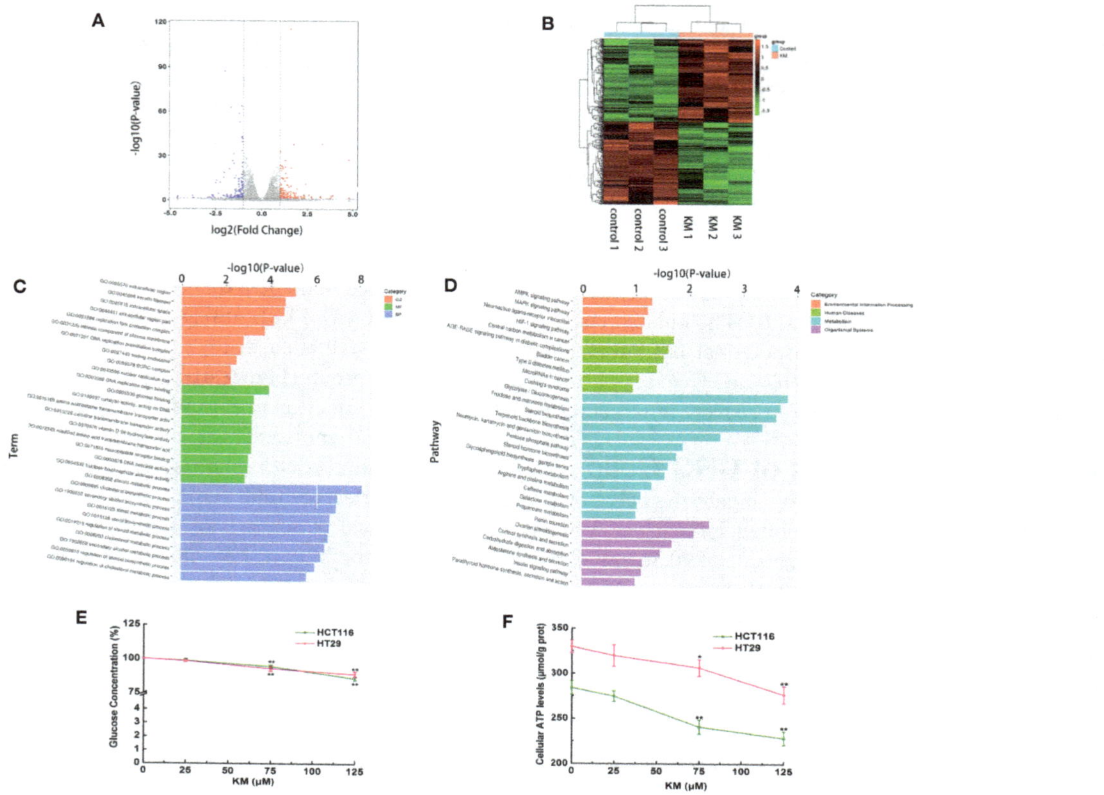

FIGURE 4 | **(A)** Volcano plot of the DEGs with FDR ≤ 0.05 and the fold change ≥ 2. Red dots indicate upregulated DEGs; blue ones indicate downregulated DEGs, and gray ones indicate no significant difference. **(B)** Heatmap of expression profile for the 306 DEGs (153 upregulated and 153 downregulated). Each row represents a mRNA and each column represents a sample. **(C)** Gene ontology (GO) enrichment analysis of DEGs. **(D)** Kyoto Encyclopedia of Genes and Genomes (KEGG) pathway enrichment analysis of DEGs. **(E)** Effect of KM on glucose consumption. **(F)** Effect of KM on production of cellular ATP. Data were presented as mean ± SD (n = 3); significance: $^*P < 0.05$, $^{**}P < 0.01$ *vs* control.

expressions of these genes were all consistent with the results of RNA-Seq (**Supplementary Table 6** and **Figure 2**).

To further confirm the results of RNA-Seq, glucose concentration in the medium and intracellular ATP level were examined after both HCT116 and HT29 cells were exposed to KM for 24 h. As shown in **Figures 4E, F**, the glucose uptake in KM treated cells was significantly lower than that in untreated control group ($P < 0.05$), meanwhile, the intracellular ATP generation of KM treated group was significantly decreased compared to control group ($P < 0.05$). An integrated analysis of mentioned above revealed that KM may facilitate the CRC cell apoptosis effect *via* suppression of the glycolysis process.

KM Inactivated the Akt/mTOR/HK2 Pathway and Promotes HK2 Disassociation to VDAC-1 *via* Targeting PDK1

In accordance with the suppression of tumor glycolysis, the expression of HK2 which is the key enzymes of glucose metabolism was markedly decreased in a dose-dependent manner (**Figure 5A**). In order to further understand the potential molecular mechanism by which KM modulating HK2 expression on CRC cell lines, we focused on the Akt/mTOR pathway, which is a widely acknowledged signaling cascade interacting with a wide variety of cellular processes including glucose metabolism of cancer cells and serve as a functional link between PDK1 and HK2. As shown in **Figure 5A**, phosphorylation of Akt and mTOR was dramatically downregulated, while KM had no effect on the expression levels of PDK1, total Akt, and mTOR after KM treatment. Taking these results together, KM might inhibit glycolysis through suppressing Akt/mTOR/HK2 pathway *via* targeting PDK1 in CRC cells.

HK2 is particularly important for the catabolism of glucose as it is the first enzyme of glycolysis (16). Moreover, HK2 is located on the outer membrane of the mitochondria *via* its binding to VDAC-1 to exert it biological function (17). The immunofluorescence was performed to detect the change of both HK2-mitochondria and HK2-VDAC-1 association of CRC cells. Intense green staining of HK2 was detected in the control group while HK2 staining co-localized with red Mitotracker staining in merged images. The HK2 intensities were dramatically decreased in response to KM exposure and a significant attenuation of HK2 associated with mitochondria was observed in merged images. Meanwhile, formation of the HK2

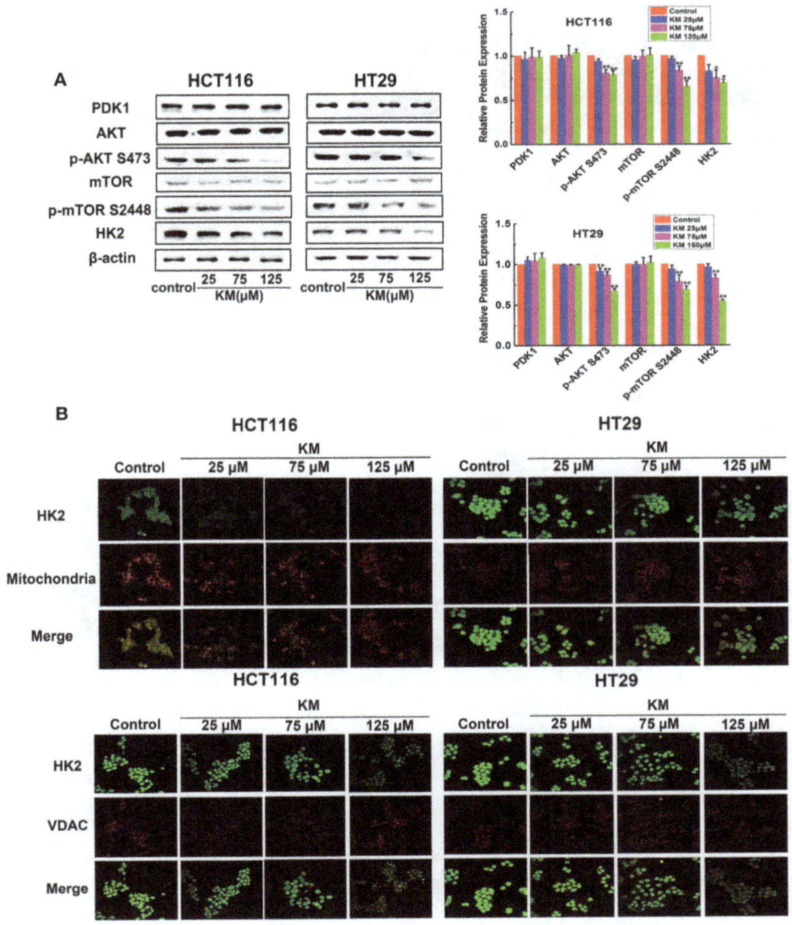

FIGURE 5 | KM repressed glycolysis and promoted the dissociation of HK2 from mitochondria and VDAC by downregulating Akt/mTOR/HK2 pathway in CRC cells. **(A)** Effect of KM on the expression level of Akt/mTOR/HK2 pathway by targeting PDK1. Protein levels were measured by Western blot analysis. **(B)** Representative immunofluorescence confocal images of CRC cells labelled with HK2, VDAC antibody and Mito-Tracker. Data were presented as mean ± SD (n = 3); significance: $^*P < 0.05$, $^{**}P < 0.01$ *vs* control.

dot-like structures became lower pronounced and less of these structures co-localized to the VDAC-1 foci (**Figure 5B**). The above observations together suggested that the suppression of Akt/mTOR pathway is responsible for the downregulation of HK2 and resulted in the disruption of HK2-VDAC combination which is conducive to metabolic activity and survival.

KM Inhibited Tumor Growth in an HCT116 Xenograft Mouse Model

To assess the effect of KM against CRC, a subcutaneous xenograft model of HCT116 cells was established in BALB/c nude mice. After 21 days treatment, the average tumor size of the control group was 1,200 ± 237 mm^3 compared with 650 ± 253 mm^3 of KM-treated group which resulted in a significant decrease in tumor volume ($P < 0.05$, **Figures 6A, B**). The average tumor weights of KM-treated group were significant smaller than those in the control group ($P < 0.05$, **Figure 6C**). Meanwhile, no obvious toxicity was observed as evaluating the change of body weight (**Figure 6D**). Moreover, immunohistochemistry staining assay showed intensity of staining of p-AKT, p-mTOR and HK2 were substantially lower after KM-treated group (**Figure 6E**) which indicated the expression of them was decreased after KM treatment. Taken together, these results indicated that 2 mg/kg KM showed effective inhibition on the xenograft tumor growth which was in accordance with the mechanisms *in vitro*.

DISCUSSION

Herbal medicine has long been recognized for their therapeutic properties and serves as an important source for chemical entities supporting drug discovery (18). Even though, the active ingredient and its mechanism have not been extensively investigated that limits their application, especially for the herbal

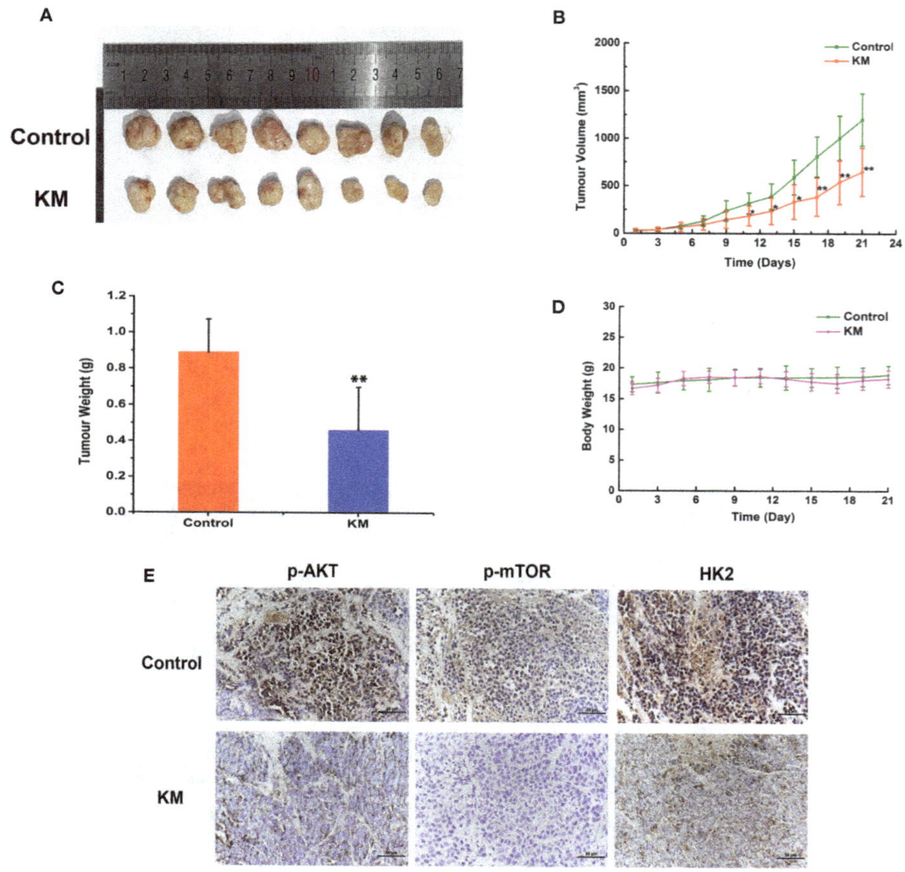

FIGURE 6 | KM inhibited colorectal tumor progression by Akt/mTOR/HK2 pathway in CRC xenograft mouse models. **(A)** Photograph of tumors in vehicle and KM treated group. **(B)** Tumor growth curve of control and KM treated group. **(C)** Tumor weight of control and KM treated group **(D)** The change of body weight of tumor bearing mice. **(E)** Immunohistochemical staining detection of p-Akt, p-mTOR and HK2 in tumor sections from control and KM-treated mice. All panels are of the same magnification. Data were shown as mean ± SD (n = 8). significance: $^{*}P < 0.05$, $^{**}P < 0.01$ *vs* control.

medicine with toxicity. The traditional methods for these studies were based on the separation and random screening with lower reproductive and throughput. It is of great significance and economic value to provide fast, efficient and high throughput approach to acquire the active ingredient and its targets of herbal medicine. The chemical constituents of *G. elegans* have been studied since the early 1930s and it has attracted a great deal of attention on cancer treatment because of their novel structures and diverse biological activities. However, the molecular mechanism of its action on CRC still was obscure. In the present study, we aimed of providing a novel, efficient and systematic strategy to identify the active ingredient and its potential molecular mechanism. Network-based pharmacology coupled with molecular docking and bioinformatics analysis were successfully applied in predicting the active ingredient and its target of *G. elegans* on CRC. As a result, KM, the most abundant molecule among the alkaloids of *G. elegans*, was deemed to be the potential effective compound with targeting PDK1.

PDK1 has been implicated in cancer progression, including proliferation, apoptosis and invasion and involved in signaling pathways altered in cancer, such as PI3K/Akt, Ras/MAPK and Myc (19). Moreover, over-expression of PDK1 was observed at both mRNA and protein levels in CRC specimens and cell lines (20). Thus, targeting PDK1 provides great therapeutic strategy for CRC. PDK1 is a soluble and globular protein composed of 556 amino acid and possesses an N-terminal Ser/Thr kinase domain and a C-terminal pleckstrin homology (PH) domain. The kinase domain contains two crucial elements for the regulation of kinase activity. One is the phosphorylation of serine 241 in the large C-terminal lobe that is catalyzed by PDK1 in *trans* and necessary for its kinase activity. Another is the PIF pocket located at the N-terminal lobe which could bind a hydrophobic motif on many PDK1 substrates (21). KM was a monoterpene indole alkaloid with a cage structure composed of six rings. Notably, KM exhibited the highest distribution in intestine *in vivo* in our previous study (22) which was consistent with the predicted results. Molecular docking result reveals that KM formed a stable complex with PDK1 at the adjacent domain of the ATP catalytic core region. The piperidine nitrogen atom establishes a hydrogen bond interaction with the backbone of Lys111. Lys111 which coordinates the α and β-phosphate of ATP with hydrogen bond has an ion pair interaction with absolutely conserved Glu130 located within the αC-helix (23). The integrity of Lys111 and Glu130 is crucial for the catalytic activity. There is another hydrogen bond interaction between the oxygen atom and Ser92. As a result, we speculated KM had a competitive interaction with ATP in the ATP catalytic site. In addition, it may also bind to the kinase domain in an allosteric pocket adjacent to the ATP-binding site. The specific mechanism remains to be further explored.

RNA-seq mainly focused on transcribed regions of genomes, serves as a powerful tool for exploring differentially expressed genes following treatment with various compounds and evaluating interactions between compounds and biological systems to reveal molecular mechanism (24). Our studies had shown that induction of apoptosis was a key molecular mechanism responsible for the anti-CRC activity of KM. To explore the possible downstream signaling of KM related to PDK1-induced CRC cell apoptosis, both RNA-seq associated with bioinformatics data-mining tools and experimental verification was performed. The DEGs were mainly enriched in the GO analysis corresponded to biological process such as the steroid metabolic and biosynthetic process and KEGG pathways related to metabolism including glycolysis/gluconeogenesis and fructose, mannose metabolism and steroid biosynthesis. The growth of malignancies including CRC prefers to metabolize glucose by glycolysis even in normoxic condition to meet high biogenetic demands in support of rapid and uncontrolled growth (25, 26). Such a reprogrammed cellular metabolism, known as "Warburg effect", is now recognized as a key hallmark of cancer which not only promotes tumor cell growth and spread but also relapse and chemotherapy resistance (27). As a result, targeting tumor glycolysis pathway has the potential to be a scientifically cancer treatment approach (28, 29). It is worth pointing out that KM determined a dramatically dose-dependent glucose uptake and ATP generation reduction. We also observed KM significantly downregulated the mRNA and protein levels of HK2, an enzyme responsible for the first step of glycolysis. These results revealed that KM has the capacity to suppress glycolysis by decreasing HK2 expression. It is generally accepted that HK2 has a dual role in tumor cells that HK2 could not only result in cell growth *via* enhanced glycolysis but also inhibit apoptosis *via* binding of VDAC-1 to the mitochondrial outer membrane. With HK2 dissociating from VDAC-1, the integrity and permeability of mitochondria membrane was disrupted which activated a release of pro-apoptotic enzyme, such as cytochrome C. It was well documented in our study that exposure to KM resulted in the decrease of the interaction between HK2 and VDAC-1, which could induce CRC cells to undergo apoptosis.

Furthermore, we investigated the pathway of KM involved in the inhibition of HK2 by targeting PDK1. Protein kinase B (Akt), one of the most defined PDK1 targets relevant in human cancer, is involved in the regulation of cellular survival through promoting glucose metabolism by stimulating the activity of hexokinase (30). Of note, studies have documented Akt/mTOR pathway has been a metabolic regulator center of cancer that could impede glycolysis and restrain cancer progression by modulating HK2 (31, 32). To further clarify whether the Akt/mTOR pathway was involved in mediating the effect of KM, the expression levels of p-Akt, Akt, p-mTOR, mTOR were assessed. With the inhibition of HK2 expression, the p-mTOR and p-Akt also reduced that indicated Akt/mTOR pathway could be of great importance during the downregulation of HK2.

Although herbal medicine has provided enormous potential lead compound to be applied to healthcare because of their structural diversity, complex scaffolds of compounds, low solubility, metabolic instability and ambiguous mechanisms of action has impeded them to achieve the final candidate drug (33, 34). It is interesting to optimize the structure of KM to increase the binding ability to receptor, raise the activity strength and selectivity. Vinyl is present in the active site which is a large space and mainly composed of hydrophobic amino acid. It is quite possible that substitution vinyl with favorable lipophilic groups, such as phenyl or benzoyl group is beneficial to better affinity as well as greater activity. Furthermore, it is also reasonable to design KM analogue by replacing the tricyclo fragment linking a vinyl group with lipophilic side chain to simplify the complicated ring system. Such further structure development and optimization of KM may contribute to the superior anti-CRC potency.

CONCLUSION

Effective ingredient and corresponding target validation are the key steps in herbal drug development chain. In this study, it adopts synthetically network pharmacology, molecular docking, transcriptomics and bioinformatics approach for mapping the anti-CRC ingredient and mechanism of *G. elegans*. It gives a novel and efficient strategy to explore the pharmacological mechanism of herbal medicine. As a result, we found that KM had a potent anti-CRC capacity through regulating glycolysis and VDAC-1 association *via* targeting PDK1. AKT/mTOR/HK2 signaling down-regulation may play an essential role in this process. Replacement of vinyl group with lipophilic group will provide rational direction for structure optimization study in the future.

ETHICS STATEMENT

The animal study was reviewed and approved by China Medical University Institutional Animal Care and Use Committee.

AUTHOR CONTRIBUTIONS

LW conducted the experiments and participated in the conception and the design of the study. HX and YD conducted the experiments and performed the analysis. LW and JL contributed to analyze the data and draft the manuscript. FM contributed to the conception, design, and analysis of the manuscript. All authors contributed to the article and approved the submitted version.

REFERENCES

1. Li L, Zhou X, Li N, Sun M, Lv J, Xu Z. Herbal drugs against cardiovascular disease: traditional medicine and modern development. *Drug Discov Today* (2015) 20:1074–86. doi: 10.1016/j.drudis.2015.04.009
2. Hu Y, Wang S, Wu X, Zhang J, Chen R, Chen M, et al. Chinese herbal medicine-derived compounds for cancer therapy: a focus on hepatocellular carcinoma. *J Ethnopharmacol* (2013) 149:601–12. doi: 10.1016/j.jep.2013.07.030
3. Rugo H, Shtivelman E, Perez A, Vogel C, Franco S, Tan Chiu E, et al. Phase I trial and antitumor effects of BZL101 for patients with advanced breast cancer. *Breast Cancer Res Treat* (2007) 105:17–28. doi: 10.1007/s10549-006-9430-6
4. Changou CA, Shiah H-S, Chen L-T, Liu S, Luh F, Liu SH, et al. A Phase II Clinical Trial on the Combination Therapy of PHY906 Plus Capecitabine in Hepatocellular Carcinoma. *Oncologist* (2020) [Epub ahead of print]. doi: 10.1002/onco.13582
5. Rujjanawate C, Kanjanapothi D, Panthong A. Pharmacological effect and toxicity of alkaloids from Gelsemium elegans Benth. *J Ethnopharmacol* (2003) 89:91–5. doi: 10.1016/s0378-8741(03)00267-8
6. Yuan Z, Matias FB, Wu J, Liang Z, Sun Z. Koumine Attenuates Lipopolysaccaride-Stimulated Inflammation in RAW264.7 Macrophages, Coincidentally Associated with Inhibition of NF-kappaB, ERK and p38 Pathways. *Int J Mol Sci* (2016) 17:430. doi: 10.3390/ijms17030430
7. Jin GL, He SD, Lin SM, Hong LM, Chen WQ, Xu Y, et al. Koumine Attenuates Neuroglia Activation and Inflammatory Response to Neuropathic Pain. *Neural Plast* (2018) 2018:9347696. doi: 10.1155/2018/9347696
8. Jin GL, Yang J, Chen WQ, Wang J, Qiu HQ, Xu Y, et al. The analgesic effect and possible mechanisms by which koumine alters type II collagen-induced arthritis in rats. *J Nat Med* (2019) 73:217–25. doi: 10.1007/s11418-018-1229-3
9. Jin GL, Yue RC, He SD, Hong LM, Xu Y, Yu CX. Koumine Decreases Astrocyte-Mediated Neuroinflammation and Enhances Autophagy, Contributing to Neuropathic Pain From Chronic Constriction Injury in Rats. *Front Pharmacol* (2018) 9:989. doi: 10.3389/fphar.2018.00989
10. Liu M, Huang HH, Yang J, Su YP, Lin HW, Lin LQ, et al. The active alkaloids of Gelsemium elegans Benth. are potent anxiolytics. *Psychopharmacology* (2013) 225:839–51. doi: 10.1007/s00213-012-2867-x
11. Yuan Z, Liang Z, Yi J, Chen X, Li R, Wu J, et al. Koumine Promotes ROS Production to Suppress Hepatocellular Carcinoma Cell Proliferation Via NF-kappaB and ERK/p38 MAPK Signaling. *Biomolecules* (2019) 9:559. doi: 10.3390/biom9100559
12. Zhang X, Chen Y, Gao B, Luo D, Wen Y, Ma X. Apoptotic Effect of Koumine on Human Breast Cancer Cells and the Mechanism Involved. *Cell Biochem Biophys* (2015) 72:411–6. doi: 10.1007/s12013-014-0479-2
13. Wang L, Wang JF, Mao X, Jiao L, Wang XJ. Gelsedine-type oxindole alkaloids from Gelsemium elegans and the evaluation of their cytotoxic activity. *Fitoterapia* (2017) 120:131–5. doi: 10.1016/j.fitote.2017.06.005
14. Jin GL, Su YP, Liu M, Xu Y, Yang J, Liao KJ, et al. Medicinal plants of the genus Gelsemium (Gelsemiaceae, Gentianales)–a review of their phytochemistry, pharmacology, toxicology and traditional use. *J Ethnopharmacol* (2014) 152:33–52. doi: 10.1016/j.jep.2014.01.003
15. Liang JW, Wang MY, Olounfeh KM, Zhao N, Wang S, Meng FH. Network pharmacology-based identifcation of potential targets of the flower of Trollius chinensis Bunge acting on anti-inflammatory effectss. *Sci Rep* (2019) 9:8109. doi: 10.1038/s41598-019-44538-z
16. Mazure NM. VDAC in cancer. *Biochim Biophys Acta Bioenerg* (2017) 1858:665–73. doi: 10.1016/j.bbabio.2017.03.002
17. Li M, Shao J, Guo Z, Jin C, Wang L, Wang F, et al. Novel mitochondrion-targeting copper(II) complex induces HK2 malfunction and inhibits glycolysis via Drp1-mediating mitophagy in HCC. *J Cell Mol Med* (2020) 24:3091–107. doi: 10.1111/jcmm.14971
18. Li FS, Weng JK. Demystifying traditional herbal medicine with modern approach. *Nat Plants* (2017) 3:17109. doi: 10.1038/nplants.2017.109
19. Gagliardi PA, Puliafito A, Primo L. PDK1: At the crossroad of cancer signaling pathways. *Semin Cancer Biol* (2018) 48:27–35. doi: 10.1016/j.semcancer.2017.04.014
20. Xu Z, Liao B, Zhang R, Yao J, Shi R, Wang L. Expression of 3-phosphoinositide-dependent protein kinase 1 in colorectal cancer as a potential therapeutic target. *Med Oncol* (2015) 32:198. doi: 10.1007/s12032-015-0645-4
21. Komander D, Fairservice A, Deak M, Kular GS, Prescott AR, Peter Downes C, et al. Structural insights into the regulation of PDK1 by phosphoinositides and inositol phosphates. *EMBO J* (2004) 23:3918–28. doi: 10.1038/sj.emboj.7600379
22. Wang L, Sun Q, Zhao N, Wen YQ, Song Y, Meng FH. Ultra-Liquid Chromatography Tandem Mass Spectrometry (UPLC-MS/MS)-Based Pharmacokinetics and Tissue Distribution Study of Koumine and the Detoxification Mechanism of Glycyrrhiza uralensis Fisch on Gelsemium elegans Benth. *Molecules* (2018) 23:1–14. doi: 10.3390/molecules23071693
23. Huse M, Kuriyan J. The conformational plasticity of protein kinases. *Cell* (2002) 109:275–82. doi: 10.1016/s0092-8674(02)00741-9
24. Gurunathan S, Qasim M, Park C, Yoo H, Kim JH, Hong K. Cytotoxic Potential and Molecular Pathway Analysis of Silver Nanoparticles in Human Colon Cancer Cells HCT116. *Int J Mol Sci* (2018) 19:2269. doi: 10.3390/ijms19082269
25. Jiang P, Du W, Wu M. Regulation of the pentose phosphate pathway in cancer. *Protein Cell* (2014) 5:592–602. doi: 10.1007/s13238-014-0082-8
26. Kitazawa M, Hatta T, Sasaki Y, Fukui K, Ogawa K, Fukuda E, et al. Promotion of the Warburg effect is associated with poor benefit from adjuvant chemotherapy in colorectal cancer. *Cancer Sci* (2020) 111:658–66. doi: 10.1111/cas.14275
27. Icard P, Shulman S, Farhat D, Steyaert JM, Alifano M, Lincet H. How the Warburg effect supports aggressiveness and drug resistance of cancer cells? *Drug Resist Updat* (2018) 38:1–11. doi: 10.1016/j.drup.2018.03.001
28. Gill KS, Fernandes P, O'Donovan TR, McKenna SL, Doddakula KK, Power DG, et al. Glycolysis inhibition as a cancer treatment and its role in an anti-tumour immune response. *Biochim Biophys Acta* (2016) 1866:87–105. doi: 10.1016/j.bbcan.2016.06.005
29. Ganapathy-Kanniappan S, Geschwind JFH. Tumor glycolysis as a target for cancer therapy_ progress and prospects. *Mol Cancer* (2013) 12:152. doi: 10.1186/1476-4598-12-152
30. Hung YP, Teragawa C, Kosaisawe N, Gillies TE, Pargett M, Minguet M, et al. Akt regulation of glycolysis mediates bioenergetic stability in epithelial cells. *ELife* (2017) 6:e27293. doi: 10.7554/eLife.27293
31. Jia L, Huang S, Yin X, Zan Y, Guo Y, Han L. Quercetin suppresses the mobility of breast cancer by suppressing glycolysis through Akt-mTOR pathway mediated autophagy induction. *Life Sci* (2018) 208:123–30. doi: 10.1016/j.lfs.2018.07.027
32. Gao X, Han H. Jolkinolide B inhibits glycolysis by downregulating hexokinase 2 expression through inactivating the Akt/mTOR pathway in non-small cell lung cancer cells. *J Cell Biochem* (2018) 119:4967–74. doi: 10.1002/jcb.26742
33. Guo Z. The modification of natural products for medical use. *Acta Pharm Sin B* (2017) 7:119–36. doi: 10.1016/j.apsb.2016.06.003
34. Yao H, Liu J, Xu S, Zhu Z, Xu J. The structural modification of natural products for novel drug discovery. *Expert Opin Drug Discov* (2017) 12:121–40. doi: 10.1080/17460441.2016.1272757

18

4-Hydroxyphenylpyruvate Dioxygenase-Like Protein Promotes Pancreatic Cancer Cell Progression and Is Associated With Glutamine-Mediated Redox Balance

Xianglai Ye[1,2,3†], Xiujuan Wei[1,2,3†], Jing Liao[1,2,3], Peipei Chen[1,2,3], Xueyun Li[1,2,3], Yulong Chen[1,2,3], Yue Yang[1,2,3], Qiongya Zhao[4], Hongwei Sun[5], Liming Pan[6], Guorong Chen[7], Xujun He[8], Jianxin Lyu[1,2,3,4,8] and Hezhi Fang[1,2,3*]*

[1] Key Laboratory of Laboratory Medicine, Ministry of Education, Wenzhou Medical University, Wenzhou, China, [2] Zhejiang Provincial Key Laboratory of Medical Genetics, Department of Cell Biology and Medical Genetics, Wenzhou Medical University, Wenzhou, China, [3] College of Laboratory Medicine and Life Sciences, Wenzhou Medical University, Wenzhou, China, [4] College of Laboratory Medicine, Hangzhou Medical College, Hangzhou, China, [5] Department of Surgery, The First Affiliated Hospital of Wenzhou Medical University, Wenzhou, China, [6] Department of Pathology, The People's Hospital of Yuhuan, The Yuhuan Branch of the First Affiliated Hospital of Wenzhou Medical University, Taizhou, China, [7] Department of Pathology, The First Affiliated Hospital of Wenzhou Medical University, Wenzhou, China, [8] Department of Laboratory Medicine, Zhejiang Provincial People's Hospital, Affiliated People's Hospital of Hangzhou Medical College, Hangzhou, China

***Correspondence:**
Jianxin Lyu
jxlu313@163.com
Hezhi Fang
fangh@wmu.edu.cn

†These authors have contributed equally to this work

Tumor cells develop a series of metabolic reprogramming mechanisms to meet the metabolic needs for tumor progression. As metabolic hubs in cells, mitochondria play a significant role in this process, including energy production, biosynthesis, and redox hemostasis. In this study, we show that 4-hydroxyphenylpyruvate dioxygenase-like protein (HPDL), a previously uncharacterized protein, is positively associated with the development of pancreatic ductal adenocarcinoma (PDAC) and disease prognosis. We found that overexpression of HPDL in PDAC cells promotes tumorigenesis *in vitro*, whereas knockdown of HPDL inhibits cell proliferation and colony formation. Mechanistically, we found that HPDL is a mitochondrial intermembrane space localized protein that positively regulates mitochondrial bioenergetic processes and adenosine triphosphate (ATP) generation in a glutamine dependent manner. Our results further reveal that HPDL protects cells from oxidative stress by reprogramming the metabolic profile of PDAC cells toward glutamine metabolism. In short, we conclude that HPDL promotes PDAC likely through its effects on glutamine metabolism and redox balance.

Keywords: mitochondria, pancreatic ductal adenocarcinoma, metabolic reprogramming, glutamine, redox balance

INTRODUCTION

Of all the cancer types, pancreatic cancers have the lowest 5-year survival rate at 9% (1). Pancreatic ductal adenocarcinoma (PDAC), as the most common type of pancreatic cancer, is a lethal cancer type as it is typically diagnosed late resulting in poor prognosis (2, 3). Increased biosynthetic demand for proliferation drives tumor cells to reprogram cellular metabolism (4). In PDAC, composed of a minority of malignant ductal cells with a dearth of blood vessels and an existence of extensive desmoplastic stroma originating from cancer-associated fibroblasts (CAFs), tumor cells live in a microenvironment of poor perfusion, poor nutrient, hypoxia and acidosis (5–7). To survive in this environment, PDAC tumor cells develop a series of metabolic reprograming mechanisms involving aerobic glycolysis, glutaminolysis, fatty acid oxidation, and protein scavenging to fuel the energy demand and biosynthetic process essential for cell growth (8–10). The oncogene *KRAS* and tumor suppressor genes *TP53*, *CDKN2A*, and *SMAD4* play a significant role in pancreatic neoplasia (11). As PDAC progresses to malignancy, called acinar-to-ductal metaplasia (ADM), oncogenic mutations of *KRAS* essentially initiate precursor lesions called pancreatic intraepithelial neoplasias (PanINs) (12).

The role of mitochondria is not typically considered important in tumor cells because they predominantly utilize glucose to generate ATP *via* aerobic glycolysis rather than mitochondrial oxidative phosphorylation (OXPHOS) (13). Since the mitochondria is the central organelle in cell metabolism where most bioenergetic and biosynthetic processes take place, they play a pivotal role in driving metabolic reprogramming (14, 15). oncogenes and tumor suppressor genes tightly regulate mitochondrial metabolism to meet metabolic need in the neoplasia process (16). Glutamine is a non-essential amino acid that can be used as a substrate in the tricarboxylic acid (TCA) cycle in mitochondria. Glutaminase (GLS), which converts glutamine to glutamate in the TCA cycle, is upregulated by the oncogene MYC-mediated mTOR pathway (17). Moreover, oncogenic mutation of *KRAS* reprograms glutamine metabolism by upregulating aspartate transaminase (GOT1) and downregulating glutamate dehydrogenase (GLUD1) at the transcription level (18).

We previously showed that the mitochondrial proteins COX6B2 and HSP60 play significant roles in the promotion of PDAC (19, 20). In addition, a recent study revealed that overexpression of the mitochondrial protein UQCRC1 from the electron transfer chain (ETC) promotes PDAC growth by enhancing OXPHOS and ATP generation (21). Since reactive oxygen species (ROS) production occurs in the ETC, redox balancing is required in all cancer cells with glutamine responsible for generating antioxidant NADPH and glutathione (GSH) (22). To account for this, a mitochondrion-localized protein SLC1A5 variant, functions as a glutamine transporter in the mitochondria, and mediates redox balancing in mitochondria (23). More and more studies have shown a close relation between PDAC and mitochondrion-localized proteins, and suggest that the role of mitochondrial proteins in the progression of PDAC cannot be ignored.

According to the subcellular map of the Human Protein Atlas (HPA), mitochondrial proteins account for 6% of all proteins and play an essential part in various cellular processes (24). There are abundant publications and experimental evidence for the function of mitochondrial proteins, but there are still 170 proteins whose functions remain to be defined (**Figure 1A**). In this study, we describe a mitochondrion-localized protein, 4-hydroxyphenylpyruvate dioxygenase like protein (HPDL). The function of HPDL has not been previously defined, apart from its association with neurodegenerative diseases (25). For this study we performed a series of experiments to test the effects of HPDL, including its effect on PDAC progression, mitochondrial function, and cellular metabolism.

MATERIALS AND METHODS

Cell Lines and Cell Culturing

Human pancreatic cell lines, PaTu 8988t, MIA PaCa-2, PANC-1, SW1990, Capan-2, and the immortalized pancreatic ductal cell line hTERT-HPNE, were obtained from the Cell Bank of the Chinese Academy of Science (Shanghai, China). Cells were cultured in Dulbecco's modified Eagle's medium (DMEM; Sigma-Aldrich, St. Louis, MO, USA) containing 4.5 g/L glucose, 4 mM glutamine, 110 mg/L sodium pyruvate, supplemented with 10% fetal bovine serum (FBS, Sigma-Aldrich), 100 U/ml penicillin (Beyotime, Shang, China), 0.1 mg/ml streptomycin (Beyotime), and 0.25 µg/ml amphotericin B (MP Biomedicals, Santa Ana, CA, USA). Cells were cultured in a CO2 incubator (Thermo Fisher Scientific, Waltham, MA, USA) at 37°C under 5% CO2.

Generation of Stable Knockdown and Overexpression Cell Lines

Stable knockdown (KD) and overexpression (OE) models were generated based on a previous protocol using second-generation lentiviruses (26). Lentiviral particles were generated by co-transfection of 5×10^5 HEK293T cells (Cell Bank of Chinese Academy of Science) in a 6-well plate with packaging vectors psPAX2 (1 µg), envelope vectors pMD2.G (0.5 µg), and shRNA sequence containing knockdown vectors pLVSHG01 (1 µg) or HPDL protein coding sequence NM_032756.3 containing overexpression vectors pLVEXP01 (1 µg) (Cyagen, Santa Clara, CA, USA). Transfection was performed using Lipofectamine 3000 (Thermo Fisher Scientific). The HPDL shRNA and scramble shRNA sequences are shown as follows: 5'-AGTCCGTACAGGAGCAATCTG-3' (HPDL), 5'-CCTAAGGTTAAGTCGCCCTCG-3' (scramble). Monoclonal selection of stable cell lines was performed based on a previously described limiting dilution method (27).

Immunohistochemical Analysis of Tissue Microarray

Immunohistochemical (IHC) analysis of tissue microarray (TMA) was performed as previously described (28). Ninety-one malignant tumor pancreatic tissue sample and 13 non-cancerous tumor pancreatic tissue samples were obtained from

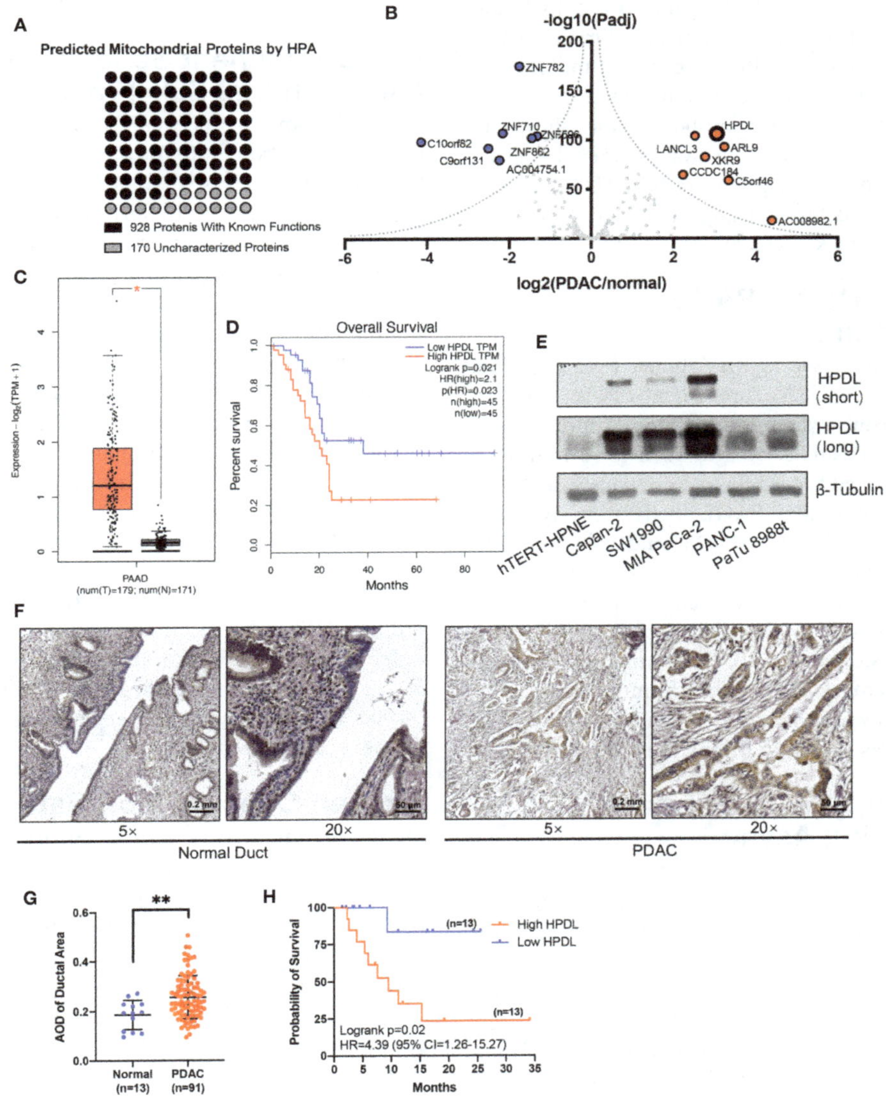

FIGURE 1 | HPDL is upregulated in pancreatic ductal adenocarcinoma and associated with poor prognosis. **(A)** Mitochondrial proteins that experimentally detected in the mitochondria by the Human Protein Atlas (http://www.proteinatlas.org). The functional definitions of these mitochondrial proteins were based on the annotation of Uniprot (https://www.uniprot.org). **(B)** Gene expression profile of function-unknown mitochondrial proteins based on the data generated by the TCGA (https://www.cancer.gov/tcga) and GTEx (https://commonfund.nih.gov/GTEx) datasets. The genes were plotted with expression of PDAC/normal duct and adjusted p-value. The red points refer to genes up-regulated in PDAC and the blue points refer to genes down-regulated in PDAC. **(C, D)** Expression plot and survival plot of HPDL in pancreatic adenocarcinoma (PAAD) made by GEPIA server (http://gepia.cancer-pku.cn). For expression plot **(C)**, threshold was set as follows: log_2FoldChange <1, p-value <0.01. For survival plot **(D)**, high and low expression groups were split by quartile, and the hazards ratio (HR) was calculated based on Cox PH model. **(E)** Western blot analysis of HPDL in different human pancreatic adenocarcinoma cell lines and human immortalized pancreatic duct cell line hTERT-HPNE. β-Tubulin was used as loading control. **(F)** Immunohistochemical (IHC) analysis of tissue microarray (TMA). TMA was incubated with anti-HPDL and stained with DAB and hematoxylin. HPDL expression in normal and malignant pancreatic ducts was shown in different zoom levels. **(G, H)** Quantitative analysis of HPDL expression in TMA. Quantification of HPDL expression was represented as average optical density (AOD). Comparisons between normal and malignant pancreatic ducts **(G)** was performed. Survival curve **(H)** was performed between low HPDL group and high HPDL group which were split by median. (*P < 0.05. **P < 0.01.)

Zhejiang Provincial People's Hospital. Experimental procedures were approved by Ethical Committee of Wenzhou Medical University (grant number: 2019-084). In short, paraffin-embedded tissues were punched into the recipient block to make the TMA, and the TMA section were then placed on a slide. After deparaffinization and hydration, endogenous peroxidase was blocked with 0.3% hydrogen peroxide (H_2O_2) and heat-induced epitope retrieval (HIER) was performed. Finally, the TMA was incubated with anti-HPDL (1:250) and stained with diaminobenzidine (DAB) and hematoxylin.

Immunofluorescence Staining

Cells in φ14mm slides were fixed with 4% paraformaldehyde and permeabilized with 0.1 mM digitonin (Sigma-Aldrich). Then, permeabilized cells were blocked with 5% goat serum, followed by primary antibodies and fluorescent-conjugated secondary antibodies. Primary and secondary antibodies was shown in **Supplementary Table 1**. The nucleus was stained by DNA binding stain 4,6-diamidino-2-phenylindole (DAPI). The fluorescence in cells was detected using an A1 confocal laser microscope (Nikon, Minato-ku, Tokyo, Japan).

SDS PAGE, Blue Native PAGE, and Immunoblotting

For SDS PAGE, cells were lysed in RIPA buffer (Cell Signaling Technology, Danvers, MA, USA) supplemented with protease inhibitor phenylmethylsulfonyl fluoride (PMSF, 1mM, Sangon Biotech, Shanghai, China), and heated to 95°C for 5 min. Blue native PAGE was performed according to a previously described protocol (29). For blue native PAGE, cells were lysed in solubilization buffer (50 mM NaCl, 50mM imidazole, 2 mM 6-aminohexonic acid, 1mM EDTA, pH 7.00) and supplemented with 2.5% digitonin (w/v, Sigma-Aldrich) and 1mM PMSF (Sangon Biotech). Proteins resolved by SDS-PAGE or blue native PAGE were transferred to a PVDF membrane (Bio-Rad, Hercules, CA, USA). Membranes were then immunoblotted with primary antibodies and secondary antibodies. Primary and secondary antibodies was shown in **Supplementary Table 1**.

Cell Proliferation, Colony Formation, and Wound Healing Assay

Cell proliferation was analyzed by counting cells in a 12-well plate with a NovoCyte flow cytometer (Agilent, Santa Clara, CA, USA). Colony formation was analyzed by seeding 1,000 cells in a 6-well plate for 10 days, and cells were fixed with 4% paraformaldehyde and stained with crystal violet (Beyotime). The size of the clones was measured using ImageJ (30). The wound healing assay was performed as previously described (31). 1×10^6 cells were seeded in a 6-well plate and the gaps were created by scratching on the monolayer of cells with a pipette tip. The gap size was measured using the Wound Healing Coherency Tool in ImageJ.

Isolation of Mitochondria

Mitochondrial isolation was performed as previously described (32). Cells was suspended in a hypotonic isolation buffer (0.1×IB, 3.5 mM Tris-HCl, 2.5 mM NaCl, 0.5 mM $MgCl_2$, pH 7.80) on ice to break the cell membrane integrity and then homogenized 20-30 strokes with a Dounce homogenizer (WHEATON, Millville, NJ, USA). The homogenate was then incorporated with 1/10 volume of hypertonic buffer (10×IB, 350 mM Tris-HCl, 250 mM NaCl, 50 mM $MgCl_2$, pH 7.80) to restore the isotonic solution. Centrifugation was performed to eliminate the contamination from nuclei, unbroken cells, and other debris. Multiple centrifugations under a low speed (1,200 × g × 3 min) were performed to remove the waste in the pellets. Finally, the mitochondria were pelleted down at 15,000 × g for 2 min and washed with homogenization buffer A (10mM Tris-HCl, 320mM sucrose, pH 7.40) to yield crude mitochondria.

Cell Component Separation and Mitochondrial Sub-Fractionation Analysis

The cell components were separated using a Nuclear and Cytoplasmic Protein Extraction Kit (Beyotime) according to the manufacturer's instructions. After treatment with hypotonic extraction buffer, cells were fully swollen, and cytoplasmic proteins were released. Nuclear pellets were obtained by centrifugation at 16,000 × g for 10 min. Nuclear extraction buffer was added to nuclei and a vortex was used several times to obtain the nuclear protein.

For mitochondrial sub-fractionation analysis, two different methods were performed as previously described (33, 34). To separate the soluble components (mitochondrial intermembrane space and matrix) and insoluble components (mitochondrial outer membrane and inner membrane), isolated mitochondria were treated with 0.1 M Na_2CO_3 on ice for 30 min, followed by ultracentrifugation (Beckman Coulter, Brea, CA, USA) at 100,000 g for 45 min. To further separate the mitochondrial components, mitochondria were treated with hypotonic buffer (10 mM HEPES/KOH, pH 7.40) on ice for 20 min to break the outer membrane. Broken mitochondria were deposited at 1,900 g for 15 min, and the supernatant was subsequently centrifuged at 50,000 × g for 30 min to separate the proteins in the outer membrane and the intermembrane space.

Oxygen Consumption Rate Assay

OCR was measured using Oxygraph-2k (OroborOSX, Innsbruck, Austria) according to the manufacturer's instructions (35). Cells (1×10^6) were added to the chamber, and the basal respiration of cells was measured. ATP synthase inhibitor oligomycin (2.5 μM, Sigma-Aldrich) and uncoupler carbonyl cyanide 4-(trifluoromethoxy) phenylhydrazone (FCCP, 5 μM, Sigma-Aldrich) were added to measure the non-phosphorylating proton leak and maximum non-coupled flux, respectively.

Adenosine Triphosphate Assay and Hydrogen Peroxide Assay

ATP determination was performed using an ATP Bioluminescent Assay Kit (Sigma-Aldrich) according to the manufacturer's instructions. Intracellular ATP was released by treating 5×10^5 cells with ATP-releasing reagent. Free ATP was detected by light produced through a luciferin-based reaction.

H_2O_2 determination was performed using a Hydrogen Peroxide Assay Kit (Beyotime) according to the manufacturer's instructions. Cells (1×10^6) were sonicated in H_2O_2 extraction buffer and intracellular H_2O_2 oxidized Fe^{2+} in xylenol orange solution to generate color. The absorbance was measured at 560 nm.

Mitochondrial DNA Copy Number Analysis

Quantitative PCR was performed using SYBR Green Supermix (Bio-Rad) with Quantagene q225 (Kubo Tech, Beijing, China).

Primers for mtDNA and nuclear DNA-encoded ACTIN are shown as follows. F: 5'-CACCCAAGAACAGGGTTTGT-3', R: 5'-TGGCCATGGGTATGTTGTTAA-3' (mtDNA). F: 5'-AGCTGTCACTCCAGGGTCC-3', R:5'-GATCCACATCTG CTGGAAGGT-3' (ACTIN).

Citrate Synthase Assay

Citrate synthase activity was determined using a previously described protocol (36). Acetyl-CoA (0.3 mM, Sigma-Aldrich) and oxaloacetic acid (0.5 mM, Sigma-Aldrich) were used as substrates for citrate synthase and 5,5-dithiobis (2-nitrobenzoic acid) (DTNB, 0.1mM, Sigma-Aldrich) were used to generate color. The reaction was activated with 10 µg snap-freeze cell lysate in reaction buffer (0.1 M Tris-HCl, pH 8.00). The absorbance was measured at 412 nm using a SpectraMax iD3 Multi-Mode Microplate Reader (Molecular Devices, Shanghai, China).

Mitochondrial Morphology Analysis

Mitochondrial morphology was analyzed by immunofluorescence staining and transmission electron microscopy (TEM). For immunofluorescence staining, analysis was performed as stated above, with HSP60 used as a mitochondrial indicator. Mitochondrial morphology was analyzed using a macro tool MINA (37) in the ImageJ software (30).

For TEM, 5×10^6 cells were fixed with 2.5% glutaraldehyde and 1% osmic acid at 4°C and stained with uranyl acetate for 1 h. Gradient dehydration was performed in 30%, 50%, 70%, 80%, 90%, and 100% acetone for 15 min each. Then, a resin-based gradient embedding was performed at 37°C followed by 65°C overnight. Finally, sectioned slides were observed under a H-7500 electron microscope (Hitachi, Chiyoda-ku, Tokyo, Japan).

Transcriptome Sequencing

RNA library construction was performed using a NEBNext Ultra RNA Library Prep Kit (New England Biolabs, Ipswich, MA, USA). mRNA was enriched with oligo(dT) beads and fragmented in fragmentation buffer. Then, reverse transcription was done using the M-MuLV system with random hexamer primer. cDNA fragments (200–250 bp) were purified with AMpure XP beads (Beckman Coulter, Beverly, CA, USA). Clustering and sequencing were performed using a TruSeq PE Cluster Kit and NovaSeq platform (Illumina, San Diego, CA, USA).

Liquid Chromatography-Mass Spectrometry Analysis

Quasi-targeted metabolic profiling analysis of cells was performed on a QTRAP6500+ mass spectrometer coupled with an ExionLC AD system (all from SCEIX, Framingham, MA, USA). Cells (1×10^7) were sonicated in 80% methanol and the centrifuged supernatant was subsequently injected into LC/MS. For the positive ion mode, samples were injected into a BEH C8 column (100×2.1 mm, 1.9 µm), and for the negative ion mode, samples were injected into an HSS T3 column (100×2.1 mm, 1.8 µm). A 25-min gradient containing flow phase A (0.1% formic acid-water) and flow phase B (0.1% formic acid-acetonitrile) was performed at a flow rate of 0.35 ml/min. For MS, the IonSpary Voltage was set at 5500V and -4500V, respectively. Metabolites were identified using multiple reaction monitoring (MRM) based on the Novogene self-built database (Novogene, Beijing, China).

Targeted metabolite analysis was performed on a Xevo G2-XS QTof mass spectrometry coupled with an ACQUITY UPLC system, and data analysis was done with Progenesis QI (all from Waters, Milford, MA, USA). Metabolites in a homogenate of 1×10^6 cells were extracted using chloroform, methanol, and water at a ratio of 8:4:3 and resuspended in 1% acetonitrile. For UPLC, samples were injected on an HSS T3 column (100×2.1 mm, 1.8 µm) using an 8-min gradient containing flow phase A (0.1% formic acid-water) and flow phase B (0.1% formic acid-acetonitrile) at a flow rate of 0.5 ml/min. For the negative ion mode, the capillary energy and sample cone were set as 2000V and 20V, respectively. Scan time was set at 0.1 s intervals for 60 s.

Bioinformatic Analysis and Statistical Analysis

Gene expression analysis and survival analysis from TCGA and GTEx databases were performed using the GEPIA server (38). The mitochondrial targeting sequence was predicted by the MitoProt server (39). Bioinformatic analysis was performed using R package. The enrichment of differentially expressed genes or metabolites was based on the KEGG pathways (40). All quantitative experiments were performed using a minimum of three independent replicates. The quantitative results are presented as mean ± SD, and the p value was calculated using a student' s *t* test with SPSS v22.0 (IBM, Chicago, IL, USA). Statistical graphs were made using Prism 8 (GraphPad Software, San Diego, CA, USA).

RESULTS

HPDL Is Upregulated in Pancreatic Ductal Adenocarcinoma and Is Associated With Poor Prognosis

We profiled gene expression in PDAC using data from TCGA and GTEx databases **(Figure 1B)**. Our results found that *HPDL* (HGNC:28242) was significantly upregulated, with considerable fold change, in PDAC. *HPDL*, also known as *GLOXD1* (Glyoxalase Domain-Containing Protein 1), is a paralog of *HPD* (4-Hydroxyphenylpyruvate Dioxygenase). It is a protein coding gene for 4-hydroxyphenylpyruvate dioxygenase like protein. Until now, the function of HPDL has been unclear.

We plotted *HPDL* expression and overall survival rate (OS) in PDAC and found upregulation was associated with poor prognosis in PDAC **(Figures 1C, D)**. In pancreatic tumor cell lines, HPDL was also detected at the protein level, especially in MIA PaCa-2, compared with immortalized normal pancreatic duct cell line hTERT-HPNE **(Figure 1E)**. We also performed immunohistochemistry (IHC) staining of 91 malignant tumor pancreatic tissue samples and 13 non-cancerous tumor pancreatic tissue samples. We quantified the staining intensity in selected ductal areas and found that the protein level of HPDL was upregulated in pancreatic malignant tumors (**Figures 1F, G**). We followed up on 26 cases and split them into two groups by median HPDL staining intensity. The survival plot showed that the high HPDL group had a lower overall survival rate (**Figure 1H**). Collectively, HPDL is upregulated in PDAC at both the mRNA and protein levels, in both tumor cell lines and tumor tissues, and high expression of HPDL is associated with poor prognosis in PDAC patients.

HPDL Promotes Pancreatic Ductal Adenocarcinoma *In Vitro*

To further investigate HPDL in PDAC, we generated two cell models in pancreatic tumor cell lines (**Figures 2A, B**). The overexpression (OE) model was generated in PaTu 8988t due to its relatively low expression among other pancreatic tumor cell lines (**Figure 1E**), which may imitate the functional effect of HPDL. For the same reason, a knockdown (KD) model was generated in the MIA PaCa-2 line which demonstrated high

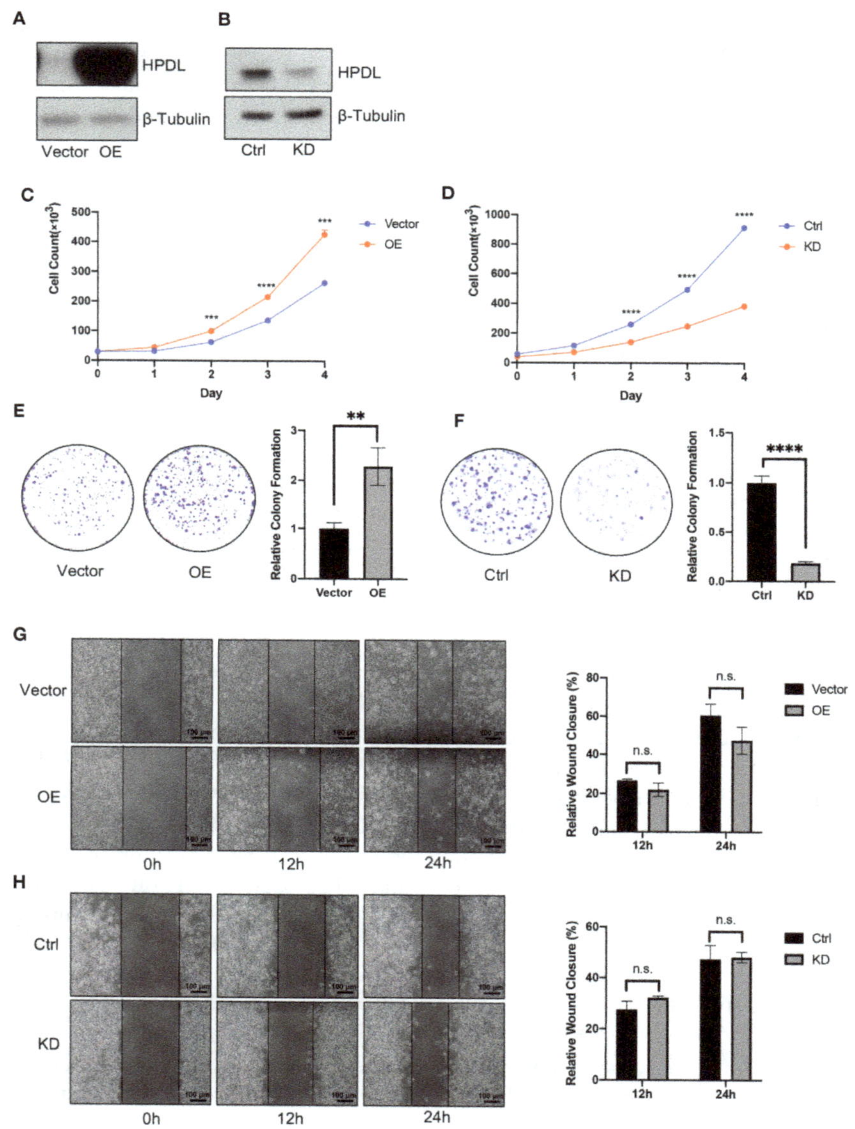

FIGURE 2 | HPDL promotes pancreatic ductal adenocarcinoma *in vitro*. **(A, B)** Validation of HPDL overexpression **(A)** and knockdown **(B)** cells with theirs paired control cells. HPDL overexpression (OE) model and its empty vector control (Vector) were generated in PaTu 8988t, HPDL knockdown (KD) model and its scramble control (Ctrl) were generated in MIA PaCa-2. Cell lysate was separated with SDS-PAGE and immunoblotted with antibodies as indicated. β-Tubulin was used as loading control. **(C, D)** Cell proliferation of HPDL OE **(C)** and KD **(D)** cells with theirs paired control cells. Cells were seeded in 12-well plate and counted for 4 days. **(E, F)** Colony formation analysis of HPDL OE **(E)** and KD **(F)** cells with theirs paired control cells. Cells were seeded in 6-well plate and stained with crystal violet after 10-day culture. **(G, H)** Wound healing analysis of HPDL OE **(G)** and KD **(H)** cells with theirs paired control cells. Cells were seeded in 6-well plate and scratched with a pipette tip. Wound closure was measured at 0, 12, and 24 h. (**$P < 0.01$. ***$P < 0.001$. ****$P<0.0001$. n.s., no significance.)

HPDL expression. In accordance with our bioinformatical analysis and IHC data, HPDL OE cells demonstrated better proliferation and HPDL KD cells had worse proliferation compared to control cells **(Figures 2C, D)**. In colony formation assays, HPDL OE and KD cells followed the same pattern **(Figures 2E, F)**.

HPDL was observed to promote PDAC growth in these two experiments, and we next tested cell migration using a wound healing assay. We found that neither OE nor KD cells were distinct from the paired control cells **(Figures 2G, H)**. These results suggest that HPDL had a positive effect on the progression of PDAC *in vitro* but did not influence migration.

HPDL Localizes to the Mitochondrial Intermembrane Space

To probe the molecular function and biological process of HPDL, we performed domain and subcellular localization analyses. A domain analysis by the Conserved Domain Database (CDD) (41) is shown in a schematic diagram **(Figure 3A)**. HPDL was predicted to contain two 4-hydroxyphenylpyruvate dioxygenase (HppD) like domains that belongs to the vicinal oxygen chelate (VOC) superfamily, which consists of structurally related metalloproteins with distinct functions (42). We further searched out active sites in HPDL and found that HPDL contained an iron biding site like other members in VOC superfamily. Moreover, there are 37 amino acid residues in the N-terminal targeting to mitochondria as predicted by the MitoProt server (39), which further strengthens our expectation that HPDL is a mitochondrial protein.

We then performed an immunofluorescence colocalization analysis in the pancreatic tumor cell lines PaTu 8988t and MIA PaCa-2. In the colocalization analysis, HSP60 was used as a mitochondrial tracker and had a strong overlap with HPDL **(Figure 3B)**. In the fractionation of cellular components, we found HPDL colocalized with cytoplasmic protein GAPDH **(Figure 3C)**. In addition, submitochondrial localization of HPDL was performed using carbonate extraction analysis, a method used to separate hydrophobic membrane proteins and soluble proteins in mitochondria (43). The carbonate extraction analysis showed HPDL localized in the aqueous compartments, including the intermembrane space (IMS) and matrix **(Figure 3D)**. To discriminate between IMS and matrix proteins, we performed hypotonic treatment to mitochondria to break the outer membrane and release the IMS proteins, following ultracentrifugation to yield IMS proteins. Finally, HPDL was found to be localized to the intermembrane space using this more delicate submitochondrial fractionation analysis **(Figure 3E)**.

HPDL Promotes Mitochondrial Respiration and Adenosine Triphosphate Generation

Having established solid confirmation of HPDL's localization in mitochondria, we next focused on understanding its possible effects on mitochondria. We first performed an oxygen consumption rate (OCR) assay with HPDL OE and KD cells **(Figures 4A, B)**. As an inhibitor of ATP synthase, oligomycin was added to disrupt OXPHOS and then the non-phosphorylation proton flux of cells can be measured. In addition, FCCP was used as an OXPHOS uncoupler to transport protons freely through mitochondrial membrane and then the maximum uncoupled respiration can be measured. As a result, overexpression of HPDL enhanced basal respiration and knockdown of HPDL diminished basal respiration and maximum uncoupled respiration. Consistent with the OCR results, cellular ATP was also increased in OE cells and decreased in KD cells **(Figures 4C, D)**. Considering the ATP generated in glycolysis, we further deprived glucose in the culture medium and added pyruvate or glutamine instead. Unlike glucose, pyruvate and glutamine will directly enter the TCA cycle in mitochondria and generate ATP. As a result, a consistent pattern was observed in the glutamine group **(Figures 4F, H)**, but not in the pyruvate group **(Figures 4E, G)**, indicating that glutamine-dependent ATP generation was promoted by HPDL.

To further determine the effect of HPDL on mitochondrial respiration, we also performed blue native PAGE (BNG) analysis with digitonin-permeabilized cells to determine the steady level of mitochondrial OXPHOS complexes and supercomplexes. In BNG, HPDL only had a modest effect on respiratory complexes and supercomplex assembly **(Supplementary Figures 1A, B)**, suggesting that the promotive effects of HPDL on OCR are separate from OXPHOS complexes. Moreover, the mitochondrial DNA (mtDNA) copy number was shown to be unchanged in the results of quantitative PCR **(Supplementary Figures 1C, D)**. Additionally, a cellular citrate assay, a quantitative marker for the cellular mitochondria number, was performed to exclude the possible change in mitochondrial number **(Supplementary Figures 1E, F)**. Confocal and transmission electron microscopy used to investigate mitochondrial morphology found that neither individual mitochondria nor mitochondrial networks showed any significant differences **(Supplementary Figure 2)**. Taken together, these results showed that HPDL promotes mitochondrial respiration and ATP generation in PDAC but does not affect the steady level of OXPHOS complexes. Furthermore, HPDL does not affect mtDNA or mitochondrial morphology.

HPDL Reprograms Metabolic Profiles in PDAC Cells

To obtain a general understanding of HPDL, we performed gene expression profiling on HPDL OE cells. Gene expression profiling revealed 6838 differentially expressed genes (DEGs), of which 3,088 were upregulated and 3,750 were downregulated **(Figure 5A)**. To identify and interpret these DEGs, gene set enrichment analysis (GSEA) was performed to enrich common pathways of DEGs **(Figure 5B)**. As expected, we found that HPDL was strongly associated with genes associated with in mitochondria, including the TCA cycle, OXPHOS, and a series of metabolic diseases with mitochondrial dysfunction, such as Parkinson's disease, Alzheimer's disease, nonalcoholic fatty liver disease(NAFLD), and Huntington's disease (44–47). Moreover, genes involved in amino acid metabolism and carbon metabolism were enriched, indicating a possible change in the cellular metabolism of HPDL OE cells. Apart from GSEA, we also found 23 DEGs in the pancreatic cancer pathway of KEGG,

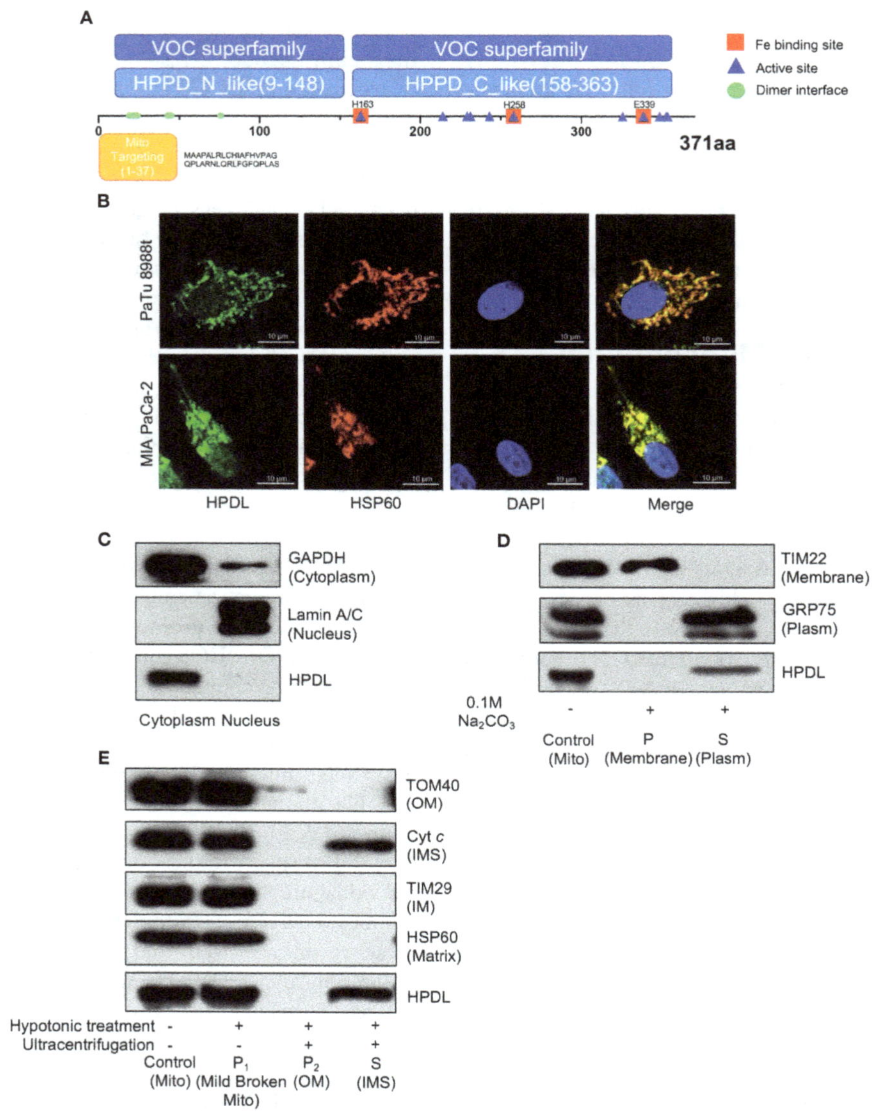

FIGURE 3 | HPDL localizes to mitochondrial intermembrane space. **(A)** Schematic diagram of HPDL protein domain structure. HPPD_N_like and HPPD_C_like, C-terminal or N-terminal domain of 4-hydroxyphenylpyruvate dioxygenase (HppD) and hydroxymandelate synthase (HmaS). **(B)** Immunofluorescence colocalization analysis of HPDL in PaTu 8988t and MIA PaCa-2. Cells were immunolabeled with HPDL (Alexa flour 488, green) and HSP60 (Alex flour 594, red), and nuclear was stained with DAPI (blue). **(C)** Subcellular fractionation analysis of HPDL in MIA PaCa-2. Cytosolic and nuclear protein was extracted and immunoblotted with antibodies as indicated. **(D)** Carbonate extraction analysis of HPDL in MIA PaCa-2. Isolated mitochondria were subjected to 0.1 M Na_2CO_3. Mitochondrial proteins in membrane and plasm was separated with ultracentrifugation. Proteins were separated with SDS-PAGE and immunoblotted with antibodies as indicated. Mito, isolated crude mitochondria. P, pellet. S, supernatant. **(E)** Submitochondrial fractionation analysis of HPDL in MIA PaCa-2. Isolated mitochondria were subjected to hypotonic buffer (10 mM HEPES/KOH, pH 7.40) to break the integrity of mitochondrial outer membrane. Mild broken mitochondria were separated with low-speed centrifugation. Proteins in mitochondrial outer membrane and intermembrane space were subsequently separated with ultracentrifugation. Proteins were separated with SDS-PAGE and immunoblotted with antibodies as indicated. Mito, isolated crude mitochondria. P_1, pellet in first centrifugation. P_2, pellet in second centrifugation. OM, outer membrane. S, supernatant in second centrifugation. IMS, intermembrane space.

including 17 oncogenes and 5 tumor suppressor genes, demonstrating the promotive effect of HPDL on PDAC (**Supplementary Figure 3**).

Pancreatic cells develop metabolic reprograming in the malignant progression of PDAC (9). To further determine the metabolic effect of HPDL, we performed metabolomic profiling on HPDL OE cells and found 91 differential metabolites (**Figure 5C**). Metabolite set enrichment analysis (MSEA) is a method designed to analyze metabolomic data (48). In line with the results of GSEA, we also found an association between HPDL and metabolites in glutamate and glutamine metabolism in MSEA (**Figures 5B, D**). It has been reported that PDAC cells

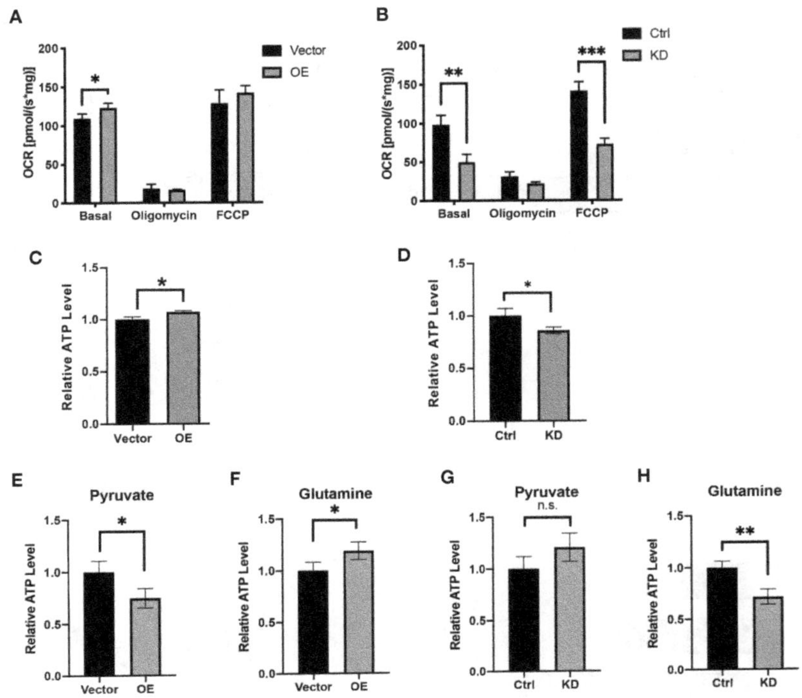

FIGURE 4 | HPDL promotes mitochondrial respiration and ATP generation. **(A, B)** Oxygen consumption rate of HPDL OE **(A)** and KD **(B)** cells with theirs paired control cells. Basal, basal respiration with endogenous substrates solely. Oligomycin, respiration in the presence of ATP synthase inhibitor oligomycin (2.5 μM). FCCP, respiration in the presence of uncoupler FCCP (5 μM). **(C, D)** Relative ATP level of HPDL OE **(C)** and KD **(D)** cells with theirs paired control cells. **(E–H)** Relative ATP level of HPDL OE **(E, F)** and KD **(G, H)** cells with theirs paired control cells in different culture conditions. Cells were cultured in medium supplemented with 5 mM pyruvate only **(E, G)** or 4 mM glutamine only **(F, H)** for 12 h and subsequently the cellular ATP was measured. (*$P < 0.05$. **$P < 0.01$. ***$P < 0.001$. n.s., no significance.)

increase glutamine utilization in ATP generation (49). Together with our data on ATP generation **(Figures 4F, H)**, it is likely that HPDL is associated with glutamine utilization in mitochondria, however, we found that glutamine and glutamate shuttle machineries including SLC1A5_variant (23) and SLC25A12/13 (50), respectively, were not interact with HPDL (**Supplementary Data Sheet 2**). This result indicates that HPDL role in glutamine metabolism is independent of classic mitochondrial glutamine and glutamate shuttle machineries.

We also found differential metabolites in glutathione metabolism and nicotinate metabolism. Together with DEGs in glutathione metabolism, these data strongly suggest that HPDL may be associated with redox balance **(Figures 5B, D)**. Collectively, our results support HPDL's role in reprograming metabolic profiles in PDAC, especially glutamate and glutamine metabolism as well as the metabolism of cellular antioxidants in PDAC.

HPDL Regulates Redox Balance *via* a Glutamine-Dependent Antioxidative Pathway

GSH is an antioxidant and acts as a scavenger of ROS in cells. In the progression of tumor cells, GSH is positively associated with tumor proliferation (51). Looking to our metabolomic data generated from HPDL OE and vector cells, we found that GSH and its oxidized form glutathione disulfide (GSSG) underwent a dramatic change **(Figures 6A, B)**. Increased GSH level and GSH/GSSG ratio in HPDL OE cells may suggest that HPDL plays a positive role in redox balance. We also found that H_2O_2 levels decreased in OE cells and increased in KD cells **(Figures 6C, D)**. Glutamine is used as a material for glutathione synthesis (52). In the presence of the glutamine antagonist 6-diazo-5-oxo-l-norleucine (DON), the H_2O_2 level remained unchanged in both HPDL OE and KD cells **(Figures 6E, F)**. In short, our data showed that HPDL is involved in the maintenance of redox balance, which is dependent on glutamine-derived GSH. In the biosynthesis of GSH, nicotinamide adenine dinucleotide phosphate ($NADP^+$) and reduced $NADP^+$ (NADPH) act as cofactors for glutathione reductase (GR) (53). Glutamine-derived aspartate is essential for generating NAPDH, and aspartate partially maintains redox balance (18). Our data showed that aspartate levels increased in OE cells **(Figure 6E)**. We further cultured OE cells in medium supplemented with either pyruvate or glutamine as the only carbon source and tested their aspartate levels. We found that the aspartate levels of cells using glutamine increased in a similar manner to cells cultured in

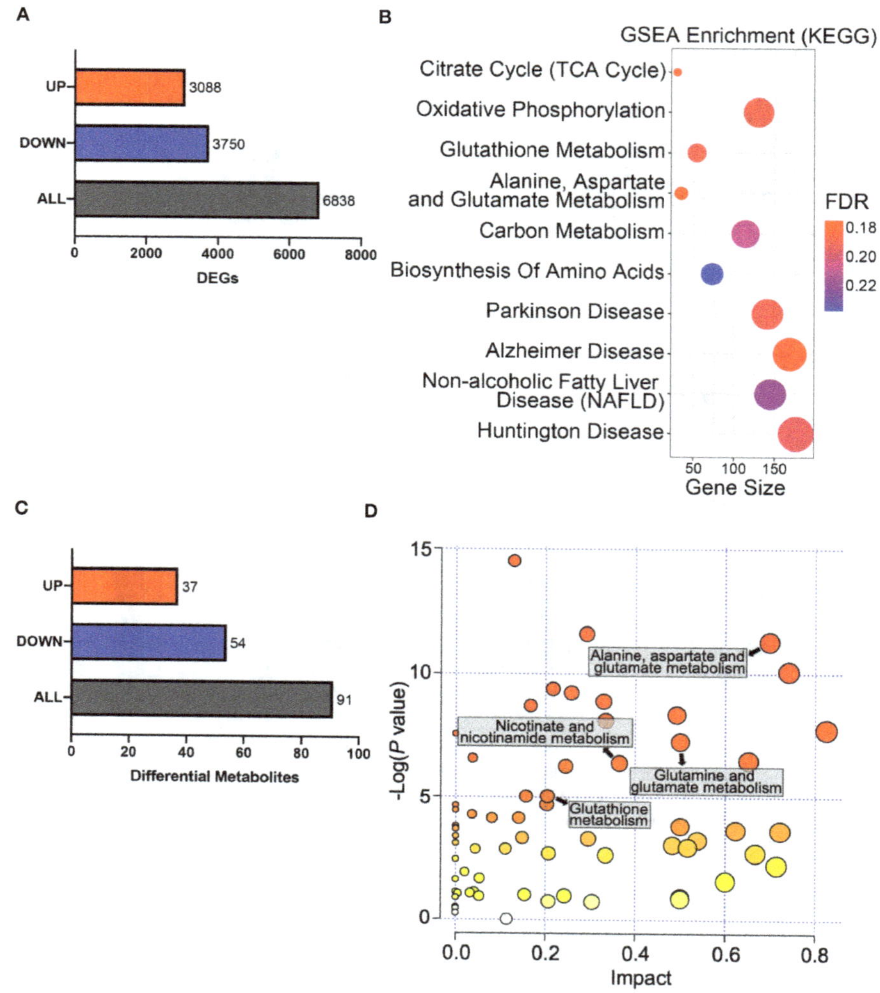

FIGURE 5 | HPDL reprograms metabolic profiles in PDAC cells. **(A)** DEGs in the gene expression profiling results of HPDL OE and control cells. Threshold was set as follows: p-adj<0.05, $|log_2(OE/Vector)|>0$. **(B)** GSEA in the gene expression profiling results of HPDL OE and control cells. Gene size refers to the count of genes enriched in certain pathways. FDR, false discovery rate. The GSEA was performed based on KEGG database (https://www.genome.jp/kegg/). **(C)** Differentially metabolites in metabolomic profiling results of HPDL OE and control cells. Threshold was set as follows: p<0.05, OE/Vector>1.2 or < 0.83. **(D)** MSEA in metabolomic profiling results of HPDL OE and control cells. Different metabolic pathways were plotted with p-value and impact. The MSEA was performed based on KEGG database (https://www.genome.jp/kegg/).

complete medium, suggesting that the increase in aspartate was derived from glutamine **(Figures 6H, I)**.

In summary, we drew a schematic overview of this glutamine-dependent antioxidative pathway. Glutamine-derived aspartate is converted to malate and subsequently convert to pyruvate following generation of NADPH. NADPH will then help to reduce GSSG to GSH, which results in the removal of H_2O_2 **(Figure 6J)**. In addition, we cultured OE cells in the presence of antioxidant N-acetylcysteine (NAC). NAC is a precursor of cysteine and helps in the biosynthesis of GSH (54). Intriguingly, HPDL only had a modest effect on cell proliferation in the presence of NAC **(Figure 6K)**. Overall, our results found that HPDL regulates redox balance *via* a glutamine-dependent antioxidative pathway, which may be the key event in explaining the positive effect on tumor proliferation of HPDL.

DISCUSSION

Over the past decade, numerous studies have reported that mitochondria are involved in tumor progression. The Warburg effect drives tumor cells to oxidize glucose *via* glycolysis but not to fuel ETC (13). However there is accumulating evidence that mitochondria still affect tumor cells pleiotropically including anabolic process, redox balance, cell signaling, and cell death (15). As hubs for metabolic processes, mitochondria also play a significant role in PDAC (55). Additionally, with regard to

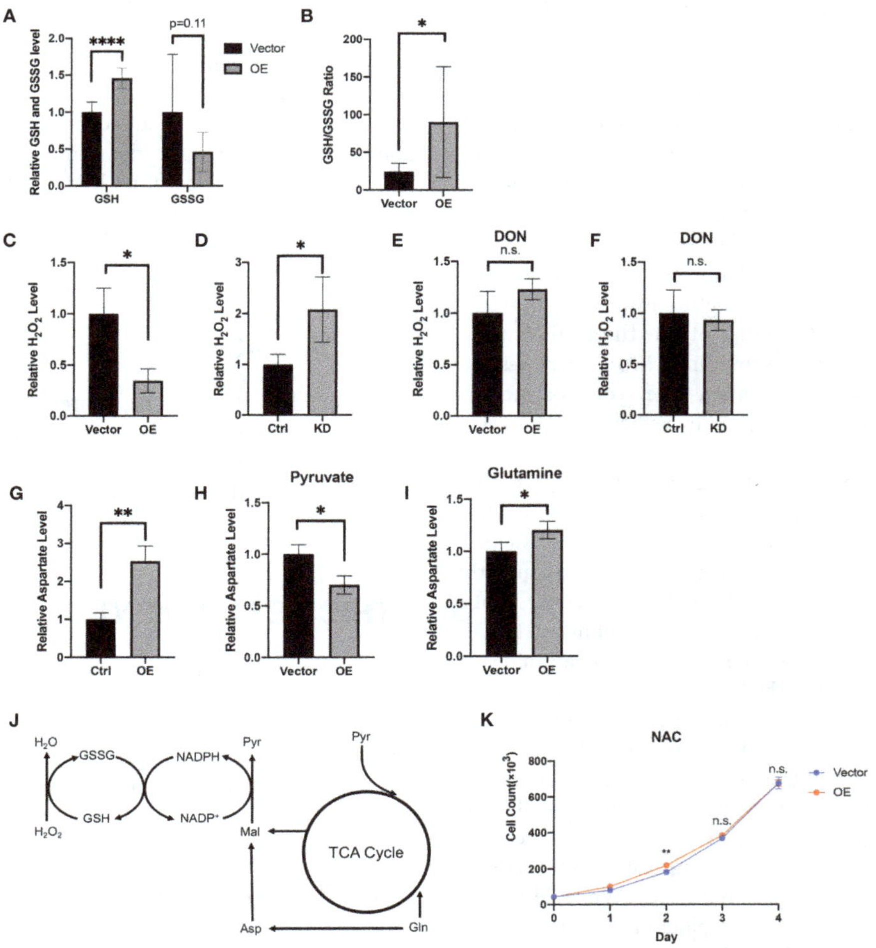

FIGURE 6 | HPDL regulates redox balance *via* a glutamine-dependent antioxidative pathway. **(A, B)** Relative GSH, GSSG level **(A)** and GSH/GSSG ratio **(B)** in metabolome results of HPDL OE and control cells. **(C, D)** Relative H_2O_2 level of HPDL OE **(C)** and KD **(D)** cells with theirs paired control cells. **(E, F)** Relative H_2O_2 level of HPDL OE **(E)** and KD **(F)** cells with theirs paired control cells in the presence of glutamine antagonist DON (5 mM). **(G)** Relative aspartate level of HPDL OE and control cells. **(H, I)** Relative aspartate level of HPDL OE and control cells in different culture conditions. Cells were cultured in medium supplemented with 5 mM pyruvate **(H)** or 4 mM glutamine **(I)** as the only carbon source for 12 h and subsequently the cellular aspartate was measured. **(J)** Schematic metabolic pathway of cellular antioxidative process. This diagram was prepared based on a previous work of Son (18). Pyr, pyruvate. Gln, Glutamine. Asp, aspartate. Mal, malate. **(K)** Cell proliferation of HPDL OE and control cells with NAC treatment. Cells were cultured in medium supplemented with 5 mM NAC. (*$P < 0.05$. **$P < 0.01$. ****$P < 0.0001$. n.s., no significance.)

PDAC's association with mitochondrial dysfunction, extensive investigation of mitochondria-targeting chemotherapeutic drugs has been performed (14). In this study, we provide a comprehensive view of HPDL, a mitochondrial protein, which has not previously been fully studied. According to bioinformatic analysis and IHC analysis, we found that HPDL was upregulated in PDAC, and high expression of HPDL was associated with poor prognosis. We also generated an overexpression model and knockdown model of HPDL on PDAC cell lines and found that HPDL promoted PDAC proliferation but not migration. To some extent, HPDL has an oncogenic effect on PDAC. This oncogenic effect was further confirmed using gene expression profiling, where the typical PDAC oncogene *KRAS* was upregulated in OE cells and tumor suppressor genes *TP53* and *CDKN2A* were downregulated in OE cells **(Supplementary Figure 3)**.

As a mitochondrial protein, HPDL also participates in the mitochondrial bioenergetic process. Our data showed that HPDL promoted mitochondrial respiration and ATP generation, suggesting a positive effect of HPDL on mitochondria. We made a preliminary attempt to explain this positive effect of HPDL on PDAC. We tested a series of possible changes in mitochondria, including the steady level of OXPHOS complexes, OXPHOS supercomplex assembly, mtDNA copy number, mitochondrial content, and mitochondrial morphology **(Supplementary Figures 1 and 2)**, but our results did not support a specific explanation. We next focused on mitochondrial metabolism. Glutamine-dependent ATP generation was observed in our data, indicating a possible effect of HPDL on metabolic reprogramming.

Tumor cells develop a series of metabolic reprogramming mechanisms to meet the anabolic and bioenergetic demands of cells in a continually changing microenvironment (4). PDAC also develops a series of metabolic reprogramming mechanisms, in which *KRAS* is considered a precursor oncogene (9). The primary effect of *KRAS* in PDAC is promoting glucose uptake and the anabolic glucose pathway (56). In the process of glutaminolysis, by which the glutamine fluxes into metabolites in the tricarboxylic acid (TCA) cycle, *KRAS* redirects glutamine flux through aspartate transaminases (GOT1) other than glutamate dehydrogenase (GLUD1). At the same time, *KRAS* increases the $NADPH/NADP^+$ ratio, which maintains the redox balance in PDAC (18). Although the mechanism by which HPDL affects mitochondrial respiration remains unknown, we still found evidence of its effect on metabolic reprogramming. In this study, we observed that glutamine-dependent ATP generation was enhanced by HPDL (**Figures 4F, H**), which could suggest that glutamine is entering the TCA cycle and subsequently contributing to mitochondrial respiration. Moreover, both gene expression profiling and metabolomic profiling of HPDL OE cells strongly implicated the metabolic reprogramming of glutamine metabolism (**Figures 5B, D**). As a carbon and nitrogen source for bioenergetic and biosynthesis process, glutamine plays a key role in cancer growth (18). GOT1 is a universally expressed enzyme that transfers nitrogen from glutamine-derived glutamate to oxaloacetate to produce aspartate and α-ketoglutarate (13). In our data, we observed a glutamine-dependent aspartate increase in HPDL OE cells (**Figure 6I**), further suggesting that HPDL reprograms glutamine metabolism in PDAC. While HPDL is not a component of classic glutamine/glutamate transporter in mitochondria (**Supplementary Data Sheet 2**), this protein may be involved in downstream glutaminolysis pathway; however, more works are required to validate this hypothesis.

According to our immunofluorescence colocalization analysis in PDAC cells, HPDL localizes to mitochondria. This result is in line with a previous study performed on mouse neuroblastoma cell line N2a (25). Meanwhile, we also found HPDL localized in the nuclear area in the immunofluorescence analysis, this was subsequently considered to be a result of fluorescence contamination, as western blotting analysis of nuclear protein showed no HPDL existence (**Figure 3C**). Through a series of submitochondrial fractionation, we have further demonstrated that HPDL is localized to the mitochondrial intermembrane space, where considerable amounts of ROS from respiratory complex III are generated (57). The redox balance in the IMS is tightly regulated (58). The IMS-localized proteins superoxide dismutase (Sod1) and cytochrome *c* peroxidase (Ccp1), together with glutathione redox buffer make up the IMS antioxidant system (58). Like other antioxidative enzymes in IMS, HPDL also contains an iron binding site, which may be the active site for its antioxidative capacity (**Figure 3A**).

In our gene expression profiling and metabolomic profiling data, we observed that HPDL OE cells experienced a metabolic alteration of glutathione (**Figures 5B, D**). Further experiments demonstrated that HPDL was associated with better regulation and control of redox balance in PDAC, which was in a glutamine-dependent pattern. The same pattern was observed by Son et al. (18), whose work on PDAC cells showed that glutamine deprivation resulted in ROS production. Moreover, Son et al. have shown that glutamine-derived NADPH that helps redox balance is critical for PDAC growth (18). Therefore, we propose this positive effect on the redox balance of HPDL may help explain its proliferative effect on tumor cells.

CONCLUSION

We conclude that HPDL has a promoting effect on PDAC, and this effect may be related to glutamine metabolism and redox balance. Although the specific pathway or enzymatic process in which HPDL participates remains unknown, we still provide a constructive direction for further study on HPDL.

ETHICS STATEMENT

The studies involving human participants were reviewed and approved by Ethical Committee of the First Affiliated Hospital of Wenzhou Medical University. Written informed consent for participation was not required for this study in accordance with the national legislation and the institutional requirements.

AUTHOR CONTRIBUTIONS

XY performed the experiments and wrote this manuscript. XW, JLi, PC, XL, YC, and YY performed the experiments. HS, LP, GC, and XH collected the tissue samples and performed the histological diagnosis. QZ performed the bioinformatics analysis. JLy and HF designed the experiments and revised the manuscript. All authors contributed to the article and approved the submitted version.

ACKNOWLEDGMENTS

We thank all the patients and their families for participating in this study. We thank Zhejiang Key Laboratory in Wenzhou Medical University for providing the experimental platform.

SUPPLEMENTARY MATERIAL

SUPPLEMENTARY FIGURE 1 | (A, B) Mitochondrial respiratory complexes analysis of HPDL OE **(A)** and KD **(B)** cells with theirs paired control cells. Cells were permeabilized with 2.5% digitonin and protein was separated by 3%-11% blue native PAGE. Mitochondrial respiratory complexes were immunoblotted with anti-Grim19 (CI), SDHA (CII), UQCRC2 (CIII), MT-CO1 (CIV) and ATP5A (CV). SCs, super complexes. CI-CV, mitochondrial respiratory complexes I-V. TOM70 was used as a loading control. Quantitative results were shown in the right panel. **(C, D)** Relative mtDNA copy number of HPDL OE **(C)** and KD **(D)** cells with theirs paired control cells. DNA was extracted from cell and mtDNA was determined by quantitative PCR. **(E, F)** Relative citrate synthase activity of HPDL OE **(E)** and KD **(F)** cells with theirs paired control cells. Cell were disrupted by snap-freeze and citrate synthase activity was determined with 0.3 mM acetyl-CoA, 0.5 mM OAA, and 0.1 mM DTNB. (n.s., no significance.)

SUPPLEMENTARY FIGURE 2 | (A, B) Mitochondrial morphology analysis of HPDL OE **(A)** and KD **(B)** cells with theirs paired control cells by immunofluorescence staining. Mitochondria were stained with green fluorescence (HSP60) using immunofluorescence staining. Median branch length of individual mitochondria and mitochondrial networks size were measured, and quantitative results was shown in lower panel. **(C, D)** Mitochondrial morphology analysis of HPDL OE **(C)** and KD **(D)** cells with theirs paired control cells by transmission electron microscopy. Mitochondria were shown in different zoom level. (n.s., no significance.)

SUPPLEMENTARY FIGURE 3 | Heatmap of oncogenes and tumor suppressor genes in HPDL OE cells. The heatmap was generated based on the data of gene expression profiling.

SUPPLEMENTARY TABLE 1 | Primary and secondary antibodies.

SUPPLEMENTARY DATA SHEET 1 | Quasi-targeted metabolomic analysis of HPDL OE cells.

SUPPLEMENTARY DATA SHEET 2 | LC-MS analysis of immunoprecipitation of FLAG-tagged HPDL proteins.

REFERENCES

1. Siegel RL, Miller KD, Jemal A. Cancer statistics, 2020. *CA Cancer J Clin* (2020) 70(1):7–30. doi: 10.3322/caac.21590
2. Adamska A, Domenichini A, Falasca M. Pancreatic Ductal Adenocarcinoma: Current and Evolving Therapies. *Int J Mol Sci* (2017) 18(7):1–43. doi: 10.3390/ijms18071338
3. Khorana AA, Mangu PB, Berlin J, Engebretson A, Hong TS, Maitra A, et al. Potentially Curable Pancreatic Cancer: American Society of Clinical Oncology Clinical Practice Guideline. *J Clin Oncol* (2016) 34(21):2541–56. doi: 10.1200/JCO.2016.67.5553
4. Pavlova NN, Thompson CB. The Emerging Hallmarks of Cancer Metabolism. *Cell Metab* (2016) 23(1):27–47. doi: 10.1016/j.cmet.2015.12.006
5. Dougan SK. The Pancreatic Cancer Microenvironment. *Cancer J* (2017) 23 (6):321–5. doi: 10.1097/PPO.0000000000000288
6. Sousa CM, Kimmelman AC. The complex landscape of pancreatic cancer metabolism. *Carcinogenesis* (2014) 35(7):1441–50. doi: 10.1093/carcin/bgu097
7. Gaustad JV, Simonsen TG, Wegner CS, Rofstad EK. Vascularization, Oxygenation, and the Effect of Sunitinib Treatment in Pancreatic Ductal Adenocarcinoma Xenografts. *Front Oncol* (2019) 9:845. doi: 10.3389/fonc.2019.00845
8. Blum R, Kloog Y. Metabolism addiction in pancreatic cancer. *Cell Death Dis* (2014) 5:e1065. doi: 10.1038/cddis.2014.38
9. Liang C, Qin Y, Zhang B, Ji S, Shi S, Xu W, et al. Metabolic plasticity in heterogeneous pancreatic ductal adenocarcinoma. *Biochim Biophys Acta* (2016) 1866(2):177–88. doi: 10.1016/j.bbcan.2016.09.001
10. Kamphorst JJ, Nofal M, Commisso C, Hackett SR, Lu W, Grabocka E, et al. Human pancreatic cancer tumors are nutrient poor and tumor cells actively scavenge extracellular protein. *Cancer Res* (2015) 75(3):544–53. doi: 10.1158/0008-5472.CAN-14-2211
11. Bailey P, Chang DK, Nones K, Johns AL, Patch AM, Gingras MC, et al. Genomic analyses identify molecular subtypes of pancreatic cancer. *Nature* (2016) 531(7592):47–52. doi: 10.1038/nature16965
12. Kanda M, Matthaei H, Wu J, Hong SM, Yu J, Borges M, et al. Presence of somatic mutations in most early-stage pancreatic intraepithelial neoplasia. *Gastroenterology* (2012) 142(4):730–3.e9. doi: 10.1053/j.gastro.2011.12.042
13. Vander Heiden MG, Cantley LC, Thompson CB. Understanding the Warburg effect: the metabolic requirements of cell proliferation. *Science* (2009) 324 (5930):1029–33. doi: 10.1126/science.1160809
14. Guerra F, Arbini AA, Moro L. Mitochondria and cancer chemoresistance. *Biochim Biophys Acta Bioenerg* (2017) 1858(8):686–99. doi: 10.1016/j.bbabio.2017.01.012
15. Vyas S, Zaganjor E, Haigis MC. Mitochondria and Cancer. *Cell* (2016) 166 (3):555–66. doi: 10.1016/j.cell.2016.07.002
16. Frezza C, Gottlieb E. Mitochondria in cancer: Not just innocent bystanders. *Semin Cancer Biol* (2009) 19(1):4–11. doi: 10.1016/j.semcancer.2008.11.008
17. Csibi A, Lee G, Yoon SO, Tong H, Ilter D, Elia I, et al. The mTORC1/S6K1 pathway regulates glutamine metabolism through the eIF4B-dependent control of c-Myc translation. *Curr Biol* (2014) 24(19):2274–80. doi: 10.1016/j.cub.2014.08.007
18. Son J, Lyssiotis CA, Ying H, Wang X, Hua S, Ligorio M, et al. Glutamine supports pancreatic cancer growth through a KRAS-regulated metabolic pathway. *Nature* (2013) 496(7443):101–5. doi: 10.1038/nature12040
19. Zhou C, Sun H, Zheng C, Gao J, Fu Q, Hu N, et al. Oncogenic HSP60 regulates mitochondrial oxidative phosphorylation to support Erk1/2 activation during pancreatic cancer cell growth. *Cell Death Dis* (2018) 9(2):161. doi: 10.1038/s41419-017-0196-z
20. Nie K, Li J, He X, Wang Y, Zhao Q, Du M, et al. COX6B2 drives metabolic reprogramming toward oxidative phosphorylation to promote metastasis in pancreatic ductal cancer cells. *Oncogenesis* (2020) 9(5):51. doi: 10.1038/s41389-020-0231-2
21. Wang Q, Li M, Gan Y, Jiang S, Qiao J, Zhang W, et al. Mitochondrial Protein UQCRC1 is Oncogenic and a Potential Therapeutic Target for Pancreatic Cancer. *Theranostics* (2020) 10(5):2141–57. doi: 10.7150/thno.38704
22. Altman BJ, Stine ZE, Dang CV. From Krebs to clinic: glutamine metabolism to cancer therapy. *Nat Rev Cancer* (2016) 16(10):619–34. doi: 10.1038/nrc.2016.71
23. Yoo HC, Park SJ, Nam M, Kang J, Kim K, Yeo JH, et al. A Variant of SLC1A5 Is a Mitochondrial Glutamine Transporter for Metabolic Reprogramming in Cancer Cells. *Cell Metab* (2020) 31(2):267–83.e12. doi: 10.1016/j.cmet.2019.11.020
24. Thul PJ, Akesson L, Wiking M, Mahdessian D, Geladaki A, Ait Blal H, et al. A subcellular map of the human proteome. *Science* (2017) 356(6340):1–12. doi: 10.1126/science.aal3321
25. Husain RA, Grimmel M, Wagner M, Hennings JC, Marx C, Feichtinger RG, et al. Bi-allelic HPDL Variants Cause a Neurodegenerative Disease Ranging from Neonatal Encephalopathy to Adolescent-Onset Spastic Paraplegia. *Am J Hum Genet* (2020) 107(2):364–73. doi: 10.1016/j.ajhg.2020.06.015
26. Campeau E, Ruhl VE, Rodier F, Smith CL, Rahmberg BL, Fuss JO, et al. A versatile viral system for expression and depletion of proteins in mammalian cells. *PLoS One* (2009) 4(8):e6529–e. doi: 10.1371/journal.pone.0006529
27. Fuller SA, Takahashi M, Hurrell JG. Cloning of hybridoma cell lines by limiting dilution. *Curr Protoc Mol Biol* (1988) 1(1):11.8. 1–.8. 2. doi: 10.1002/0471142727.mb1108s01
28. Kampf C, Olsson I, Ryberg U, Sjöstedt E, Pontén F. Production of tissue microarrays, immunohistochemistry staining and digitalization within the human protein atlas. *J Vis Exp* (2012) 63:3620. doi: 10.3791/3620
29. Wittig I, Braun HP, Schagger H. Blue native PAGE. *Nat Protoc* (2006) 1 (1):418–28. doi: 10.1038/nprot.2006.62
30. Schneider CA, Rasband WS, Eliceiri KW. NIH Image to ImageJ: 25 years of image analysis. *Nat Methods* (2012) 9(7):671–5. doi: 10.1038/nmeth.2089
31. Jonkman JE, Cathcart JA, Xu F, Bartolini ME, Amon JE, Stevens KM, et al. An introduction to the wound healing assay using live-cell microscopy. *Cell Adh Migr* (2014) 8(5):440–51. doi: 10.4161/cam.36224

32. Fernandez-Vizarra E, Ferrin G, Perez-Martos A, Fernandez-Silva P, Zeviani M, Enriquez JA. Isolation of mitochondria for biogenetical studies: An update. *Mitochondrion* (2010) 10(3):253–62. doi: 10.1016/j.mito.2009.12.148
33. Lorenzi I, Oeljeklaus S, Aich A, Ronsor C, Callegari S, Dudek J, et al. The mitochondrial TMEM177 associates with COX20 during COX2 biogenesis. *Biochim Biophys Acta Mol Cell Res* (2018) 1865(2):323–33. doi: 10.1016/j.bbamcr.2017.11.010
34. Badugu R, Garcia M, Bondada V, Joshi A, Geddes JW. N terminus of calpain 1 is a mitochondrial targeting sequence. *J Biol Chem* (2008) 283(6):3409–17. doi: 10.1074/jbc.M706851200
35. Gnaiger E. *Mitochondrial pathways and respiratory control. An introduction to OXPHOS analysis. Mitochondr Physiol Network 19.12.* Innsbruck: OROBOROS MiPNet Publications (2014).
36. Spinazzi M, Casarin A, Pertegato V, Salviati L, Angelini C. Assessment of mitochondrial respiratory chain enzymatic activities on tissues and cultured cells. *Nat Protoc* (2012) 7(6):1235–46. doi: 10.1038/nprot.2012.058
37. Valente AJ, Maddalena LA, Robb EL, Moradi F, Stuart JA. A simple ImageJ macro tool for analyzing mitochondrial network morphology in mammalian cell culture. *Acta Histochem* (2017) 119(3):315–26. doi: 10.1016/j.acthis.2017.03.001
38. Tang Z, Li C, Kang B, Gao G, Li C, Zhang Z. GEPIA: a web server for cancer and normal gene expression profiling and interactive analyses. *Nucleic Acids Res* (2017) 45(W1):W98–W102. doi: 10.1093/nar/gkx247
39. Claros MG, Vincens P. Computational method to predict mitochondrially imported proteins and their targeting sequences. *Eur J Biochem* (1996) 241 (3):779–86. doi: 10.1111/j.1432-1033.1996.00779.x
40. Kanehisa M, Goto S. KEGG: kyoto encyclopedia of genes and genomes. *Nucleic Acids Res* (2000) 28(1):27–30. doi: 10.1093/nar/28.1.27
41. Marchler-Bauer A, Derbyshire MK, Gonzales NR, Lu S, Chitsaz F, Geer LY, et al. CDD: NCBI's conserved domain database. *Nucleic Acids Res* (2015) 43 (Database issue):D222–6. doi: 10.1093/nar/gku1221
42. Armstrong RN. Mechanistic diversity in a metalloenzyme superfamily. *Biochemistry* (2000) 39(45):13625–32. doi: 10.1021/bi001814v
43. Kim H, Botelho SC, Park K, Kim H. Use of carbonate extraction in analyzing moderately hydrophobic transmembrane proteins in the mitochondrial inner membrane. *Protein Sci* (2015) 24(12):2063–9. doi: 10.1002/pro.2817
44. Park J-S, Davis RL, Sue CM. Mitochondrial Dysfunction in Parkinson's Disease: New Mechanistic Insights and Therapeutic Perspectives. *Curr Neurol Neurosci Rep* (2018) 18(5):21–. doi: 10.1007/s11910-018-0829-3
45. Moreira PI, Carvalho C, Zhu X, Smith MA, Perry G. Mitochondrial dysfunction is a trigger of Alzheimer's disease pathophysiology. *Biochim Biophys Acta (BBA) - Mol Basis Dis* (2010) 1802(1):2–10. doi: 10.1016/j.bbadis.2009.10.006
46. Nassir F, Ibdah JA. Role of mitochondria in nonalcoholic fatty liver disease. *Int J Mol Sci* (2014) 15(5):8713–42. doi: 10.3390/ijms15058713
47. Intihar TA, Martinez EA, Gomez-Pastor R. Mitochondrial Dysfunction in Huntington's Disease; Interplay Between HSF1, p53 and PGC-1α Transcription Factors. *Front Cell Neurosci* (2019) 13(103):1–10. doi: 10.3389/fncel.2019.00103
48. Xia J, Wishart DS. MSEA: a web-based tool to identify biologically meaningful patterns in quantitative metabolomic data. *Nucleic Acids Res* (2010) 38(Web Server issue):W71–7. doi: 10.1093/nar/gkq329
49. Roux C, Riganti C, Borgogno SF, Curto R, Curcio C, Catanzaro V, et al. Endogenous glutamine decrease is associated with pancreatic cancer progression. *Oncotarget* (2017) 8(56):95361–76. doi: 10.18632/oncotarget.20545
50. Amoedo ND, Punzi G, Obre E, Lacombe D, De Grassi A, Pierri CL, et al. AGC1/2, the mitochondrial aspartate-glutamate carriers. *Biochim Biophys Acta* (2016) 1863(10):2394–412. doi: 10.1016/j.bbamcr.2016.04.011
51. Traverso N, Ricciarelli R, Nitti M, Marengo B, Furfaro AL, Pronzato MA, et al. Role of Glutathione in Cancer Progression and Chemoresistance. *Oxid Med Cell Longevity* (2013) 2013:972913. doi: 10.1155/2013/972913
52. Sappington DR, Siegel ER, Hiatt G, Desai A, Penney RB, Jamshidi-Parsian A, et al. Glutamine drives glutathione synthesis and contributes to radiation sensitivity of A549 and H460 lung cancer cell lines. *Biochim Biophys Acta* (2016) 1860(4):836 43. doi: 10.1016/j.bbagen.2016.01.021
53. Xiao W, Wang RS, Handy DE, Loscalzo J. NAD(H) and NADP(H) Redox Couples and Cellular Energy Metabolism. *Antioxid Redox Signal* (2018) 28 (3):251–72. doi: 10.1089/ars.2017.7216
54. Samuni Y, Goldstein S, Dean OM, Berk M. The chemistry and biological activities of N-acetylcysteine. *Biochim Biophys Acta* (2013) 1830(8):4117–29. doi: 10.1016/j.bbagen.2013.04.016
55. Reyes-Castellanos G, Masoud R, Carrier A. Mitochondrial Metabolism in PDAC: From Better Knowledge to New Targeting Strategies. *Biomedicines* (2020) 8(8):270. doi: 10.3390/biomedicines8080270
56. Ying H, Kimmelman AC, Lyssiotis CA, Hua S, Chu GC, Fletcher-Sananikone E, et al. Oncogenic Kras maintains pancreatic tumors through regulation of anabolic glucose metabolism. *Cell* (2012) 149(3):656–70. doi: 10.1016/j.cell.2012.01.058
57. Xu X, Arriaga EA. Qualitative determination of superoxide release at both sides of the mitochondrial inner membrane by capillary electrophoretic analysis of the oxidation products of triphenylphosphonium hydroethidine. *Free Radic Biol Med* (2009) 46(7):905–13. doi: 10.1016/j.freeradbiomed.2008.12.019
58. Herrmann JM, Riemer J. The intermembrane space of mitochondria. *Antioxid Redox Signal* (2010) 13(9):1341–58. doi: 10.1089/ars.2009.3063

19

Zinc Finger Protein CTCF Regulates Extracellular Matrix (ECM)-Related Gene Expression Associated With the Wnt Signaling Pathway in Gastric Cancer

Chenbin Liu [1†], Linyi Deng [1†], Jinrong Lin [2], Jianjun Zhang [1], Shu Huang [1], Jinglin Zhao [1], Peipei Jin [1], Peiqing Xu [1], Peihua Ni [1], Dakang Xu [1], Le Ying [1,3,4*] and Yiqun Hu [1*]*

[1] Faculty of Medical Laboratory Science, Ruijin Hospital, School of Medicine, Shanghai Jiao Tong University, Shanghai, China, [2] Department of Sports Medicine, Huashan Hospital, Fudan University, Shanghai, China, [3] Centre for Innate Immunity and Infectious Diseases, Hudson Institute of Medical Research, Clayton, Victoria, Hudson Institute of Medical Research, Clayton, VIC, Australia, [4] Department of Molecular and Translational Science, Monash University, Clayton, VIC, Australia

***Correspondence:**
Yiqun Hu
ichunhu@126.com
Le Ying
le.ying@hudson.org.au
Dakang Xu
dakang.xu@monash.edu

†These authors have contributed equally to this work

Gastric cancer (GC), a leading cause of cancer-related death, is a heterogeneous disease. We aim to describe clinically relevant molecular classifications of GC that incorporate heterogeneity and provide useful clinical information. We combined different gene expression datasets and filtered a 7-gene signature related to the extracellular matrix (ECM), which also exhibited significant prognostic value in GC patients. Interestingly, putative CCCTC-binding factor (CTCF) regulatory elements were identified within the promoters of these ECM-related genes and were confirmed by chromatin immunoprecipitation sequencing (ChIP-Seq). CTCF binding sites also overlapped with histone activation markers, indicating direct regulation. In addition, CTCF was also correlated with the Wnt signaling pathway. A comparison of human GC cell lines with high or low expression of ECM-related genes revealed different levels of tumor aggressiveness, suggesting the cancer development-promoting functions of ECM-related genes. Furthermore, CTCF regulated COL1A1 and COLA31 expression *in vitro*. Silencing CTCF or COL1A1/COL1A3 markedly inhibited cell growth and migration in the metastatic GC cell line BGC823. Collectively, this ECM-related 7-gene signature provides a novel insight for survival prediction among GC patients. The zinc finger protein CTCF regulates ECM-related genes, thereby promoting GC cell growth and migration.

Keywords: gastric cancer, zinc finger protein CTCF, extracellular matrix (ECM), Wnt signaling, histone modification

INTRODUCTION

Gastric cancer (GC) is the fourth most common cancer in the world and causes approximately 738,000 deaths each year, making it the third leading cause of cancer-related death worldwide (1–4). East Asia is recognized as a high-risk region probably due to the high incidence of *Helicobacter pylori* (*H. pylori*) infection and cancer-associated dietary habits. The 5-year relative GC survival rate of all Surveillance, Epidemiology, and End Results (SEER) stages combined is approximately 32%. Early detection and reliable screening are of vital importance in improving the survival rate. Although there are more new insights into the molecular basis of GC than ever before, currently available diagnostic and therapeutic methods do not significantly improve the overall survival (OS) of GC patients. The use of disease risk stratification (tumor-node-metastasis (TNM) stage) and histological grade based on tumor size, lymph node or distant metastasis is not sufficient to determine the prognosis of a given GC patient. The discovery and identification of molecular subtypes and novel biomarkers play an important role in clinical decision making for more effective and selective treatment. Molecular biomarkers have potential values as diagnostic and prognostic tools in GC. It is worthwhile to investigate the molecular mechanisms of GC and to identify novel and specific biomarkers and targets.

Significant progress has been made in identifying novel molecular subtypes of GC over the last few years. The mechanism of GC pathogenesis in these subsets remains unclear and relies on multiple factors. Activation of multiple oncogenic signaling pathways, including the Wnt/β-catenin, PI3K/Akt, ERK/MAPK, and JAK/STAT3 pathways, is common in the process of carcinogenesis. Among these abnormal carcinogenic signaling pathways, the Wnt/β-catenin signaling pathway has attracted considerable attention, and its dysregulation plays an important role in the tumorigenesis of GC. The Wnt signaling pathway is a central regulatory pathway that regulates gene expression. The pathway has an essential role in embryonic development but also functions in a variety of cellular processes, including proliferation, differentiation, migration, and stemness. The Wnt family currently contains 19 members and regulates three pathways: the canonical pathway, the planar cell polarity pathway, and the Ca^{2+} pathway (5). Genomic statistics indicate that deregulation of the Wnt/β-catenin pathway is noted in 46% of gastric tumors (6). Studies have demonstrated that WNT6 and Cav1 together react positively in the chemoresistance of cells to DNA-damaging anthracycline drugs through the activation of the canonical Wnt/β-catenin pathway (7). Cancer generally demonstrates rapid and anomalous growth through extracellular matrix (ECM) remodeling by collagen type I α 1 (COL1A1) and its collagen family members, and the ECM is also highly activated by the Wnt pathway (8, 9). Cell surface receptors transduce signals into cells from the ECM, which regulate diverse cellular functions, such as survival, growth, migration, and differentiation, and are vital for maintaining normal homeostasis; dysregulation of the ECM could lead to cancer progression. However, the underlying Wnt-regulated ECM target gene expression programs in GC are unknown. Further, there is a lack of knowledge regarding how Wnt regulates target gene expression *via* transcription factors (TFs) and histone modifications (HMs).

CTCF, a well-known transcription factor that is essential in organizing chromatin into highly self-interacting, topologically associated domains, has recently become of great interest to researchers in the cancer field (10). CTCF overexpression has been identified in breast cancer (11), cervical cancer (12), ovarian cancer (13), and hepatocellular carcinoma (14). Some mutations are related to tumors (15). In particular, hotspot binding site mutations occur at quite a high frequency (25%) in GC, and these mutations are associated with alterations in gene expression (16). However, the expression pattern of CTCF and its target genes and its roles in GC growth and metastasis remain unknown. Thus, work sought to identify and characterize the initiating molecular subtypes for GC tumors. Indeed, a recent chromatin profiling study to identify enhancers revealed molecular subtypes in other cancers, but no comparable dataset currently exists for GC.

In the current study, we systematically integrated RNA sequencing (RNA-Seq), chromatin immunoprecipitation sequencing (ChIP-Seq) and tissue microarray (TMA) data to identify ECM subtype gene signatures regulated by the zinc finger protein CTCF transcription factor, which is also linked to the Wnt signaling pathway. CTCF target genes that have an important impact on tumor phenotype and prognosis were validated using GC cell line experiments. Cell viability and migration assays showed that silencing CTCF, COL1A1, and COL1A3 inhibited the growth and migration of GC tumor cells.

MATERIALS AND METHODS

Gene Expression Profile Data

The microarray dataset GSE79973 was downloaded from the GEO database (Gene Expression Omnibus (GEO), RRID : SCR_005012). This dataset contained 10 paired GC tissues and adjacent nontumor tissues from GC patients who underwent radical gastrectomy for GC at Zhejiang Provincial People's Hospital from May 2011 to June 2012.

Raw RNA sequencing data were downloaded from the TCGA (The Cancer Genome Atlas, RRID : SCR_003193). A total of 375 GC samples and 32 matched nontumor samples were obtained for further analysis. Clinical parameters, including age, gender, grade, *H. pylori* infection status and TNM stage (8th edition in 2016), were also downloaded.

Identification of DEGs

For analysis of the validation cohort from the GEO GC dataset, the LIMMA (17) package (LIMMA, RRID: SCR_010943) of the Bioconductor project in R software was applied to screen the differentially expressed genes (DEGs). We set the cut offs as $|\log2$ fold change (FC)$| \geq 1$ and false discovery rate (FDR) < 0.01 for filtering the DEGs. To analyze the validation cohort from the TCGA GC dataset, we used the edgeR (18) Bioconductor project package (edgeR, RRID : SCR_012802). Genes with $|\log2FC| \geq 2$ and FDR < 0.01 were considered to be significantly differentially expressed. The overlapping DEGs between the GEO dataset and the TCGA dataset were retained for further study.

Kyoto Encyclopedia of Genes and Genomes (KEGG) Enrichment, Protein-Protein Interaction (PPI) Network and Module Analyses

KEGG analysis was conducted using the Database for Annotation, Visualization and Integrated Discovery (DAVID) (DAVID, RRID : SCR_001881). The PPI network was constructed using a widely used online database, the Search Tool for the Retrieval of Interacting Genes (STRING) (STRING, RRID : SCR_005223). Cytoscape software was used to visualize the PPI networks (19). The molecular complex detection (MCODE) (MCODE, RRID : SCR_015828) plugin with degree cutoff = 2, node score cutoff = 0.2, k-score = 3, and max depth = 100 was utilized for subset clustering (20).

Survival Analysis of Hub Genes

The Kaplan-Meier method was used for survival analysis and was performed using the Gene Expression Profiling Interactive Analysis (GEPIA) (Gene Expression Profiling Interactive Analysis, RRID : SCR_018294) web server (21).

Transcription Factor Binding Site Prediction

Profiles of the transcription factor binding sites were retrieved from the JASPER database. CiiiDER was used to predict transcription factor binding sites across regions of interest (22). Overlapping genes were analyzed to identify common regulatory transcription factors with an upstream scan limit=2,000 bases, a downstream scan limit=500 bases, and deficit threshold=0.15.

Mapping Transcription Factor Binding Sites

We downloaded the call set from the Encyclopedia of DNA Elements (ENCODE) portal (https://www.encodeproject.org/) (Encode, RRID : SCR_015482) with the following identifiers: ENCBS630AAA. UCSC Browser (http://genome.ucsc.edu/) (UCSC Genome Browser, RRID : SCR_005780) was used to visualize the mapping results.

Single-Sample Gene Set Enrichment Analysis (ssGSEA) of Transcription Factors

CTCF gene expression was input into the GSEA tool (http://www.broadinstitute.org/gsea/index.jsp) (Gene Set Enrichment Analysis, RRID : SCR_003199) to calculate the separate enrichment score.

Pathology Analysis of Hub Genes

The immunohistochemistry (IHC) staining images of COL3A1, SPP1, and THBS2 from GC tumor and normal gastric tissues were downloaded from the Human Protein Atlas (HPA) (HPA, RRID : SCR_006710) database (http://www.proteinatlas.org/) for further analysis (23–25). QuPath software (QuPath, RRID : SCR_018257) is used for image analysis (26).

Cell Culture and Transfection with siRNA

The human GC cell lines HGC27, TGBC11TKB, LMSU, NCC-StC-K140, FU97, MKN45, AGS, HGC27, and BGC823 were purchased from the American Type Culture Collection (ATCC; Manassas, VA, USA) (ATCC, RRID : SCR_001672), CellBank Australia, or Sigma-Aldrich and cultured in RPMI 1640 medium (Invitrogen, CA, USA) supplemented with 10% fetal bovine serum (Invitrogen, CA, USA) and incubated at 37°C and 5% CO_2. CTCF, COL1A1, and COL3A1 were selected from the upregulated gene groups. A commercially available RNA interfering panel targeting the above genes using SMARTpool siRNA, non-target siRNA, and negative control siRNAs were purchased from GenePharma (Shanghai, China). Individual siRNA sequences are presented in **Supplementary Table 1**. siRNA was used at a concentration of 50 pM and transfected into HGC27 and BGC823 cells to account for the influence of transfection itself. Real-time qRT-PCR was performed to detect the expression of the above genes to verify the effectiveness of knockdown.

Quantitative Real-Time PCR Analysis

Total RNA was extracted using TRIzol reagent (Invitrogen, USA) according to the instructions. The concentration and quality of RNA were determined using a Nanodrop spectrophotometer (Thermo Fisher Scientific, USA). Reverse transcriptional mRNA expression was analyzed using PrimeScript RT Master Mix (TaKaRa, Japan). For RNA expression analysis, total RNA was first transcribed using the Mir-X™ RNA first-strand synthesis kit (TaKaRa, Japan). Real-time PCR SYBR Premix Ex Taq (TaKaRa, Japan) was replicated thrice in a 7900 HT Real-Time PCR system (Applied Biosystems, USA), and GAPDH expression levels were used as an endogenous control. The results were determined using the $2^{-\Delta\Delta ct}$ calculation method. See **Supplementary Table 2** for primer information.

MTT Assay

The cells were plated in culture plates and incubated in a CO_2 incubator. Next day, according to the experimental requirement, at respective time points, 50 µl MTT solutions from the stock (5 mg/ml) was added, and cells were incubated in a CO_2 incubator in the dark for 2 h. The medium was removed, and formazan crystals that formed in the cells were dissolved using 500 µl of DMSO followed by transfer to a 96-well plate. Metabolically active cells reduced the MTT to blue formazan crystals, which were dissolved in DMSO. Absorbances were measured at 560 nm. Cell viability was calculated as a percentage of vehicle control using GraphPad Prism v.5.0.

Cell Wound Healing Assay

Cells were plated at confluence in 24-well plates. A wound was created by scraping the confluent monolayer with a p200 pipette tip, and cells were grown in medium supplemented with 1% FBS. The migration of the cells was recorded at 0, 24, and 48 h using a MicroFire camera fitted to an Olympus Inverted Phase Microscope (Olympus) at 10X magnification. The area of the uncovered wound gap was measured using ImageJ software, and details are described in our previous studies (27, 28). All experiments were repeated in triplicate.

Statistical Analysis

All statistical analyses were performed in R software (version 3.6.3) and GraphPad Prism 7 software. All statistical tests with $P < 0.05$ were statistically significant.

RESULTS

Workflow to Identify Key Genes and Pathways in GC

We aimed to identify the DEGs between tumor and normal tissues, establish clinically relevant molecular subtypes and identify significant signatures for GC. First, RNA-Seq data from the GEO and TGCA databases were used to identify DEGs. The overlapping DEGs from two databases were used for KEGG pathway and PPI network analyses. The top 12 up-regulated pathways from TCGA and GEO datasets as well as the pathways from KEGG pathway and PPI network were further analyzed to filter two shared up-regulated pathways. Seven genes (COMP, COL10A1, COL11A1, COL3A1, THBS2, and COL1A1) that were shared by both pathways were defined as hub genes. Next, the correlation among the seven key genes and clinicopathological features were evaluated. The expression of the seven key genes was validated using immunohistochemistry staining and qPCR assays. Then, we used CiiiDER to identify the common transcription factor binding sites of the seven hub genes. Further *in vitro* experiments were applied to validate the role of CTCF in tumorigenesis and regulating these key genes (**Figure 1**).

Gene Expression Programs in Tumors Recapitulate Clinically Distinct ECM Subtypes

The GSE79973 gene expression profile and the TCGA GC dataset were used to identify the shared key genes and pathways that may play a pivotal role in the development of GC (**Supplementary Table 3**). A total of 869 DEGs were

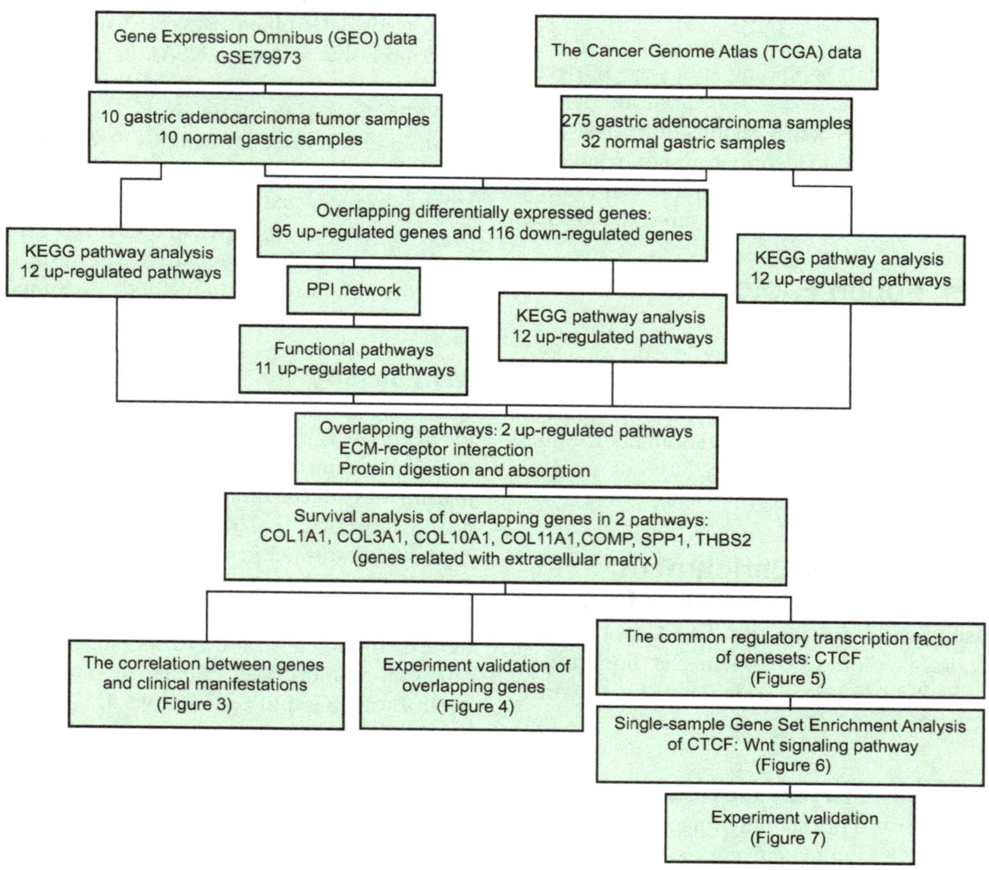

FIGURE 1 | Flow chart of the systematic comprehensive analysis of differentially expressed genes (DEGs) from The Cancer Genome Atlas (TCGA) cohort and the Gene Expression Omnibus (GEO) series of gastric cancer (GC) patients and correlation of DEG expression with overall survival (OS). Further investigation revealed that the extracellular matrix (ECM) signature regulates gastric cancer (GC) progression through the Wnt pathway, and this result was validated by mRNA expression, cell viability and migration assays using a siRNA strategy in aggressive GC cell lines.

obtained from the GSE79973 dataset, which contains 10 gastric tumor samples and 10 paired adjacent normal samples. These 869 DEGs included 425 upregulated genes and 444 downregulated genes. The DEGs acquired from the TCGA GC dataset consisted of 1,019 upregulated and 1031 downregulated genes. A total of 221 DEGs were present in both the GSE79973 and TCGA GC datasets, including 95 upregulated genes and 116 downregulated genes (**Figure 2A**). To explore the potential biological effects of these genes, KEGG pathway analysis was conducted using the DEGs from each dataset. KEGG analysis showed that a total of 26 pathways were enriched in the GC group (**Figure 2B**). The DEGs from the GSE79973 dataset were significantly enriched in 10 pathways, including human papillomavirus infection, PI3K-Akt signaling, focal adhesion, ECM-receptor interaction, and protein digestion and absorption (**Figure 2C, Supplementary Table 4**). The top 10 upregulated enriched pathways from TCGA GC dataset included cytokine-cytokine receptor interaction, neuroactive ligand-

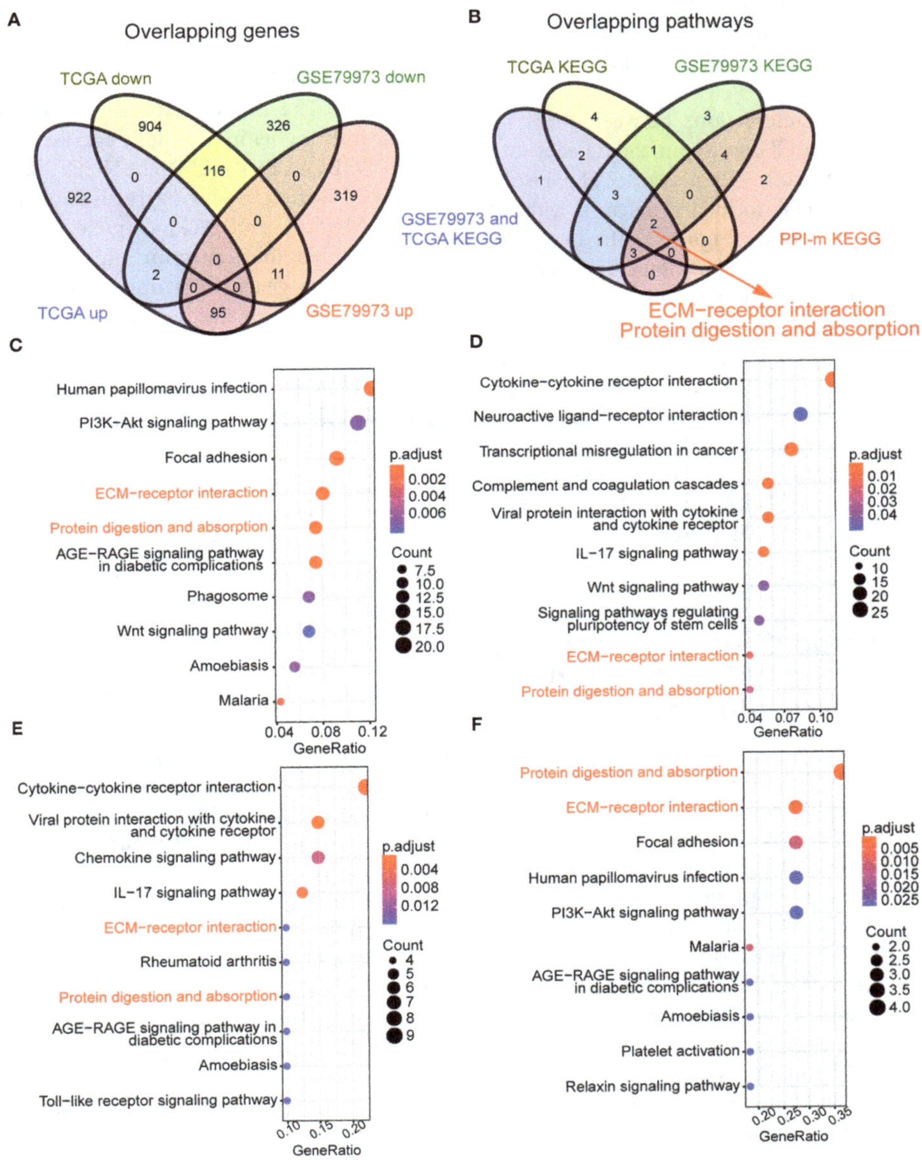

FIGURE 2 | Identification of the extracellular matrix (ECM) subtype. **(A)** Venn diagrams of the differentially expressed genes (DEGs) between the GSE79973 dataset and the The Cancer Genome Atlas (TCGA) gastric cancer (GC) dataset. Ninety-five DEGs were upregulated and 116 DEGs were downregulated in the two datasets. **(B)** Venn diagrams of the overlapping pathways. A total of two enriched pathways overlapped the two datasets: ECM-receptor interaction and protein digestion and absorption. **(C)** Kyoto Encyclopedia of Genes and Genomes (KEGG) pathway enrichment analysis of the DEGs in the GSE79973 dataset. **(D)** KEGG pathway enrichment analysis of the DEGs in TCGA GC dataset. **(E)** KEGG pathway enrichment analysis of overlapping DEGs between the GSE79973 dataset and the TCGA dataset. **(F)** KEGG pathway enrichment analysis of the genes in the protein-protein interaction (PPI) module. The overlapping pathways are marked in red.

receptor interaction, transcriptional dysregulation in cancer, complement, and coagulation cascades, viral protein interaction with cytokine and cytokine receptor, the IL-17 signaling pathway, the Wnt signaling pathway, signaling pathways regulating pluripotency of stem cells, ECM-receptor interaction and protein digestion and absorption (**Figure 2D, Supplementary Table 5**). We further assessed the pathways in which the 95 upregulated overlapping DEGs were enriched. Interestingly, the results indicated that the ECM-receptor interaction and protein digestion and absorption pathways were significantly upregulated in GC samples compared to normal samples (**Figure 2E, Supplementary Table 6**). These two pathways were also listed among the most enriched pathways in the individual GSE79973 and TCGA DEGs (**Figures 2C–D**).

To determine the potential interactions between these 95 upregulated overlapping genes in GC, we input these genes into the STRING website to construct a PPI network. The results showed that the upregulated DEGs formed a network with 92 nodes and 326 edges (**Supplementary Figure 1**). In total, two modules were enriched by protein–protein interaction network analysis, which included 20 genes (**Supplementary Figure 2**). KEGG pathway enrichment analysis of the genes from the PPI module revealed 10 upregulated enriched pathways (**Figure 2F, Supplementary Table 7**). Interestingly, ECM-receptor interaction and protein digestion and absorption were the only two shared up-regulated pathways across all the pathway analyses. By filtering the significant DEGs in these two pathways, a total of seven hub genes, including COL1A1, COL3A1, COL10A1, COL11A1, COMP, SPP1, and THBS2, were identified. These seven genes are all ECM-related genes.

Elevated ECM Subtype Gene Expression is Significantly Correlated With Advanced Clinicopathological Indicators and Poor Prognosis

We next evaluated whether these seven genes could be used as a gene signature for predicting prognostic results in GC patients. Based on the median gene expression, we divided all GC samples from the TCGA into two groups (high score versus low score). Intriguingly, GC patients with high gene signature score exhibited significantly ($P=0.028$) poorer survival outcomes compared to patients with low gene signature score (**Figure 3A**). We then asked whether each of these seven genes exhibited a high correlation with patients' clinical features. As shown in **Figure 3B**, significantly higher expression of COL1A1, COL3A1, COL10A1, COL11A1, COMP, and THBS2 was observed in GC with advanced clinical and TNM stage compared with early-stage GC. In contrast, SPP1 expression only correlated with TNM stage, not clinical stage. This finding was further validated by one-way ANOVA in **Figure 3C**. The expression of these genes only significantly correlated with clinical stage and T stage but did not significantly correlate with patients' age, gender, grade, M/N stage or *H. pylori* infection status.

Validation of the Expression of ECM-Related Genes at the Protein Level Between GC Tissues and Normal Tissues and at the Transcriptional Level Between Aggressive and Less Aggressive GC Cells

To validate the expression of the 7 genes in GC samples, we further confirmed the IHC staining results of COL1A1, COL3A1, SPP1, and THBS2 in both GC tumor and adjacent normal tissues using the HPA website (**Figures 4A–D**). The quantification results suggested that COL1A1, COL3A1, SPP1, and THBS2 protein levels were significantly increased in GC tumor tissues compared to normal adjacent tissues. We further investigated the mRNA levels of these genes in seven different GC cell lines (HGC27, TGBC11TKB, LMSU, NCC-StC-K140, FU97, MKN45, and AGS). The mRNA expression levels of these genes were significantly higher in the highly aggressive gastric carcinoma cell lines TGBC11TKB, LMSU, NCC-StC-K140, and HGC27 compared with the less aggressive adenocarcinoma cell lines FU97, MKN45 and AGS (**Figure 4E**). Overall, our results suggested that the transcript and protein expression levels of ECM subtype genes were upregulated in GC tumor samples, which validated our findings from the above analyses.

ECM Subtype Genes Exhibit Unique CTCF Binding Motif and Histone Modification Patterns

CTCF is a well-known transcription factor that is essential in organizing chromatin and regulates target genes related to cancer (29). To explore the upstream transcription factors of the above hub genes, CiiiDER, a tool for predicting and analyzing transcription factor binding sites, was utilized to analyze mutual transcription factors of these hub genes. CiiiDER operates through an intuitive graphical user interface with interactive, high-quality visual output that makes it accessible to all researchers. CiiiDER predicts transcription factor binding sites (TFBSs) in different regulatory regions, such as promoters and enhancers from any species. CiiiDER can be used to identify TFs that are significantly under- or overexpressed compared to customized background sets; thus, it is useful to identify gene sets of pathophysiological importance (22). We scanned 2 kb upstream and 500 bp downstream from the transcription start site (TSS) for CTCF binding sites. Overlapping genes, including COL1A1, COL3A1, COL10A1, COL11A1, COMP, SPP1, and THBS2, were analyzed to identify common regulatory transcription factors based on three criteria: an upstream scan limit=2,000 bases, a downstream scan limit=500 bases, and deficit threshold=0.15. Moreover, the profiles of the transcription factor binding sites were retrieved from the JASPER database (**Figure 5A**). Given that these six key genes were significantly upregulated in GC, we wanted to understand whether the active histone modifications were associated with these genes. CHIP-Seq data of two common active markers, H3K27Ac and H3K4me3, were visualized using the ENCODE platform (**Figure 5B**). The results confirmed that H3K27Ac and

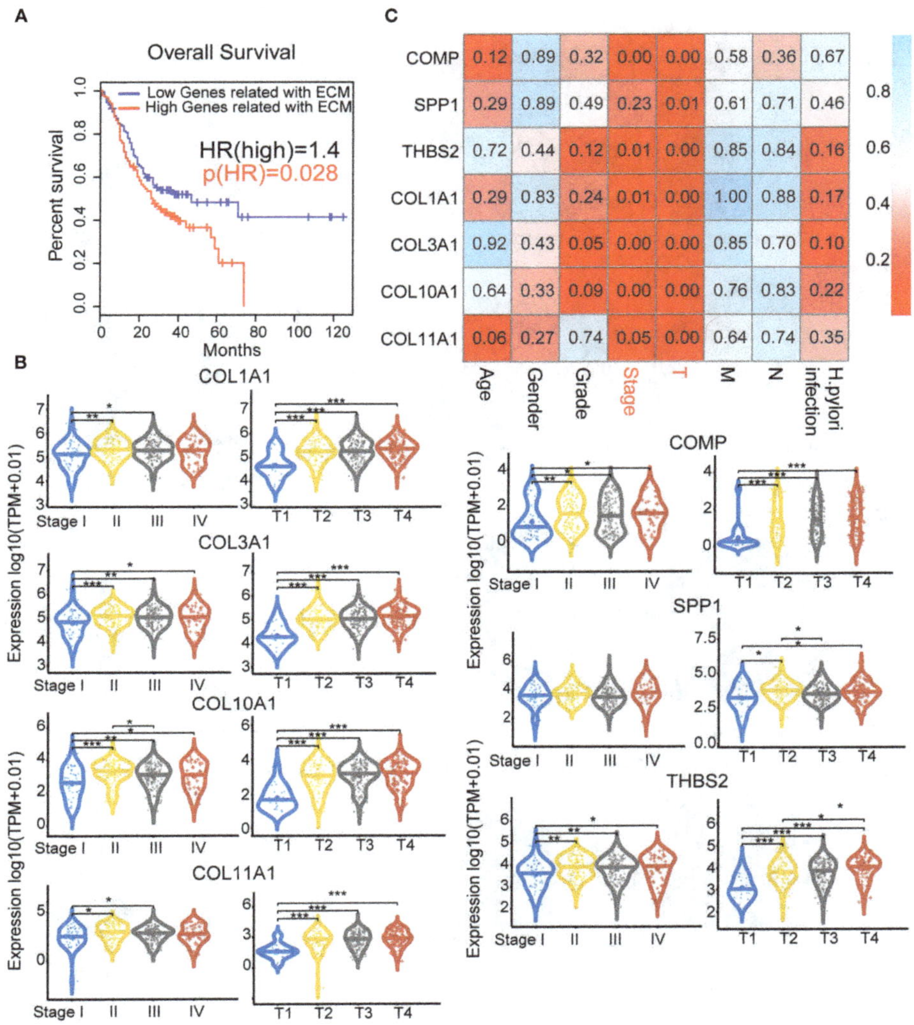

FIGURE 3 | Clinical pathological indicators and prognostic characteristics of elevated extracellular matrix (ECM) subtype genes: Analysis of the correlations between ECM subtype gene expression and survival and clinical characteristics. **(A)** Survival analysis for the ECM subtype genes COMP, SPP1, THBS2, COL1A1, COL3A1, COL10A1, and COL11A1. **(B)** Correlations between the seven hub genes and clinical characteristics. The numbers in each small rectangle indicate the P-value for the correlation. **(C)** The relationship between the hub genes and clinical stage and T stage. *$P < 0.05$, **$P < 0.01$, ***$P < 0.001$.

H3K4me3 peaks were present in the promoter regions of COL1A1, COL3A1, COL10A1, COL11A1, SPP1, and THBS2 and overlapped with CTCF binding sites, indicating that the upregulation of these genes might be associated with H3K27Ac and H3K4me3.

CTCF Expression Was Correlated With the Wnt Signaling Pathway

CTCF expression in GC was assessed using Gene Expression Profiling Interactive Analysis (GEPIA) and verified with the TCGA database. CTCF was significantly overexpressed in GC tissues compared to adjacent normal tissues (**Figure 6A**). To explore the molecular mechanisms of CTCF in GC, ssGSEA analysis was performed to identify the enriched pathways related to CTCF. The top six enriched pathways were cell cycle, ubiquitin-mediated proteolysis, oocyte meiosis, insulin signaling, lysine degradation, and Wnt signaling (**Figure 6B**, **Supplementary Table 8**). In addition, we analyzed the DEGs in the whole Wnt signaling pathway and classified the GC patients into two groups. We found that patients with low expression (relative to the median) of Wnt signaling pathway proteins exhibited significantly better survival outcome compared with those with high expression (**Figure 6C**). Therefore, the Wnt signaling pathway could be an important pathway involved in the progression of GC. The heatmaps in **Figure 6D** illustrated the expression levels of individual genes involved in the Wnt pathway correlated to high CTCF expression. Further analyses showed CTCF expression was correlated with some keys genes in the Wnt pathways, including

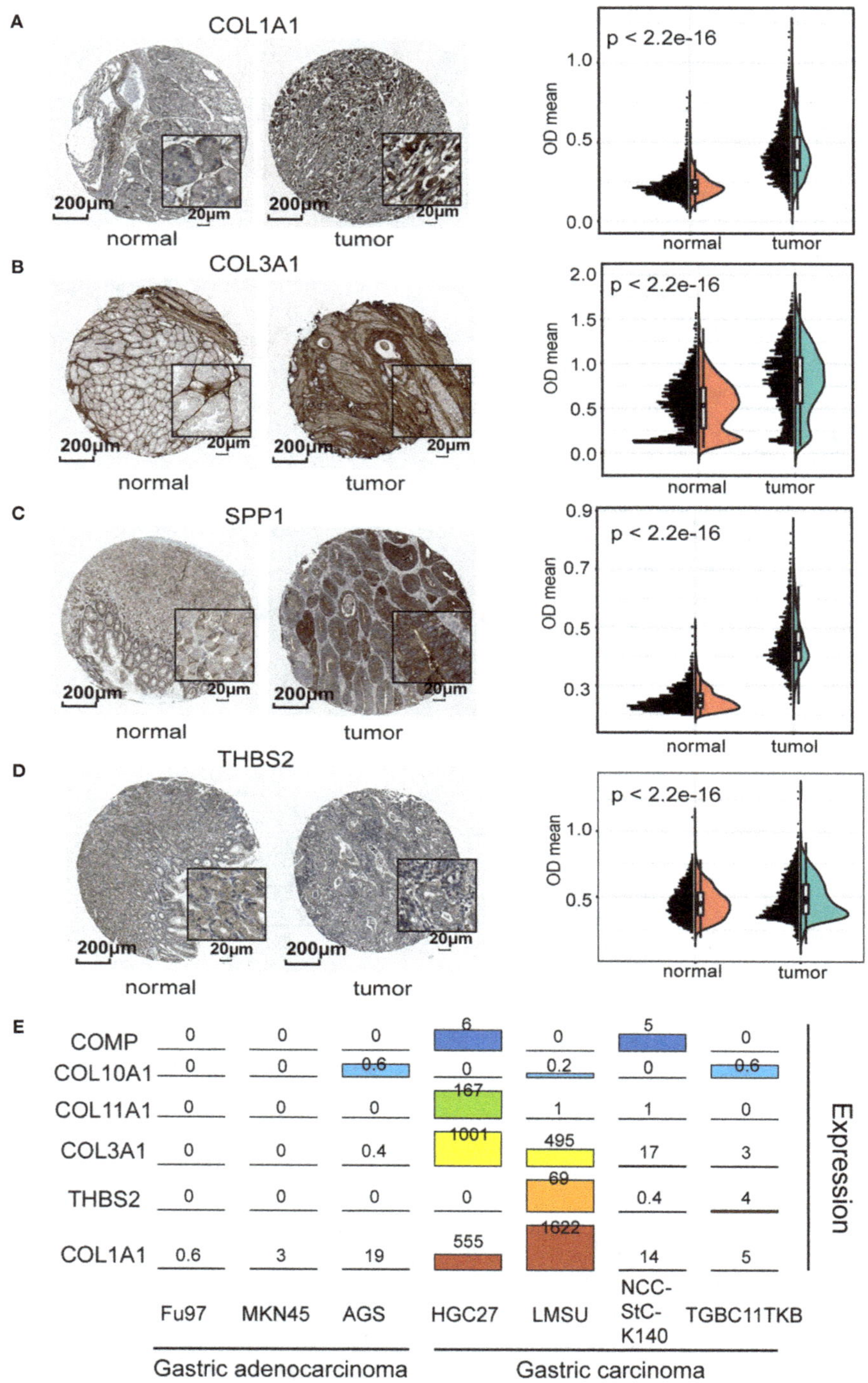

FIGURE 4 | Exploration of the biological relevance of expression differences in the extracellular matrix (ECM) subtype genes: **(A–D)** Representative immunohistochemistry (IHC) images of ECM subtype genes in gastric cancer (GC) tissues and normal tissues [Human Protein Atlas (HPA) database]. The quantification results suggested that the protein levels of COL1A1, COL3A1, SPP1, and THBS2 were significantly increased in GC tumor tissues compared to normal gastric tissues. **(E)** Expression levels of the ECM subtype genes were determined in seven GC cell lines (aggressive cell lines: BGC823, HGC27, LMSU, and NCCStCK140; and less aggressive cell lines: FU97, MKN45, and AGS).

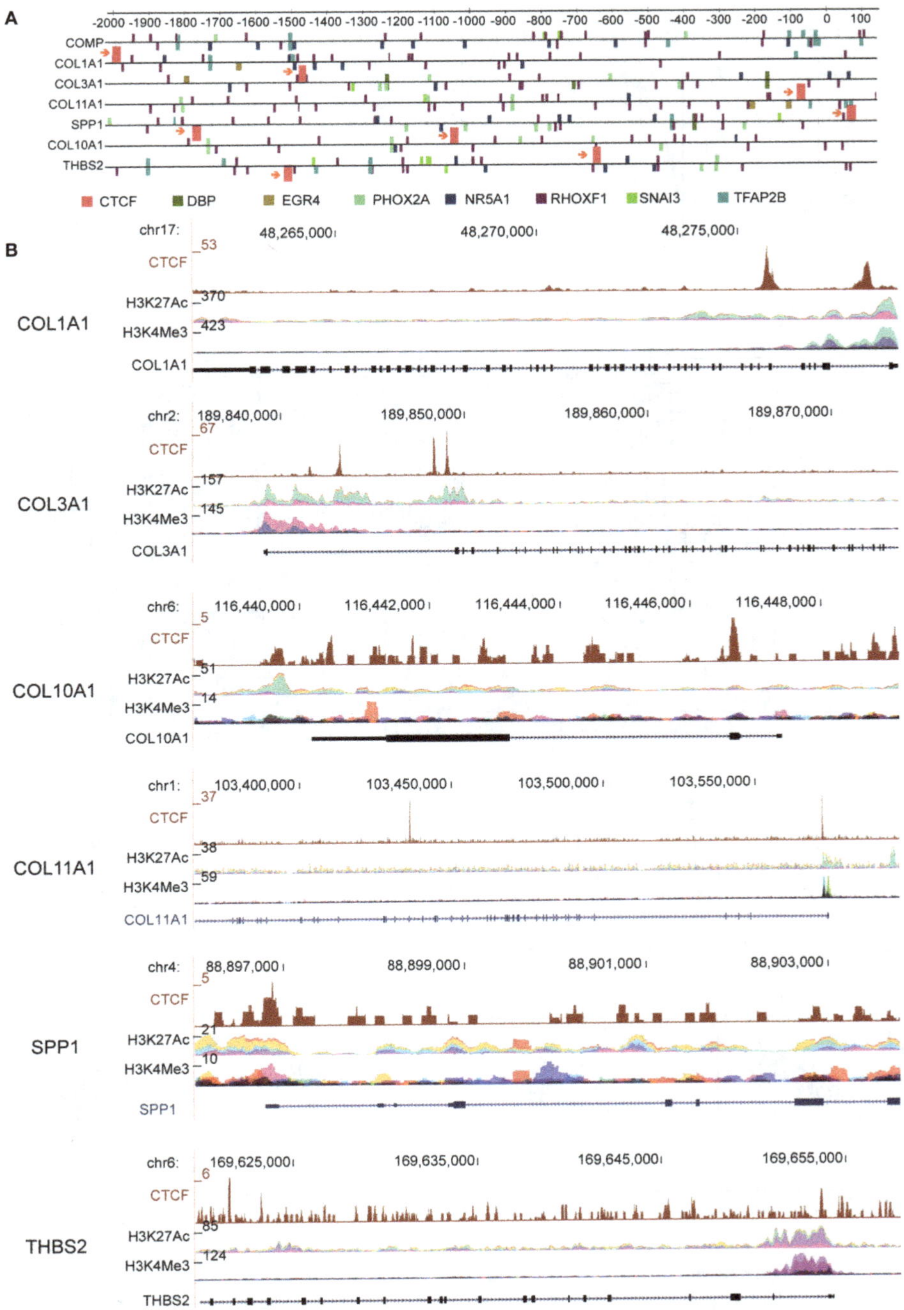

FIGURE 5 | CCCTC-binding factor (CTCF) transcription factor binding motifs are present in a subset of extracellular matrix (ECM) candidate genes. **(A)** Computational predictions of binding sites of CTCF and other transcription factors are shown upstream of the ECM-related gene transcription factor binding sites (TFBSs); COL1A1, COL3A1, and COL11A1 genes have a common transcription factor: CTCF. **(B)** ChIP-Seq data of two common active markers, H3K27Ac and H3K4me3, in the promoter region of ECM subtype genes that overlapped with the CTCF binding sites.

GSK3B, LRP6, NLK, APC, SMAD4, DVL3, TCF7L2, and AXIN1 (**Figure 6E**). The top three genes co-expressed with CTCF were (a) SMAD4 (R = 0.61), (b) NLK (R = 0.55), and (c) LRP6 (R = 0.5) (**Figure 6E**). Our data shown the CTCF expression correlated APC expression in the one of most affected pathways.

CTCF Regulates ECM-Related Genes and Contributes to Promoting Cell Growth and Migration in GC Cell Lines

The ECM regulates diverse cellular functions, including cell survival, migration, and dysregulation of the ECM could lead

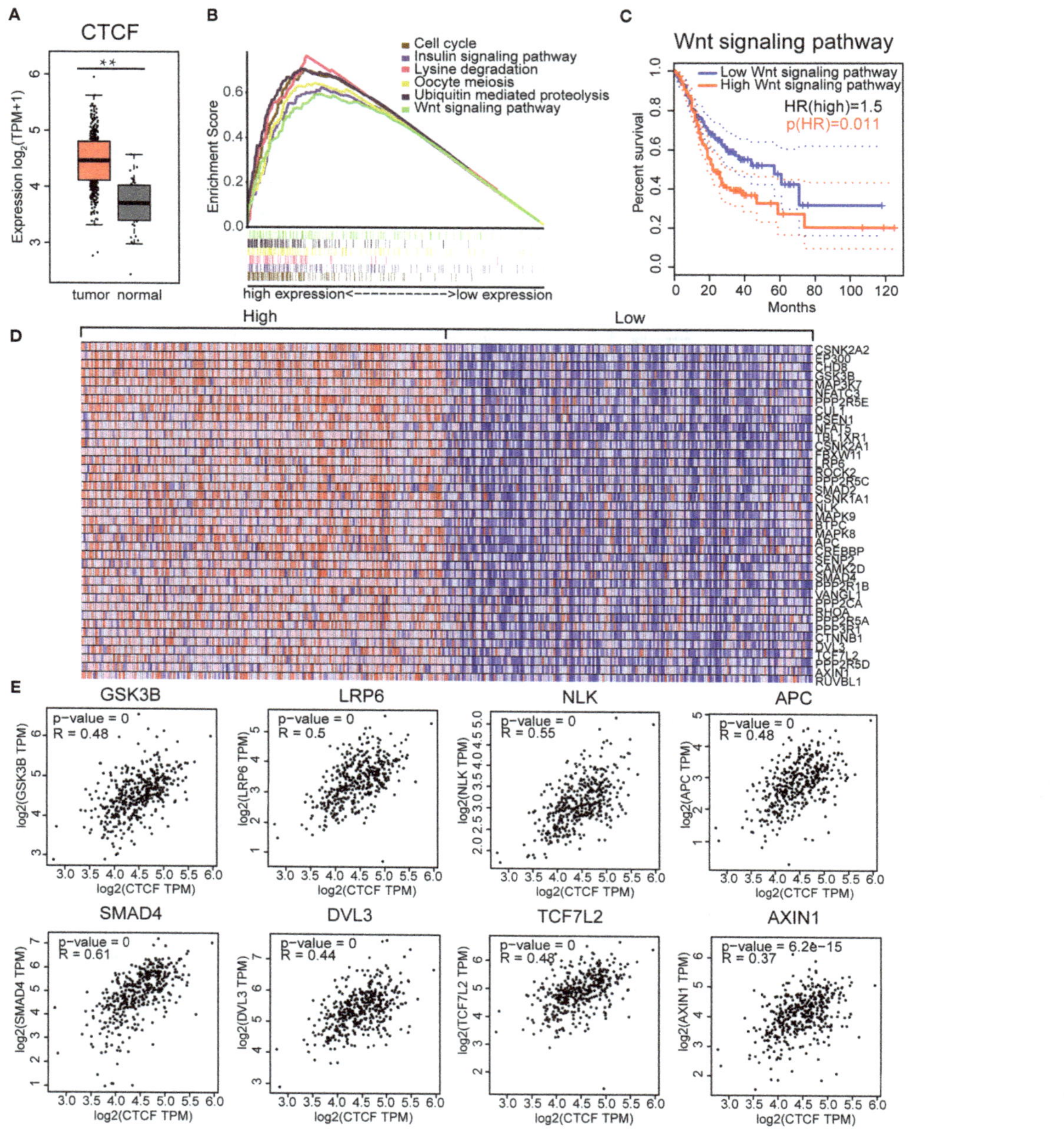

FIGURE 6 | CCCTC-binding factor (CTCF) expression correlated with the Wnt signaling pathway: **(A)** The CTCF transcript was highly expressed in GC tissues compared with normal tissues. **(B)** The top six enriched pathways in GC samples with high CTCF expression were identified by gene set enrichment analysis (GSEA). **(C)** The prognostic value of the Wnt signaling pathway in gastric cancer (GC). Kaplan-Meier curves demonstrate the correlation between Wnt signaling protein expression and overall survival. **(D)** Gene Set Enrichment Analysis (GSEA)-generated heat map for highly enriched genes in samples with high CTCF expression vs. those with low CTCF expression. **(E)** Pearson's correlation analysis of CTCF and Wnt pathway-related genes. We used the service provided by the website Gene Expression Profiling Interactive Analysis (GEPIA) (http://gepia.cancer-pku.cn/index.html) to examine the correlations among GSK3B, LRP6, NLK, APC, SMAD4, DVL3, TCF7L2, AXIN1, and CTCF.

to cancer progression (30). First, we selected the human gastric cell lines BGC-823 and HGC27 based on their cell migration, invasion and epithelial-mesenchymal transition (EMT) features to represent aggressive tumor cell lines. To evaluate the potential clinical relevance of CTCF and these ECM-related genes, we first examined the mRNA expression of CTCF and other two key ECM-related genes COL1A1 and COL3A1 in BGC823 and HGC27 human GC cell lines (**Figure 7A**). Given that the BCG823 cell line exhibited increased CTCF, COL1A1, and COL3A1 expression, we generated single siRNA to interfere with CTCF signaling in the BGC823 cell line. CTCF siRNA interference not only significantly reduced CTCF mRNA levels but also resulted in reduction of COL1A1 and COL1A3 mRNA expression in BCG823 cells (**Figure 7B**). This finding further

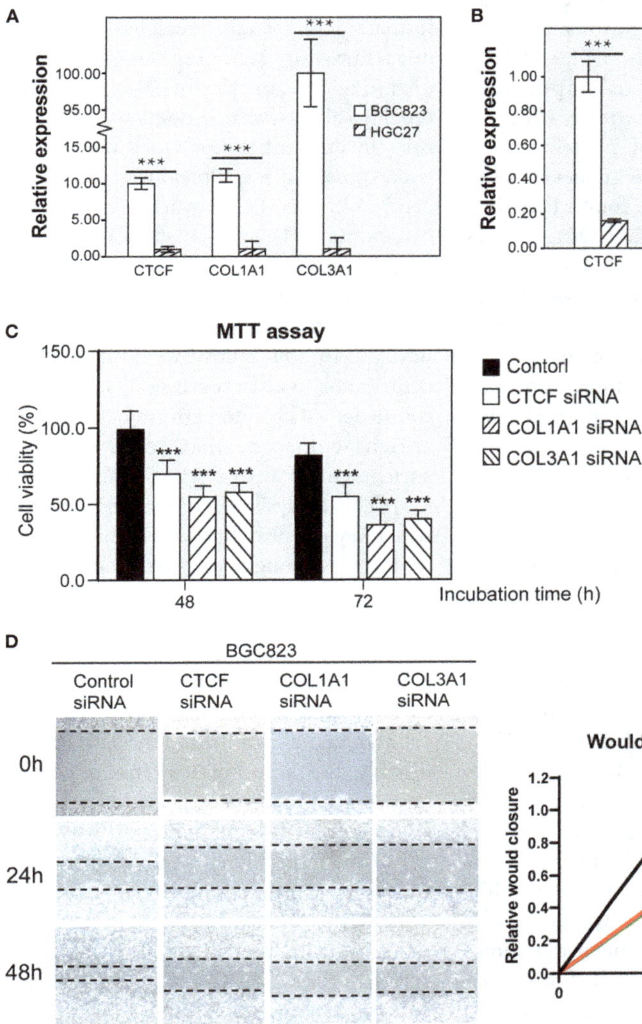

FIGURE 7 | CTCF, COL1A1, and COL3A1 promote gastric cancer (GC) cell viability and migration *in vitro*. **(A)** Comparison of CTCF, COL1A1, and COL3A1 mRNA expression between BGC823 and HCG27 by RT-qPCR. **(B)** Real-time qRT-PCR was performed to detect the expression of the indicted genes to verify the effectiveness of knockdown. **(C)** BGC823 cells were treated with siRNA for 24, 48, and 72 h, and the MTT index was measured based on the MTT assay. The result is presented as fold change of metabolic viability/cell and normalized with respect to control. **(D)** Wound-healing assays were used to determine the effects of single siRNAs targeting CTCF, COL1A1, or COL3A1 on BGC823 cell migration. The bar chart represents the wound width (%) at 24 or 48 h divided by the width at 0 h. Data are presented as the mean ± SD of three independent experiments. **P < 0.001.

demonstrated that CTCF might regulate COL1A1 and COL1A3 expression in GC cells *in vitro*. To explore the cellular function of CTCF, COL1A1, and COL1A3, we further used siRNA to interfere with CTCF, COL1A1, and COL1A3 expression, respectively, in BGC823 cells. MTT assay results demonstrated that BGC823 cell viability was significantly decreased in cells transfected with CTCF siRNA, COL1A1 siRNA or COL1A3 siRNA when compared with siRNA control cells after 48 or 72 h (**Figure 7C**). Similarly, the migration ability of cells transfected with CTCF siRNA, COL1A1 siRNA, or COL1A3 siRNA was decreased compared to siRNA control cells (**Figure 7D**). Overall these results indicated that CTCF could regulate the expression of COL1A1 and COL1A3 *in vitro* and silencing CTCF, COL1A1, and COL3A1 expression led to decreased cell viability and migration in BGC823 cells.

DISCUSSION

GC is a leading cause of cancer-related death due to a lack of knowledge about the relevant molecular classification of subtypes in pathogenic development. Thus, identifying key transcription factors that regulate the molecular signature associated with GC progression will definitely be useful. Here, an integrative strategy was used to comprehensively analyze the variable patterns of GC based on RNA-Seq, ChIP-Seq, gene profiling and molecular signature studies. We discovered a key molecular subtype, namely, a 7-gene signature related to ECM subtype that is linked to distinct patterns of molecular alterations and to disease progression and prognosis. In addition, ECM-related genes in this subtype are regulated by an important transcription factor, the zinc finger protein CTCF. Furthermore, we validated the expression of proteins and mRNAs related to CTCF and the ECM in tumor tissues and in aggressive and less aggressive GC cell lines. We found that the silencing of CTCF decreased mRNA expression of COL1A1 and COL1A3, two key ECM-related genes included in the 7-gene signature. Furthermore, silencing CTCF and two ECM-related genes caused reductions in cell viability and migration. These results reveal that the ECM-related 7-gene signature could be a useful prognostic factor for survival. The zinc finger protein CTCF regulates ECM-related genes and plays an important role in promoting GC cell growth and migration *in vitro*.

The combination of ChIP-Seq and transcriptomic analysis is gradually becoming the standard for molecular spectrum analysis of various cancers. The challenge is now to combine these different molecular biological data to obtain a more comprehensive and informative view of key biological processes in cancer progression. Our objective was to systematically analyze RNA-Seq, ChIP-Seq, gene map, and molecular marker data in GC to understand the major regulatory factors and target genes in this disease. Our study identified differences in mRNA expression between tumors and adjacent normal tissues from different clinical cohorts. The identified DEGs were filtered through KEGG, PPI network and functional pathway analyses. We were the first to identify a key molecular subtype, referred to as the ECM subtype, and provide prognostic factors. The expression of ECM-related genes was also correlated with the clinical status of cancer progression. GC pathway analysis results were consistent with known processes in GC, such as ECM-receptor interaction and protein digestion and absorption. Furthermore, our ChIP-Seq and histone modification analysis results suggested that the expression of these target ECM-related genes is influenced by the distance from the transcription start site (TSS) to their CTCF binding sites. Of note, KEGG pathway analysis identified transcription factor binding site motifs and histone modification markers, demonstrating that DEGs with CTCF-binding motif modifications exhibiting functional enrichment during cancer development. The expression of these target genes is closely related to OS in GC patients. Kaplan-Meier survival analysis confirmed this findings (**Figures 3** and **6**). We found that CTCF may modulate previously unreported ECM target genes and mediate their possible roles. In summary, combining data from different sources is a promising strategy for identifying major regulators and target genes for cancer.

The chromatin-organizing CCCTC-binding factor (CTCF) encodes a transcription regulator protein with 11 highly conserved zinc finger domains that binds to more than 20,000 DNA loci in the human genome (31). CTCF plays indispensable roles in transcriptional inhibition/activation, insulation, gene imprinting, and regulation of 3D chromatin structure (32). Studies have previously demonstrated that chromosomal architecture is largely mediated by the CTCF/cohesin complex (33, 34) because it is of vital importance in promoting the formation of cohesin-mediated loops and boundaries that are necessary for gene regulation. This process enables the organization of chromatin into highly self-interacting topologically associated domains (10). Its expression pattern and roles in different tumor types vary greatly. For instance, CTCF overexpression was previously reported in breast cancer (11), cervical cancer (12), ovarian cancer (13), and hepatocellular carcinoma (14) and is often related to tumor features with adverse prognostic impacts. Additionally, mutations in CTCF or defects in CTCF function have been observed in GC (16). However, the clinical impact of CTCF expression in GC is unclear. In this study, we identified CTCF as an important contributor to GC progression, survival and prognosis. Then, we conducted ssGSEA to perform hallmark analysis, which defines an enrichment score that represents the degree of absolute enrichment of a gene set in each sample within a given dataset (35). This analysis demonstrated that the Wnt/signaling pathway was a key pathway that was highly related to CTCF.

Here, we sought to determine whether CTCF was regulated by a signaling pathway or associated with another pathway involved in gastric cancer. The Wnt signal transduction pathway is a highly conserved extracellular signal transduction pathway that is implicated in many vital cellular functions, such as stem cell regeneration and organogenesis. Several intra-cellular signal transduction pathways are induced by Wnt, notably the Wnt/beta-catenin dependent pathway, which is known as the canonical pathway, and the non-canonical or beta-catenin-independent pathway. The latter includes the Wnt/Ca^{2+} and Planar Cell Polarity pathway (PCP) (36–39). Colorectal cancers exhibit evidence of Wnt signaling pathway activation associated with loss of function of the tumor regulator APC. Our data also demonstrated that CTCF expression correlated with APC expression in the one of most affected pathways (**Figure 6**). This finding indicated the some ECM genes are linked to the Wnt signaling pathway through the CTCF transcription factor. Taken together, these data confirm that Wnt signaling is an important mechanism driving GC metastasis and can therefore be considered an attractive therapeutic target.

Major efforts have been made to elucidate the molecular mechanisms that regulate the Wnt signaling pathway and its role in development, homeostasis, and cancer. However, there is a lack of understanding about the relationships between Wnt signaling and ECM adhesion. WNT7A depletion in 5637 HMI and T24 cells reduced urinary bladder cancer (UBC) cell invasion and decreased the levels of active β-catenin and its downstream target genes involved in ECM degradation, but these studies lacked detail on the regulatory mechanism between Wnt and ECM. ECM is an important component of the tumor microenvironment and plays critical roles in cancer development and metastasis, in which collagen is the major structural protein. Collagen type I alpha 1 (COL1A1) reportedly promotes cancer cell migration. In our study, knockdown of COL1A1 or COL3A1 inhibited GC cell metastasis with low levels of CTCF and WNT5 or CTCF and WNT3 (**Supplementary

Figure 3), which is independent of the epithelial-mesenchymal transition (EMT) process. Our results have identified a CTCF/WNT axis that controls GC migration through ECM regulation *via* the canonical Wnt/β-catenin signaling, which may offer prognostic and therapeutic opportunities.

There are several limitations in this study. First, although the Wnt signaling pathway was highly correlated with CTCF expression, we did not have sufficient experimental evidence to elucidate the detailed relationships between CTCF and the Wnt signaling pathway. Second, more experiments were needed to double-confirm whether CTCF could regulate the expression of other ECM-related genes besides COL1A1 and COL1A3. Protein level validations should be performed. Third, more experiments were needed to determine whether CTCF-mediated regulation of COL1A1/COL1A3 occurred directly or indirectly.

CONCLUSION

In the present study, we systematically analyze the RNA-Seq, ChIP-Seq, gene profiling, and molecular signature data of GC and performed experimental validation to obtain insight into the main regulators and target genes in GC. We identified that the zinc finger protein CTCF regulates the ECM-related genes COL1A1 and COL1A3 *via* a novel mechanism and that this pathway could be used to evaluate GC progression. Overall, using a combination of multiple omics analyses and wet lab experimental data, the present study provides a potential prognostic factor for survival prediction among GC patients.

ETHICS STATEMENT

Ethical review and approval were not required for the study on human participants in accordance with the local legislation and institutional requirements. Written informed consent for participation was not required for this study in accordance with the national legislation and the institutional requirements. Written informed consent was not obtained from the individual(s) for the publication of any potentially identifiable images or data included in this article.

AUTHOR CONTRIBUTIONS

YH, LY, and DX made a substantial contribution to the concept and design of the work. CL, LD, JiaZ, JL, PJ, JinZ, and SH performed the acquisition, analysis, and interpretation of the data. CL, LD, YH, LY, and DX drafted the article. PX, PN, LY, DX, and YH revised it critically for important intellectual content. All authors contributed to the article and approved the submitted version.

REFERENCES

1. Ferro A, Peleteiro B, Malvezzi M, Bosetti C, Bertuccio P, Levi F, et al. Worldwide trends in gastric cancer mortality (1980-2011), with predictions to 2015, and incidence by subtype. *Eur J Cancer* (2014) 50(7):1330–44. doi: 10.1016/j.ejca.2014.01.029
2. Jemal A, Center MM, DeSantis C, Ward EM. Global patterns of cancer incidence and mortality rates and trends. *Cancer Epidemiol Biomarkers Prev* (2010) 19(8):1893–907. doi: 10.1158/1055-9965.EPI-10-0437
3. Bray F, Ferlay J, Soerjomataram I, Siegel RL, Torre LA, Jemal A. Global cancer statistics 2018: GLOBOCAN estimates of incidence and mortality worldwide for 36 cancers in 185 countries. *CA Cancer J Clin* (2018) 68(6):394–424. doi: 10.3322/caac.21492
4. Siegel RL, Miller KD, Jemal A. Cancer statistics, 2018. *CA Cancer J Clin* (2018) 68(1):7–30. doi: 10.3322/caac.21442
5. Katoh M, Katoh M. WNT signaling pathway and stem cell signaling network. *Clin Cancer Res* (2007) 13(14):4042–5. doi: 10.1158/1078-0432.CCR-06-2316
6. Ooi CH, Ivanova T, Wu J, Lee M, Tan IB, Tao J, et al. Oncogenic pathway combinations predict clinical prognosis in gastric cancer. *PloS Genet* (2009) 5 (10):e1000676. doi: 10.1371/journal.pgen.1000676
7. Yuan G, Regel I, Lian F, Friedrich T, Hitkova I, Hofheinz RD, et al. WNT6 is a novel target gene of caveolin-1 promoting chemoresistance to epirubicin in human gastric cancer cells. *Oncogene* (2013) 32(3):375–87. doi: 10.1038/onc.2012.40
8. Ferrari N, Ranftl R, Chicherova I, Slaven ND, Moeendarbary E, Farrugia AJ, et al. Dickkopf-3 links HSF1 and YAP/TAZ signalling to control aggressive behaviours in cancer-associated fibroblasts. *Nat Commun* (2019) 10(1):130. doi: 10.1038/s41467-018-07987-0
9. Liu Y, Xu J, Xu L, Wu T, Sun Y, Lee YW, et al. Cystic fibrosis transmembrane conductance regulator mediates tenogenic differentiation of tendon-derived stem cells and tendon repair: accelerating tendon injury healing by intervening in its downstream signaling. *FASEB J* (2017) 31(9):3800–15. doi: 10.1096/fj.201601181R
10. Debaugny RE, Skok JA. CTCF and CTCFL in cancer. *Curr Opin Genet Dev* (2020) 61:44–52. doi: 10.1016/j.gde.2020.02.021
11. Docquier F, Farrar D, D'Arcy V, Chernukhin I, Robinson AF, Loukinov D, et al. Heightened expression of CTCF in breast cancer cells is associated with resistance to apoptosis. *Cancer Res* (2005) 65(12):5112–22. doi: 10.1158/0008-5472.Can-03-3498
12. Velazquez-Hernandez N, Reyes-Romero MA, Barragan-Hernandez M, Guerrero-Romero F, Rodriguez-Moran M, Aguilar-Duran M, et al. BORIS and CTCF are overexpressed in squamous intraepithelial lesions and cervical cancer. *Genet Mol Res* (2015) 14(2):6094–100. doi: 10.4238/2015.June.8.7
13. Zhao L, Yang Y, Yin S, Yang T, Luo J, Xie R, et al. CTCF promotes epithelial ovarian cancer metastasis by broadly controlling the expression of metastasis-associated genes. *Oncotarget* (2017) 8(37):62217–30. doi: 10.18632/oncotarget.19216
14. Zhang B, Zhang Y, Zou X, Chan AW, Zhang R, Lee TK, et al. The CCCTC-binding factor (CTCF)-forkhead box protein M1 axis regulates tumour growth and metastasis in hepatocellular carcinoma. *J Pathol* (2017) 243 (4):418–30. doi: 10.1002/path.4976
15. Filippova GN, Qi CF, Ulmer JE, Moore JM, Ward MD, Hu YJ, et al. Tumor-associated zinc finger mutations in the CTCF transcription factor selectively alter tts DNA-binding specificity. *Cancer Res* (2002) 62(1):48–52.
16. Guo YA, Chang MM, Huang WT, Ooi WF, Xing MJ, Tan P, et al. Mutation hotspots at CTCF binding sites coupled to chromosomal instability in gastrointestinal cancers. *Nat Commun* (2018) 9(1):1–14. doi: 10.1038/s41467-018-03828-2
17. Ritchie ME, Phipson B, Wu D, Hu Y, Law CW, Shi W, et al. limma powers differential expression analyses for RNA-sequencing and microarray studies. *Nucleic Acids Res* (2015) 43(7):e47. doi: 10.1093/nar/gkv007

18. Robinson MD, McCarthy DJ, Smyth GK. edgeR: a Bioconductor package for differential expression analysis of digital gene expression data. *Bioinformatics* (2010) 26(1):139–40. doi: 10.1093/bioinformatics/btp616
19. Shannon P, Markiel A, Ozier O, Baliga NS, Wang JT, Ramage D, et al. Cytoscape: A software environment for integrated models of biomolecular interaction networks. *Genome Res* (2003) 13(11):2498–504. doi: 10.1101/gr.1239303
20. Bader GD, Hogue CW. An automated method for finding molecular complexes in large protein interaction networks. *BMC Bioinf* (2003) 4(1):1–27. doi: 10.1186/1471-2105-4-2
21. Tang Z, Kang B, Li C, Chen T, Zhang Z. GEPIA2: an enhanced web server for large-scale expression profiling and interactive analysis. *Nucleic Acids Res* (2019) 47(W1):W556–W60. doi: 10.1093/nar/gkz430
22. Gearing LJ, Cumming HE, Chapman R, Finkel AM, Woodhouse IB, Luu K, et al. CiiiDER: A tool for predicting and analysing transcription factor binding sites. *PloS One* (2019) 14(9):e0215495. doi: 10.1371/journal.pone.0215495
23. Uhlen M, Fagerberg L, Hallstrom BM, Lindskog C, Oksvold P, Mardinoglu A, et al. Proteomics. Tissue-based map of the human proteome. *Science* (2015) 347(6220):1260419. doi: 10.1126/science.1260419
24. Thul PJ, Akesson L, Wiking M, Mahdessian D, Geladaki A, Ait Blal H, et al. A subcellular map of the human proteome. *Science* (2017) 356(6340). doi: 10.1126/science.aal3321
25. Uhlen M, Zhang C, Lee S, Sjostedt E, Fagerberg L, Bidkhori G, et al. A pathology atlas of the human cancer transcriptome. *Science* (2017) 357(6352). doi: 10.1126/science.aan2507
26. Bankhead P, Loughrey MB, Fernandez JA, Dombrowski Y, McArt DG, Dunne PD, et al. QuPath: Open source software for digital pathology image analysis. *Sci Rep* (2017) 7(1):16878. doi: 10.1038/s41598-017-17204-5
27. Yuan X, Yu L, Li J, Xie G, Rong T, Zhang L, et al. ATF3 suppresses metastasis of bladder cancer by regulating gelsolin-mediated remodeling of the actin cytoskeleton. *Cancer Res* (2013) 73(12):3625–37. doi: 10.1158/0008-5472.CAN-12-3879
28. Yan F, Ying L, Li X, Qiao B, Meng Q, Yu L, et al. Overexpression of the transcription factor ATF3 with a regulatory molecular signature associates with the pathogenic development of colorectal cancer. *Oncotarget* (2017) 8 (29):47020–36. doi: 10.18632/oncotarget.16638
29. Das S, Shah R, Dimmeler S, Freedman JE, Holley C, Lee J-M, et al. Noncoding RNAs in Cardiovascular Disease: Current Knowledge, Tools and Technologies for Investigation, and Future Directions: A Scientific Statement From the American Heart Association. *Circ: Genom Precis Med* (2020) 13(4):e000062. doi: 10.1161/hcg.0000000000000062
30. Nissen NI, Karsdal M, Willumsen N. Collagens and Cancer associated fibroblasts in the reactive stroma and its relation to Cancer biology. *J Exp Clin Cancer Res* (2019) 38(1):115. doi: 10.1186/s13046-019-1110-6
31. Ohlsson R, Renkawitz R, Lobanenkov V. CTCF is a uniquely versatile transcription regulator linked to epigenetics and disease. *Trends Genet* (2001) 17(9):520–7. doi: 10.1016/S0168-9525(01)02366-6
32. Liu FM, Wu DJ, Wang XD. Roles of CTCF in conformation and functions of chromosome. *Semin Cell Dev Biol* (2019) 90:168–73. doi: 10.1016/j.semcdb.2018.07.021
33. Hnisz D, Day DS, Young RA. Insulated Neighborhoods: Structural and Functional Units of Mammalian Gene Control. *Cell* (2016) 167(5):1188–200. doi: 10.1016/j.cell.2016.10.024
34. Merkenschlager M, Nora EP. CTCF and Cohesin in Genome Folding and Transcriptional Gene Regulation. *Annu Rev Genomics Hum Genet* (2016) 17:17–43. doi: 10.1146/annurev-genom-083115-022339
35. Barbie DA, Tamayo P, Boehm JS, Kim SY, Moody SE, Dunn IF, et al. Systematic RNA interference reveals that oncogenic KRAS-driven cancers require TBK1. *Nature* (2009) 462(7269):108–12. doi: 10.1038/nature08460
36. Semenov MV, Habas R, Macdonald BT, He X. SnapShot: Noncanonical Wnt Signaling Pathways. *Cell* (2007) 131(7):1378. doi: 10.1016/j.cell.2007.12.011
37. MacDonald BT, Tamai K, He X. Wnt/beta-catenin signaling: components, mechanisms, and diseases. *Dev Cell* (2009) 17(1):9–26. doi: 10.1016/j.devcel.2009.06.016
38. Nusse R, Clevers H. Wnt/beta-Catenin Signaling, Disease, and Emerging Therapeutic Modalities. *Cell* (2017) 169(6):985–99. doi: 10.1016/j.cell.2017.05.016
39. Rao TP, Kuhl M. An updated overview on Wnt signaling pathways: a prelude for more. *Circ Res* (2010) 106(12):1798–806. doi: 10.1161/CIRCRESAHA.110.219840

Permissions

All chapters in this book were first published by Frontiers; hereby published with permission under the Creative Commons Attribution License or equivalent. Every chapter published in this book has been scrutinized by our experts. Their significance has been extensively debated. The topics covered herein carry significant findings which will fuel the growth of the discipline. They may even be implemented as practical applications or may be referred to as a beginning point for another development.

The contributors of this book come from diverse backgrounds, making this book a truly international effort. This book will bring forth new frontiers with its revolutionizing research information and detailed analysis of the nascent developments around the world.

We would like to thank all the contributing authors for lending their expertise to make the book truly unique. They have played a crucial role in the development of this book. Without their invaluable contributions this book wouldn't have been possible. They have made vital efforts to compile up to date information on the varied aspects of this subject to make this book a valuable addition to the collection of many professionals and students.

This book was conceptualized with the vision of imparting up-to-date information and advanced data in this field. To ensure the same, a matchless editorial board was set up. Every individual on the board went through rigorous rounds of assessment to prove their worth. After which they invested a large part of their time researching and compiling the most relevant data for our readers.

The editorial board has been involved in producing this book since its inception. They have spent rigorous hours researching and exploring the diverse topics which have resulted in the successful publishing of this book. They have passed on their knowledge of decades through this book. To expedite this challenging task, the publisher supported the team at every step. A small team of assistant editors was also appointed to further simplify the editing procedure and attain best results for the readers.

Apart from the editorial board, the designing team has also invested a significant amount of their time in understanding the subject and creating the most relevant covers. They scrutinized every image to scout for the most suitable representation of the subject and create an appropriate cover for the book.

The publishing team has been an ardent support to the editorial, designing and production team. Their endless efforts to recruit the best for this project, has resulted in the accomplishment of this book. They are a veteran in the field of academics and their pool of knowledge is as vast as their experience in printing. Their expertise and guidance has proved useful at every step. Their uncompromising quality standards have made this book an exceptional effort. Their encouragement from time to time has been an inspiration for everyone.

The publisher and the editorial board hope that this book will prove to be a valuable piece of knowledge for researchers, students, practitioners and scholars across the globe.

List of Contributors

Zhijian Zheng, Dan Hong, Yixin Chang, Ning Sun, Zhenni Lin, Ruirui Zhang and Honglei Jin
Zhejiang Provincial Key Laboratory of Medical Genetics, Key Laboratory of Laboratory Medicine, Ministry of Education, School of Laboratory Medicine and Life Sciences, Wenzhou Medical University, Wenzhou, China

Hongyan Li and Haishan Huang
Zhejiang Provincial Key Laboratory of Medical Genetics, Key Laboratory of Laboratory Medicine, Ministry of Education, School of Laboratory Medicine and Life Sciences, Wenzhou Medical University, Wenzhou, China
Key Laboratory of Laboratory Medicine, Ministry of Education, School of Laboratory Medicine and Life Sciences, Wenzhou Medical University, Wenzhou, China

Xiaodong Zhang
Department of Colorectal Anal Surgery, The First Affiliated Hospital of Wenzhou Medical University, Wenzhou, China

Shirui Huang and Qipeng Xie
Department of Clinical Laboratory, The Second Affiliated Hospital & Yuying Children's Hospital of Wenzhou Medical University, Wenzhou, China

Cong Wang, Xueli Jiao, Zihui Jin, Yujie Zhu, Ziling Fang and Lingling Zhao
Key Laboratory of Laboratory Medicine, Ministry of Education, School of Laboratory Medicine and Life Sciences, Wenzhou Medical University, Wenzhou, China

Lei Wu
Department of General Surgery, Heze Municipal Hospital, Heze, China

Haipeng Zhu
Precision and Personalized Cancer Treatment Center, Division of Cancer Diagnosis & Therapy, Ciming Boao International Hospital, Boao Lecheng International Medical Tourism Pilot Zone, Qionghai, China
Stem Cell and Biotherapy Technology Research Center, Xinxiang Medical College, Xinxiang, China

Xiaojun Liu
Division of Cellular & Biomedical Science, Ciming Boao International Hospital, Boao Lecheng International Medical Tourism Pilot Zone, Qionghai, China

Yan-Ru Chen
State Key Laboratory of Organ Failure Research, Guangdong Province Key Laboratory of Molecular Tumor Pathology, Department of Pathology, Nanfang Hospital, School of Basic Medical Sciences, Southern Medical University, Guangzhou, China
Department of Research and Teaching, Huizhou Municipal Central Hospital, Huizhou, China

Wan-Ying Feng
State Key Laboratory of Organ Failure Research, Guangdong Province Key Laboratory of Molecular Tumor Pathology, Department of Pathology, Nanfang Hospital, School of Basic Medical Sciences, Southern Medical University, Guangzhou, China

Yuan-Xiong Cheng
Department of Respiratory and Critical Care Medicine, The Third Affiliated Hospital, Southern Medical University, Guangzhou, China

Yi Gao
General Surgery Center, Department of Hepatobiliary Surgery II, Guangdong Provincial, Research Center for Artificial Organ and Tissue Engineering, Guangzhou Clinical Research and Transformation Center for Artificial Liver, Institute of Regenerative Medicine, Zhujiang Hospital, Southern Medical University, Guangzhou, China

Wei-Jie Zhou
State Key Laboratory of Organ Failure Research, Guangdong Province Key Laboratory of Molecular Tumor Pathology, Department of Pathology, Nanfang Hospital, School of Basic Medical Sciences, Southern Medical University, Guangzhou, China
Department of Respiratory and Critical Care Medicine, The Third Affiliated Hospital, Southern Medical University, Guangzhou, China
General Surgery Center, Department of Hepatobiliary Surgery II, Guangdong Provincial, Research Center for Artificial Organ and Tissue Engineering, Guangzhou Clinical Research and Transformation Center for Artificial Liver, Institute of Regenerative Medicine, Zhujiang Hospital, Southern Medical University, Guangzhou, China
Microbiome Medicine Center, Zhujiang Hospital, Southern Medical University, Guangzhou, China
Bioland Laboratory (Guangzhou Regenerative Medicine and Health Guangdong Laboratory), Guangzhou, China

Chengxing Wang, Xiaoping Li, Weijun Liang, Shangren Li, Qunying Tan and Yaoming He
Department of Gastrointestinal Surgery, Jiangmen Central Hospital, Affiliated Jiangmen Hospital of Sun Yat-sen University, Jiangmen, China

Jinglin Zhao
Department of Gastrointestinal Surgery, Jiangmen Central Hospital, Affiliated Jiangmen Hospital of Sun Yat-sen University, Jiangmen, China
Faculty of Medical Laboratory Science, Ruijin Hospital, School of Medicine, Shanghai Jiao Tong University, Shanghai, China

Liangliang Ren, Meimei Wu and Xin Zhang
Clinical Experimental Center, Jiangmen Key Laboratory of Clinical Biobanks and Translational Research, Jiangmen Central Hospital, Affiliated Jiangmen Hospital of Sun Yat-sen University, Jiangmen, China

Changyi Ma
Department of Radiology, Jiangmen Central Hospital, Affiliated Jiangmen Hospital of Sun Yat-sen University, Jiangmen, China

Yuehua Liao and Lixia Sun
Department of Pathology, Jiangmen Central Hospital, Affiliated Jiangmen Hospital of Sun Yat-sen University, Jiangmen, China

Hongwei Jin
Xiamen Key Laboratory of Biomarker Translational Medicine, Medical Laboratory of Xiamen Humanity Hospital Fujian Medical University, Xiamen, China

Wei Zheng, Jingjing Hou and Huiqin Zhuo
Department of Gastrointestinal Surgery, The Affiliated Zhongshan Hospital, Xiamen University, Xiamen, China
Department of Gastrointestinal Surgery, Xiamen Municipal Key Laboratory of Gastrointestinal Oncology, Xiamen, China

Huifang Peng
Department of Endocrinology, The First Affiliated Hospital and College of Clinical Medicine of Henan University of Science and Technology, Luoyang, China

Yuqiong Wang
Department of Gastroenterology, the Hospital of 92608 People's Liberation Army of China (PLA) Troops, Shanghai, China

Dan Wang, Yunxia Fan and Jun Gao
Institute of Oncology, Second Affiliated Hospital, Xi'an Medical University, Xi'an, China

Yanmiao Dai, Yaodong Wang and Hongwei Xu
Department of Gastroenterology, Kunshan Affiliated Hospital of Nanjing University of Chinese Medicine, Suzhou, China

Xiangyu Kong, Xian Zhu, Hongyu Wu, Jing Jin and Kaixuan Wang
Department of Gastroenterology, Changhai Hospital, Second Military Medical University, Shanghai, China

Wenzhu Yao
Bureau of headmaster, Xi'an Medical University, Xi'an, China

Qingjie Kang, Xudong Peng, Xiangshu Li, Denghua Hu, Guangxu Wen and Zhengqiang Wei
Department of Gastrointestinal Surgery, The First Affiliated Hospital of Chongqing Medical University, Chongqing, China

Baohong Yuan
Department of Anesthesiology, The First Affiliated Hospital of Chongqing Medical University, Chongqing, China

Zhengqi Wen
Department of Oncology, The First Affiliated Hospital of Kunming Medical University, Kunming, China

Dun Xiong
Department of Oncology, The People's Hospital of Puer City, Puer, China

Shurong Zhang, Jiankun Liu and Raomei Li
Department of Gastroenterology, The 920th Hospital of the Joint Logistics Support Force, PLA, Kunming, China

Bitao Li
Department of Prevention and Health Care, The First Affiliated Hospital of Kunming Medical University, Kunming, China

Hushan Zhang
The Medical Department, 3D Medicines Inc., Shanghai, China

Lin Dai
Cancer Prevention Center, Sun Yat-sen University Cancer Center, Guangzhou, China
State Key Laboratory of Oncology in South China, Guangzhou, China
Collaborative Innovation Center for Cancer Medicine, Guangzhou, China

Hao Zhu and Hong-Juan Liu
Department of Bioinformation, School of Basic Medical Sciences, Southern Medical University, Guangzhou, China

Zilin Huang and Wang Li
Department of Medical Imaging and Interventional Radiology, Sun Yat-sen University Cancer Center, Guangzhou, China

Miao Yu
Shandong Provincial Third Hospital, Cheeloo College of Medicine, Shandong University, Jinan, China
Department of Clinical Laboratory, Shandong Cancer Hospital and Institute, Shandong First Medical University and Shandong Academy of Medical Sciences, Jinan, China
Department of Clinical Laboratory, Jinan Qilu Medical Inspection Co., Ltd., Jinan, China

Xing-guo Song, Ya-jing Zhao, Xiao-han Dong, Li-min Niu, Xiao-ling Shang, You-yong Tang and Li Xie
Department of Clinical Laboratory, Shandong Cancer Hospital and Institute, Shandong First Medical University and Shandong Academy of Medical Sciences, Jinan, China

Zhi-jun Zhang
Department of Clinical Laboratory, Tai'an City Central Hospital, Tai'an, China

Xian-rang Song
Department of Clinical Laboratory, Shandong Cancer Hospital and Institute, Shandong First Medical University and Shandong Academy of Medical Sciences, Jinan, China
Shandong Provincial Key Laboratory of Radiation Oncology, Shandong Cancer Hospital and Institute, Shandong First Medical University and Shandong Academy of Medical Sciences, Jinan, China

Pengping Li
Department of General Surgery, First Affiliated Hospital of Anhui Medical University, Hefei, China
Department of General Surgery, First People's Hospital of Xiaoshan, Hangzhou, China

Wei Cao, Mengqiu Cheng, Xin Xu, Sihan Chen, Bo Chen, Guodong Cao and Maoming Xiong
Department of General Surgery, First Affiliated Hospital of Anhui Medical University, Hefei, China

Rui Ding
Department of General Surgery, First Affiliated Hospital of Anhui Medical University, Hefei, China
Department of Emergency, the Lu'an Affiliated Hospital of Anhui Medical University, Lu'an, China

Shuang Zhao and Hua-chuan Zheng
Department of Oncology and Experimental Center, The Affiliated Hospital of Chengde Medical University, Chengde, China

Chang-lai Hao
Department of Hematology, The Affiliated Hospital of Chengde Medical University, Chengde, China

En-hong Zhao
Department of Surgery, The Affiliated Hospital of Chengde Medical University, Chengde, China

Hua-mao Jiang
Department of Urology, The First Affiliated Hospital of Jinzhou Medical University, Jinzhou, China

Rilei Jiang, Xiaolei Chen and Jiatuo Xu
School of Basic Medicine Science, Shanghai University of Traditional Chinese Medicine, Shanghai, China

Shaohua Ge, Yichang Liu, Haijun Chen and Jiang Wu
Department of Oncology, Kunshan Hospital of Traditional Chinese Medicine Affiliated to Nanjing University of Chinese Medicine, Kunshan, China

Qin Wang
First Clinical Medical College, Nanjing Medical University, Nanjing, China

Hang Xue
Department of Oncology and Experimental Center, The Affiliated Hospital of Chengde Medical University, Chengde, China

Duilia Brex, Cristina Barbagallo, Federica Mirabella, Angela Caponnetto, Rosalia Battaglia, Davide Barbagallo, Cinzia Di Pietro, Michele Purrello and Marco Ragusa
Department of Biomedical and Biotechnological Sciences – Section of Biology and Genetics "Giovanni Sichel," University of Catania, Catania, Italy

Rosario Caltabiano and Giuseppe Broggi
Department of Medical, Surgical Sciences and Advanced Technologies G.F. Ingrassia, University of Catania, Catania, Italy

Lorenzo Memeo
Department of Experimental Oncology, Mediterranean Institute of Oncology (IOM), Catania, Italy

Xianglai Ye, Xiujuan Wei, Jing Liao, Peipei Chen, Xueyun Li, Yulong Chen, Yue Yang and Hezhi Fang
Key Laboratory of Laboratory Medicine, Ministry of Education, Wenzhou Medical University, Wenzhou, China
Zhejiang Provincial Key Laboratory of Medical Genetics, Department of Cell Biology and Medical Genetics, Wenzhou Medical University, Wenzhou, China
College of Laboratory Medicine and Life Sciences, Wenzhou Medical University, Wenzhou, China

Lin Wang, Hai-li Xu, Jing-wei Liang, Ying-ying Ding and Fan-hao Meng
School of Pharmacy, China Medical University, Liaoning, China

Qiongya Zhao
College of Laboratory Medicine, Hangzhou Medical College, Hangzhou, China

Hongwei Sun
Department of Surgery, The First Affiliated Hospital of Wenzhou Medical University, Wenzhou, China

Liming Pan
Department of Pathology, The People's Hospital of Yuhuan, The Yuhuan Branch of the First Affiliated Hospital of Wenzhou Medical University, Taizhou, China

Guorong Chen
Department of Pathology, The First Affiliated Hospital of Wenzhou Medical University, Wenzhou, China

Xujun He
Department of Laboratory Medicine, Zhejiang Provincial People's Hospital, Affiliated People's Hospital of Hangzhou Medical College, Hangzhou, China

Jianxin Lyu
Key Laboratory of Laboratory Medicine, Ministry of Education, Wenzhou Medical University, Wenzhou, China
Zhejiang Provincial Key Laboratory of Medical Genetics, Department of Cell Biology and Medical Genetics, Wenzhou Medical University, Wenzhou, China
College of Laboratory Medicine and Life Sciences, Wenzhou Medical University, Wenzhou, China
College of Laboratory Medicine, Hangzhou Medical College, Hangzhou, China
Department of Laboratory Medicine, Zhejiang Provincial People's Hospital, Affiliated People's Hospital of Hangzhou Medical College, Hangzhou, China

Chenbin Liu, Linyi Deng, Jianjun Zhang, Shu Huang, Peipei Jin, Peiqing Xu, Peihua Ni, Dakang Xu and Yiqun Hu
Faculty of Medical Laboratory Science, Ruijin Hospital, School of Medicine, Shanghai Jiao Tong University, Shanghai, China

Jinrong Lin
Department of Sports Medicine, Huashan Hospital, Fudan University, Shanghai, China

Le Ying
Faculty of Medical Laboratory Science, Ruijin Hospital, School of Medicine, Shanghai Jiao Tong University, Shanghai, China
Centre for Innate Immunity and Infectious Diseases, Hudson Institute of Medical Research, Clayton, Victoria, Hudson Institute of Medical Research, Clayton, VIC, Australia
Department of Molecular and Translational Science, Monash University, Clayton, VIC, Australia

Index

www.ingramcontent.com/pod-product-compliance
Lightning Source LLC
LaVergne TN
LVHW082128200926
848484LV00008B/2022